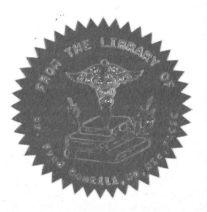

Obstetrics and Gynecology

Obstetrics and Gynecology

J. Robert Willson, M.D.

Professor of Obstetrics and Gynecology,
The University of Michigan Medical School, and
Chairman of the Department of Obstetrics and
Gynecology, The University of Michigan Medical Center,
Ann Arbor, Mich.

Clayton T. Beecham, M.D.

Director of Gynecology and Obstetrics,
The Geisenger Medical Center,
Danville, Pa.

Elsie Reid Carrington, M.D.

Professor of Obstetrics and Gynecology and
Chairman of the Department of Obstetrics and
Gynecology, Medical College of Pennsylvania,
Philadelphia, Pa.

FOURTH EDITION

With 525 illustrations

The C. V. Mosby Company

Saint Louis   1971

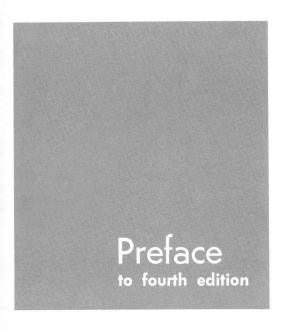

Preface
to fourth edition

In preparing the fourth edition of *Obstetrics and Gynecology* we have attempted to maintain the concept that the book serves best as a text for medical students and as a reference on the basic principles of reproduction for physicians in all fields. We resisted the temptation to expand it to an all-purpose text because we believe there is real need for a textbook in obstetrics-gynecology directed primarily toward medical students, most of whom will practice in other areas, but all of whom should be familiar with the basic facts of reproductive physiology and the methods for detecting and treating the more common disorders of the female reproductive organs. We have attempted to replace and update material rather than to expand the size of the book by adding to it. In some areas, however, it was impossible simply to rewrite the text because new and important information in addition to that already included in previous editions has become available during the last few years. We had to include this without deleting other equally essential material.

We have attempted to respond to the increasing need for information concerning social problems relating to reproduction. The material on abortion, contraception, prematurity, prenatal care, and infection in particular has been rewritten with this in mind.

New diagnostic methods, particularly those relating to hormone assays and their interpretation, laparoscopy, methods for determining fetal status, genetic disorders, and others of equal importance have been included, and improvements in the more standard methods have been described. We have covered in some detail diagnostic methods that can be performed by the physician in his own office. The material on hormone assays was reviewed and revised by Uwe T. Goebelsmann, Associate Professor of Obstetrics and Gynecology and Director of the Departmental Endocrine Laboratories, The University of Michigan Medical School, Ann Arbor.

The sections on normal and abnormal labor have been extensively revised as a result of our experience with the use of the labor graph as a standard method for charting the course of labor. The principles for the recognition and management of abnormalities in each of the several phases of labor have been discussed in detail.

Other areas that have been revised extensively or added include those concerned with puerperal and nonpuerperal pelvic infections, evaluation of fetal status during labor, placental and fetal physiology, and diabetes, heart disease, and other medical conditions complicating pregnancy.

The chapters on psychology, life periods, sexual response, dysmenorrhea, and premenstrual tension have also been rewritten. Dr.

v

M. J. Daly, Associate Professor of Obstetrics and Gynecology, and Harold Winn, Clinical Assistant Professor of Psychiatry, both of the Temple University School of Medicine, Philadelphia, continue to be responsible for these important areas that are overlooked or rejected by so many obstetrician-gynecologists. Some of the social and sexual pressures that have been steadily increasing in recent years are described.

We hope that this edition of *Obstetrics and Gynecology* will continue to serve its basic purpose, that of a textbook for medical students, while it is also a source of information on reproduction for physicians in all fields of medicine.

J. Robert Willson
Clayton T. Beecham
Elsie Reid Carrington

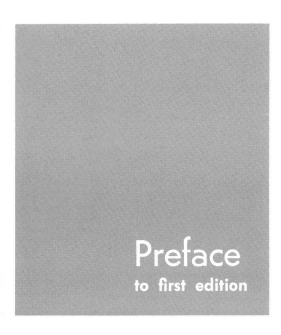

Preface
to first edition

In 1949 we first prepared a mimeographed summary of the contents of the courses in obstetrics and gynecology given to the third- and fourth-year students in the Temple University School of Medicine. The original was revised and expanded many times, each revision being larger and more complete than the previous one. As the notes became more inclusive, many of the students used them in preference to the recommended standard textbooks which they were intended to supplement. Since our mimeographed volume, though relatively comprehensive, was completely inadequate to serve as a text, we were forced to decide whether to eliminate it entirely or to expand it into a true textbook. After considerable deliberation we chose the latter course.

Our next problem concerned the type of book which would best serve the purpose of the student. There are excellent outlines and synopses of obstetrics and gynecology and many costly encyclopedic texts in which are included the details of anatomy, physiology, pathology, and laboratory and operative techniques necessary to diagnose and treat almost any condition the obstetrician-gynecologist might encounter in his practice. Existing outlines and synopses are usually complete, but the material is presented so concisely that many of the steps necessary for arriving at a diagnosis or for establishing a plan for treat-

ment are of necessity omitted. These are better suited for rapid reference or for review rather than as a basic student text. The authors of the costly encyclopedic books discuss obstetric and gynecologic conditions in great detail. They present numerous theoretical ideas concerning etiology, complicated procedures for diagnosis, and several plans for treatment, some of which are diametrically opposed to each other, and many of which can be applied only by highly trained specialists. Such books are excellent for graduate students and physicians in practice but are confusing and often discouraging to the medical student who does not as yet even understand the basic clinical problems. We therefore agreed to prepare a textbook of obstetrics and gynecology which would fit somewhere between these two extremes; one in which the emphasis is placed upon the changes produced in body structures and their function by various obstetric and gynecologic conditions; a book emphasizing methods of diagnosis and treatment which can be utilized by the family physician, as well as by the specialist, in his own office or in the hospital. We have indicated the conditions under which he should seek consultation with a more experienced individual. The details of diagnostic and surgical procedures which require specialized training and experience (forceps delivery, cesarean section, breech extractions, etc.) are omitted, but the indications for these operations and their contra-indications are discussed.

Those interested in more detailed study of any specific condition or of operative techniques can refer to the articles listed in the bibliographies. Most of the references were selected either because of their historic interest or because we believed their coverage of a particular subject or their bibliographies were especially good. Few references to recent experimental work, particularly that which is as yet unproved, are included. Such material is better covered in small group discussions.

Some of our colleagues were of the opinion that a book of this type, even though it describes widely accepted methods currently in use in the Temple University Medical Center, would serve a too limited purpose because those who wished to learn more about the subject during residency training or in practice could not use it. This argument is not valid. The book can serve as a reference for the family physician because it does contain specific recommendations for diagnosis and treatment which are well within his ability. Those who go into specialty training will need several books concerning various aspects of obstetrics and gynecology; no resident or practicing obstetrician-gynecologist could possibly be satisfied with an old edition of any one textbook as a reference.

Several years ago we stopped teaching obstetrics and gynecology as individual subjects, except on the wards, and attempted to arrange all the material concerning the functions and disorders of the female reproductive organs into a systematic sequence. In introductory courses we now present a sequential story of the life history of normal women and their diseases from birth through puberty, maturity, the climacteric, and senescence. Normal and abnormal pregnancies are considered as a unit, although certain gynecologic problems are introduced at what we

consider to be appropriate points in the obstetric discussions. For instance, puerperal infection, acute and chronic gonorrhea, tuberculosis, and miscellaneous infections are all discussed together. This permits the student to compare and contrast all the infections at once rather than to learn about puerperal infection during the obstetric portion of the course and gonorrhea several months later during the gynecologic portion. The acute childbirth injuries and the subsequent relaxation of the pelvic supporting structures which often occur as an aftermath of delivery trauma are also considered together. Since this approach has been most satisfactory for teaching, we have arranged the material in the text in a similar manner. An exception is pediatric gynecology, which is presented near the end of the book rather than at the beginning. It would be impossible for the student to understand the gynecologic lesions in children without first having basic information concerning similar lesions as they occur in adults.

We have discussed the emotional, as well as the physical, aspects of obstetric and gynecologic problems whenever it is appropriate and have indicated the importance of emotional factors in the management, as well as in the etiology, of certain conditions. We hope that this will stimulate students to consider the patient's background, family situation, and environment, as well as the physical manifestations of the disturbance. Preventive aspects of obstetrics and gynecology are also stressed; if an abnormality can be prevented, it need never be treated. This is of particular importance in potentially lethal conditions such as hemorrhage, eclampsia, infections, etc.

It is our hope that this volume will not only provide students with a sound background of basic information concerning obstetrics and gynecology, but also stimulate a few to undertake a more comprehensive study of the subject.

J. Robert Willson
Clayton T. Beecham
Isador Forman
Elsie Reid Carrington

Contents

Obstetrics and Gynecology

Introduction

It might appear that the physician who confines his professional activities to the treatment of pregnant women (obstetrics) and patients with dysfunctioning genital organs (gynecology) is limiting his practice rather severely. On the contrary, the obstetrician and gynecologist must be familiar with many fields of medicine because his patients vary in age from those newly born to senescent women. It is possible for women with medical conditions such as hypertension, tuberculosis, rheumatic heart disease, diabetes, multiple sclerosis, and a host of others to conceive, and all manner of acute medical and surgical conditions may develop during pregnancy. As a gynecologist the physician must be a pediatrician, internist, endocrinologist, and surgeon, since he treats females of all ages and often is the first person consulted because of symptoms that actually arise in structures other than the genital organs. He must also be familiar with the basic principles of psychiatry and must be able to recognize the emotional problems that so frequently manifest themselves in sexual disorders. The specialist who has little knowledge of general physiologic function and of disease processes in other parts of the body thinks only in terms of the pelvis and, as a consequence, tends to attribute most symptoms, whatever their nature, to some presumed dysfunction of a pelvic structure. A comprehensive approach, by which the emotional and physical functions of the patient as a whole are considered, is more important when dealing with pregnant women and those with gynecologic disorders than in almost any other branch of medicine.

Most women in the United States are still delivered by general practitioners, but more and more are seeking care from obstetrician-gynecologists as the number of specialists increases. There is no reason why the general practitioner should not do obstetrics if he is willing to devote enough time to his pregnant patients. He should be able to manage normal pregnancy and many of the complications perfectly satisfactorily if he works in a well-equipped hospital and has competent consultants to assist him with the more serious problems. Unfortunately many doctors who practice obstetrics are so busy that they neglect their expectant mothers; they may fail to examine pregnant patients completely because they have no definite symptom other than the pregnancy; they may leave the prenatal care to the office nurse; they may fail to discuss diet and other important problems with their patients; and they may make other less qualified persons assume responsibility for care during labor. The end results cannot possibly be as good as those attained by either family physicians or specialists who take a genuine interest in the welfare of the women who consult them for care during pregnancy.

Family physicians as well as obstetricians and gynecologists share the responsibility for reducing the mortality and morbidity in infants and their mothers and in women with various gynecologic disorders. Despite the remarkable decrease in maternal mortality during recent years, too many deaths are still avoidable. The change in infant mortality has been less spectacular, but it too can be improved by closer supervision during pregnancy and by applying methods for delivery and for the treatment of complications that have been proved safe as well as effective. Many children are handicapped by serious birth injuries, some of which occurred because of inadequate supervision or treatment during labor and at delivery.

Most gynecologic conditions can be corrected by medical rather than surgical treatment, and many can be managed by the family physician who will take time to examine his patients and make accurate diagnoses. In gynecology, as in obstetrics, consultation is necessary for complicated diagnostic problems and before performing an operation. Accurate diagnoses can usually be made with a minimum of laboratory study, but there are many helpful diagnostic tests that can be performed by the physician himself. Unfortunately the busy practitioner sometimes treats symptoms without making an examination and may therefore overlook cancer, abnormal pregnancy, and other serious conditions, all of which can usually be diagnosed without difficulty.

More and more women are consulting physicians for periodic physical examinations. Much of the responsibility for such examinations falls upon the obstetrician-gynecologist because he may have delivered their babies or operated upon them; but this need not be strictly his province. There is no reason why periodic examinations cannot be performed by family physicians and internists as well as by obstetrician-gynecologists. Such examinations should be designed to detect general physical abnormalities, not isolated ones such as pelvic cancer. The family physician and the internist must, therefore, examine the pelvis and make use of the tests designed to detect the first evidences of pelvic disease. By the same token the obstetrician-gynecologist must perform a complete examination and must not focus his attention on the pelvis while he overlooks hypertension or some other equally important medical condition.

■ **Birthrates**

The *birthrate,* the number of live births per 1,000 population, varies from year to year, depending upon a multitude of factors. The rate fell progressively from 30 in 1910 to 18.4 in 1933. It is interesting that this low rate was attained before the present sophisticated contraceptive methods were available and undoubtedly represents a calculated

mass decision to prevent pregnancy because of the severe financial depression.

Most couples were forced to delay starting their families because of World War II, but the birthrate started upward in 1940 and rose precipitously after 1945, reaching a peak of 26.6 in 1947. It was 25 with 4,254,784 births in 1957 and 23.3 with 4,268,326 births in 1961. After this it again fell, reaching an all-time low of 17.8 with 3,520,959 births in 1967.

Everyone has expected the number of births to begin to increase in 1969 because of the large numbers of young people who will be marrying and starting families. The numbers actually did increase during that year. The birthrate probably also will rise. It is not clear whether the present low birthrate indicates a trend toward smaller families or simply a greater interval between births.

A better indication of what is happening is the *fertility rate,* the births per 1,000 women between the ages of 15 and 44 years. In 1967 this was 87.6, the lowest since 1936 when it was 75.8. The fertility rate in 1957 was 122.9. In 1967 the fertility rate for whites was 83.1 and for nonwhites, 119.8.

Birthrates by age of the mother in 1967 were as follows:

AGE (years)	BIRTHRATE
10-14	0.9
15-19	67.9
20-24	174
25-30	142.6
31-34	79.3
35-39	38.5
40-44	10.6
45-49	0.7

■ **Illegitimacy**

In 1967 there were 318,100 *illegitimate births.* The ratios per 1,000 live births were as follows: total 90.3, white 48.7, and nonwhite 293.8.

The ratios of illegitimate births by age of the mother were as follows:

AGE (years)	ILLEGITIMACY RATIO
15-19	18.7
20-24	38.6
25-29	41.4
30-34	29.8
35-40	15.3
40-44	4

Table 1

Age (years)	Total deaths	Ratio	
		Legitimate	Illegitimate
<15	25.5	20.6	26.5
15-19	14.1	12.3	19.4
20-24	11.6	10.8	20.8
25-29	12.6	12	25.7
30-34	18.6	17.6	41
35-39	27.4	26.3	51.5
40+	40.3	39.5	57.8

There is no way of knowing how many women conceived before marriage, and were married as a consequence, or how many illegitimate births were not reported as such.

The significance of illegitimate pregnancy, in addition to the effect on the mother herself, is its major contribution to perinatal mortality. The proportion of illegitimate pregnancies that terminate in premature delivery is much higher than that for married mothers. To a large extent this is a result of teen-age pregnancy and pregnancy in women of low socioeconomic status.

The effect of maternal age and marital status on *fetal death* is significant. The ratios of fetal deaths for various age groups in 1967 are listed in Table 1.

Since the curves for neonatal mortality are similar to those for fetal deaths, it is evident that the best reproductive results are obtained when married women have their babies between the ages of 20 and 30 years.

■ **Maternal mortality**

A *maternal death* is the death of any woman from any cause while she is pregnant or within 42 days of the termination of pregnancy, irrespective of the duration of pregnancy or its site. A *direct obstetric death* is one resulting from a complication of pregnancy itself—from intervention, from omissions of or incorrect treatment, or from a chain of events resulting from any of the preceding. An *indirect obstetric death* is one resulting from a disease that had existed previously or that developed during pregnancy, but the course of which was aggravated by the physiologic effects of pregnancy. An example is serious rheumatic heart disease with decompensation during the period of maximum cardiac stress. A *nonobstetric death* is one resulting from an incidental cause unrelated to pregnancy. An example of a nonobstetric death is one resulting from injuries sustained in an automobile accident or death from a brain tumor.

Maternal death rates vary considerably in different parts of the country and with different classes of patients. The mortality is higher in nonwhite patients than in either white nonprivate or white private patients. This undoubtedly occurs because the nonwhite patients include the most impoverished and least well-educated people in the United States. There is a higher incidence of medical complications such as essential hypertension, anemia, malnutrition, and toxemia among this group of patients, and these conditions often remain untreated. These patients frequently do not seek prenatal care, entering the hospital only after labor has begun, and if they do register in clinics, they often appear late in pregnancy, attend irregularly, and cannot afford adequate diets and medications. The death rate is highest in urban communities and in the southeastern states, where the concentration of nonwhite patients and those of low economic status is greatest. It is of interest that the largest proportion of home deliveries and of births that are not attended by physicians also occurs in the deep South. Maternal mortality is lowest in the Northwest, parts of New England, and the upper Midwest,

Table 2

Cause		Total
Toxemia		189
Eclampsia	77	
Preeclampsia	18	
Hypertension	14	
Renal disease	6	
Abortion		187
Hemorrhage		142
Post partum	72	
Retained placenta	14	
Antepartum	56	
Infection		127
Ectopic pregnancy		67
Other causes		304

where the population is more homogeneous with fewer blacks and less poverty and malnutrition. Reduction in maternal mortality therefore must be a concern of educators, sociologists, and economists as well as of physicians.

The *maternal death rate,* the number of direct obstetric deaths per 10,000 live births, was 58 in 1935; by 1967 the rate had been reduced to 2.8. In 1967 the rate for white women was 1.95 and for nonwhite women, 6.95. See Table 2 for the causes of the 987 direct obstetric deaths registered in 1967.

There is considerable overlapping of causes, which is not evident in a table because a specific cause of death must be assigned. For example, most deaths after abortions are caused by infection, and many of the women who die of puerperal sepsis have had postpartum hemorrhage.

Indirect and nonobstetric deaths are classified under the specific cause, such as heart disease, rather than as a maternal death. A most disturbing fact is the increasing number of deaths from anesthesia, almost all of which are caused by errors in the choice of the agent or in its administration.

The reduced maternal death rate is a result of many factors, which include an increase in hospital deliveries, the availability of blood, and the ability to treat infection effectively. In addition, there are many more highly trained and skillful obstetricians in all parts of the country with whom general practitioners can consult when a complication develops. Most hospital staffs are organized and have established rules by which obstetric practice in the institution is governed. Those without special training and experience are required to seek consultation for serious complications and for abnormalities of labor. This is in contrast to the previous situation, when any staff member, regardless of his ability, was permitted to perform any type of operative procedure or manage any complication without seeking help.

Maternal mortality can be reduced even further: It should be possible at least to eliminate deaths from hemorrhage and infection, both of which can be prevented or treated if they do occur. Deaths from abortion can be eliminated or reduced to a minimum by making reliable contraceptive methods and legal hospital abortion available to everyone who wants them. There may be an irreducible minimum of obstetric deaths, but it can only be reached if every physician concentrates on preventing or detecting and correcting potentially lethal abnormalities and if the facilities in which pregnant women are treated are optimal.

■ Perinatal mortality

A *fetal death* is the death of a fetus weighing 500 grams or more before or during birth. No heartbeat, respiratory activity, or movement of voluntary muscle can be detected after birth. If the weight is unknown, fetal death is diagnosed if the pregnancy is of 20 weeks or more duration as measured from the first day of the last normal menstrual period. A *neonatal death* is the death of a live-born infant weighing 500 grams or more within the first 28 days of life. The term *perinatal death* is an inclusive one, indicating the deaths of fetuses weighing 500 grams or more before or during birth and of live-born infants of the same weight within the first 28 days of life. The *perinatal mortality rate* is the number of fetal deaths plus the number of neonatal deaths per 1,000 live-born infants.

Most states require that the deaths of all infants born after 20 or more weeks of pregnancy be reported; in some states it is necessary to report deaths from pregnancies of less than 20 weeks' duration. The total perinatal mortality when calculated on this basis—*perinatal mortality rate* I—will include many infants who are too immature to survive even though they are born alive. A more realistic method is to base the calculation on infants who are likely to live. *Perinatal mortality rate* II includes the deaths of fetuses weighing 1,001 grams or more (over 28 weeks' gestation) and liveborn infants of the same weight who live less than 7 days. This does not mean, of course, that the large number of deaths of smaller infants can be ignored because spontaneous abortions and immature births constitute one of the most important causes of infant loss.

There are many reasons for perinatal deaths; some, such as those associated with toxemia and other acute and chronic diseases in the mother, complications of labor, infections, and birth injuries, can often be avoided. Those due to congenital malformation, cord entanglement, and certain disorders of placental function cannot yet be controlled. The latter, however, are in the minority. If a postmortem examination is performed on every infant who dies and if the attending obstetrician will review his management of the pregnancy and delivery, he may find an obvious cause for the death of the baby. The application of this information to similar situations in the future may help him to prevent another death. Most hospitals hold regular mortality conferences in which the obstetricians, pediatricians, and pathologists participate; interested individual physicians can accomplish the same things by reviewing the deaths of their own patients.

Fetal deaths. The World Health Organization has recommended the term *fetal death* to replace the older terms, "stillbirth" and "abortion." Fetal deaths are classified as follows:

Group I: Early fetal deaths—less than 20 completed weeks of pregnancy
Group II: Intermediate fetal deaths—20 through 27 completed weeks of pregnancy
Group III: Late fetal deaths—28 or more completed weeks of pregnancy
Group IV: Unclassified

In 1967 there were 54,934 fetal deaths. The *fetal mortality ratio* was 15.6 per 1,000

live births. The total number of fetal deaths cannot be determined accurately because most states do not require the reporting of deaths from pregnancies of less than 20 weeks' duration; 10% to 15% of all pregnancies terminate in spontaneous abortion. Perhaps half of these occur because of unpreventable factors, such as chromosomal abnormalities, but some of the rest might have been prevented. An additional million or more pregnancies are terminated by nontherapeutic abortion each year. These, and the maternal deaths resulting from them, could also be prevented by adequate conception control and legal hospital abortion.

The most common causes of fetal deaths are *anoxia* (many of which are associated with abruptio placentae, placenta previa, toxemia, maternal diabetes, prolapsed cord, and abnormal labor), *congenital anomalies,* and *infection* associated with premature rupture of the membranes and prolonged labor. In one third to one half of fetal deaths no cause can be determined, even though an autopsy is performed.

Neonatal deaths. In 1967, 58,127 liveborn infants died during the first 28 days after birth. Of these, 52,650 were less than 7 days old when they died and 27,331 died during the first 24 hours. The *neonatal mortality rates* were as follows: total 16.5, white 15, and nonwhite 23.8. This figure indicates that the neonatal death rate has been reduced but less spectacularly than the maternal death rate. Neonatal mortality was 20 in 1951, 28.8 in 1940, and 39.7 between 1920 and 1924.

The main causes of neonatal death in 1967 were as follows:

CAUSE	NEONATAL DEATHS
Postnatal asphyxia and atelectasis	12,536
Congenital malformations	7,850
Birth injury	6,555
Pneumonia	2,219
Erythroblastosis fetalis	1,186

Prevention of neonatal mortality. Approximately half of all neonatal deaths occur in premature infants who are unable to cope with the hazards of an independent existence. The most obvious way to reduce neonatal mortality, therefore, is to reduce the premature delivery rate. Although it is possible to accomplish this in certain patients, our understanding of many of the causes of premature labor is as yet incomplete, and we cannot always prevent it. An example of the importance of prematurity is that 9,283 of the 12,536 infants who died of postnatal asphyxia and atelectasis were immature, as were 7,948 of the 9,821 infants who died of ill-defined disorders peculiar to early infancy and 4,168 of 6,555 infants who died of birth injuries. In an additional 11,842, immaturity was the only obvious cause of death.

Most of the deaths occur with *high-risk pregnancies;* therefore, it is essential that women with conditions associated with increased perinatal mortality be given special attention during pregnancy and labor. Examples of high-risk pregnancies are those complicated by diabetes mellitus, hypertensive disorders, hydramnios, multiple fetuses, and antepartum bleeding. The principal problems of delivery are breech and other malpresentations, prolapsed cord, placenta previa, and abruptio placentae.

Illegitimate pregnancies and pregnancies at the extremes of the reproductive years are accompanied by increased prematurity and fetal and neonatal death rates. It is essential, therefore, that sexually active teenagers and women who want no more children be provided with reliable contraceptive methods. The perinatal mortality rates in socioeconomically deprived women, regardless of race, are high. They also need protection against too many and too frequent pregnancies.

■ Nonlethal effects of the birth process

Not all infants who are born alive are normal. Approximately 7% of all live-born infants have structural or functional defects. Less than half of these defects are diagnosed during the early postnatal period; the rest appear weeks or even years later.

According to Apgar, at least 15 million people in the United States have one or more congenital defects that affect their lives. Among these, 1 million have congenital orthopedic conditions, 750,000 have hearing defects, 500,000 are blind, 350,000 have congenital heart lesions, and 100,000 have speech defects; 2.9 million are mentally deficient.

It is difficult to determine how many of these conditions could have been prevented by better obstetric care because many must be due to unrecognized chromosomal conditions or to teratogenic stimuli during pregnancy. Many, however, particularly those who are mentally defective, might have been normal had they not been born prematurely, injured during labor and delivery, or suffered hypoxia. Improvements in these figures must await more information concerning the prevention of premature labor, sensitive instruments that will detect early intrauterine hypoxia, precise methods for determining the need for delivery, and improvements in the treatment of postdelivery respiratory distress.

References

Anderson, G. W., and Nesbitt, R. E. L., Jr.: The clinical and pathologic aspects of premature perinatal death, Bull. Hopkins Hosp. **97:**113, 1955.

Apgar, V.: Birth defects, their significance as a public health problem, J.A.M.A. **204:**79, 1968.

Arey, J. P., and Dent, J.: Causes of fetal and neonatal death with special reference to pulmonary and inflammatory lesions, J. Pediat. **42:**1, 1953.

Babson, S. G., and Benson, R. C.: Primer on prematurity and high-risk pregnancy, St. Louis, 1966, The C. V. Mosby Co.

Nesbitt, R. E. L., Jr., and Anderson, G. W.: Perinatal mortality; clinical and pathologic aspects, Obstet. Gynec. **8:**50, 1956.

Potter, E. L.: Pathology of the fetus and newborn, Chicago, 1952, Year Book Medical Publishers, Inc.

Windle, W. F.: Brain damage at birth; functional and structural modifications with time, J.A.M.A. **206:**1967, 1968.

2

Diagnostic methods in obstetrics and gynecology

An accurate medical history and a careful general physical examination are at least as important for pregnant women and those with gynecologic disorders as for medical and surgical patients. In obstetric patients, abnormalities in other organs may influence the course of pregnancy adversely, and many gynecologic patients, who are likely to be in the older age groups, have medical conditions such as hypertension, diabetes, heart lesions, etc., of which they may be unaware. The principles of history taking and examination do not differ from those for other patients except that the complaints usually concern the genital organs; consequently, more emphasis must be placed on the details of their function and structure. Changes in the other organs and systems must not be overlooked, however.

Few women enjoy pelvic examinations, and most find it somewhat difficult to discuss the details of menstrual and sexual function candidly with a strange man. Nevertheless, the gynecologist can obtain a far better survey of the patient's life in general and her emotional reactions in particular than can most physicians because so many problems of all sorts manifest themselves in disturbed sexual and genital response. Women who have made up their minds to consult a physician because of a pelvic complaint are also more willing to discuss it and genital function in general than are those with disturbances in other parts of the body. Despite this, it may be difficult for them to give a satisfactory history and to permit the examinations necessary to make a diagnosis.

■ History

The patient should be encouraged to tell her story in her own words, even though this may be a prolonged process in some instances. Details can be filled in by questions that will provide the additional information necessary to complete the recital. It usually is better to ask questions after she has given an account of her illness rather than to interrupt frequently. Direct questions concerning sexual functions and her relationships with her husband, children, and parents will sometimes provide a clue as to the basis of her symptoms or may lead to the discovery of more serious emotional situations. Too often these questions are deliberately avoided because the physician feels inadequate to cope with such problems or because he knows that they may precipitate a long, tearful session which will interrupt his daily schedule. Questions should be phrased simply in words the patient can comprehend easily; too many will answer "no" to questions they cannot understand rather than display what they presume to be ignorance. No one except the doctor and the patient should be present while the history is being recorded.

The family history, past medical history, menstrual history, history of vaginal discharge, obstetric history, marital history, and present illness should provide adequate information concerning both obstetric and gynecologic patients.

Family history. Particular reference to medical conditions such as diabetes and

7

vascular disease, to emotional problems, and to the patient's relationships with her parents and siblings should be made.

Past medical history. Serious illnesses and the details of operative procedures should be noted. In the systemic review particular interest should be directed toward endocrine disorders, cardiovascular diseases, diseases and dysfunctions of the urinary tract (infection, urinary control, etc.), and symptoms of pelvic relaxation.

Menstrual history. The menstrual history should include the age at which periods began and the type of flow at onset (regular, irregular, etc.), preparation for menstruation and reaction to its onset, frequency and duration of periods and amount of bleeding (number of well-saturated or stained pads, clots, etc.), pain (type, when it began, how long it lasts, how much interference with activity, what medications required for relief), date of last *normal* menstrual period and previous *normal* period, intermenstrual bleeding (duration, amount, pain, relation to trauma), and relationship of other symptoms to menstruation.

Vaginal discharge. Information concerning vaginal discharge should include how long it has been present; its relation to menses, coitus, or other stimuli; bleeding; irritation; and previous treatment.

Obstetric history. List each pregnancy chronologically with information concerning prenatal complications, duration and termination, type of termination, complications of labor, and puerperium; sex and weight of infants and their subsequent development; and patient's reactions to pregnancy and her evaluation of labors.

Marital history. Note the number of marriages and the duration of each and reason for termination and frequency of sexual relations and response to them, contraceptive method, and patient's evaluation of husband in psychosexual problems.

Present illness. The chronologic account of the problem should be obtained, including the applicable details of menstrual disturbance, symptoms referable to pelvic structures, vaginal discharge, etc.

■ Physical examination

A general physical examination should be performed on new patients except those referred from other physicians only for pelvic

evaluation. The *gynecologic examination* itself includes recording the weight and blood pressure, palpation of the breasts, and abdominal and pelvic examination. The general survey does not differ from that usually made, except that particular attention is directed toward abdominal masses or tenderness which might be caused by enlarged, displaced, or improperly functioning pelvic structures. In most instances the abdominal tenderness caused by painful lesions of the pelvic structures is located low in the abdomen and just above the pubis, unless the organs are abnormally enlarged. Tenderness in the upper abdomen, near the umbilicus, in the region of the cecum, and along the course of the descending colon is seldom associated with disease in the pelvic organs.

Pelvic examination. The pelvic examination is performed with the patient in lithotomy position, suitably draped with a sheet, her feet in stirrups, and her buttocks hanging just over the lower end of the table. Unless the physician wishes to obtain a specimen of urine by catheter or to check for urinary control, the patient should void immediately before being examined. The external genitals are inspected in a good light and palpated for evidence of developmental anomaly or of change due to disease. A note should be made of hair distribution, clitoral size, skin changes, discharge, irrigation, new growths, and enlargements of Bartholin's glands.

A *speculum,* moistened with water when necessary, is gently inserted into the vagina to expose the cervix and the vaginal mucosa. Lubricating jelly should not be used if the physician intends to obtain a sample of the vaginal or cervical secretions for cytologic examination or to study for infection. After the exposed cervix has been wiped clean with dry cotton, a note is made of its color, size, and configuration, and any obvious lesions are described minutely. Material is collected from the cervical canal for cytologic examination, and when indicated, a sample of the fluid from the vaginal canal is obtained for culture or for microscopic study. The canal is probed in an attempt to provoke bleeding, and a biopsy of the cervix is performed when indicated. As the speculum is slowly withdrawn, the vaginal walls are inspected.

Two fingers are then inserted into the vagina to depress the posterior wall as the patient holds her breath and "bears down."

If the muscular supports of the bladder and rectum have been damaged, these structures will bulge through the open introitus as intra-abdominal pressure is increased. The uterus also may be forced downward if its supports have been weakened.

Although it is not possible to visualize the body of the uterus and the adnexal structures, their size, shape, position, mobility, and sensitivity can usually be determined with reasonable accuracy if the patient is able to relax sufficiently and if there is no painful lesion present. This information can be obtained by *bimanual examination,* in which the fingers of one hand are inserted into the vagina while those of the other hand palpate through the abdominal wall. Vaginal examination is embarrassing at best, and it is difficult enough for patients to relax, but if the palpatory motions produce pain, it is impossible for patients to keep from contracting the abdominal and pelvic muscles. This limits the accuracy of the examination. Most women, even virgins, can be examined vaginally with little discomfort if only the index finger is inserted.

The consistency of the cervix and the direction in which it points are determined, and the cervix and uterus are pushed upward and from side to side to detect pain produced by motion. The body of the uterus is located, and its size, shape, and consistency

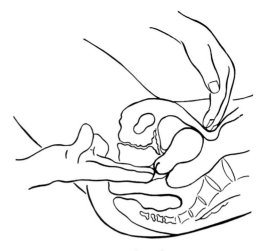

Fig. 2-2. Bimanual palpation of uterus.

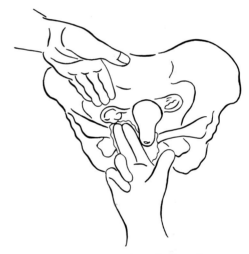

Fig. 2-3. Bimanual palpation of adnexal structures.

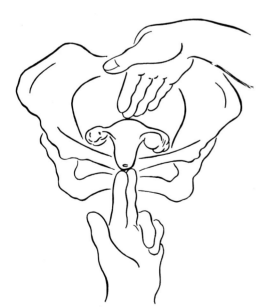

Fig. 2-1. Bimanual palpation of uterus.

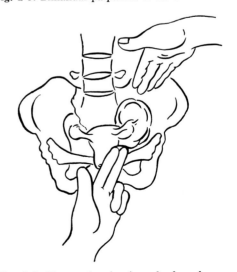

Fig. 2-4. Bimanual palpation of adnexal mass.

are determined by palpating it between the finger in the vagina and the fingers pushing the abdominal wall structures inward. An attempt is then made to feel each tube and ovary between the fingertips of the two hands. The right adnexus can be outlined most accurately with the fingers of the right hand in the vagina and those of the left hand palpating abdominally. The left adnexus can be felt best with the fingers of the left hand in the vagina. The normal tube and ovary usually cannot be outlined, except that the patient may experience momentary discomfort as the ovary is squeezed between the fingers on the abdomen and those in the vagina. Adnexal masses can usually be felt if they are large enough and if the patient is not too obese.

The posterior surface of the uterus and broad ligaments, the uterosacral ligaments, the posterior cul-de-sac, and the structures on the lateral pelvic walls can be felt more accurately by rectal than by vaginal palpation. Rectocele and other lower bowel lesions such as polyps and carcinoma can also be felt. Rectal or rectovaginal examination should be performed as a part of every pelvic examination.

■ Diagnostic tests

In many women the information obtained from the history and the physical examination is enough to indicate what treatment, if any, is required. In others further study is necessary before a treatment plan can be developed. Most organic gynecologic disorders are caused by infection, endocrine dysfunction, injury, and tumor growth; of these the last two can usually be diagnosed without difficulty, but it often is necessary to perform certain laboratory studies to identify the infecting organism or the hormone disorder. Many diagnostic tests are simple and can be performed in the physician's office, little equipment other than a microscope and stains for bacteria being necessary. A few tests can be done only in elaborate and specialized laboratories.

Urine examination. The microscopic examination of a catheterized or clean voided specimen of urine often is helpful because infections occur so frequently in women. The physician should perform urine tests in his own office because the examination of the sediment of freshly collected urine is far

more revealing than that which has stood for several hours awaiting transportation to the laboratory. There is little point in performing a microscopic examination on voided urine in women unless special precautions are taken to prevent contamination by vulvar debris.

Blood examination. Hemoglobin and hematocrit determinations may aid in the diagnosis of certain gynecologic conditions, but they are seldom necessary. One must occasionally differentiate between a minor pelvic disorder and appendicitis or between tubal pregnancy and salpingo-oophoritis; in such patients a white blood cell count may be useful. As a general rule, however, the white blood cell count is of little help in gynecologic conditions.

Smears and suspensions of vaginal secretions. It is often helpful to identify the organism responsible for the various types of pelvic infection. In some instances this can be accomplished in the physician's office, but in others it is necessary to send the specimens to a laboratory. The material for study should be obtained directly from the infected area and transported to the laboratory as rapidly as possible. The cotton swabs or small fragments of infected tissue should be placed in nutrient broth immediately, and under no circumstances should they be permitted to dry out. Crusts or exudates covering the lesions should be removed so that the material for culture can be obtained directly from the affected tissue.

Smears. Smears for bacteriologic examination are most informative in the study of localized infections and ulcerated areas and are least helpful in the evaluation of ordinary chronic cervicitis and vaginitis. Material should be obtained from the urethra and cervical canal of every woman suspected of having *gonorrhea.* Culture is far more accurate than examination of a stained smear. For greatest accuracy the material must be collected from the gland openings. The gonococci in free pus in the vagina are likely to be dead. A swab is inserted through the urethral meatus, and the urethra is milked from above downward by finger pressure through the vagina to evacuate the glands. The cervix is then exposed and wiped clean, and a dry swab is inserted into the canal and rotated. Infected material can be expressed from the glands by closing the blades of the

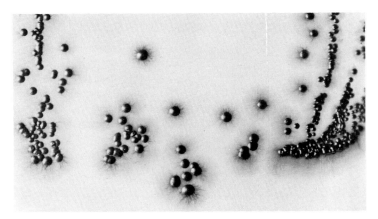

Fig. 2-5. Colonies of yeastlike organisms on Nickerson's medium.

speculum and squeezing the cervix while the applicator is left in the canal. A more accurate result can be obtained, particularly in chronic quiescent gonorrheal cervicitis, by gently scraping the cervical canal with a small sharp curet.

Smears are also helpful in the diagnosis of *vaginal candidiasis*. The material is obtained with a dry swab from the inflamed vaginal wall and streaked on suitable culture medium for bacteriologic examination. *Candida* can be grown in the physician's office on Nickerson's medium or Pagano-Levin medium without special equipment. The surface of the commercially prepared slant is streaked with the discharge, and within 48 hours characteristic colonies will appear. Bacteria do not grow, and the tubes can be kept at room temperature. Yeastlike organisms can also be identified by Gram's stain and in an unstained saline suspension. With Gram's stain the branching mycelia stain blue, the spore capsule is red, and its center is blue. The addition of 2 to 3 drops of a 10% aqueous solution of potassium hydroxide to a saline suspension will dissolve the epithelial, white, and red cells, leaving the mycelia and spores.

Suspensions. If a small amount of vaginal discharge is examined under the microscope without staining, *trichomonads* can be detected if they are present. An unlubricated speculum is inserted into the vagina, and a specimen of the secretion is collected with a dry cotton swab, which is immediately placed in a test tube containing about ½ inch of warm physiologic saline solution and agitated. A drop of the suspension is placed on a clean glass slide covered with a coverslip and examined under the microscope without staining. The trichomonads are actively motile and slightly larger than a leukocyte.

■ Hormone assay

There are few gynecologic conditions, other than menstrual disorders and infertility, in which hormone assays are particularly helpful. The physician must often decide whether a woman ovulates, and if she does not, whether she produces estrogens. This can be determined by reliable hormone assays, which are more elaborate and costly than simple office procedures that can be performed more rapidly. These office procedures are generally based upon the effects that certain hormones exert upon the patient's vaginal epithelium, cervical mucus, and endometrium. Such tests are at best semi-quantitative, and their lack of accuracy is further compounded by insufficient specificity. This results from the well-known fact that cells do not have many ways of responding to a variety of stimuli. As a result, such office procedures, at best, allow the physician to distinguish between low, normal, or elevated hormone levels of estrogenic and/or progestogenic activity. Nevertheless, this information is sufficient for a proper diagnosis and therapy in a good number of patients.

TESTS FOR ESTROGENIC ACTIVITY

Examination of vaginal smears. The presence of systemic estrogen activity may be assumed when a smear of cellular material collected from the upper vagina and stained

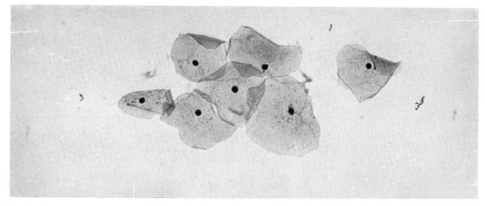

Fig. 2-6. Strong estrogenic effect. Large, flat squamae with pyknotic nuclei and acidophilic cytoplasm (cornified cells) are present universally here. Smear has "clean" appearance.

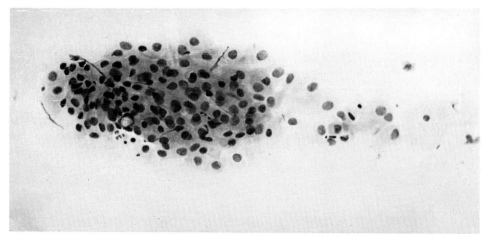

Fig. 2-7. Lack of estrogenic effect. Clump of cells demonstrating moderately advanced atrophy of vaginal epithelium. Vaguely outlined basophilic "deep" cells with large nuclei predominate.

by the Papanicolaou technique, or simply with methylene blue, reveals true cornified cells and/or precornified cells. Estrogenic effect can be considered absent when the smear is composed predominantly of basal and parabasal cells.

A rough measure of estrogenic effect is the *maturation index:* the proportions of parabasal, precornified (intermediate), and cornified (superficial) cells in each 100 vaginal mucosal cells counted. Absence of estrogen is indicated by a predominance of parabasal cells (100:0:0). With a small amount of estrogen there is cellular stimulation and more precornified cells (10:80:10). At ovulation the numbers of precornified and cornified cells are about equal (0:40:60), and with increasing estrogen stimulation the

percentage of cornified cells increases even more. Similar measurements can be made by determining the percentage of acidophilic staining cells *(eosinophilic index)* and the percentage of cells with pyknotic nuclei *(karyopyknotic index);* both eosinophilia and pyknotic nuclei increase with increasing estrogen stimulation.

Examination of cervical mucus. Papanicolaou (1945) described an interesting pattern of arborization, or ferning, in cervical mucus spread on a clean glass slide and allowed to dry. This phenomenon is most pronounced during the midinterval of the menstrual cycle, near the time of ovulation; it is absent immediately before and after menstruation and cannot be demonstrated in cervical mucus of castrated, postmeno-

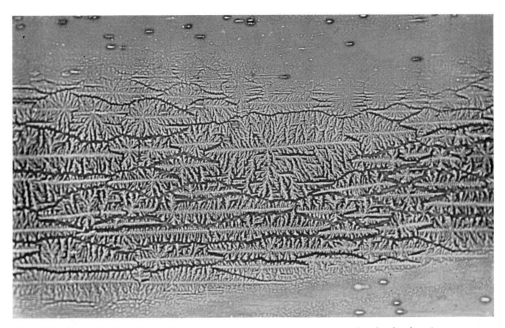

Fig. 2-8. Arborization of cervical mucus, 2 plus fern, a layer of arborization between two cellular areas. This type of smear indicates moderate estrogen activity.

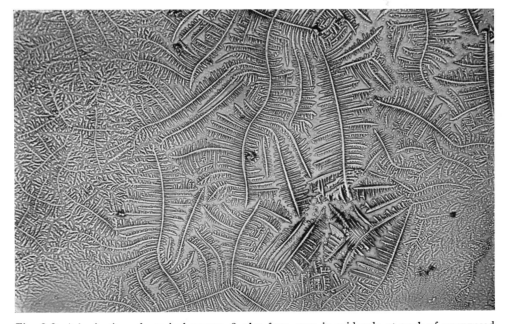

Fig. 2-9. Arborization of cervical mucus, 3 plus fern, seen in midcycle at peak of unopposed estrogen activity. (×164.)

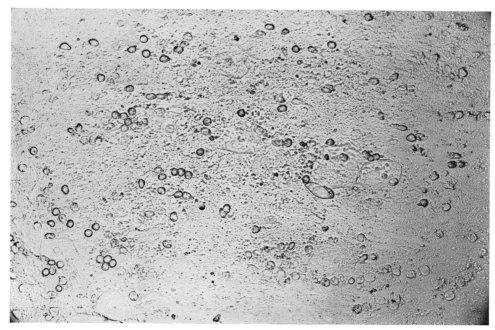

Fig. 2-10. Arborization of cervical mucus. Negative smear. Cellular elements and mucous debris seen during premenstrual and postmenstrual phases of cycle. (×153.)

pausal, or normally pregnant women. Zondek was able to induce arborization in the mucus of castrated and postmenopausal women by administering 1 mg. of estrone, thus demonstrating that ferning is a result of estrogen activity. A negative test may indicate either the absence of estrogen (postmenopause, castration, etc.) or the presence of fern-inhibiting progesterone (premenstrually and during pregnancy).

To obtain mucus an unlubricated speculum is inserted into the vagina, exposing the cervix, from which the visible discharge is wiped. A cotton-tipped applicator is gently inserted into the cervical canal and rotated. The mucus that adheres to the cotton swab is then spread on a clean glass slide and allowed to dry at room temperature or by heating over a flame. The dried, unstained spread is then scanned under the low power of the microscope. Moderate (2 plus) or strongly positive (3 plus) arborization is quite evident under this magnification, but if it is minimal (1 plus) or questionable, the field should be studied under higher magnification.

Not infrequently the cervical mucus is so scant and tenacious that it is difficult to obtain an adequate quantity by means of the cotton-tipped applicator. When this occurs,

a uterine dressing forceps or, preferably, a specially designed cervical mucus forceps (Fig. 2-11) is employed. A drop of mucus is grasped by this instrument and is deposited on the slide by opening the jaws of the forceps while they are in contact with the glass slide.

The slides used for examination of cervical mucus should be washed and the instruments sterilized in distilled water, since the electrolytes in tap water may produce a false arborization. Also, in obtaining cervical mucus the physician should be careful not to traumatize the cervix because blood mixed with the mucus may inhibit arborization.

Endometrial biopsy. Since estrogen produces characteristic endometrial proliferation, the physician can detect estrogenic activity by studying the histologic pattern of endometrium obtained with a biopsy curet. This procedure is more difficult and costly than the study of vaginal smears and no more accurate; therefore, it is rarely used for this purpose.

Biologic and chemical estrogen assays. Estrogens can be extracted from plasma and urine and may be separated from other lipids and steroid hormones. The isolated estrogens may then be quantitated by a variety of biologic and chemical methods.

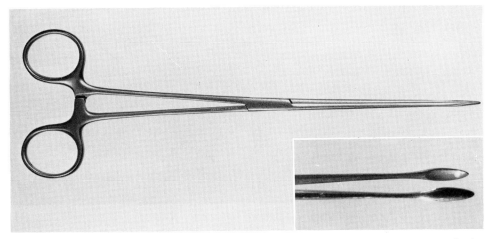

Fig. 2-11. Cervical mucus forceps (Palmer) for obtaining cervical mucus for arborization smear and postcoital test. Inset shows detail of spoon-shaped ends.

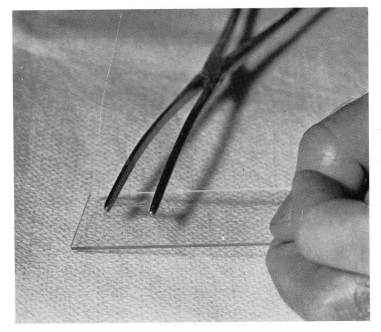

Fig. 2-12. Fern test. Recommended technique for cervical mucus smear.

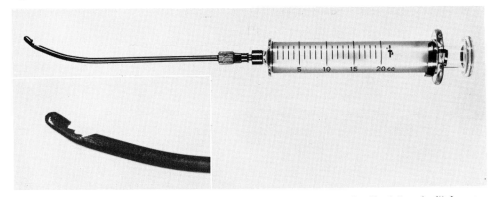

Fig. 2-13. Endometrial biopsy suction curet (Novak). Inset shows detail of "toothed" fenestration.

Biologic assays are carried out by injecting estrogen extracts into immature rats or mice. The quantity of estrogens injected is reflected by the degree of vaginal epithelial cornification or by the increase in uterine weight. Even if several animals are used for a single assay, bioassays are relatively inaccurate, since the injected extracts represent usually a mixture of several estrogens with pronounced differences in estrogenic activity.

Chemical methods have been developed for the measurement of unfractionated ("total") estrogens, fractionated estrogens (estrone, estradiol, and estriol), and urinary estriol in pregnancy; colorimetry, fluorometry, and gas chromatography are used to quantitate the isolated estrogens. Milligram

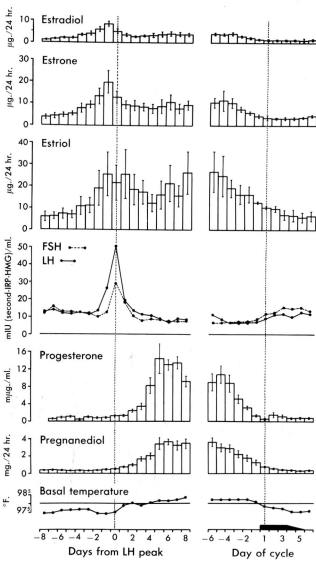

Fig. 2-14. Means of serum LH and FSH levels, serum progesterone concentrations, 24-hour urinary estrone, estradiol, estriol, and pregnanediol excretions, and basal body temperatures in 5 normal women. The data are plotted both in terms of days from the midcycle LH and FSH peak, from the approximate time of ovulation, and from the onset of menstruation. Vertical bars indicate standard errors. (From Goebelsmann, U., Snyder, D. L., and Jaffe, R. B.: Unpublished data.)

quantities of estriol are excreted during pregnancy, and estriol measurements may be used as a method of assessing placental function and fetal status. During the menstrual cycle, estrogen excretion amounts to microgram quantities and is subject to typical changes. Estrogen excretion is low during the early follicular phase of the normal cycle, where it is hardly distinguishable from low estrogen values encountered in amenorrheic and postmenopausal women. Estrogen excretion rises rapidly at midcycle and is elevated during the luteal phase, dropping prior to the onset of menstruation (Fig. 2-14). Estrogen excretion varies widely among different "normally ovulating" women. The method described by Brown (1955) is the most widely used procedure to measure urinary estrogens in nonpregnant women.

TESTS FOR PROGESTERONE

Basal body temperature charts. Since progesterone has a thermogenic property, a sustained rise in the basal body temperature during the latter half of the menstrual cycle is presumptive evidence of progesterone activity. A monophasic curve is suggestive of absent or deficient progesterone secretion.

Premenstrual endometrial biopsy. Histologic examination of tissue removed for curettage or for endometrial biopsy several days before the onset of the flow or even on the first day of menstruation is a most accurate method for the determination of progesterone activity. A late secretory endometrium is indicative of an adequate progesterone effect, whereas an endometrium in the proliferative or early secretory phase during the premenstruum indicates absent or inadequate progesterone secretion.

Examination of cervical mucus. Examination of cervical mucus may be of value in determining progesterone activity. If arborization is adequate at midcycle and tends to disappear in the premenstrual phase, it can be assumed that the change was brought about by the fern-inhibiting effect of progesterone.

Examination of vaginal smears. Vaginal smears may be of help in determining progesterone activity if they are examined daily during the menstrual cycle. However, the

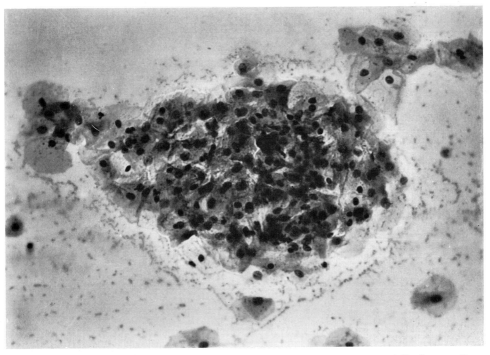

Fig. 2-15. Moderately advanced progestogenic effect. Acidophilic and basophilic intermediate, undifferentiated squamous-type cells predominate in this typical clump. Some cornified cells persist. Mucus and bacteria create a "smudgy" picture.

cytologic changes may be so indefinite that only a trained cytologist can interpret them properly.

Assays for progesterone and pregnanediol. Competitive protein-binding and radioimmunoassay procedures have recently been developed for the determination of plasma progesterone levels, which increase from low follicular phase levels (0.4 to 1 ng./ml.) to significantly elevated concentrations (5 to 15 ng./ml.) during the luteal phase (Fig. 2-14). These luteal phase progesterone levels drop prior to the onset of the next menstruation or rise sharply in early pregnancy under the stimulus of chorionic gonadotropin. Plasma progesterone concentration increases throughout the course of pregnancy.

Since plasma progesterone assays have just become available in a few laboratories, progesterone secretion is generally assessed by pregnanediol determinations. Pregnanediol is the chief urinary excretion product, although not an exclusive metabolite, of progesterone. Using a gas-chromatographic procedure, the urinary pregnanediol excretion during the follicular phase on days 7, 8, or 9 ranged from 0.2 to 0.6 mg./ 24 hr. (average: 0.4 mg.) and during the luteal phase on days 23, 24, or 25 ranged from 1.6 to 4.7 mg./24 hr. (average: 2.6 mg.) in 20 women. Pregnanediol excretion increases during gestation, reaching 40 mg./ 24 hr. at term.

TESTS FOR GONADOTROPINS

Until recently, pituitary gonadotropin secretion could only be assessed by measuring urinary gonadotropins by bioassay. Urine extracts are prepared and injected into immature female mice. The gonadotropins present in the extract stimulate the ovaries to produce estrogens, which effect uterine growth. As a result, uterine weight increases parallel the amount of gonadotropins injected. These bioassays are not very accurate and do not distinguish between follicle-stimulating hormone (FSH) and luteinizing hormone (LH) but measure principally FSH. In most patients, however, bioassays provide enough information for an accurate clinical diagnosis. The urinary gonadotropin excretion during the reproductive years ranges from 6 to 48 units/24 hr. and is characterized by a midcycle peak

at the time of ovulation, by higher values in the follicular phase, and by lower values in the luteal phase. In postmenopausal women, gonadotropin excretion is greatly elevated.

Plasma LH and FSH levels ranging from a few milli-international units (mIU) to less than 100 mIU in normally ovulating women can now be measured by radioimmunoassay. As these specific and accurate assays become more readily available, pituitary gonadotropin secretion can be assessed more conveniently than by bioassay of urinary extracts.

TESTS FOR ANDROGENS

Testosterone assays in plasma or urine require specialized procedures and are not readily available. Recently, competitive protein-binding methods have been described for the measurement of plasma testosterone levels, simplifying testosterone assays. Urinary 17-ketosteroid determinations in general do not reflect elevated levels of plasma testosterone, since even elevated testosterone levels that cause virilization do not significantly raise the 17-ketosteroid excretion. In women the 17-ketosteroid excretion averages 8 mg./24 hr. (range: 5 to 15 mg.) as compared to men with 15 mg./24 hr. (range: 8 to 20 mg.). More than 10% of the 17-ketosteroid excretion measured in a normal woman is caused by unspecific urinary pigments, and about 75% is of adrenal origin secreted mainly in the form of dehydroisoandrosterone, whereas the remainder, less than 20% of the total 17-ketosteroids, reflects ovarian androgen secretion.

TESTS FOR OVULATION

Without ovulation, reproduction is impossible. This makes it important for us not only to be able to detect ovulation but also to time its occurrence with some degree of accuracy. The only certain method for ascertaining this would be the inspection of an ovary or the recovery of an ovum. This is obviously impractical. There are, however, a number of fairly reliable presumptive evidences that ovulation has occurred which may be used to determine and to time this event.

Mittelschmerz. A few women experience varying degrees of lower abdominal pain at the time of ovulation. The pain is usually unilateral and may be accompanied by a mucoid or mucosanguineous vaginal discharge. It occurs so infrequently and so sporadically that it has very limited clinical applicability.

Cervical mucus. Examination of cervical mucus near midcycle and again just prior to menstruation may be used as a presumptive test for ovulation. The mucus at midcycle is abundant, watery, glassy, and elastic and shows typical arborization only when sufficient amounts of estrogenic hormone are produced. If the second examination 1 to 2 days before the onset of menstruation shows scanty mucus with an abundance of cells but with inhibition of the previously observed arborization, this is proof of corpus luteum formation and adequate progesterone production. If the midcycle examination is omitted, the physician might diagnose ovulation and corpus luteum formation on the basis of a negative fern reaction when what actually occurred was a hypoestrogenic cycle with complete failure of ferning. Since there is a progressive increase in the amount of arborization as the ovulatory phase nears, one may, by correlating this phenomenon with the appearance of the basal body temperature chart, predict the day of ovulation with a fair degree of accuracy.

Vaginal smear. During the normal cycle, ovulation is marked by maximum estrogenic effect on the vaginal epithelium. At the height of the follicular phase the vaginal smear is "clean," showing little mucus and few leukocytes (Fig. 2-6). Superficial, cornified, acidophilic-staining vaginal cells predominate. After ovulation the smear changes in character under the influence of progesterone. The desquamated cells become curled and folded, and the cytoplasm loses its acidophilic-staining property (Fig. 2-15). Unfortunately even an experienced cytologist cannot always detect ovulation or determine by cytologic studies when it actually occurred.

Endometrial biopsy. Histologic examination of a piece of endometrium removed either by curettage or by biopsy 3 to 5 days before the onset of a menstrual period should demonstrate a late secretory endometrium. This is probably the most reliable evidence that ovulation has occurred. The limitations in this method are that it indicates only what has happened in one isolated cycle and that the discomfort incident

to obtaining the tissue and the expense involved make it impractical to repeat the test during several cycles.

Unless contraceptives are used during the cycle in which a premenstrual biopsy is to be performed, there is always the danger of interfering with an early pregnancy. To obviate this possibility some authors have suggested that the endometrial biopsy be obtained during the first few hours of the menstrual flow. This is not always practicable, and furthermore, the histologic picture of the endometrium during the bleeding phase is not nearly so well defined as it is during the premenstruum.

The tissue can be obtained in the physician's office without anesthesia. The patient is placed in lithotomy position, and a bimanual examination is performed to determine the status of the pelvic viscera and, particularly, the position of the uterus. The cervix is exposed, cleansed, its anterior lip is grasped with a tenaculum forceps, and a sound is passed into the uterine cavity. A narrow suction tube-curet is inserted to the fundus of the uterus, pressed firmly against the anterior wall, and suction is applied as the instrument is slowly withdrawn. An attempt is then made to obtain specimens from the posterior and lateral walls, but this is not always successful. The strips of tissue are placed in 10% formalin solution and are submitted to the pathologist for histologic examination.

Basal body temperature charts. The occurrence and timing of ovulation can be determined by recording daily the basal body temperature (BBT) throughout a cycle. During the preovulatory estrogen phase the basal temperatures remain at a relatively low level. A slight drop, as compared with the waking temperature of the preceding day, and a sharp rise of about 0.6° F. on the following day are typical of ovulation. The rise is maintained with minor fluctuations until a day or two prior to the onset of menstruation, at which time it drops. When these daily fluctuations are charted, they produce a typical *biphasic curve,* which is indicative of progesterone production and, presumably, of ovulation. The degree of corpus luteum function may be roughly gauged by its thermogenic effect; normal function is presumed if the rise in temperature is abrupt, and inadequate pro-

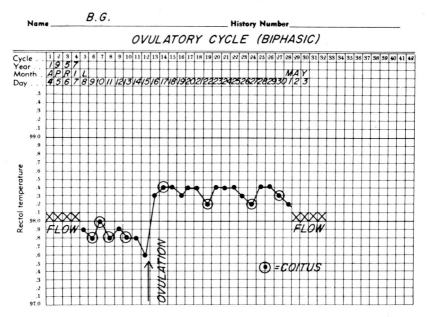

Fig. 2-16. Basal body temperature chart showing biphasic curve indicative of ovulatory cycle. Note the drop and sharp rise at the time of ovulation.

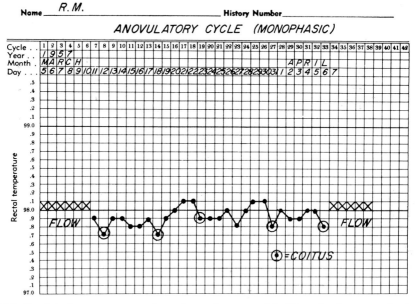

Fig. 2-17. Basal body temperature chart (anovulatory cycle). Note the flat monophasic curve.

gesterone secretion is suspected if the rise is gradual or steplike, but this is not invariable. A curve in which the rise is of short duration, lasting perhaps only 8 or 9 days instead of 12 or 13 days, is less frequently seen but is more indicative of a deficiency of progesterone secretion.

A *monophasic curve,* which indicates complete failure of ovulation, is produced when the temperature level remains low throughout the cycle. In cycles in which ovulation and fertilization have occurred, the secondary rise is maintained past the date of the expected menstrual period. This often provides the earliest evidence of the presence of pregnancy.

The patient is provided with a chart simi-

lar to the one illustrated in Fig. 2-16 and with a special thermometer that is graduated in tenths of degrees and that records a temperature range of only 3.5° F. (96° to 99.5° F.). The thermometer is kept at the bedside, and the temperature is taken immediately upon awakening at approximately the same time each morning. The thermometer is allowed to remain in place for 5 minutes, is read, and is shaken down after the reading is recorded on the chart. For proper evaluation, accurate temperature recordings should be kept over a period of at least three menstrual cycles.

The basal body temperature curve is a simple, inexpensive method for determining ovulation. It may not be as accurate as pre-

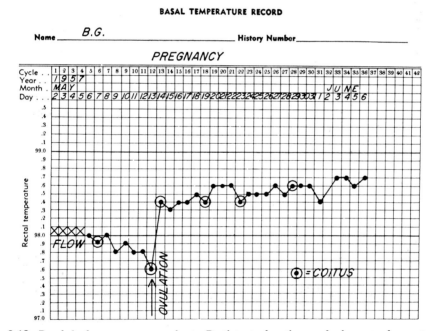

Fig. 2-18. Basal body temperature chart. Persistent elevation and absence of menstruation are suggestive of pregnancy.

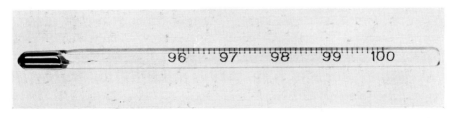

Fig. 2-19. Special thermometer for recording basal body temperature.

menstrual endometrial biopsy in establishing an ovulatory cycle, but it has the advantage of simplicity and the feasibility of repeated observations over a period of several months. In addition it is a fairly accurate guide to the timing of ovulation. However, in spite of these advantages, this method should not be employed over unduly long periods of time, since it may become a source of irritation and anxiety to the patient and her husband.

Menstrual history (Ogino-Knaus principle). Ogino and Knaus independently demonstrated that menstruation occurs about 14 days after ovulation. Therefore, in regularly menstruating women the ovulation day can be estimated fairly accurately. Rock has reckoned that this occurs 14 plus or minus 2 days before menstruation.

Hormone assay. The luteinization of the follicle after ovulation is intimately connected with a pronounced increase in ovarian *progesterone* secretion. Consequently, serum progesterone levels are significantly increased during the luteal phase (Fig. 2-14). The use of plasma progesterone determinations to assess ovulation and corpus luteum function seems very promising.

Together with the midcycle surge of plasma LH, FSH, and progesterone levels the urinary *pregnanediol* excretion rises, and for a period of about 10 days commencing with the fourth day after the midcycle LH and FSH peak and ending with the day prior to the onset of the next menstruation, pregnanediol excretion remains above 1 mg./24 hr. as compared to 0.4 ± 0.1 mg./24 hr. (standard deviation in 20 normal women) prior to ovulation. This very distinct increase in urinary pregnanediol excretion over the next 2 or 3 days following ovulation explains why pregnanediol, even as a single assay, is such a valuable test for assessing ovulation and corpus luteum function.

Urinary *estrogen* excretion is always higher during the luteal phase than during the first 8 or 10 days of the follicular phase of the menstrual cycle, but the increase in estrogen excretion is not as distinct as that of pregnanediol, there is a large individual variation in estrogen excretion (Fig. 2-14), and estrogen secretion is not a unique feature of the corpus luteum. Thus estrogen determinations would be useless as an indicator of ovulation and corpus luteum function.

■ Tests for pregnancy

Soon after the ovum is fertilized the trophoblast begins to secrete a hormone called human chorionic gonadotropin (HCG), which shares certain biologic and immunologic properties with pituitary LH. Using the highly sensitive technique of radioimmunoassay, HCG has been detected as early as 9 days after the midcycle surge of LH and FSH. The production of HCG increases rapidly, and as early as 1 week after the first missed period it may be detected in serum and urine with the commonly available immunologic and biologic pregnancy tests. Serum levels and urinary excretion of HCG rise to a peak at about 8 to 10 weeks' gestation and decline toward a lower plateau, which is maintained throughout the second and third trimesters. Pregnancy tests remain positive throughout gestation or as long as viable trophoblastic tissue is in contact with the maternal circulation. A negative pregnancy test, however, may occasionally be encountered during the second half of a normal pregnancy. Thus a negative pregnancy test during the latter half of gestation does not necessarily indicate intrauterine fetal death. Urinary estriol determinations may be a more valuable hormonal measurement for assessing fetal viability.

Aschheim-Zondek test. The Aschheim-Zondek test (1928) is the original chorionic gonadotropin test for pregnancy. It is too cumbersome, however, for routine laboratory diagnosis. The test requires five test animals (immature mice), multiple injections, and 4 to 5 days for completion. The appearance of hemorrhagic follicles or corpora lutea indicates the presence of chorionic gonadotropin in the test urine and is interpreted as a positive pregnancy reaction.

Friedman test. In 1931 Friedman and Lapham described a modification of the Aschheim-Zondek reaction that has proved more practical and almost as accurate as the original test. A positive test is indicated by the presence of corpora hemorrhagica in the ovaries of an adult, isolated female rabbit 36 to 48 hours following the intravenous injection of 10 ml. of urine of a pregnant woman. This test is quite reliable and simple but has been replaced in many laboratories because of its expense and the time necessary (36 to 48 hours) to obtain a result.

Rat ovarian hyperemia test. The rat ovarian hyperemia test is a more rapid test, based on the appearance of a deep red color in the ovary of the immature rat. It represents the earliest detectable ovarian reaction to HCG. A positive result is observed 4 to 24 hours following the intraperitoneal injection of 1 or 2 ml. of urine or serum containing at least 2 I.U. of the hormone. This test requires some experience to interpret the end point accurately, but it has the advantages of simplicity and speed. The rat ovarian hyperemia test can be used for serum, which should not be used in immunologic pregnancy tests.

Immunologic tests. Immunologic pregnancy tests are based on the reaction of urinary HCG with antiserum to chorionic gonadotropin (rabbit anti-HCG). Most pregnancy tests utilize the agglutination inhibition principle as an indicator. Either latex particles (slide tests) or sheep erythrocytes (test tube assay) are employed.

In the former tests 1 drop of urine to be tested and 1 drop of antiserum against chorionic gonadotropin are stirred together for 30 seconds on a glass slide. Two drops of a suspension of latex particles that have been coated with HCG are added and mixed. The slide is then rocked gently for 2 minutes to assure complete exposure of the latex particles to the fluid. Urine from a nonpregnant woman contains no chorionic gonadotropin, therefore the antiserum is free to react with the latex particles coated with HCG, causing them to agglutinate (negative test). This agglutination appears as a fine flocculation. If the women is pregnant, the HCG in the urine will neutralize the antiserum, thus preventing agglutination of the latex particles (positive pregnancy test).

In the hemagglutination inhibition test a small volume of urine is mixed with the antiserum, and a suspension of sheep erythrocytes coated with HCG is added. Within 2 hours, either a mat of agglutinated red cells has settled to the bottom of the test tube (negative test), or a ring of nonagglutinated red cells has formed (positive test).

Although the hemagglutination inhibition test is a 2-hour test as compared to the 2-minute slide tests, it is more accurate and sensitive than currently available slide tests. Slide tests may fail to detect very early pregnancies, when the rat ovarian hyperemia test and hemagglutination inhibition procedures are already positive.

Basal body temperature charts. A persistent elevation of the basal body temperature for 7 to 10 days following a missed menstrual period is quite suggestive of early pregnancy. Therefore, when basal temperatures are being kept, as in cases of infertility, a sustained high level for a period of 3 weeks may be considered as a presumptive positive test for pregnancy.

Evaluation of pregnancy tests. Ordinarily the diagnosis of pregnancy can be made without the laboratory procedures described. However, there are situations in which the history and physical findings are inconclusive or in which a complication such as threatened abortion or ectopic pregnancy is suspected but cannot be confirmed. Under these circumstances properly performed tests for pregnancy may prove an invaluable aid in diagnosis.

The hormone tests for pregnancy are about 98% accurate when carried out by hemagglutination inhibition procedures or by the rat ovarian hyperemia test and when done properly and not before 6 weeks have elapsed since the first day of the last menstruation. Slide tests are less accurate in early pregnancy. False negative tests are encountered more frequently than false positive tests. False negative tests may result under the following conditions: performing the test too early in pregnancy before there is sufficient circulating hormone; a highly dilute urine; technical errors, either in handling or storing of the test urine, or in the use of an unresponsive test animal. Negative pregnancy tests are encountered in intrauterine fetal death unless viable trophoblast tissue is present. In ectopic pregnancies, negative pregnancy tests are not infrequent: A negative pregnancy test never excludes the possibility of an ectopic pregnancy. False positive tests may be obtained early in the menopause or in other gonadal deficiencies in which there is an overproduction of pituitary gonadotropin and because of errors in technique. False positive tests may be encountered in patients who have been taking tranquilizing drugs, notably promazine or one of its derivatives.

It must be emphasized that all of these tests demonstrate the production and excretion of chorionic gonadotropin and do not necessarily indicate the presence of a normal pregnancy. The only thing we can conclude from a positive test is that there is a source of gonadotropin which may be a normal pregnancy.

■ Tests for cancer

Some of the common benign cervical lesions look much like cancer grossly and can only be differentiated by special tests, all of which require highly trained personnel for their interpretation. The specimens must be properly collected and carefully handled so that they will provide the maximum amount of information.

Schiller test. Normal cervical epithelium contains much glycogen and is immediately stained dark brown when painted with Lugol's iodine solution. Abnormal epithelial cells are devoid of glycogen and therefore do not stain. The Schiller test, which is performed by painting the cervix with iodine solution, is based upon the ability of iodine to stain glycogen. It is not diagnostic of cancer of the cervix, but it does indicate areas of abnormal epithelium from which tissue for microscopic study can be obtained.

Cytologic examination. A trained cytologist can detect abnormal cervical and endometrial cells in specially prepared and stained spreads from the cervix. The most accurate results are obtained when the material is collected from the cervical canal (endometrial and endocervical secretions) and from the junction of the squamous and columnar epithelium at or near the external cervical os. The former specimen is obtained by rotating a dry cotton swab within the cervical canal or by aspirating the secretion with a pipet. Material from the cervix is collected by scraping and abrading the area with a special wooden spatula or with a dry cotton swab and transferring the material to a clean glass slide, which is then stained and read by the cytologist.

Cytologic examination is a screening rather than a diagnostic procedure and can serve only to indicate those patients in whom further study is necessary. Whenever

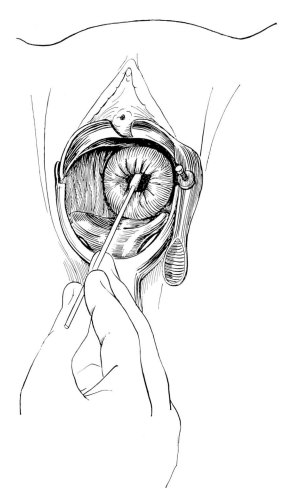

Fig. 2-20. Cytologic examination. The cervix is exposed with a speculum, and the secretions to be examined are obtained by rotating a dry cotton swab in the canal.

abnormal cells are found on a cytologic spread, more precise investigation, usually by cone biopsy and curettage, is necessary. Cytologic studies should be obtained as a part of the periodic examination, even though the cervix appears normal because the earliest carcinomas are not obvious clinically.

Cervical biopsy. Histologic examination of tissue removed from the cervix is an important part of the study of cervical lesions because it permits more precise diagnosis than that by either gross inspection or cytologic examination. Small bites of tissue can be removed with a *punch biopsy instrument* in the physician's office without causing undue pain or alarming bleeding. This procedure is most valuable when a small lesion such as polyp can be removed completely, but it also is helpful in the study of larger lesions, particularly those having the gross appearance of cancer. If several bites of tissue are taken from such a lesion and invasive carcinoma is diagnosed, the physician may proceed directly to treatment. If carcinoma in situ, cervicitis, or some similar condition is diagnosed, further study with cone biopsy is indicated.

Cone biopsy, with which the visible cervical lesion, the squamocolumnar junction, and most of the cervical canal are removed, must be performed in the hospital operating room under anesthesia. This procedure is indicated in women with abnormal cytologic examinations, particularly if the cervix looks normal, and in those with atypical epithelial proliferation and carcinoma in situ diagnosed by punch biopsy. If multiple sections are cut from the removed cone of tissue, the pathologist can make a more exact diagnosis than he can from the small bites obtained by punch biopsy.

Endometrial biopsy. Endometrial biopsy is quite satisfactory for evaluation of the endometrial pattern, but it is totally inadequate as a means of eliminating endometrial cancer, although occasionally the diagnosis can be made from fragments of tissue removed in the office.

Vulvar disease. Carcinoma of the vulva is likely to be multicentric and in its earliest phase presents no characteristic gross appearance. Malignant areas can be detected by applying 1% aqueous toluidine blue solution to the vulva, permitting it to dry and then sponging the vulva with 1% acetic acid. Malignant, excoriated, or abraded tissue retains a dark blue stain, which indicates quite obviously the areas from which tissue should be removed for histologic study.

■ X-ray examination

X-ray examination may be helpful in the evaluation of pelvic masses; areas of calcification may be seen in fibroid tumors and in ovarian neoplasms; and bowel and urinary tract lesions can be differentiated from those in the genital organs. The most important use of x-ray examination in gynecology, however, is for hysterosalpingography, by which small intracavitary uterine lesions as well as abnormalities in the tubes can be detected. The technique is described in Chapter 11.

The most important uses of diagnostic x-ray examination during pregnancy are to determine the age, size, position, and number of fetuses, to localize the placenta, to determine the size and shape of the pelvic cavity, and to aid in the evaluation of abnormal labor.

Although the physician cannot deny the value of x-ray examinations in obstetric and gynecologic patients, he also cannot ignore their potential dangers. The genetic effects of radiation on *Drosophila* are well known, and there is no reason to doubt that similar changes can be produced in human beings by appropriate exposure to radioactive materials. Such genetic changes may be produced through an effect either on the maternal or the fetal gonads. Since it is the opinion of most geneticists that mutations are undesirable and offer a distinct threat to future generations, we must be cautious in our use of diagnostic and therapeutic radiation during the reproductive years.

The Genetics Committee of the National Academy of Sciences has recommended that the maximum cumulative dosage to the gonads that can safely be administered during the first 30 years of life is 10 r (roentgens) from all sources. Of this, about 5 r will come from background and cosmic radiation that cannot be avoided. If background and cosmic radiation increases from year to year, that which will be administered by diagnostic roentgenography must be reduced. It is wise, therefore, to be certain that any particular x-ray examination will be of help in establishing a diagnosis and that the one which will provide the necessary information with the least amount of radiation be selected. For example, when a chest x-ray examination is indicated, a 14 by 17 film is preferable to a miniature photofluorogram, primarily because the gonadal dose with the film is 0.00025 r and with the photofluorogram, 0.005 r.

X-ray studies during the first few weeks of pregnancy are more likely to disturb fetal growth than are those during the second and third trimesters, when the organs are reasonably well formed. The tissues are particularly susceptible from the second to the fourth or fifth week after conception, when it may be impossible to diagnose pregnancy.

Both the physician who requests an examination of the abdomen or pelvis and the radiologist who performs it should question the patient concerning the date her last period began. If her anticipated period is overdue, the examination should be postponed. After the primary organ systems have developed and the embryonic cells are transformed to those with adult characteristics, it is unlikely that ordinary diagnostic procedures will influence embryonic growth.

As a general rule, x-ray examinations during pregnancy and particularly those in which the gonads receive large amounts of radiation should be avoided unless they are essential to proper management of a patient. If they must be performed, the gonads should be properly protected and the technique should be one that will provide the necessary information with the minimum exposure. The physician cannot afford to be unduly concerned about possible effects on future generations if the life or health of a mother or her baby is at stake.

■ Ultrasound

High-frequency sound waves send back echoes whenever there is a change in density of the tissues through which they are passing. Studies with this technique indicate that it may be useful in diagnosing early pregnancy, in identifying multiple pregnancy, in differentiating hydatidiform moles from normal pregnancy, in measuring the biparietal diameter of the fetal skull, and in the differential diagnosis of various uterine and ovarian enlargements. Diagnostic sound waves appear to have no deleterious effect on maternal or fetal tissues.

■ Culdoscopy

Culdoscopy (the visualization of pelvic structures through a tubular instrument similar to a cystoscope that is introduced through a small incision in the posterior vaginal cul-de-sac) is not strictly an office procedure. This examination is accurate and relatively safe when performed by a physician experienced in its technique; otherwise it is dangerous.

■ Laparoscopy

The development of high-intensity, fiber-optic light sources has led to a reevaluation of an old method of examining the peritoneal cavity. The instrument, the laparoscope, is inserted through the anterior abdominal wall after pneumoperitoneum has been established. With this instrument it is possible to inspect the contents of the pelvis and the upper abdomen. The view of the pelvic organs is better than that provided by the culdoscope because one looks down from above and can see the bladder, the anterior surface of the uterus, and the posterior cul-de-sac, none of which can be seen by culdoscopy.

The principal *indications* for laparoscopy are the evaluation of pelvic pain, for inspection of small uterine or ovarian masses, infertility, endocrinopathies, amenorrhea, congenital anomalies, and ascites and for a "second look" after treatment of ovarian cancer. The main *complications* are hemorrhage from punctured blood vessels and perforation of a hollow viscus.

References

Aschheim, S., and Zondek, B.: Die Schwangerschaftsdiagnose aus dem Harn durch Nachweis des Hypophysenvorderlappenhormons, Klin. Wschr. **7**:1404, 1928.

Brown, J. B.: A chemical method for the determination of oestriol, oestrone and oestradiol in human urine, Biochem. J. **60**:185, 1955.

Fear, R. E.: Laparoscopy; a valuable aid in gynecologic diagnosis, Obstet. Gynec. **31**:297, 1968.

Forman, I.: Cervical mucus arborization; aid in ovulation timing, Obstet. Gynec. **3**:287, 1956.

Friedman, M. H., and Lapham, M. E.: A simple rapid procedure for the laboratory diagnosis of early pregnancies, Amer. J. Obstet. Gynec. **31**:405, 1931.

Goebelsmann, U., Midgley, A. R., Jr., and Jaffe, R. B.: Regulation of human gonadotropins. VII. Daily individual urinary estrogens, pregnanediol and serum luteinizing and follicle stimulating hormones during the menstrual cycle, J. Clin. Endocr. **29**:1222, 1969.

Griem, M. L.: The effects of radiation on the fetus, Lying-in: J. Reprod. **1**:367, 1968.

Hodges, P. C.: Health hazards in diagnostic use of x-ray, J.A.M.A. **166**:577, 1958.

Jaffe, R. B., and Midgley, A. R., Jr.: Current status of human gonadotropin radioimmunoassay, Obstet. Gynec. Survey **24**:200, 1969.

Papanicolaou, G.: General survey of vaginal smear and its use in research and diagnosis, Amer. J. Obstet. Gynec. **51**:316, 1946.

Paschkis, K. E., Rakoff, A. E., and Cantarow, A.: Clinical endocrinology, New York, ed. 3, 1967, Paul B. Hoeber, Inc., Medical Book Department, Harper & Row, Publishers.

Roland, M.: A simple test for the determination of ovulation, estrogen activity and early pregnancy, using the cervical mucus secretion, Amer. J. Obstet. Gynec. **63**:81, 1952.

Taylor, E. S., Holmes, J. H., Thompson, H. E., and Gottesfeld, K. R.: Ultrasound diagnostic technics in obstetrics and gynecology, Amer. J. Obstet. Gynec. **90:**655, 1964.

Tompkins, P.: The use of basal temperature graphs in determining the date of ovulation, J.A.M.A. **124:**698, 1944.

Venning, E. H., and Browne, J. S. L.: Studies in corpus luteum function; urinary excretion of sodium pregnanediol glucuronidate in human menstrual cycle, Endocrinology **21:**711, 1937.

Whitehouse, W. M., Simons, C. S., and Evans, T. N.: Reduction of radiation hazard in obstetric roentgenography, Amer. J. Roentgen. **80:**690, 1958.

Wilson, D. G.: Vaginal candidiasis during pregnancy; its diagnosis with Nickerson's medium and its treatment with Gentersal and ORM-1, Western J. Surg. **64:**180, 1956.

Zondek, B., and Cooper, K. L.: Cervical mucus in pregnancy; inability of estrogen to produce arborization in pregnancy and its clinical significance, Obstet. Gynec. **4:**484, 1954.

Zondek, B., and Rozin, S.: Cervical mucus arborization; its use in the dtermination of corpus luteum function, Obstet. Gynec. **3:**463, 1954.

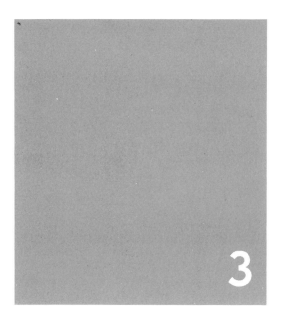

3

Pediatric gynecology

Genital disorders most frequently encountered in girls from infancy to adolescence include various local infections, injuries, congenital anomalies, and abnormal sexual development. Those disorders occurring during the adolescent years are chiefly concerned with menstrual function. The differences in adult and adolescent anatomy and physiology alter the method of examination and the interpretation of findings.

Pelvic examination can be performed in girls at any age from infancy on, usually without anesthesia and without psychic trauma. *Normal variations from adult genitals* include a more anterior location of the introitus and a relative prominence of the clitoris, which may measure 1 to 1.5 cm. For 10 to 14 days after birth the external genitals appear somewhat swollen and moistened with a mucoid discharge, and as estrogen levels drop, slight vaginal bleeding may occur. Maternal estrogen effects disappear in the newborn infant after 2 or 3 weeks. From this time until puberty the thin uncornified epithelium imparts a redness to the vaginal mucosa, frequently interpreted as inflammation. The vaginal pH becomes neutral or alkaline, and the vaginal smear is made up of atrophic basal and intermediate cells. Fine, short pubic hairs may be noted in young girls as a result of sensitive end-organ response to normal levels of androgens. The hymen is redundant and with strain may protrude beyond the surrounding parts. The hymenal opening changes little in size throughout the prepubertal period and is adequate for passage of the same instruments in the infant as in the girl of 10 years of age. Glandular structures in Bartholin's, paraurethral, and cervical regions are rudimentary and virtually functionless.

The cervical os is flattened and often pouched out as an ectropion, the endocervical epithelium extending for a short distance over the surface. This should not be interpreted or treated as an erosion. Since the posterior fornix is short and the cul-de-sac almost nonexistent, it is difficult to advance the examining finger high enough vaginally to outline pelvic structures. Rectal palpation is more informative. The uterus occupies a horizontal rather than an anterior position in the pelvis. The total size is 2.5 to 3 cm. with reversal of the adult cervix-corpus ratio, the cervix in the immature female comprising two thirds the size of the entire organ. Complete reversal of the ratio does not occur until full maturation, which can be within a few months or as long as several years after the menarche.

Visualization of the vaginal vault and cervix can be readily accomplished with a small, well-lubricated vaginoscope or urethroscope. If vaginal smears or cultures are to be obtained, a combined rectovaginal examination is better tolerated than instrumentation of the vagina alone. While the patient's attention is diverted by rectal examination, a cotton-tipped applicator moistened in sterile saline solution is rolled through the hymenal opening. The thin rectovaginal septum makes possible a clear outline of the vaginal tract between the examining finger and the applicator.

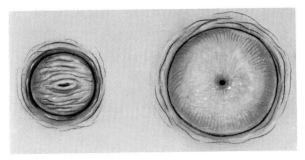

Fig. 3-1. Appearance of the immature cervix compared with the mature nulliparous cervix.

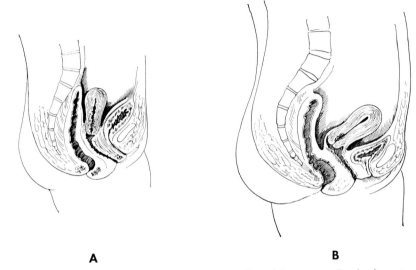

A   B

Fig. 3-2. Comparison of immature, **A**, and mature, **B**, pelvic organs. In the immature organs the uterus is horizontal, the cervix comprises two thirds of the organ, and the vaginal fornices are short.

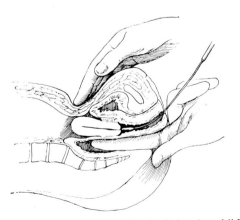

Fig. 3-3. "Combined examination" in the child. Rectal palpation and vaginal sound or applicator.

■ Gynecologic problems in preadolescents

Vulvovaginitis. Investigation of infections involving the external genitals should include pelvic examination, culture of the discharge, perianal examination, particularly for pinworm ova, and urinalysis to exclude urinary tract infection and diabetes.

Acute gonorrheal vulvovaginitis. Acute gonorrheal vulvovaginitis produces an intense inflammatory reaction, edema of the vulva, and a profuse purulent vaginal discharge. Cervical, paraurethral, and Bartholin's glands are poorly developed and rarely involved, but an associated specific proctitis is not uncommon. Upper genital tract infections are extremely rare. Systemic reactions are minimal. Parenteral penicillin, 300,000 units daily for 3 days, will generally effect a cure. Estrogen therapy need be employed only in resistant cases.

Hemolytic streptococcal vaginitis. Hemolytic streptococcal vaginitis is more often the cause of bloody or serosanguineous discharge than is a foreign body, although the possible presence of the latter should not be overlooked. Evidence of genital infection generally appears 2 to 4 weeks after a streptococcal infection elsewhere, particularly in the throat or skin, or after scarlet fever. Malek has suggested that this type of discharge may be of significance in the epidemiology of scarlet fever. Diagnosis is made by culture. Antibiotic therapy is indicated for 5 to 7 days.

Nonspecific vaginitis. Nonspecific vaginitis is characterized by a relatively low-grade, often persistent mixed infection. Local irritation by scratching or manipulation is a common cause. Intestinal *pinworm infestations* should be suspected in any persistent or recurrent nonspecific vaginitis, and examination should be made for ova and parasites. *Treatment* consists of good local hygiene and removal of irritation. The use of antibiotics is unnecessary and should be avoided. Pinworm infestations, when present, must be eradicated. Sitz baths two or three times a day, the application of a protective ointment (plain Lassar's paste, one-half strength), then good local cleansing once a day is usually sufficient. When inflammation of the vulvovaginal tissues is intense, the oral administration of sulfonamides gives more prompt relief than local measures alone. *Estrogen* therapy is indicated for persistent or recurrent vaginitis. Cornification of the epithelium and reduction of the vaginal pH increases local tissue resistance. Stilbestrol, 0.1 to 0.5 mg., depending on the age of the patient, is usually given daily for 21 days. Oral preparations are as effective as suppositories and far more readily accepted. Breast stimulation occurs but is reversed when the hormone is discontinued.

Monilial vaginitis. Candidiasis is uncommon except in diabetic children. It may also follow antibiotic administration. A urine or blood glucose determination is indicated in every case.

Trichomonas. Trichomonas infections are rare, but when present, trichomonads are usually found in the urine as well as in the vaginal discharge, and treatment is difficult. The use of oral trichomonacides should be advantageous to attack both the cystitis and the vaginitis. Those recently available need further evaluation with respect to their use in the pediatric patient.

Vaginal foreign body. The presence of a persistent vaginal discharge, generally accompanied by pain, suggests a foreign body. Endoscopic visualization and combined rectovaginal palpation offer the best means of localization. X-ray examination is necessary if the foreign body has migrated into adjacent tissues. A nonspecific vaginitis occurs secondarily and requires treatment preceding and after removal of the foreign body.

Lichen sclerosus et atrophicus. At the onset, lichen sclerosus et atrophicus is a white papular lesion that later tends to coalesce and cover the vulvar and perianal regions. It is not a common lesion but does occur in children and must be differentiated from leukoplakia. Diagnosis can be made by biopsy, which shows superficial hyperkeratosis, but the rest of the epidermis is atrophic, elastic tissue is absent, and there is a characteristic sclerotic change in the connective tissue just beneath the epidermis. The etiology is unknown, but the lesion is benign and usually disappears spontaneously. There are reports of several cases of lichen sclerosus et atrophicus in adolescents treated by vulvectomy. It should therefore be stressed that surgery, other than biopsy, is contraindicated. Restraint needs to be reemphasized because local treatment with vitamins A and D, hydrocortisone, or estrogen compounds is likely to provide only minimal relief from pruritus, and thus repeated reassurance to the parents of its benign nature and self-limited course is necessary.

Labial agglutination. Labial agglutination may occur congenitally or as the result of irritation, denuding the thin membrane and leading to adhesion of the labia minora in the midline. A characteristic livid line, extending vertically down the center of the membrane, distinguishes agglutination from the less commonly encountered imperforate hymen or vaginal atresia. This condition is self-limited and disappears as puberty approaches and estrogen levels rise. The ag-

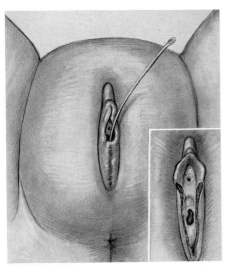

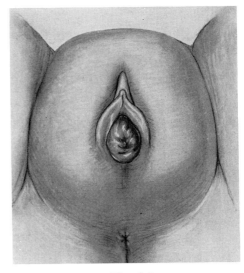

Fig. 3-4   Fig. 3-5

Fig. 3-4. Labial agglutination. Means of separation by pressure upon well-lubricated probe.
Fig. 3-5. Prolapsed urethra.

glutination encourages pocketing of urine, irritation, and infection. Application of an estrogen cream induces cornification of the epithelium, and spontaneous separation will often occur. Otherwise correction can be carried out in the office without anesthesia. A lubricated probe is inserted into the anterior opening, and quick firm pressure readily separates the labia. Bleeding is slight. A bland ointment or an estrogen cream that will cornify the epithelium should be applied for 2 weeks to prevent reagglutination.

Prolapsed urethra. The symptoms of vaginal bleeding, the appearance of a mass at the vaginal orifice, and pain, particularly with micturition, suggest prolapse of the urethral mucosa. The congested edematous mass occupies the entire area between the labia, occludes the vagina, and is likely to be misinterpreted as vaginal prolapse or genital tumor. Although no lumen is visible, a lubricated catheter inserted in the center of the mass will seek the bladder and confirm the diagnosis. Reduction of the prolapse can be accomplished occasionally, but usually necrosis is present, and excision of the redundant tissue at the meatal line of demarcation is necessary. An indwelling catheter should be left in place overnight. Recurrences or late sequelae are unusual.

Trauma. Injuries to the female genitals rarely produce any permanent damage. Bleeding can usually be controlled by pressure. Deep lacerations requiring suture heal with little scarring. The location of the urethra provides protection against actual injury, but urinary retention as a result of spasm is not uncommon. Reassuring the parents that local genital injuries will not interfere with future functions is one of the most important aspects of treatment.

Trauma caused by rape results in circumferential tears, abrasions, and ecchymosis. These evidences or the demonstration of sperm about the genitals are indications for prophylactic penicillin therapy. A single 2 ml. injection of long-acting penicillin containing 600,000 units per milliliter should provide protection against either gonorrhea or syphilis. Since normal variations in patency of the hymenal ring can be misleading to the most experienced examiner, the diagnosis of rape should not be made in the absence of characteristic signs.

■ Congenital anomalies

Because of the close embryologic relationship of the genital and urinary tracts developmental anomalies noted in one system warrant thorough examination of both. The mechanisms involved in their development are discussed in Chapter 10.

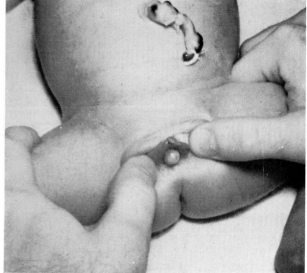

Fig. 3-6. Ectopic ureter with ureterocele.

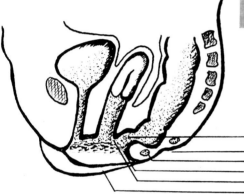

Rectovaginal communication
Anal dimple
Sphincter
Vestibule
Hymen
Vulva

Fig. 3-7. Vaginal ectopic anus.

Imperforate hymen. Imperforate hymen is an exception in that it usually occurs as an isolated anomaly. Surgical correction is desirable when the diagnosis is made but is imperative at puberty. Simple puncture of the membrane will heal over and is inadequate. Crucial incisions across the membrane will maintain patency.

Vaginal atresia. Complete vaginal atresia is generally associated with absent or rudimentary development of the uterus and tubes. Ovarian development usually is normal. It is unlikely that a rudimentary uterus will respond to stimulation, and the need for providing a menstrual outlet arises only on the rare occasion when the uterus is normal. Periodic examinations during adolescence will clarify this issue and at the same time offer opportunities to assist the young girl's social adjustment when necessary and to make psychologic preparation for future

treatment. It is advisable to defer surgical correction until the structures are well developed.

Ectopic ureter with vaginal terminus. Because ectopic ureter in the female most often terminates in the vaginal vault or the vestibule, attention is focused primarily upon the genital tract. If the terminus is closed, the *ureterocele* thus formed appears as a cystic mass that protrudes from the vagina. This is the most common "vaginal cyst" in infants. If the ectopic ureter is patent, constant irritation from urine promotes infection, and a vaginitis may be the first sign. Direct visualization of a vaginal ureteral orifice is frequently impossible, even under anesthesia. Instillation of methylene blue into the bladder will rule out a vesicovaginal communication. X-ray examination after the instillation of radiopaque media into the vagina and into the ectopic channel, if possible, along

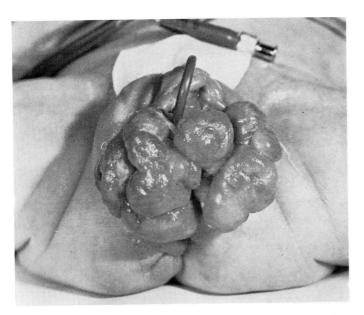

Fig. 3-8. Sarcoma botryoides.

with intravenous pyelography will outline both tracts most effectively. It is imperative that the entire urinary system be visualized before surgery is carried out. Removal of the ectopic ureter and the associated portion of the kidney is the treatment of choice.

Vaginal ectopic anus. Imperforate anus associated with a rectovaginal communication in the female infant represents erratic migration of the hindgut, occurring by 6 to 8 weeks of embryonic life. A skin dimple is visible at the normal anal site, surrounded by an intact external sphincter muscle. The rectum ends blindly above this area, and a fistulous tract passes forward to the genital region at various levels from the posterior fornix to the perineum. A few muscle fibers usually surround the opening and prevent gross incontinence. If the fistulous tract and its orifice provide an adequate lumen, correction should be deferred until definitive measures are feasible. Mobilization of the rectum downward and backward through the external sphincter can then be carried out.

■ Neoplasms

Tumors of the genital tract are of importance not because of their frequency but because of their highly malignant potentiality. The least likely but most significant cause for vaginal bleeding in the young girl is a malignant tumor. *Sarcoma botryoides* arises from mesenchymal tissue of the cervix or vagina and appears as an edematous grape-like mass of tissue that bleeds readily on touch. Extension proceeds locally, involving all pelvic structures. Distant metastasis is not characteristic. The neoplasm is resistant to x-ray or radium therapy and curable only by early radical extirpation.

Ovarian neoplasms are occasionally encountered in preadolescents. Dermoid cyst is the most common type and is more likely to cause symptoms as a result of torsion rather than size. Karrer and Swenson reported a case of twisted ovarian cyst in a newborn infant and reviewed 25 cases of ovarian cysts in infants under 1 year of age. Feminizing tumors must be considered in connection with precocious puberty in the young girl, but masculinizing ovarian tumors are almost nonexistent before 15 years of age. Abell and Holtz studied 188 primary ovarian neoplasms from patients under the age of 20 years. Forty percent of these were of nongerm cell origin, the majority arising from coelomic epithelium or its derivatives. The behavior of these and 113 germ cell neoplasms found in young girls is discussed in detail by the authors.

■ Abnormal sexual development

Classification of intersexual states is based on morphologic criteria including the following: (1) sex chromatin, (2) sex chromosomal constitution, (3) structure of the gonads, (4) structure of internal genital organs, and (5) structure of external genital organs. Management of intersexual problems, however, is influenced by the hormonal status evoked by the disorder and by psychologic factors, the sex of rearing, and the gender role.

Diagnosis, prognosis, and management of abnormalities in sexual development are dependent first and foremost on clear understanding of the dynamics of hormonal and morphologic interaction, particularly during four critical periods: conception, intrauterine life, the newborn period, and puberty. The genetic sex is determined at the time of fertilization. Abnormalities in sex chromosomal complements originate at this moment. Whereas the sex of the undifferentiated gonad is thus determined by sex-controlling genes in the X and Y chromosomes, endocrine activity of the fetal gonad directs sexual development along male or female lines. Differentiation always tends to proceed along female lines in the absence of a male gonad. A nonsteroidal material "organizer substance," produced solely by the embryonic testes, is required in order to suppress the müllerian system and to stimulate development of the wolffian system. Thus the genitals are phenotypically female if the gonad is ovary and the chromosomal complement is XX. It is also female if the fetal gonads are absent (Turner's syndrome XO) or if the embryonic testes are deficient in production of testicular organizer substance (testicular feminizing syndrome or male pseudohermaphroditism XY).

During intrauterine life, masculinization of the female fetus due to androgen excess may alter the external genitals, but the internal genitals remain distinctly female (congenital adrenal hyperplasia, effects of maternal androgenic drugs, or masculinizing tumors).

Certain intersex states are not evident until puberty, when hormonal effects on secondary sex characteristics are inappropriate or lacking. These include gonadal dysgenesis without other physical stigmata, testicular feminization, Klinefelter's syndrome, and mild forms of congenital adrenal hyperplasia with postpubertal virilization.

SEXUAL AMBIGUITY OF THE NEWBORN

The proper assignment of sex of the newborn infant is one of the first obligations of the obstetrician. Cases of doubtful sex noted at birth involve abnormalities in development of the external genitals, and these fall into four main groups as follows: (1) congenital adrenal hyperplasia, (2) nonadrenal masculinization due to maternal environmental factors, (3) male pseudohermaphroditism with incomplete development of the external genitals, and (4) true hermaphroditism.

Congenital adrenal hyperplasia is the most frequent cause of distinct virilization of the newborn infant. The disorder is an inborn error in metabolism and may be hereditary. There is impairment or block of the synthesis of cortisol due to specific defects in steroid hydroxylating enzyme. In order of frequency, deficits occur in C-21 hydroxylase, C-11 hydroxylase, and 3-beta-ol dehydrogenase. Impairment of C-21 hydroxylation of the 17-alpha-hydroxyprogesterone is followed by diminution in the biosynthesis of deoxycortisol (compound S) and in turn by reduction in cortisol. Since the rate of adrenocorticotropic hormone (ACTH) secretion by the pituitary is regulated by cortisol feedback, diminution of this hormone results in excessive ACTH secretion and overstimulation of the adrenal glands with resultant hyperplasia of the zona reticularis. Overproduction of androgenic hormones ensues in response to ACTH stimulation, since the metabolic pathway for these end products remains unimpaired. When deficits of C-21 hydroxylase is incomplete, the condition is known as compensated congenital adrenal hyperplasia, and the clinical characteristics are limited to virilization. In approximately one third of the cases the deficit is so great that virilization is accompanied by the salt-losing syndrome due to critical reduction in corticosterone. This aspect of congenital adrenal hyperplasia may be temporary or permanent in nature in contrast to the virilization that is always progressive if untreated.

The clinical characteristics in the newborn are shown in Fig. 3-9. These include relative persistence of the urogenital sinus, accentuation of the labial folds, and enlargement of the clitoris. A small vagina usually communicates with the urethra. The single opening is located at the base of the enlarged clitoris and suggests hypospadias. The appearance can be so perplexing that determination of sex on the basis of external examination alone is impossible. Chromosome studies for determination of sex, rectal palpation of the uterus, and visualization of the cervix by endoscopy or the urinary and genital tracts by x-ray examination after radiopaque instillation aid in diagnosis. Elevated 17-ketosteroid and pregnanetriol levels are diagnostic. Amounts of pregnanetriol normally excreted by the female are insignificant up to the age of 1 year and less than 1 mg. before the age of 10 years.

Treatment poses difficult problems. Partial adrenalectomy fails to control viriliza-

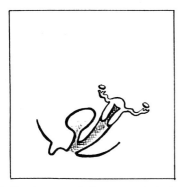 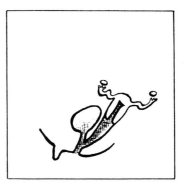

Fig. 3-9. Persistence of the urogenital sinus in females with congenital adrenal hyperplasia; these are the usual sites of communication between urethra and vagina.

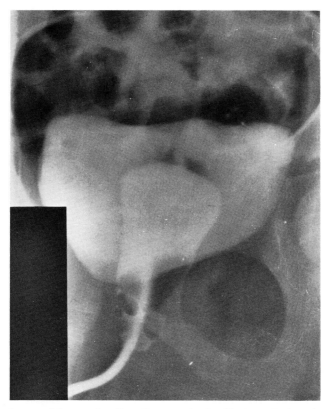

Fig. 3-10. Female pseudohermaphrodite. Retrograde instillation of dye through persistent urogenital sinus. Vagina and lower urinary tracts are visualized separately above the common perineal opening.

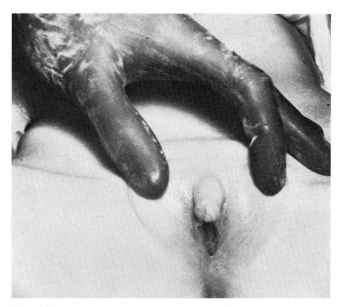

Fig. 3-11. Nonadrenal pseudohermaphroditism.

tion. Administration of female sex hormones is ineffective, but cortisone will reverse the symptoms in some of these patients. Early diagnosis of sex and the establishment of a plan for the child's future are of the utmost importance. Surgical correction includes excision of the clitoris, which should be done before the age of 3 or 4 years, and reconstruction of the vagina when the need arises after maturity. Cortisone therapy must be continued, and at puberty oral estrogens can be added to the therapeutic regimen to improve development of the secondary sex characteristics.

Virilizing symptoms appearing after infancy in the child whose urinary and genital systems were previously normal are more frequently caused by *adrenal tumor* than by hyperplasia. Administration of cortisone is of aid in the differential diagnosis. Cortisone will reduce the levels of 17-ketosteroids in patients with hyperplasia but has little or no effect on high levels when a tumor is present.

Nonadrenal virilization. Masculinization of the female fetus can occur when certain progestins are administered to the expectant mother during early pregnancy. Except for the importance of accurate diagnosis, this type of masculinization does not pose a serious problem, since effects are limited to the external genitals. The clitoris is enlarged, and the labial folds may be firmly fused in the midline, giving an ambiguous impression of the sex (Fig. 3-11). There is no interference with differentiation of the müllerian and wolffian ducts, and therefore the vagina, uterus, and tubes are normal. The fetal ovary is unaffected. In contrast to adrenal female pseudohermaphroditism, progressive virilization does not occur. Instead, growth and development are normal; secondary sex changes and menstrual and reproductive functions are not affected, although the latter aspect deserves further exploration as most of these individuals reach maturity.

Diagnosis is made by (1) buccal smear, which should show chromatin-positive nuclei characteristic of normal females, (2) normal 17-ketosteroid and pregnanetriol excretion, and (3) a history of oral or intramuscular administration of progestins to the expectant mother before the twelfth and through the fifteenth or sixteenth week of gestation, usually for threatened or habitual abortion. Treatment is first of all the reassurance of the parents. Removal of the large clitoris and surgical correction of the fused labia are not difficult and should be done before the age of 3 years. There is no need for hormone therapy.

Male pseudohermaphroditism. The physical characteristics of individuals with male pseudohermaphroditism show gradations of abnormality. The external genitals may appear feminine, doubtful, or masculine. The feminine type, *testicular feminizing syndrome,* is most common. In this type the external genitals give the appearance of a normal female, but the vagina ends as a blind pouch. Internal genitals are absent or rudimentary. The testicles, although usually undescended, have occasionally been found in the labia. When feminization is incomplete, extreme caution in the assignment of sex is particularly urgent in this condition. A buccal smear for sex chromatin analysis is negative, since the chromosomal complement is usually 46 XY, and one is tempted to make an assignment of male sex on this cursory examination. However, the presence of a vagina, the fact that the hormonal effects of the malfunctioning testes become evident during adolescence when breast development and body configuration proceed along female lines, and the fact that there is frequently a defective end-organ response to androgen, which is reflected by remarkably little response to exogenous testosterone, are good reasons why these patients are appropriately raised as females.

The assignment of a contradictory sex at birth is a difficult commitment for both the physicians and the family. In difficult problems such as this the final solution should not be reached without recourse to the many sources of information now available in the fields of cytogenetics, endocrinology, and psychosexual development.

True hermaphroditism, in which both male and female gonads are present, is rare. In the newborn infant there are no distinguishing physical chromosomal or hormonal changes that can be considered diagnostic of true hermaphroditism. Since the organizer substance in the fetal testes is responsible for masculinization of the external genitals and since testicular tissue is present in true hermaphroditism, it is not surprising that male external genital configuration predominates in a ratio of approximately 3:1. Yet it is of the utmost importance to establish the dominant sex as soon after birth as possible in order that the optimal choice of gender may be made. Both the confirmation of diagnosis and the treatment require laparotomy. Treatment consists of removal of the contradictory gonad. Hormone therapy may be necessary at puberty if the appearance of appropriate secondary sex characteristics is delayed.

SEXUAL PRECOCITY

Manifestations of precocious puberty are either isosexual or heterosexual. Isosexual types in the female child are dependent upon early or abnormal estrogen stimulation that may be pituitary (constitutional), neurogenic, or ovarian in origin. Effects are entirely feminizing. Heterosexual types, resulting in virilization, are usually caused by increased adrenocortical activity.

Isosexual precocity. The onset of puberty has a wide normal range. In the absence of vaginal bleeding, early appearance of secondary sex characteristics usually represents *sensitive end-organ response* to minimal hormone stimulation, but the occurrence of the menarche before the age of 10 years deserves investigation.

The most common type of isosexual precocious puberty is "constitutional," in which *idiopathic pituitary activation* occurs. No abnormalities other than early maturity are associated. Pituitary, ovarian, and adrenal hormones reach normal adult levels, menstruation is ovulatory, and pregnancy is possible. Rarely, *central nervous system lesions* may produce pituitary stimulation and result in a similar precocious development with normal hormonal relationships.

Social adjustment poses the most serious problem for these children. Sexual awakening and receptivity are far in advance of mental maturity. Management must be aimed chiefly at offering guidance to the parents as well as to the young patient with this problem.

Collipp reported the results obtained in treating 10 girls with constitutional isosexual precocious puberty with medroxyprogesterone acetate in doses of 100 mg. intramuscularly every 2 weeks. The cessation of bleeding and the inhibition of ovulation are the most important effects. In addition, reduction of breast development and possibly a delay in epiphyseal closure may be added benefits.

Precocious sexual development and uterine bleeding resulting from *feminizing tumors of the ovary* are estrogen induced and anovulatory. Hence pregnancy does not occur, but in other respects the clinical features of this type of precocity do not differ from other isosexual varieties. Examination under anesthesia may reveal an ovarian mass, but in some instances actively functioning feminizing tumors are too small to be outlined. Under these circumstances it may be difficult to differentiate ovarian and constitutional types. In ovarian types the vaginal smear shows a more pronounced unopposed estrogen effect with consistent cornification throughout the cycle, and gonadotropin excretion is low or absent. In association with constitutional precocious puberty the vaginal smear usually shows less pronounced cornification with cyclic changes, and gonadotropin excretion attains mature levels. When the diagnosis cannot be otherwise made, laparotomy is indicated. Removal of the involved ovary and biopsy of the opposite ovary to rule out bilateral involvement results in cessation of bleeding, but regression of secondary sex characteristics may be incomplete.

Heterosexual precocity. Virilization is the striking manifestation of heterosexual precocity and is usually due to an adrenal lesion. When evident at birth, congenital adrenal hyperplasia is most likely, whereas after the first year of life the onset of an adrenogenital syndrome is usually due to an adrenal tumor or a mild delayed type of adrenal hyperplasia. Virilization appearing in puberty and in early adulthood is associated with adrenal or ovarian tumors, the incomplete form of male pseudohermaphroditism, and delayed or acquired adrenal hyperplasia. These disorders and their management are discussed earlier in this chapter and in Chapters 6 and 48.

■ Gynecologic problems in adolescent girls

Menarche. The sequence of events leading up to the menarche, or first menstrual period, is illustrated in Fig. 3-12. Characteristic bodily changes precede the menarche by several years. There is increasing evidence that the primary stimulus for initiation of these changes originates in the hypothalamus and is mediated through the pituitary gland. Harris transplanted the pituitary from prepubertal rats into adult female hypophysectomized hosts and found that estrus cycles were resumed and pregnancies achieved. In the human being pituitary hormones that are low before puberty show a sharp rise 1 to 4 years before the menarche. Increasing amounts of estrogenic and androgenic hormones are secreted, and secondary sex changes become apparent. Growth spurt is

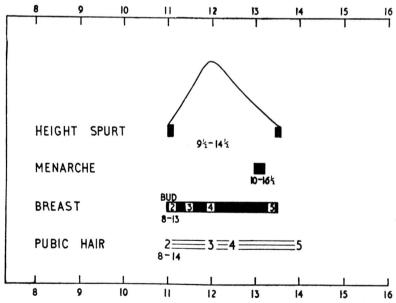

Fig. 3-12. Diagram of sequence of events at adolescence in girls. An average girl is represented; the range of ages within which some of the events may occur is given by the figures placed directly below them. (From Tanner, J. M.: Growth at adolescence, ed. 2, Oxford, England, 1962, Blackwell Scientific Publications.)

greatest during this time, the protein requirement being three times that of the adult. Growth continues for another 3 years or so after the onset of menstruation, but the rate is slower and rarely exceeds 2 inches. Ossification centers gradually disappear and growth is complete. Thus girls in whom the menarche occurs at an early age are likely to be shorter as adults than those in whom its appearance is late.

There is apparently considerable variation in the sensitivity of breast tissue and the pubic hair follicles to stimulation by estrogen and androgen, respectively. This phenomenon explains the early appearance of breast development and pubic hair growth in many girls in whom endocrine function and onset of menstruation are normal.

Early menarche. The onset of menstruation before the age of 10 years is precocious and should be investigated. This problem was discussed under abnormal sexual development, earlier in this chapter.

Late menarche. Absence of menstruation beyond the sixteenth year should be considered abnormal, and the possibility of a disorder of genetic origin should be given careful consideration in all such cases. Chromosomal abnormalities are found in approximately 40% of phenotypic females in whom the symptoms of primary amenorrhea extend beyond the sixteenth year. There are instances in which the menarche has occurred as late as the twenties, but these are rare.

DIAGNOSTIC PROCEDURES. The first step in seeking out a central nervous system, a systemic, or an anatomic cause of early or late menarche is a careful history and general physical and pelvic examinations. When these are normal, endocrine function, including thyroid, ovarian, pituitary, and adrenal, must be assessed.

1. *General.* Blood count, urine for protein and sugar determinations, 2-hour postprandial blood glucose, and chest x-ray films should be taken.

2. *Thyroid function.* Studies of the protein-bound iodine or basal metabolism rate should be made. (If true hypothyroidism is found, the amenorrhea can often be treated successfully with thyroid replacement.)

3. *Ovarian function.* *Vaginal smears* showing cornified and intermediate cells provide gross indication of estrogenic activity. *Vaginal pH* should be acid unless infection is present. Cytologic examination of *urinary sediment* should show cellular cornification, similar to that in vaginal smears. Arborization, or ferning, of *cervical mucus* also provides good evidence of estrogen secretion. *"Medical curettage"* after intramuscular injection of 100 mg. of progesterone, if followed by withdrawal bleeding, provides evidence of an intact estrogen-primed endometrium. When bleeding occurs under these circumstances, prognosis for establishing a normal menstrual cycle is good. Stimulation with progesterone or one of the progestational agents during the last half of the stimulated cycle should be repeated for a total of 3 months. If bleeding does not occur after progesterone administration, *endometrial biopsy* and 24-hour urine estrogen levels should be obtained.

4. *Pituitary function.* Low values for 24-hour urinary gonadotropic excretion suggest primary pituitary hypofunction; if high, they suggest primary ovarian failure. Either of these disorders is generally refractory to treatment. The part played by the hypothalamus in pituitary hypofunction is the most difficult to assess and the most unpredictable in behavior. We have seen 2 cases of delayed menarche in which pituitary follicle-stimulating hormone (FSH) levels were low or absent, yet physical development appeared normal. Spontaneous activation of the pituitary-ovarian-endometrial axis took place at ages 24 and 26 years, respectively, and pregnancies were achieved. On the other hand, ovarian failure in young women, as revealed by high FSH excretion, has less chance for spontaneous or even therapeutic correction, since it implies gonadal agenesis or destruction by x-ray therapy, surgery, or disease.

5. *Adrenal function.* High values for 24-hour, urinary 17-ketosteroid and pregnanetriol excretion during adolescence are most commonly found in association with congenital adrenal hyperplasia. Genital defects are usually present, as noted previously in this chapter. Adrenal or functioning ovarian tumors must be considered in the differential diagnosis.

Adolescent dysfunctional uterine bleeding. Menstrual irregularities, so common at this time of life, are usually the result of unopposed estrogen production by the immature, nonovulating ovary, but even in young girls the possibility of systemic or pelvic lesions must be eliminated before the diagnosis of dysfunctional uterine bleeding is made. Although a reasonable time must be allowed for the establishment of a full ovulatory cycle, adolescent dysfunctional uterine bleeding is not necessarily self-limited. In a long-range study of 538 adolescents with menstrual disorders conducted by Southam and Richart, 291 were diagnosed as dysfunctional uterine bleeding. The follow-up period was as long as 25 years. These authors showed that if symptoms persist for a period of 4 years or more, there is a fifty-fifty chance of future irregularities, a diminution in reproductive potential, and an increased risk of uterine neoplasm. Since ovulation occurs in only about 2% of young women in the first 6 months of menstrual experience and only about 18% by the end of the first year after the menarche, at least this amount of time should be given for maturation.

In this group cyclic treatment is discussed in Chapter 7.

Dysmenorrhea. Primary dysmenorrhea, the most common menstrual disorder in adolescent girls, is discussed in detail in Chapter 8.

References

Abell, M. R., and Holtz, F.: Ovarian neoplasms in childhood and adolescence. II. Tumors of non-germ cell origin, Amer. J. Obstet. Gynec. **93**:850, 1965.

Bongiovanni, A. M., and Eberlein, W. R.: Symposium: Adrenal steroids; defects in steroidal metabolism of subjects with adrenogenital syndrome, Metabolism **10**:917, 1961.

Carrington, E. R.: Gynecologic problems in infants and prepubertal girls, Surg. Clin. N. Amer. **34**:1615, 1954.

Carrington, E. R.: Laboratory examination of the pediatric gynecologic patient, Symposium on Pediatric and Adolescent Gynecology, Ann. N. Y. Acad. Sci. **142**:623, 1967.

Collipp, P. J., Kaplan, S. A., Boyle, D. C., Plachte, F., and Kogut, M. D.: Constitutional isosexual precocious puberty; effects of medroxyprogesterone acetate, Amer. J. Dis. Child. **108**:399, 1964.

Costin, M. E.: Ovarian tumors in infants and children, Amer. J. Dis. Child. **76**:127, 1948.

Hahn, H. B., Hayles, A. B., and Albert, A.: Medroxyprogesterone and constitutional precocious puberty, Mayo Clin. Proc. **39**:182, 1964.

Harris, G. W.: Neutral control of the pituitary gland, London, 1955, E. Arnold, Ltd., p. 298.

Jones, G. S.: Diagnostic evaluation of patients with intersexuality, Symposium on Pediatric and Adolescent Gynecology, Ann. N. Y. Acad. Sci. **142**:729, 1967.

Jones, H. W., and Heller, R. H.: Pediatric and adolescent gynecology, Baltimore, 1966, The Williams & Wilkins Co.

Karrer, F. W., and Swenson, S. A.: Twisted ovarian cyst in a newborn infant, Arch. Surg. (Chicago) **83**:143, 1961.

Lang, W. R.: Pediatric vaginitis, New Eng. J. Med. **253**:1153, 1955.

Lawrence, W. D.: Lichen sclerosus et atrophicus of the vulva, Obstet. Gynec. **14**:65, 1959.

Malek, J.: Streptocoques béta-hémolytiques du niveau des organes génitaux infantils au cours de la scarlatine, Schweiz. med. Wschr. **78**:402, 1948.

Paschkis, K. E.: Precocious puberty and pseudopuberty, Med. Clin. N. Amer. **36**:1711, 1952.

Schauffler, G. C.: Pediatric and adolescent gynecology, Obstet. Gynec. **5**:390, 1955.

Shackman, R.: Sarcoma botryoides of the genital tract in female children, Brit. J. Surg. **38**:26, 1951.

Simmons, K., and Greulick, W. W.: Menarcheal age and the height, weight and skeletal age of girls age seven to seventeen years, J. Pediat. **22**:518, 1943.

Southam, A. L.: Dysfunctional uterine bleeding in adolescence, Obstet. Gynec. **3**:241, 1960.

Southam, A. L., and Richart, R. M.: Prognosis for adolescents with menstrual abnormalities, Amer. J. Obstet. Gynec. **94**:637, 1966.

Tanner, J. M.: Growth at adolescence, ed. 2, Oxford, 1955, Blackwell Scientific Publications.

Taylor, E. S., and Snow, R. H.: Adrenal virilism in the female child and adult, Amer. J. Obstet. Gynec. **67**:1307, 1954.

Wilkins, L.: The diagnosis and treatment of endocrine disorders in childhood and adolescence, ed. 3, Springfield, Ill., 1966, Charles C Thomas, Publisher.

Wilkins, L.: Masculinization of female fetus due to use of orally given progestins, J.A.M.A. **172**:1028, 1960.

4

Psychology and life periods of women

The physician who is consulted by a woman is entrusted with the care of her whole being. The management of obstetric and gynecologic problems requires a knowledge of the emotions as well as of anatomy, physiology, and pathology. Sexuality and pregnancy, which are integral parts of obstetrics and gynecology, are areas of great emotion. An evaluation of the personality of women therefore allows us to make a more accurate diagnosis and to direct our therapeutic efforts in a more effective way.

■ The woman and her physician

The proper management of any patient is based upon an understanding of her personality and anxieties. The patient consults the physician because she is fearful about her condition; this anxiety motivates the patient in therapy. It is the relief of the symptoms and anxiety that the patient inter-

prets as improvement. The primary area of interest of the physician, the cause of the illness, is of minor importance to most patients. This divergence of interest is easily overcome, since the very act of coming to the physician, because of his knowledge and position, puts the patient in a parent-child relationship. The patient transfers to her physician the trust and faith that were originally attached to the parents and expects this parent figure to understand and treat her anxiety.

It is not often sufficiently recognized that almost every form of diagnosis and therapy is dependent upon the goodwill and cooperation of the patient, who must return for treatment, studies, and medication. To obtain her cooperation and to establish a plan of management from which the patient will derive maximum benefit the physician must understand her personality. Often this is done on the basis of intuition, but a scientific approach to the understanding of the patient's personality clearly benefits both parties. Many physicians hesitate to delve into a patient's emotions because they fear a negative reaction from the patient or even that their questions might make the patient worse. If the physician questions the patient gently and watches for signs of great resistance, no harm can be done. Certainly the patient who responds with great anger or disgust should be allowed to keep her own confidences, but this response in itself indicates to the physician that an emotional problem exists. Many physicians interpret the doctor-patient relationship in a social sense and believe that an interest in their patients' emotions is not proper. Such confusion and insecurity on the physician's part can arouse similar feelings in the patient. Therefore, any discussion of emotions should be frank and open, the physician showing by his approach that his interest in these areas is a part of an adequate evaluation.

The examination of the patient's personality need not be a lengthy matter. It should begin as the patient enters the consultation room and sits opposite the physician. By the patient's dress, walk, makeup, and attitude in answering questions, a judgment of her personality begins. The physician notices whether the patient is reacting to the interview in a feminine way or whether she is domineering, demanding, masculine, aggressive, or passive in her attitude. These initial impressions can be confirmed by further observation or history.

There are some areas in the history that are of particular significance. The date of the patient's first menstrual period should be asked and an effort made to find out how the patient felt about it, where she got her information, and the attitudes toward menstruation of significant people such as her parents, siblings, and friends. Many parents show little hesitation or embarrassment in discussing sexual problems but have difficulty in discussing menstruation because it has a connotation of being dirty and unacceptable. This is not surprising when we consider that to the immature girl menstrual blood comes from the same area as feces and urine; this causes her to transfer to menstruation the feelings she has toward these excretions.

The patient should be questioned about the sexual aspects of her life. Questioning should not stop at the frequency of coitus but should continue to finding out the degree of satisfaction obtained. If there is a problem in this area, the patient's attitude toward sexuality should be traced back to that of significant people in her past (her mother, father, and siblings). The young girl learns about sex and men from her mother, with an assist from father, siblings, and friends. Her feelings about previous pregnancies should be elicited, with special attention to anxieties and depressions.

The patient's reactions during the physical examination should be observed closely. The problem of the pelvic examination can be a difficult one for women and some doctors. By approaching the examination in a confident manner the doctor reassures the patient that the social and sexual implications that are influencing her anxiety are not important at the moment. A more thorough pelvic examination is obtained if the patient is relaxed. The physician should let the patient know that he recognizes her anxiety and that he will pay attention to her concern about modesty. If the patient is unduly anxious or tense, the physician should stop and discuss the source of tension. Occasionally the doctor is challenged by the problem of treating a woman who refuses a pelvic examination. This type of behavior necessitates careful discussion of the patient's emotions about this area of the body. No physician can assume the responsibility of caring for a patient when she insists that he be blindfolded. A continued refusal is an indication that a psychiatric referral and/or refusal to treat the patient is in order.

■ Periodic health examination

Periodic medical consultation is advisable for females of all ages, either to prevent illness or to detect the earliest signs of disease processes. To guard the health and to observe the development of the growing young girl throughout childhood and adolescence, the family doctor or pediatrician usually sees the patient at definitely stated intervals. During the childbearing period, problems of sex hygiene, fertility, and pregnancy bring the woman to the doctor more or less regularly. Prenatal and postnatal consultations provide an opportunity for instruction in regard to diet, sex hygiene, and good general health habits. As the end of the childbearing period approaches, the average woman tends to discontinue her more or less regular visits to her physician unless she is encouraged to return for periodic reexamination. This is particularly advisable during the premenopausal and postmenopausal periods because of the frequent occurrence of benign and malignant genital tumors and also because of the development of systemic disease in women in these age groups. Patients usually are most grateful when this service is offered to them and are quite eager to avail themselves of it. Many women resist the idea of the periodic examination. The most common causes for this are lack of knowledge and anxiety about the pelvic examination or the possibility of discovering a serious condition.

The procedure in the periodic consultation is as follows: The patient is weighed and her blood pressure is taken before she is admitted to the examining room. She is then instructed to disrobe and to empty her bladder, submitting a sample of the voided urine for examination for albumin and sugar content. Before proceeding with the actual examination the patient is questioned regarding her health in general and especially whether there has been any unusual discharge, bleeding, or menstrual irregularity since her last visit. A simple, general physical survey that stresses careful palpation of the neck, axillae, breasts, and abdomen is performed. The patient's feet are then placed in stirrups, and the vulva is carefully inspected. An *unlubricated* speculum is inserted into the vagina and the cervix is inspected; material is obtained from the endocervical canal and portio for cytologic examination. The next step is a careful bimanual and rectal examination. After this the patient is ushered into the consultation room for discussion of any positive findings or symptoms. During this part of the consultation she is encouraged to ask questions relating to sex hygiene, contraception, the significance of minor symptoms, etc. These points are discussed, and the patient is given an appointment for another examination, which is usually in 12 months unless there is an indication for more frequent observation.

■ Douching

Women often ask the question, "How often should I take a douche and what should I use?" To the patient who has no evidence of vaginitis or cervicitis our answer usually is, "You need never douche except perhaps immediately after a menstrual period." Some women will protest that they feel cleaner after a douche, and a few will hesitantly tell us that they are aware of an unpleasant odor unless they douche regularly. Both of these reasons express a psychologic rather than a physical need for cleanliness. The physician should explain to these patients that unless there is an abnormal discharge from the vagina, that organ is neither unclean nor malodorous. The objectionable odor in most instances is caused by the secretions of the glands of the skin of the vulva, the mons veneris, and the crural regions and can be adequately treated by thorough cleansing of those parts. This explanation is particularly helpful to the obsessive woman who tends to think of the vagina as a "dirty cavity" that needs careful cleansing once or several times each day.

When a cleansing douche is indicated, warm water, physiologic saline solution, or a mildly acid solution (vinegar, 50 ml. to 2 L. of water) should be employed. Strong antiseptics such as iodine, permanganate, or Lysol should never be prescribed. Medicated and aromatic powders are preferred by some patients for aesthetic reasons. These are harmless, but they are expensive and accomplish nothing more than the simple saline douche that we ordinarily recommend.

■ The feminine core

The essence of every woman's personality falls somewhere within a continuum of traits ranging from the masculine to the feminine. The traits that compose the core of the female personality are feminine narcissism, masochism, and passivity. The male traits of masculine narcissism, aggression, and activity lie at the other end of this spectrum.

The sexual and aggressive instincts with which all individuals are born develop in their particular way in the female according to three influences. These influences tend to turn the female's aggressions, narcissism, and activity in an inward direction. The first influence is physiologic: The woman is not as active or aggressive as the male because of her constitution and lesser muscular development. Her sexual organ is receptive and cannot easily be used actively or aggressively. The second influential situation is in the family. The young girl both desires her father (oedipal feelings) and loves her mother; to attract her father and please her mother she assumes feminine traits. Both parents consciously and unconsciously encourage the little girl not to be active, aggressive, or narcissistic in a masculine manner. Finally, our culture rigidly prescribes what is acceptable behavior for the female. When these three influences take the same general direction, a harmonious personality, which has the inner strength to cope with the traumas of life, develops.

Feminine narcissism. Women tend to love in a different way from men. The woman falls in love with the idea of being loved; whereas the man loves an object for the pleasure it will give. The woman receives gratification from the idea of being loved and bases an increased sense of her own value on her image of the person who loves her. She says, "I am valuable, important, etc. because he loves me." This type of narcissism finds expression in many aspects of a woman's life, the most obvious being her interest in clothes, personal appearance, and beauty. Such interest is normal and entirely feminine if its main object is to have someone admire and love her. It is subverted when it becomes an end in itself.

Every phase of a woman's life is influenced by narcissism. To an adolescent and young woman it gives impetus to her efforts to attract a man. As a wife it allows her to be gratified by the success and achievements of her husband. In pregnancy and labor it expands her conception of herself in that she is going to reproduce and give her husband a gift of a child. As she raises the child, her feminine narcissism rewards her by the pleasure she feels in the accomplishments of the child. All individuals have a mixture of masculine and feminine narcissism. The man loves an object that gratifies and gives pleasure. The woman takes pleasure in the idea of being loved and measures importance in terms of the person who loves her.

Feminine masochism. Feminine masochism may be differentiated from neurotic masochism by an understanding of the goals involved. In neurotic masochism the goal is the suffering itself as a means of pacifying the superego. Feminine masochism is quite different. The woman is willing to suffer and sacrifice, but only in order to achieve certain rewards. The idea of suffering is an essential part of her life, since every woman has to face the fear of childbirth and the fear of the pain that is attached to this. Pain is not an integral part of the male's concept of his role. He can fantasy a life without physical pain that does not produce a conflict in his sexual identity. The woman cannot do this.

Every aspect of a woman's life is colored by her ability to accept the masochism that is a part of her feminine role. As a young girl being courted she must *allow* herself to be won by the man she chooses. In the role of a wife she often must submit her own needs to build up the personality and strivings of her husband and family. Sexually there is always an element of rape in that the male organ penetrates. As a mother she sacrifices her own needs to those of her children. Finally, she must accept her children's marriage and separation from her.

What is essential to her continued mental well-being is the reward she receives from her narcissism, that is, her ability to identify with the accomplishments of her loved ones—husband and child. She is protected from excessive sacrifice by a sense of her own identity and importance and by a need to receive as well as give.

Feminine passivity. The woman's passivity is activity that is turned inward toward herself, her home, children, and husband. It is not the passivity that allows others to assume responsibility and action.

It is feminine passivity that permits the woman to put great efforts into making herself attractive so that the male will pursue her while she seemingly waits. As a wife she must show interest in the home and in the well-being of its occupants. She must accept the idea that she is given things by her husband and even by her children, rather than assuming an active and aggressive role in attaining these things for herself. Sexually she must be passive and receptive to the male.

Feminine passivity therefore is activity directed toward construction and enhance-

Table 3. Components of mature feminine personality

Feminine core	Courtship (young woman)	Wife	Sexuality	Pregnancy	Mother
Feminine narcissism	Concern with beauty to attract men	Pride in husband's accomplishments	Efforts to make self alluring	Pride in ability to reproduce; reward of having a child	Pride in accomplishments of children and their growth to maturity
Feminine masochism	Allows male to conquer	Sacrifices own personality to build up that of husband	Allows self to be conquered	Accepts discomfort of prenatal period and labor	Sacrifices self to benefit of children
Feminine passivity	Allows self to be pursued	Makes home	Passive, receptive	Waiting of 40-week gestation	Homemaking

ment of the home and the family. It is an active assumption of the responsibility for these roles. The woman gives up her outwardly oriented active and aggressive strivings for the rewards involved in identification with her family.

Feminine maturity. The three personality traits that make up the essentials of the woman's personality must in the mature woman be in balance with each other. Too much feminine narcissism without masochism and passivity produces a self-centered woman interested only in attaining love and admiration from those around her. There is no element of giving. Too much feminine masochism without the protective narcissism produces a woman who sacrifices herself without idea of rewards. The overly passive woman is continually waiting to receive without any willingness to give of herself in a masochistic or narcissistic manner. These traits must not only be in balance with each other but also with the opposing masculine elements of the personality. If the masculine traits are stronger than the feminine traits, a masculine woman develops.

The mature woman is a delicate balance of both masculine and feminine traits in continually changing interplay, all freely available for use when called upon by the various stresses of her life (Table 3).

■ Life periods of the female

The function of the genital system is the preservation of the species by reproduction —a function that is intimately interrelated with the psychology of the woman. The reproductive system, although present at birth, does not begin its job until some years later. It is relatively inactive during childhood, is stimulated to activity during puberty, continues its activity during the reproductive years, and becomes relatively inactive during the menopause and the postmenopause period. Thus we divide the sexual life cycle of the human female into the following phases: (1) childhood, (2) puberty-adolescence, (3) maturity, (4) climacteric-menopause, and (5) postmenopause (senescence).

CHILDHOOD

During childhood, a period of general body growth and relatively little genital development, the basic personality of the in-

dividual is established. The psychologic development during this period is divided into the oral, anal, phallic, and latency phases. The *oral phase,* which lasts from birth to about 1½ years of age, is the period when the infant's primary interest is centered around satisfaction-dissatisfaction of the gastrointestinal system. During this phase the female child begins to learn to differentiate herself from the world around her. The memories of the pleasure of being mothered make the adult woman react positively to mothering her own child. The *anal phase,* which lasts from 1½ to 3 years, is one in which mastery of the musculature is of concern to the child. It centers around mastery of the anal-urethral sphincters because this is the first major area in which the parents expect the child to control himself. Many of the woman's attitudes toward her genitals and sexuality have their roots in this phase of her own life because of the physical closeness of all three organs. During the *phallic phase* (3 to 6 years of age) the child becomes interested in the genital organs and the differences between the sexes. Young girls feel envy and regret over not having a penis and being like boys. The feeling is more deeply buried, but young boys may feel the same toward the girl's ability to be a mother and all that is associated with motherhood. The young girl is attempting to solve her oedipal conflicts. It is during this period that future adult acceptance or rejection of sexuality is established. Masturbation is evident during this phase in both sexes, and parents need to be helped to understand that this is a natural phenomenon unless it is excessive. The *latency phase,* which is from 6 years of age to puberty, is one in which the young child begins to apply her mastery of her body and her interpersonal relationships within the family to the outside world, mainly school and friends. Heterosexual interests become dormant and are sublimated into games, studies, and other social activities.

ADOLESCENCE

Adolescence is a period that begins with the onset of menses and sexual development in the woman. The sexual endocrine system slowly becomes active, bringing about many anatomic and psychologic changes. The more significant physical changes are growth of pubic and axillary hair, development of the breasts, and the occurrence of the first menstrual period. These physical changes cause an upsurge in sexual feelings. Because of her anxieties, the young girl seeks the support of friends and the group. The group establishes rigid standards within which the girl can practice being an adult. She can no longer accept as much direction as before from her parents because of her increased drive for independence. The young women looks outside the home for women with whom she can identify and who can help her to establish her own feminine core on a firm footing.

The menarche usually occurs between the ages of 11 and 14 years. A young girl reacts to it as a result of the way she has been prepared and of how she feels about her own femininity. If she has not been prepared, she may believe that she has an internal injury. Some may be unable to accept menstruation because they cannot accept their own femininity or its signal as the beginning of adulthood. Others may be very disappointed because of nonappearance of the miraculous changes they expected with this first sign of adulthood. Occasionally an inexperienced young girl may believe that she is pregnant because her first periods are so irregular.

The deeply emotional nature of menstruation is reflected in its nicknames—"the curse," "being unwell," or "falling off the roof." None of these is a wonderful experience. In most primitive societies there is an element of taboo connected with menstruation.

Many disorders of menstruation arise from emotional factors rather than from pituitary or ovarian failure. Excessive tension such as that in young girls going away to school can cause her to miss a period. It has been demonstrated that postmenopausal women who have been separated from the significant men in their lives, such as father or husband, may have vaginal bleeding. A woman with strong conflicts about becoming pregnant may develop amenorrhea as in pseudocyesis. To manage this syndrome the physician must understand that the patient's unconscious wish not to become pregnant is mixed with a strong unconscious drive for the secondary gains of pregnancy.

Physicians can help mothers to transmit to their daughters that menstruation is not a sickness but a normal function. There need be no restrictions in physical activity. It is also during this period that the young woman will be concerned about douching. The young patient who has no evidence of vaginitis or cervicitis need not douche. Some patients may feel a need to do this because of psychologic problems; that is, they believe the discharges are dirty or foul. Objectionable odors in most instances are caused by the secretions of the glands of the skin of the vulva, mons veneris, and crural regions and can be adequately treated by thorough cleaning of those parts (see discussion of douching, earlier in this chapter).

It is during adolescence that the young girl is in most need of sexual education. It is the warmth and understanding as much as the factual data that are of importance in sexual education. Many parents are unable to provide this education and will bring the adolescent girl to the physician for instruction. The best approach is first to find out what the young girl knows and believes; thus misconceptions and unpleasant emotional reactions can be specifically examined and dispelled. Adolescence is the time that young girls reevaluate themselves as women. This period of life also affords the physician a good opportunity to correct physical and emotional problems that these adolescents may present, thus strengthening the maturing female so that she may be better able to have a rewarding experience in the reproductive years.

MATURITY

Maturity is the phase in which reproduction and regular menstruation are the chief functions of the genital system. This phase lasts about 35 years and is often spoken of as the child-bearing period. Sex education, preparation for marriage and childbirth, and information regarding control of conception should be made available to all women in this phase of life.

Pregnancy. One of the central impulses in a woman's life is her desire to reproduce. The ability to have children of her own is important for many reasons. To a woman, children can represent her status in society. In various cultures it is the number, accomplishments, or sex of the children that is important. In almost every society and religion the woman's status is enhanced by her ability to have children. This is also reflected in her relationship with her husband; a child is a gift to him. It also represents a milestone on the road to maturity. There is also a deep emotional drive to reproduce something of herself and thus attain some assurance of immortality.

Pregnancy can also create deep emotional conflicts. Children are a challenge to the woman's ability to give and act in a mature fashion. They force her to fall back upon her own experiences, with her mother as a model to be copied or rejected, in rearing them. Pregnancy arouses a woman's fears of physical pain or injury. It is a challenge that increases her maturity if she responds, but it may also arouse feelings of inadequacy and fear. She may not be able to accept the pain and discomfort that accompany the pregnancy because of her sensitization in the past or the feeling that the reward of a child is not worth it. All of the conflicting emotions that can be aroused by the idea of pregnancy make it necessary for the physician to observe his pregnant patient closely. Her positive feelings toward the pregnancy cause little difficulty. It is the negative reactions, which the patient may be afraid or ashamed to express, that cause symptoms. The desire not to have a child, which the patient may repress, often finds expression in somatic or emotional symptoms. Ptyalism, hyperemesis, headache, and extreme lethargy all may be symptoms of the woman's fear of pregnancy or her attempt to eliminate the fear.

In the first trimester the expectant mother's feelings are inward. The child-to-be is not a reality to her. The child is in a sense a part of her. The patient's involvement with her conflicting feelings about the child may cause her to lose interest in her husband, family, and the world around her. During the middle trimester of pregnancy the advent of fetal movements, her increasing size, and other factors begin to give the woman the awareness that the child is a separate entity that she will have to give up to the world. She begins to have many fantasies about the child. It is important that the physician help the women to establish the child's individuality. He can help her in this emotional transition by his response to the fetal movements, by allowing her to hear the heart sounds, and by his general attitude. During the last trimester the patient feels a mounting tension that culminates with the delivery. She is increasingly uncomfortable and wishes "to get it over with." It is during this stage that the patient may have fears of death during childbirth. This may cause insomnia and depression. Patients should be allowed to express their fears. Some fear is normal, but excessive fear may be caused by guilt. As to any important rewarding event in life, past guilts can be attached to pregnancy and cause the fear that the reward will be damaged or denied because of past sins.

The physician responsible for his patient's prenatal care must change his attitude with the changes of the pregnancy. In the patient's early visits he must gradually get to know her and attempt to develop her feeling of trust in him. His concern for the patient and her diet, weight, and vitamin and iron intake, as well as his interest in any medical complications, is usually sufficient.

During the second trimester, when the child is more of a reality, the physician can discuss breast-feeding, and the patient should be allowed to make her choice. The overanxious mother will be unable to do the job of breast-feeding, and the infant will feel her anxiety. It is during this middle period that the mother-to-be acts out her feelings by making baby clothes and planning for the baby in many other ways.

During the third trimester a wish "to get it over with" develops. Most women will ask, "Do you think the baby will come early, Doctor?" Occasionally the patient will complain of insomnia. Her physical condition may be the most obvious cause, but upon closer examination it may be found to be caused by *dreams* of death. Since the darkness of night is associated with loneliness and death, this same patient may be able to sleep easily during the day.

During labor the patient faces the reality of having a baby, with the accompanying fear of injury and death. These realistic fears can be augmented by neurotic problems, which may interfere with the natural progress of labor. Upon entering the hospital the contractions may stop (Selye's fear and flight reaction). The arrival of the physician and the transference of her fears to him coupled with the judicious use of medication will in most patients reestablish labor. The physician is usually the one familiar object in the strange environment of the hospital. He is also the person the patient has built up in her mind to represent security.

As the labor progresses, the patient has many worries that are not concerned directly with childbirth. She is concerned about how much she should let herself go or how much she should move about or ask for assistance. She is often worried about cleanliness and getting messy. She is likely to feel that she is animal-like and thinks that the personnel are treating her as such. At full dilatation there is often a shift in mood, in which the patient reports that she cannot go on. She seems to lose most of her control. During the delivery anything the physician can do that can produce a feeling of cooperation and participation in the act will add to the patient's sense of well-being and accomplishment afterward. Throughout the labor a calm and reassuring attitude that transmits to the patient the idea that the physician is aware of what is happening both physically and mentally and is capable of handling this will allow the labor to progress in a comfortable fashion. He need only intervene when complications arise.

After the delivery the mother may feel, for varying lengths of time, a sense of unreality about the infant. She is not sure this is really her baby, especially if she has not seen the baby immediately after birth. For 9 months the baby has been primarily an imaginary symbol; the mother has difficulty progressing from this imaginary symbol to the real infant. This feeling soon disappears in the normal woman as she cares for the child. The new mother has many preconceived feelings and ideas in connection with her infant. On the deepest level they are connected with her relationship to her own mother. If this relationship has been good, very little conflict arises; but if the patient thinks of her mother with anger or hate and cannot approve of how her mother treated her, many problems arise. This is because so many of the "instinctive" things the mother does for her child have been picked up from the actions of her own mother. If the new mother cannot accept her mother's action, she must then doubt her own actions toward her child.

On about the third day post partum most patients report a short period of depression. In one study 67% cried for at least 5 minutes some time during the first few days following the birth of the baby. This occurs because the rewards of motherhood have been built to such great proportions before labor that the reality of having a baby rarely meets these expectations.

A feeling of lack of support from her husband or other significant figures can be of importance at this time. Another factor is that the relationship to the infant revives the new mother's own childhood experiences. Deep, latent problems can be stirred up that can result in psychosis. When this occurs, psychiatric aid should be sought promptly. The patient with postpartum psychosis usually has a good prognosis, especially if the previous personality has been a relatively mature one.

Gynecologic problems. The studies of Selye on the general adaptation syndrome and the response of endocrine glands to stress have led many investigators to appreciate the importance of emotions in producing body changes. The effects of feelings can be transmitted in many ways to the female organs and the endocrine system. There is a direct pathway from the hypothalamus to the autonomic nervous system. There can be an indirect neurologic influence through the cerebral cortex, the hypothalamus, and the pituitary gland, affecting the rest of the endocrine system. The influence of the emotions on the female endocrine system is demonstrated in a study by Benedek and Rubenstein, in which the psychoanalyst was able to predict ovarian function on the basis of her understanding of the female personality, especially the unconscious processes and dreams.

When an emotional conflict is discharged through the mechanisms just related, physical symptoms may arise. For example, the patient may consult a physician because of vaginal discharge. A saline suspension reveals the presence of *Trichomonas,* and a diagnosis can be made. Is it a complete one? Prescribing treatment is usually insufficient. These parasites are found in many women without symptoms. When we study the problem, we find it is during periods of stress and sexual tension that the patient becomes symptomatic. A warm, sympathetic physician who shows a genuine interest in the problems of the patient can be of great assistance to the patient at this time.

A woman who comes to a gynecologist often wishes to talk about problems of sexual relations. The complaint she presents may be a simple nonsexual one. The patient may seem to bring up the sexual problem as an afterthought. No matter when or how a patient presents her problem about the lack of enjoyment of coitus, dyspareunia, or frigidity, it is of great significance in her life. The cause of these symptoms may be relatively minor, but it can also be a serious emotional disturbance. The interested physician can solve many of the superficial problems. When the patient fails to respond and seems to be unduly emotional about the discussion, her transfer to a psychiatrist is indicated.

The infertile couple is a difficult problem for the physician. The inability to conceive has many organic, etiolgic factors, but not infrequently emotional problems may be associated or may even be the cause. This is readily apparent in the case of previously infertile women who become pregnant after dilatation and curettage that has been done for diagnostic reasons. The physician has reassured and helped her in her emotional conflict. As he continues to care for this woman, he should be aware that an emotional problem exists and that this woman is under additional emotional strain during her pregnancy.

Any operation can have symbolic meaning to the patient. This is especially true of surgery performed in the pelvic region. Many patients believe that the source of their sexual desires is located in this area. This is a common belief of black patients, who think that it is in the uterus; white patients think that it is in the ovaries. A surgeon operating in this area must be aware that the patient may believe she will lose her femininity when these organs are approached. It is important to discuss her feelings before surgery and to reassure her. If the problem is not handled well, the patient may develop postoperative frigidity or other psychophysiologic complaints. Surgery may also affect the husband after his wife has had a hysterectomy. Depression is also a frequent occurrence in the posthysterectomy patient because of the danger of operation and the feeling of loss of sexuality. A comprehensive approach is therefore of great importance for this patient.

CLIMACTERIC

The climacteric period, like adolescence, is a transitional stage. Its chief manifestation, menopause (the cessation of menstruation), is preceded by several months of irregular ovulation. The physical menopause usually occurs at from 45 to 50 years of age and is an indication of the waning of ovarian function. The menses may cease suddenly, but as a rule the cessation of menstruation is a gradual process and may display the same irregularities as were seen in the adolescent girl. Normally the cycles become longer and the flow scantier. However, excessive and more frequent bleeding is experienced by a considerable number of women early in the menopause. Since in this age group irregular bleeding may be a symptom of cancer of the uterus, a diagnostic curettage should be performed in all women who bleed excessively. Other physical complaints that may arise are the hot flush, joint pains, and a feeling of fatigue.

The psychologic menopause arises whenever the woman begins to believe that she is approaching the end of her childbearing stage. Women take this as a significant milestone, indicating that they are getting old, approaching death, and losing their position of value in the world. Many women develop depressions during this period that may be difficult to diagnose because they appear as symptoms of fatigue, anorexia, insomnia, irritability, constipation, and hypochondriasis. The patient may seek treatment for all of these conditions without realizing that her basic problem is emotional. She may be helped by being shown that she is useful and by encouragement to participate in the activities in her environment. The woman who has dedicated her life to bearing and caring for children may be the one who is hardest hit by the menopause. This patient must be helped to channel her interest into new areas —work, hobbies, organization, or grandchildren. The patient must regain the feeling of being needed and valued.

SENESCENCE

Senescence is the stage that begins with the complete cessation of menstruation and continues to the end of the woman's life. It is marked by progressive atrophy of the genital structures as well as the rest of the body. Loss of physical beauty may be very disturbing, especially to the woman who has put great emphasis on her attractiveness. Pelvic relaxations that had previously produced little discomfort now tend to become symptomatic and often require surgical correction because of the loss of estrogenic stimulation to the supporting structures. Cancer of the uterus and of the vulva frequently develops in this age group. Periodic examination is recommended.

Psychologically this is also a period of change in the woman's life. She has to give up many things that are of great importance to her, such as her home, her children who are growing up and moving away, a job, social prestige when her husband retires, and a decrease in her economic status. All of these things lead to great insecurity. The woman who has been dependent upon a rigidly scheduled existence during most of her lifetime will find it most difficult to adjust to these changes and thus may develop psychologic or psychophysiologic symptoms.

■ Summary

The total patient should be evaluated in every case. Evaluation of her personality should not be ignored because the physician believes it will be time consuming. An evaluation can be made swiftly if the physician is aware of its importance, notices the patient's attitude and behavior, and asks a few key questions. All of this may be accomplished during the history taking and physical examination. Emotional and organic problems cannot be separated, and a diagnosis should not be made by a process of exclusion. The diagnosis should be based on a total evaluation and on the presence of positive findings. Therapy will then be more effective, and most problems may be managed either emotionally and/or physiologically by an interested physician.

References

Benedek, T.: Psychosexual functions in women, New York, 1952, The Ronald Press Co.

Benedek, T., and Rubenstein, B. B.: The sexual cycle in women, Psychosomatic Medicine Monographs 3; nos. 1 and 2, 1942.

Caplan, G.: Concepts of mental health, United States Department of Health, Education, and Welfare, Washington, D. C., 1959, Government Printing Office.

Deutsch, H.: The psychology of women, vols. I and II, New York, 1944-1945, Grune & Stratton, Inc.

Donovan, J.: Some psychosomatic aspects of obstetrics and gynecology, Amer. J. Obstet. Gynec. 75:72, 1957.

Freud, S.: Female sexuality (collected papers), vol. V, London, 1950, Hogarth Press, Ltd.

Freud, S.: On narcissism; an introduction (collected papers), vol. IV, London, 1948, Hogarth Press, Ltd.

Gardiner, S. H.: Motivation for obstetrical care, Obstet. Gynec. 33:306, 1969.

Kroger, W. S., and Freed, S. C.: Psychosomatic gynecology, Chicago, 1956, Free Press.

Mondy, A. J., and Mondy, T. E.: The emotional aspects of obstetrics and gynecologic disorders, Amer. J. Obstet. Gynec. 60:605, 1950.

Mann, E.: Habitual abortion, Amer. J. Obstet. Gynec. 77:706, 1959.

Watson, A.: Prolonged labor, Obstet. Gynec. 13:598, 1959.

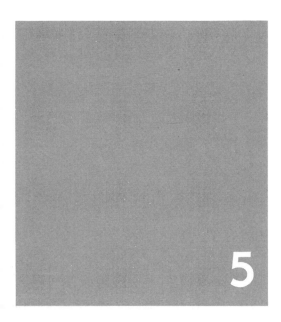

5

Normal menstruation

Menstruation is the periodic discharge of blood and of disintegrating uterine mucosa that has been built up for the reception of a fertilized ovum but has not been utilized. This is the bleeding phase or menstrual period. The term *menstruation* cannot properly be applied to anovulatory or dysfunctional bleeding, to the discharge of blood during pregnancy, or to bleeding caused by the presence of neoplasms or other abnormalities. The *menstrual cycle* is the interval between the onset of one period and the onset of the next. The average length of the menstrual cycle is 26 to 30 days.

Because menstruation is the hallmark of the reproductive function of the adult human female, a clear concept of the physiology of this phenomenon is necessary for the proper understanding and intelligent management of the abnormalities of the menstrual function.

Precise knowledge of menstruation was impossible until the epoch-making discoveries of Allen and Doisy (1923) and of Corner and Allen (1929). These investigators demonstrated the presence of ovarian hormones in the urine of pregnant women and succeeded in isolating and identifying them. The role of the pituitary in regulating ovarian function was definitely established by the discoveries of Smith and Engle and Aschheim and Zondek. Evidence of the importance of the hypothalamus and higher centers became available when Markee, Everett, and Sawyer demonstrated a neurohormonal mechanism influencing ovulation in the rabbit. More recently the eixstence of such a mechanism has become a certainty. Harris transplanted the pituitary gland from immature rats into adult hypophysectomized hosts and found that estrus cycles were resumed and, in fact, pregnancies were achieved. That stimuli from the cerebral cortex mediated through the hypothalamus can influence menstrual function is clearly seen in instances in which amenorrhea and other menstrual irregularities are directly related to fear of pregnancy or various emotional crises.

■ Physiology of the menstrual cycle

The cyclic events of menstruation reflect delicate balance in the neuroendocrine control mechanisms. Influences of the central nervous system are mediated by nerve fibers in the hypothalamus that liberate substances into the capillary plexus of the median eminence. These substances (releasing factors) are carried via the portal vessels to the anterior lobe of the pituitary, where they exert neurohumoral control. At puberty, activation of the hypothalamus results in production and release of follicle-stimulating releasing factor (FSRF) and luteinizing hormone releasing factor (LHRF) as the first step in sexual maturation. A third factor, prolactin or luteotropic hormone inhibiting factor (PIH), whose action is inhibitory rather than stimulatory, resides in the hypothalamus and is released at this time.

The functional role of the hypothalamus in reproduction is demonstrated in classic stimulation and ablation studies. Electrical stimulation of the hypothalamus will evoke ovulation and increase luteinizing hormone (LH) release in rabbits. Transplantation of the anterior pituitary to a distant site results in a gradual loss in capacity of the pituitary to secrete follicle-stimulating hormone (FSH) and LH but no loss in capacity to secrete prolactin. Reimplantation under the median eminence results in return of capacity to secrete FSH and LH and restoration of fertility. These experiments confirm the hypothesis that the hypothalamic controlling mechanisms are stimulatory for pituitary FSH and LH and inhibitory for lactogenic hormone.

Apart from the influence of the hypothalamus and higher centers, normal menstruation depends mainly on the functional integrity of three organs: the anterior lobe of the pituitary gland, the ovary, and the uterus. Thus at puberty, secretion of gonadotropic hormone becomes sufficient to stimulate the more or less dormant ovary and ultimately to induce ovulation and secretion of the normal ovarian hormones, estrogen and progesterone. These, in turn, stimulate the growth and secretory activity of the uterus in preparation for the reception of a fertilized ovum. This implies a well-regulated ebb and flow of activity between the hypophysis and the ovary and profound anatomic and functional changes in the reproductive organs during each cycle.

HORMONES OF MENSTRUATION

Estrogenic hormone. The "classic estrogens" are estrone, estradiol, and estriol; the first two are elaborated by the ovary, whereas estriol is their major degradation product. A considerable number of other estrogens have been identified, but except for 16-epiestriol, their amounts are extremely small and their biologic activity insignificant. Estradiol possesses the greatest biologic activity (100 times that of estrone and 500 times that of estriol). Estrogens in the circulation are in part bound to protein. Inactivation is carried out at a relatively rapid rate by the liver, and excretion is via the urine and feces chiefly in conjugated forms (glucuronates and sulfates). Histochemical studies by McKay and his co-workers point to the cells of the theca interna as being the site of estrogen production in the maturing follicle and those of the corpus luteum as being the site of both estrogen and progesterone production. The peak of estrogenic hormone secretion is reached at the time of ovulation, after which a brief fall occurs followed by a second peak near midluteal phase that is slightly less than the ovulatory peak.

The main effect of biologically active estrogen is on the genital tissues, but it also exerts a specific constitutional action on the entire organism. In addition to providing a growth stimulus to the endometrium and the endometrial spiral arterioles, estrogen has the following effects: It stimulates myometrial growth and sensitizes the muscle to stimulation by oxytocin; induces rhythmic contractions of the fallopian tubes; stimulates cervical mucus secretion; causes proliferation of vaginal epithelium; stimulates growth of the duct system of the breasts; and is responsible for the development of feminine body contours. High levels of estrogen inhibit the release of FSH from the anterior pituitary gland.

Progesterone. Progesterone is secreted by the corpus luteum of the ovary during the latter half of the cycle. The peak of its activity is reached about 7 days after ovulation. Its chief function is to induce secretory activity in the endometrial glands previously primed by estrogen and to induce decidual hypertrophy of the endometrial stromal cells, thereby preparing a favorable site for nidation of a fertilized ovum. Progesterone also desensitizes the myometrium to oxytocic activity, modifies the histologic appearance of the vaginal epithelium that has been primed previously by estrogen, and inhibits the secretory activity of the cervical glands. This hormone stimulates the development of the alveolar system of the breast and causes an increase in basal body temperature. Progesterone also inhibits the secretion of LH and probably stimulates the release of FSH from the anterior pituitary gland. In large amounts progesterone may produce an androgenic effect, probably because of the close chemical relationship between progesterone and androgenic substances. The conversion of progesterone to androgenic metabolites may explain the virilizing phenomena in certain ovarian tumors.

Gonadotropic principals. The gonadotropic principals are the *follicle-stimulating hormone* (FSH), which is responsible for the ripening of the graafian follicle, the *luteinizing hormone* (LH), which induces ovulation and the luteinization changes in

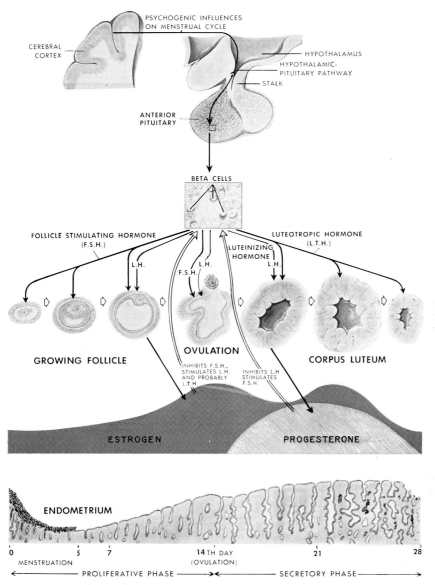

Fig. 5-1. Hormone interrelationships in normal menstrual cycle. (From Behrman, S. J., and Gosling, J. R.: Fundamentals of gynecology, New York, 1959, Oxford University Press, Inc.)

the ovary, and the *luteotropic hormone* (LTH), whose function is to maintain the corpus luteum. Both FSH and LH are glycoprotein substances secreted by basophilic cells of the anterior pituitary, whereas LTH contains no carbohydrate and is secreted by acidophilic cells. Both FSH and LH have been isolated in purified form from human pituitary glands and are present throughout the menstrual cycle, but the balance, or ratio, of one to the other is altered in a pattern

shown in Fig. 5-1. LTH has been isolated in purified form from the pituitary glands of lower animals, but in the human it has not been separated from the growth hormone in purified form. Nalbandov's work supports the concept that pituitary LTH is released shortly after ovulation in amounts sufficient to maintain the corpus luteum for its normal life-span. The hypothalamus exerts an inhibitory effect upon anterior pituitary secretion of LTH, and conditions resulting in persistent galactorrhea such as the Chiari-Frommel syndrome or certain brain tumors may represent a block of the normal inhibitory action.

There is a reciprocal functional relationship between the ovary and the pituitary gland. Pituitary gonadotropin secretion may be inhibited by high levels of ovarian hormones, and there may be an oversecretion when the ovaries cease to function, for instance during the menopause. There is some evidence to suggest that high levels of estrogen that depress the production of FSH may improve the secretion of LH.

CHANGES IN THE PITUITARY GLAND AND THE OVARY DURING MENSTRUAL CYCLE

Early in each cycle primordial ovarian follicles are stimulated by the FSH. Several begin to grow, but for some unknown reason one outstrips its fellows and rapidly develops

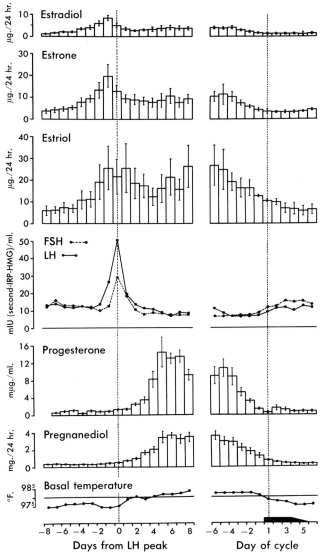

Fig. 5-2. Means of serum LH and FSH levels, serum progesterone concentrations, 24-hour urinary estrone, estradiol, estriol, and pregnanediol excretions, and basal body temperatures in 5 normal women. The data are plotted both in terms of days from the midcycle LH and FSH peak, from the approximate time of ovulation, and from the onset of menstruation. (From Goebelsmann, U., Snyder, D. L., and Jaffe, R. B.: Unpublished data.)

into a *graafian follicle*. The remainder regress and eventually become *atretic follicles*. As the graafian follicle matures, its lining of granulosa cells becomes cuboidal and multilayered and develops a central cavity, or antrum, which is filled with fluid *(liquor folliculi)* containing the ovum. At this point, midway in the cycle, the second gonadotropic hormone (LH) induces follicular rupture and *ovulation*. LH is present in small amounts during the first half of the cycle, but apparently a critical level must occur between the existing level of LH and the diminishing quantity of FSH before the LH can perform its special function of inducing ovulation. This occurs about the twelfth to the fifteenth day in the average menstrual cycle.

The rupture of the follicle is attended by capillary bleeding. The blood replaces the spilled follicular fluid, and a *hemorrhagic follicle* is formed. Through the continued action of luteinizing hormones, the granulosa cells soon become luteinized and a *corpus luteum* results. The corpus luteum, under the influence of the LTH, continues to grow and function until about the twenty-third or twenty-fourth day of the cycle, when it begins to regress. If the ovum, which was discharged at the time of ovulation, is fertilized, this regression does not take place; the corpus luteum continues to function as the corpus luteum of pregnancy.

During the preovulatory phase the granulosa and theca cells of the growing follicle secrete increasing quantities of *estrogen*. After ovulation the cells lining the hemorrhagic follicle and the corpus luteum continue to secrete estrogen as well as gradually increasing amounts of the corpus luteum hormone *progesterone*. The secretion of both of these hormones depends on an intact corpus luteum. When the corpus luteum has regressed completely, about the twenty-sixth to the twenty-eighth day of the cycle, the estrogen and progesterone levels drop sharply.

CHANGES IN THE UTERUS DURING MENSTRUAL CYCLE

The cervical mucosa, the myometrium, and the blood vessels of the uterus are all influenced by the cyclic changes in the levels of the hormones of the ovary, but the endometrium shows the most dramatic effect of the influence of estrogen and progesterone control and release. The changes are divided into four phases.

Postmenstrual phase. Immediately after menstruation the endometrium is thin, the epithelium is cuboidal, and the glands are straight and narrow. The stroma is compact. This stage lasts for about 5 days, that is, until the ninth day of the cycle.

Interval or proliferative phase. The continued action of estrogen brings about an increased thickness of the mucosa in the interval phase. The epithelium becomes columnar. As the phase progresses, the stroma becomes looser, more abundant, and more vascular. This phase lasts until about the eighteenth day of the menstrual cycle.

Premenstrual or secretory phase. During the premenstrual stage the progesterone from the corpus luteum stimulates the proliferative endometrium to secretory activity. The mucosa becomes thick and velvety. The glands become widened and assume a corkscrew pattern, and the stroma becomes edematous and very loose. The individual cells undergo hypertrophy and begin to resemble decidual cells. Early in the secretory phase the nuclei appear to move away from the basement membrane, leaving a characteristic area of subnuclear vacuolization. Secretion within the lumen of the glands is maximal by the twenty-fifth day. Special staining techniques reveal that secretions are rich in glycogen. There is an increased coiling of arterioles. At this stage the three distinct layers of endometrium can be distinguished, the *basalis, spongiosa,* and *compacta*. If the ovum is fertilized during the cycle and the corpus luteum persists, this phase progresses to the formation of the *decidua*.

Menstrual or bleeding phase. Because of the sudden withdrawal of the ovarian hormones upon the regression of the corpus luteum, the stimulative effect on the endometrium is removed. This, together with the ischemia produced by excessive constriction of the coiled arterioles, causes a breakdown of the endometrium with a discharge of blood and cellular debris from the uterus. Markee's observation of endometrial implants in the anterior chamber of the eye of a monkey disclosed several mechanisms of bleeding, the most frequent of which were rhexis of a blood vessel wall,

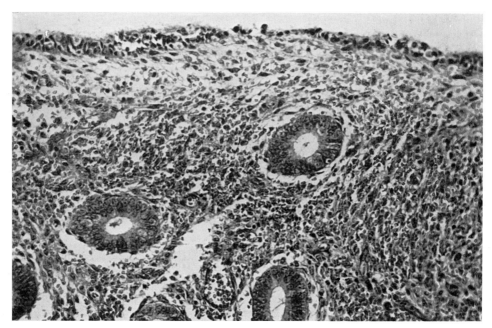

Fig. 5-3. Early proliferative endometrium. Abundant, compact, lymphoid-appearing stroma and a few small, narrow, straight glands are present. (×255.)

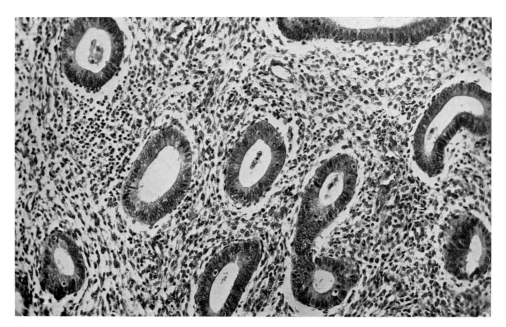

Fig. 5-4. Advancing proliferative endometrium. Note increase in number and size of glands and compactness of stroma. Although some of the glands are elongated, they are not tortuous. (×197.)

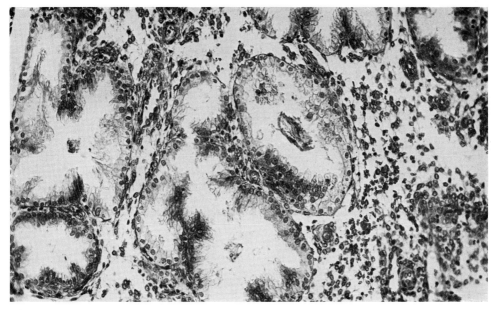

Fig. 5-5. Secretory endometrium. The stroma is scanty and loose, and the dilated, tortuous glands show intraluminal tufting and secretory activity. (×220.)

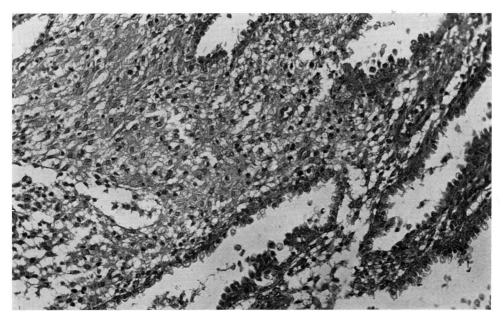

Fig. 5-6. Secretory endometrium with pseudodecidual stroma (tubal pregnancy). Note the compact pseudodecidual stroma and the dilated secretory glands. (×220.)

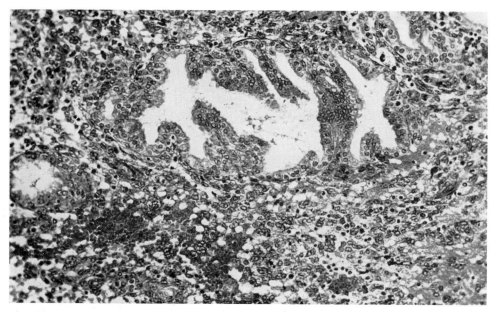

Fig. 5-7. Menstrual endometrium. The stratum compactum is edematous. Recent hemorrhage and cellular infiltration are evident. (×220.)

hematoma formation, and subsequent rupture of the hematoma.

The most controversial aspect of the entire process is the specific nature of the agent that acts directly on the endometrial arterioles, causing the intense vasoconstriction. An interesting observation is the appearance of leukocytes within the endometrial stroma while hormonal support is failing but in advance of necrosis and hemorrhage. It is apparent that some chemical or enzymatic activity is initiated by hormone withdrawal, but its nature is elusive.

CHANGES IN THE CERVICAL MUCUS DURING MENSTRUAL CYCLE

In the immediate postmenstrual phase the cervical mucus is scant, viscid, and opaque. During the follicular ovarian phase, because of the stimulating effect of estrogen, the columnar cells become taller, and the cervical glands begin to secrete increasing quantities of thin, clear, watery mucus, which exhibits the physical properties of *spinnbarkheit* (the ability to form long thin threads) and arborization (Chapter 2).

In the normal menstrual cycle the peak of estrogen activity is reached in the immediate preovulatory phase. The cervical mucus at this point is greatly increased in amount, is quite watery, and exhibits maximum

spinnbarkheit and *arborization*. This remarkable change in the amount of character of the mucus favors sperm motility and survival and enhances its penetrability.

After ovulation, under the influence of increasing progesterone production, the cervical mucus gradually decreases in amount and becomes viscid and tenacious; the arborization phenomenon tends to diminish and disappears entirely a few days before menstruation.

CHANGES IN THE VAGINA DURING MENSTRUAL CYCLE

The effect of the ovarian hormones on the vaginal epithelium of laboratory animals was observed and reported many years ago. Allen and Doisy demonstrated cyclic changes in the vaginal epithelium of rodents in response to changing levels of estrogen. Similar changes occur in the vagina of the adult human female. In a newborn girl the vaginal epithelium has a well-developed, thick structure because of the high levels of estrogen transferred from the maternal blood. Within a few days the estrogenic hormone is completely excreted, and the vaginal lining gradually regresses to a thin membrane and remains so throughout childhood. With the increase of ovarian function at puberty the epithelium becomes thicker and develops into a mature vaginal mucosa after the menarche.

The adult vaginal epithelium is composed of three main layers: a superficial *functional* zone, consisting of flattened, poorly staining squamous cells; beneath this is an *intermediate* zone of transition cells; and finally is the deepest *basal* layer, which consists of one or several rows of deeply staining, round and oval basal cells. The degree of proliferation of the vaginal epithelial cells parallels the rise of estrogen levels during the cycle; and maximum growth occurs at the time of ovulation.

After the menopause, with the decrease in ovarian function, the epithelium of the vagina again becomes thin and eventually may resemble that of the prepubertal girl. This is usually a gradual process and may not be evident for many years after the complete cessation of menstruation.

■ Anovulatory cycles

Cyclic menstrual bleeding that is not preceded by ovulation and corpus luteum formation is caused by an imbalance in the normal cyclic reciprocity in the hypothalamic-pituitary-gonadal axis. The ovaries produce estrogen but no progesterone because the ovarian cycle is incomplete. The progesterone-deprived endometrium has a proliferative pattern throughout the entire anovulatory cycle. Anovulation occurs frequently at the two extremes of menstrual life and less often during the active childbearing period. The adolescent girl may bleed quite regularly and yet ovulate infrequently, if at all. Similarly, as women approach the end of their reproductive life, many anovulatory cycles occur. This accounts for the relative infertility of women in the premenopausal period.

■ Clinical aspects of normal menstruation

The length of the menstrual cycle and the duration and amount of flow vary considerably among normal women, but pronounced deviations from the accepted norms should suggest the possibility of functional or anatomic abnormality. The characteristics of the menses that are clinically significant are the *age at onset, periodicity, duration* and *amount of flow, character of flow,* and *associated symptoms.*

Age of onset. The first period usually occurs at about 13 years of age, but the menses may appear at age 9 or may be delayed until age 16 without being considered abnormal. Many factors are responsible for this wide variation. The most significant are race, heredity, and the general health and nutritional status of the individual girl. If the periods start before the age of 9 years, it is spoken of as *precocious menstruation;* if they are delayed past the age of 16 years, it is spoken of as *delayed menstruation.*

Periodicity. The theoretic normal interval from the beginning of one period to the onset of the next is 28 days, but few women menstruate absolutely regularly. There are many variations from this ideal normal, even in women who insist that they menstruate regularly within this cycle. Intervals of 21 to 35 days may be considered normal. Cycles shorter than 3 weeks or longer than 5 weeks may indicate some disturbance of menstrual function, but even this may not be of a serious nature. Patients with short cycles are said to have *polymenorrhea.* If the cycles are unusually long (40 to 60 days), we designate the condition as *oligomenorrhea.*

Duration. The usual length of flow is 3 to 5 days, but periods may last as long as 7 or 8 days or stop after 2 days and yet be within normal limits. Very short or scant periods are designated as *hypomenorrhea,* whereas unusually long or profuse menses are referred to as *hypermenorrhea.*

Amount of flow. The amount of blood lost at each period varies greatly. The average is about 50 ml. and may be as little as 20 ml. or as much as 150 ml. without being considered abnormal. Actually it is almost impossible to determine with any degree of accuracy the amount of menstrual flow. In practice, estimates are based on the number of pads used daily or during the entire period. Most women soil from four to five napkins daily during the height of the flow and two to three on the first and last days of menstruation, a total of twelve to fifteen pads.

Character of flow. The menstrual discharge consists of blood, mucus, and desquamated particles of endometrium. It is usually dark red and has a characteristic, musty odor. An interesting feature of menstrual blood is its failure to clot under normal circumstances. If bleeding is very free, the discharged blood may be bright red and may contain clots of varying size.

Symptoms. A characteristic group of symptoms may appear several days preceding the menstrual flow. These symptoms, which include weight gain, edema, breast fullness and discomfort, heaviness of the legs, and irritability or depression, are referred to as *menstrual molimina*. Because irritability is the most consistent of these complaints, the syndrome is usually termed *premenstrual tension*. Its etiology is controversial. The sodium- and water-retaining properties of the sex steroids may be contributory factors, but physiologic increases in these hormones do not appear to be sufficient to induce these changes. The work of Thorn suggests that cyclic edema along with other related manifestations is caused by a more complex disturbance of hormone balance in which hyperaldosteronism plays the leading role. Aldosterone output has been shown to increase in anxiety and tension states.

Even though menstruation is a normal function and should be free from disturbing symptoms, most women experience some degree of discomfort during the period of bleeding. A sense of weight in the pelvic region, mild backache, and cramping are such common complaints that they may be considered as normal accompaniments of the menses. When these symptoms become more severe, the patient is said to be suffering from *dysmenorrhea*.

■ Hygiene of menstruation

Women need not restrict their usual daily routine in any way during the menstrual flow; this includes work and social and athletic activities. Most couples abstain from sexual intercourse during menstruation because of aesthetic reasons, based mainly on the ancient tabu of uncleanliness. There is no medical reason for sexual abstinence during the period.

A daily bath or shower is not only permissible but most helpful in eliminating the characteristic odor that is present during the menstrual period.

Most women employ external pads to absorb the menstrual discharge, but an ever-increasing number of women are turning to the intravaginal tampon for protection. These are much more convenient and may be used by women who are free from abnormal vaginal or cervical discharge. The internal tampon is not applicable in virgins with small hymenal openings or in multiparous women with marked vaginal relaxations. During a very free flow it may be necessary for the woman to wear both a tampon and a pad.

References

Allen, E., and Doisy, E. A.: An ovarian hormone; preliminary report on its localization, extraction, partial purification, and action in test animals, J.A.M.A. **81:**819, 1923.

Bartelmez, G. W.: Factors in the variability of the menstrual cycle, Anat. Rec. **115:**101, 1953.

Brown, J. B., Kloffer, A., and Loraine, J. A.: The urinary excretion of oestrogens, pregnanediol and gonadotropins during the menstrual cycle, J. Endocr. **17:**401, 1958.

Corner, G. W., and Allen, W. M.: Production of a special uterine reaction by extracts of the corpus luteum, Amer. J. Physiol. **88:**326, 1929.

Davis, M. E., and Fugo, N. W.: Causes of physiologic basal temperature changes in women, J. Clin. Endocr. **8:**550, 1948.

Harris, G. W.: Neural control of the pituitary gland, London, 1955, E. Arnold, Ltd.

Lamson, E. T., Elmadjian, F., Hope, J. M., Pincus, G., and Jorjorian, D.: Aldosterone excretion of normal, schizophrenic and psychoneurotic subjects, J. Clin. Endocr. **16:**954, 1956.

McArthur, J. W., Worcester, J., and Ingersoll, F. M.: The urinary excretion of interstitial-cell and follicle-stimulating hormone activity during the normal menstrual cycle, J. Clin. Endocr. **18:**1186, 1958.

McKay, D. G., Pinkerton, J. H. M., Hertig, A. T., and Danziger, S.: The adult human ovary; a histochemical study, Obstet. Gynec. **18:**13, 1961.

Markee, J. E.: Menstruation in intraocular endometrial transplants in the rhesus monkey, Contrib. Embryol. **28:**219, 1940.

Markee, J. E., Everett, J. W., and Sawyer, C. H.: The relationships of the nervous system to the release of gonadotrophin and the regulation of the sex cycle, Recent Progr. Hormone Res. **7:**139, 1952.

Papanicolaou, G. N.: General survey of vaginal smear and its use in research and diagnosis, Amer. J. Obstet. Gynec. **51:**316, 1946.

Ratner, A., Dhariwal, A. P. S., and McCann, S. M.: Hypothalamic factors in gonadotropic hormone regulation. In Jaffe, R. B., editor: Hormones in reproduction, Clin. Obstet. Gynec. **10:**106, 1967.

Roger, J.: Menstrual disorders, New Eng. J. Med. **270:**356, 1964.

Rosemberg, E., and Keller, P. J.: Studies on the urinary excretion of follicle-stimulating and luteinizing hormone activity during the menstrual cycle, J. Clin. Endocr. 25:1262, 1965.

Smith, P. E., and Engle, E. T.: Experimental evidence regarding role of anterior pituitary in development and regulation of the genital system, Amer. J. Anat. 40:159, 1927.

Thorn, G. W.: Cyclical edema, Amer. J. Med. 23: 507, 1957.

Zondek, B., and Aschheim, S.: Das Hormon des Hypophysenvorderlappens; Testobjekt zum Nachweis des Hormons, Klin. Wschr. 6:248, 1927.

Amenorrhea

6

The term *amenorrhea* indicates the absence of menstruation. This is a symptom not a disease entity and may be caused by a variety of physiologic and pathologic processes. *Oligomenorrhea* means infrequent menstruation or short periods of amenorrhea. Since the etiologic factors in this disorder are essentially the same as those in amenorrhea, we shall consider them together. Amenorrhea is considered to be *primary* if a normal, spontaneous period has not occurred at age 16 years. *Secondary amenorrhea* indicates cessation of menstruation after a variable period of normal function.

■ Etiology

Since amenorrhea may be brought about by a variety of physiologic, anatomic, pathologic, or constitutional factors, our primary concern whenever we are confronted with this symptom is to determine which of these is the basis of the disorder. This is important for two reasons. First, although the amenorrhea may be physiologic or perhaps caused by a minor and negligible systemic or psychic disturbance, it also may be an early symptom of a serious constitutional disease or endocrinopathy. Second, the determination of the cause will often lead to appropriate and successful therapy of the symptom as well as of the disease. For these reasons the following systemic classification of the possible etiologic factors involved in amenorrhea and an anatomic classification are offered as a guide to the diagnostic study of this symptom.

ETIOLOGIC FACTORS

I. Physiologic factors
  A. Amenorrhea during adolescence
  B. Pregnancy
  C. Lactation
  D. Premenopausal factors

II. Anatomic causes
  A. Congenital absence of vagina
  B. Congenital absence of uterus
  C. Hysterectomy
  D. Congenital hypoplasia of uterus
  E. Gynatresia (cryptomenorrhea)
  F. Destruction of endometrium
    1. Irradiation
    2. Disease (tuberculosis)
    3. Trauma (surgical, chemical)
  G. Castration
    1. Irradiation
    2. Surgical
    3. Disease (rare)

III. Genetic factors
  A. Ovarian dysgenesis (Turner's syndrome)
  B. Testicular feminizing syndrome (male pseudohermaphroditism)
  C. Congenital adrenal hyperplasia (female pseudohermaphroditism)
  D. Poly-X syndromes (superfemale syndrome)
  E. Minor chromosomal abnormalities (isochromosomes, deletion)
  F. True hermaphroditism

IV. Endocrinopathic factors
  A. Pituitary
    1. Lesions
      a. Basophilic adenoma
      b. Chromophobe adenoma
      c. Acidophilic adenoma
      d. Destructive (Simmonds' disease and Sheehan's syndrome)
    2. Hypofunction
      a. Fröhlich's syndrome
  B. Ovarian
    1. Hypofunction
    2. Nonfunctioning cysts—luteal
    3. Stein-Leventhal syndrome
    4. Functioning tumors
      a. Arrhenoblastoma
      b. Adrenal rest
      c. Hilus cell
      d. Germinoma

C. Thyroid
  1. Hypofunction
  2. Hyperfunction
D. Adrenal
  1. Hyperplasia
  2. Neoplasm
    a. Adenoma
    b. Adenocarcinoma
  3. Insufficiency (Addison's disease)
V. Constitutional factors
  A. Malnutrition
  B. Tuberculosis
  C. Diabetes
  D. Obesity
  E. Anemias
  F. Drug addiction
VI. Psychogenic factors
  A. Psychoneurosis
  B. Psychosis
  C. Pseudocyesis
  D. Anorexia nervosa

ANATOMIC CLASSIFICATION

I. Uterovaginal
  A. Congenital malformations
  B. Atrophy of endometrium
  C. Hysterectomy
II. Ovarian
  A. Complete ovarian failure
    1. Agenesis
    2. Castration
    3. Premature menopause
  B. Dysfunction
    1. Follicle cytosis
    2. Functioning cysts
    3. Functioning tumors
III. Pituitary
  A. Fröhlich's syndrome
  B. Simmonds' disease
  C. Hypopituitarism of malnutrition
  D. Destructive tumors
  E. Chiari-Frommel syndrome
IV. Thyroid
  A. Hypothyroidism
  B. Hyperthyroidism
V. Adrenal
  A. Hyperplasia
  B. Neoplasm
VI. Hypothalamic
  A. Psychogenic
  B. Pseudocyesis

■ Physiologic factors

Amenorrhea during adolescence. Whereas the average healthy American girl usually experiences her first menstrual period at about the age of 12 years, it is not at all unusual for the menarche to be delayed until 15 or 16 years of age. Similarly, although many girls bleed quite regularly after the onset of the first period, many will exhibit considerable irregularity with frequent prolonged periods of amenorrhea during the first few years. This so-called "dodging" period during adolescence is so common that it may be considered quite normal.

If the first menstrual period does not appear by the age of 16 years, the girl is considered to have a *delayed menarche*. This may have a variety of causes, the most common being a constitutional or biologic variant with a slow rate of maturation. However, failure to menstruate may result from anatomic causes or from serious endocrine or genetic abnormalities. The complaint of primary amenorrhea in a young woman will occasionally provide the first opportunity to uncover one of these conditions.

Pregnancy. Pregnancy is the most common cause for amenorrhea and should *always* be considered as the immediate etiologic factor in all patients in the childbearing period. Instances of cyclic uterine bleeding during pregnancy are probably caused by a disturbance of pregnancy or by an organic lesion rather than by menstrual periods.

Lactation. The first menstrual period after delivery usually occurs within 10 weeks unless the infant is breast-fed, in which event menstruation may be delayed until it is weaned. Follicle-stimulating hormone (FSH) and luteinizing hormone (LH) secretion is suppressed by the lactogenic hormone. Ovarian function is thereby reduced in nursing mothers. In nonnursing mothers Cronin found that ovulation occurs before the first menstrual period in one third of cases, whereas ovulation in lactating mothers is rare before the tenth week post partum, unless a menstrual period occurs before that time. These facts underscore the importance of counseling in family planning early in the puerperium because occasionally ovulation, and even pregnancy, may occur in lactating amenorrheic women.

Premenopausal factors. Variable periods of amenorrhea may occur for a number of years preceding the final cessation of menstruation. This is frequently a source of considerable anxiety to the middle-aged woman, who may consider the amenorrhea as a symptom of pregnancy. Since most women of this age period do not ovulate, conception is most unlikely, but it occasionally does occur, and it may need to be ruled out by appropriate diagnostic procedures.

ANATOMIC CAUSES OF AMENORRHEA

Primary amenorrhea may be caused by congenital malformations that preclude the possibility of menstruation. These abnormalities are rather rare and account for about 2% of all amenorrhea not caused by pregnancy.

Absence of the uterus and vagina. The most commonly encountered structural malformation is absence of the uterus and associated complete or partial absence of the vagina. Young girls with uterine aplasia usually have normal or near-normal ovarian function, consequently skeletal growth and secondary sex characteristics appear in proper sequence. The condition should be suspected whenever well-developed young women fail to menstruate. Examination of the genitals usually is sufficient to disclose the cause of the amenorrhea.

Rarely a uterus and a vagina are present at birth, but they fail to develop normally at puberty and remain hypoplastic. If the cervix is relatively longer than a tiny corpus, the physician is justified in making the diagnosis of an *infantile uterus*. Skeletal growth and secondary sex characteristics are normal if the ovaries are present and functioning. Hormone studies, vaginal smears, and basal body temperature charts indicate adequate endocrine function, but for some reason the uterus remains unresponsive to the stimulus of the ovarian hormones.

Atresia of the vagina and imperforate hymen. Atresia of the vagina and imperforate hymen, too, is a rather uncommon condition that is responsible for failure of the menarche to appear in young girls who are in good health and show no evidence of endocrinopathy. Absence of menstruation results from an obstruction at some point in the vagina or cervix. Most often the congenital malformation is an *imperforate hymen*. Since the ovaries and endometrium in these patients are perfectly normal, a discharge of blood from the uterus does occur at the time of the menarche, but it is retained and hidden in the vagina *(cryptomenorrhea)*. This process is repeated from month to month and leads to a progressive distention of the vagina with old blood *(hematocolpos)*. If the situation is unrecognized, the uterus and even the fallopian tubes may become filled with this material, resulting in *hematometra* and *hematosal-*

pinx, episodes of lower abdominal pain and backache are characteristic. Inspection of the vulva and rectal examination will readily confirm the diagnosis. Simple incision of the hymen will usually solve the problem.

Destruction of endometrium. Secondary amenorrhea is often caused by either surgical removal or irradiation of the uterus, endometrium, or ovaries. Rarely a disease process may be destructive enough to produce a similar result. Obviously if the uterus is completely removed, menstruation is permanently abolished. However, if a subtotal hysterectomy or, as in some instances, a high amputation of the uterus is performed, periodic bleeding may continue from the remaining portion of the endometrium. If periods cease after subtotal hysterectomy and subsequently recur, the physician should suspect a cancer in the cervical stump rather than a resumption of menstrual function.

Irradiation of the pelvis results in either temporary or permanent amenorrhea, depending on the dose employed. This effect is produced by the destructive action of either radium or the roentgen ray on the endometrium and/or ovaries. If periods recur after a long period of irradiation-induced amenorrhea, an intrauterine malignancy must be ruled out as a cause of bleeding.

Traumatic uterine adhesions. Amenorrhea may develop after repeated or too strenuous curettage, particularly in the postpartum and postabortal uterus. Asherman has demonstrated cervical and uterine corpus adhesions that partially or completely block the canal. There is no accumulation of menstrual blood behind this stricture. For some obscure reason the endometrium is unresponsive to hormone stimulation, yet dilatation of the cervix and breaking up of adhesions result in the resumption of ovulatory menstruation and the restoration of fertility.

GENETIC FACTORS

Gonadal dysgenesis (Turner's syndrome). Classic features of Turner's syndrome include congenital webbed neck, low-set ears, cubitus valgus, shortness of stature, and sexual infantilism. Other anomalies such as congenital heart disease, particularly coarctation of the aorta, renal malformation, and impaired intellect occur more frequently in

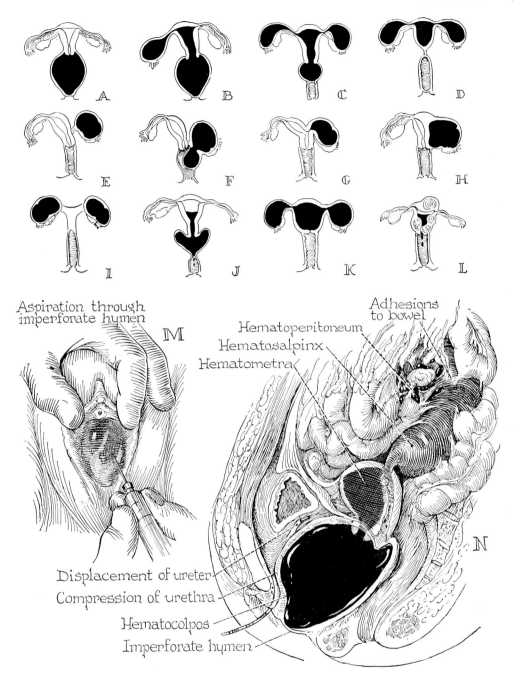

Fig. 6-1. Cryptomenorrhea. **A,** Imperforate hymen, hematocolpos. **B,** Imperforate hymen, hematocolpometra, right hematosalpinx. **C,** Congenital atresia of the cervix, hematocolpometra, bilateral hematosalpinx. **D,** Congenital atresia of the cervix, hematometra, bilateral hematosalpinx. **E,** Uterus bicornis unicollis, lateral hematometra in a blind, rudimentary horn. **F,** Uterus didelphys, lateral hematocolpometra due to blind left vagina. **G,** Uterus bicornis unicollis, lateral hematometra in blind left horn. **H,** Uterus septus duplex, lateral hematometra in a blind left uterine cavity. **I,** Uterus didelphys, two rudimentary horns, hematometra due to gynatresia. **J,** Acquired atresia of the cervix, intermittent hematocolpometra. **K,** Acquired atresia of the cervix, hematometra, bilateral hematosalpinx. **L,** Cervical fibromyoma, intermittent hematometra. (From Ball, T. L.: Gynecologic surgery and urology, ed. 2, St. Louis, 1963, The C. V. Mosby Co.)

patients with this disorder. The complete picture of this syndrome, including all the foregoing anomalies, is relatively rare, whereas sexual infantilism and short stature are quite consistent findings. It is not unusual for the patient to present herself with amenorrhea as the first complaint. About 80% to 90% of these patients are chromatin negative and show a sex chromosome constitution of XO. The chromosome number therefore is 45 instead of 46 because of the loss of the second X chromosome. These individuals, who are basically female despite the chromatin-negative smear, have no male Y chromosome and only half the number of female X chromosomes. The chromosomal constitution in others may show mosaicism such as XO/XX, XO/XXX, XO/XX/XXX. Thus the chromosomal number of the majority is 45, whereas some have chromosomal counts of 46 or even 47. An XO/XY form has also been described.

This condition represents primary and complete ovarian failure. At laparotomy no ovarian tissue is found except for elongated, whitish ridges or streaks on the broad ligament. Histologic examination shows no evidence of primordial follicles or germ cells, but the stromal tissue is similar to that of the ovary. The absence of estrogen secretion is reflected in lack of breast development, genital hypoplasia, amenorrhea, and a high titer of FSH.

Diagnosis is made by examination of the buccal smear for nuclear sex evaluation, determination of chromosomal constitution, high FSH excretion, and ovarian biopsy. Estrogenic hormone replacement should be deferred until after growth is complete. These patients rarely achieve more than 4 feet 8 inches in height, and early administration of estrogen will hasten epiphyseal closure. Cyclic therapy using estrogen and progesterone may be used to induce menstrual cycles and is of importance in improving genital development and preventing osteoporosis. Synthetic progestins with anabolic properties may be given with estrogen because of their potential for increasing growth.

Testicular feminizing syndrome (male pseudohermaphroditism). Individuals suffering from testicular feminizing syndrome are chromatin-negative or genotype males, but the phenotype is female. The breasts are well developed and a small vagina is present, but there are no other female genital structures. The testes are usually found as swellings in the inguinal region. Pubic and axillary hair is sparse.

The gonad produces both estrogen and androgen. Urinary estrogens correspond in values to those found in normal women. The FSH level is at about that found in premenopausal women, and if the gonad is removed these values increase to levels found in menopausal women. The 17-ketosteroid excretion is normal or slightly elevated. Thus the androgen produced by the gonad may be less active than normal, or there may be some defect in the metabolism of androgen that interferes with its peripheral effect. Wilkins demonstrated that large doses of testosterone may fail to stimulate facial or other hair growth.

Despite the female phenotype, the sex chromatin is negative and the chromosomal number is 46, as might be expected in the normal male. Furthermore, the chromosomal constitution is XY, but it is possible that one or the other of these components is abnormal. An attempt has been made to incriminate excessive estrogen stimulation during gonadogenesis as a causative factor. However, mosaicism has been found with this condition, and therefore a genetic background seems probable.

Because the abdominally or inguinally located testes are likely to undergo malignant change and because the feminization is often incomplete the gonads should be removed. Most authorities suggest waiting until puberty to gain the full advantage of endogenous estrogen effect. Estrogen replacement is indicated thereafter.

Poly-X (superfemale syndrome). The chromosomal pattern in poly-X syndrome is 47 XXX or 48 XXXX. The term *superfemale* refers only to the number of sex chromosomes. Clinically the patient shows infantile sexual structures, amenorrhea, or infertility and is frequently mentally retarded.

Isochromosomes and the sex chromosomes with other morphologic changes as described in Chapter 10 are believed to be responsible for some cases of amenorrhea that have been otherwise unexplained.

ENDOCRINOPATHIC FACTORS

The most frequent cause of amenorrhea is some disturbance of one or more of the endocrine glands directly or indirectly involved in the menstrual function. The menstrual cycle is dependent on the cooperative action of the pituitary and ovary and, secondarily, of the thyroid and adrenal glands. Amenorrhea may result from a functional defect or disease of any of these because of the reciprocal functional relationship among all of them. Since higher centers in the brain exert control over pituitary activity, central nervous system lesions, especially those within or adjacent to the hypothalamus, cause disturbances in reproductive physiology. Also, nonendocrine constitutional disease or psychogenic factors may impair the function of the endocrine glands and cause amenorrhea.

Pituitary gland. About 70% of all cases of endocrinopathic amenorrhea are caused by dysfunction of the anterior lobe of the pituitary gland.

Pathologic lesions of the pituitary gland. Amenorrhea may be the first symptom of an adenoma of the pituitary gland, and recognition of this fact may lead to early diagnosis and prompt and appropriate treatment. The tumor may arise from the basophilic, acidophilic, or chromophobe cells of the anterior lobe.

The *basophilic adenoma* (Cushing's disease) was first recognized and described by Harvey Cushing. The syndrome is characterized by amenorrhea, obesity, hirsutism, abdominal striae, glycosuria, hypertension, and osteoporosis. The causative factor is the excessive secretion of ACTH by the anterior pituitary gland. Cushing's syndrome is now recognized to be far more commonly associated with hyperplasia or tumors of the adrenal cortex. The symptoms result from an overproduction of 11-oxysteroids and 17-hydroxycorticosteroids primarily. The androgenic 17-ketosteroids are normal or only slightly elevated. The same symptoms can be provoked by excessive or prolonged administration of cortisone or ACTH.

Diagnosis is made by x-ray examination of the skull and examination of the visual fields for evidence of pituitary adenoma. The typical response to ACTH stimulation test is a threefold to fivefold elevation above normal of the blood and urinary corticoids in Cushing's syndrome secondary to adrenal hyperplasia but no rise in the secretion rate of cortisol or its metabolites if adrenal neoplasm is the cause.

Treatment is surgical removal of adrenal neoplasm, bilateral adrenalectomy with subsequent replacement therapy for hyperplasia, or irradiation for pituitary adenoma.

Chromophobe adenoma is the most common type of pituitary adenoma. It is characterized by amenorrhea, sterility, headache, and progressive optic atrophy. X-ray examination of the skull usually reveals distortion and enlargement of the sella turcica.

Acidophilic adenoma produces giantism or acromegaly, depending on the age at which the tumor develops. Amenorrhea is not an early symptom of this disease but may develop as the tumor enlarges and destroys the anterior lobe of the pituitary gland.

Pituitary necrosis (Sheehan's syndrome) is produced most often after a severe postpartum hemorrhage or severe puerperal infection. Normally the pituitary gland becomes enlarged during pregnancy and for some reason is quite susceptible to hemorrhage, thrombosis, and infection in the immediate postpartum period.

The clinical picture usually has in its background a history of a traumatic delivery with hemorrhage and shock. If a considerable portion of the anterior lobe is destroyed, the patient fails to lactate during the puerperium; the genital organs atrophy, and she is amenorrheic. Premature aging is evidenced by loss of axillary and pubic hair, emaciation, and hypometabolism. The excretion of 17-ketosteroids is greatly reduced (less than 5 mg./24 hr.). Eventually symptoms of adrenal failure develop, and the patient may die during an addisonian crisis unless she is treated with adrenocortical hormones.

Less complete destruction of the anterior lobe also occurs. There may be no evidence of hypopituitarism, and the patient may even conceive. If ACTH production is selectively impaired, the patient may die of adrenal insufficiency during periods of stress such as complicated pregnancy or after a surgical operation.

Pituitary hypofunction. Adiposogenital dystrophy (Fröhlich's syndrome) results from a disturbance of function of the anterior lobe of the pituitary gland. The lesion in some instances is a craniopharyngioma, as in Fröhlich's original patient. An identical picture of adiposogenital dystrophy is also seen in the hypothalamic obesity of childhood and adolescence and occasionally in adults without evidence of tumor. The causative factor in such patients is believed to be a disorder of the metabolic center in the hypothalamus.

Adiposogenital dystrophy is characterized by amenorrhea, obesity, and occasionally facial hirsutism. The distribution of the obesity is quite typical. The adipose tissue is deposited mainly about the hips, shoulders, breasts, and abdomen. The amenorrhea may occur suddenly but usually develops gradually over a period of time, whereas the obesity is usually abrupt in onset. The urinary excretion of both gonadotropins and estrogens is greatly reduced. In patients who develop hypertrichosis of the face, the 17-ketosteroid values may be slightly elevated. The sugar tolerance is usually high in these patients. Endometrial biopsy usually discloses an atrophic or proliferative pattern, but occasionally a hyperplastic or even secretory endometrium is encountered in patients with amenorrhea.

Ovary. Endocrinopathic factors may cause ovarian failure, resulting in amenorrhea.

Functional defects. Primary ovarian failure is a rather rare condition in which the gonads, although present, are genetically immature and do not respond adequately to stimulation by gonadotropins. Occasionally the defect may be acquired through either disease or irradiation. The ovaries are rather flat, smooth, and show no evidence of follicular growth. The patient complains of amenorrhea and presents evidence of poorly developed secondary sex characteristics. The breasts are flat, the bones of the extremities are unusually long, and axillary and pubic hair is scant. Frigidity, dyspareunia, and infertility are very common complaints. The most significant laboratory finding is the presence of high titers of FSH in the blood and urine, whereas estrogens are either very low or not demonstrable. Studies of the endometrium show an atrophic epithelium with little glandular development.

Keettel and Bradbury carried out extensive studies of 24 young women with secondary amenorrhea resulting from premature ovarian failure in which none of the usual precipitating causes could be found. The diagnosis is of great consequence to the patient, since there is as yet no means of reversing the process. Therefore diagnosis should be made with due caution and only after repeated analysis, including inspection of the ovaries. Ovarian resection is of course of no value in ovarian failure, whereas hormone replacement will prevent atrophy of the genital organs and other remote effects of hypoestrogenism.

Nonneoplastic ovarian cysts. A follicular cyst of the ovary may be responsible for varying periods of amenorrhea, but as a rule this type of ovarian cyst either produces no menstrual disturbance or is associated with dysfunctional bleeding. *Corpus luteum cysts* (corpus luteum persistens) may induce a short period of amenorrhea followed by irregular bleeding. These symptoms and the presence of an adnexal mass often lead the physician to suspect ectopic pregnancy. The situation becomes even more confusing when the endometrium presents the picture of a pseudodecidual reaction in response to the high progesterone output. Most so-called persistent corpus luteum cysts probably represent pregnancy with early spontaneous abortion.

Stein-Leventhal syndrome. The classic features of the complete symptom complex originally described by Stein and Leventhal in 1935 were amenorrhea, infertility, and facial hirsutism. The ovaries were described as oysterlike in appearance with a thick grayish capsule, numerous tiny cysts beneath the thickened tunica, and an enlargement amounting to approximately two to three times their normal size. A typical finding in polycystic ovarian syndrome, hyperplasia and luteinization of the theca interna (hyperthecosis) and a relatively scanty granulosa layer, was described later. Stein recognized that some of the symptoms were inconstant; hirsutism occurred in only about 50% of the cases, and instead of amenorrhea, menstrual irregularities with episodes of menometrorrhagia were not uncommon. The amenorrhea tends to develop gradually over a period of years. Obesity is not always present. However, bilateral polycystic ovaries with thick fibrous tunica and infertility are consistent findings.

Determination of the primary etiologic factor in the polycystic ovary syndrome has been controversial, probably because of the difficulty in discriminating between two basic disorders that result in the same ovarian changes and the same symptomatology.

The most common is primarily an ovarian disorder, whereas the second is primarily adrenal in origin. It can be stated with certainty that in the primary ovarian disorder the polycystic ovary produces significantly more androgen than the normal ovary.

Plasma testosterone levels are often increased, although the 17-ketosteroid values remain within normal levels or are only slightly elevated. Kase incubated tissue homogenates of resected portions of polycystic ovaries from women with the Stein-

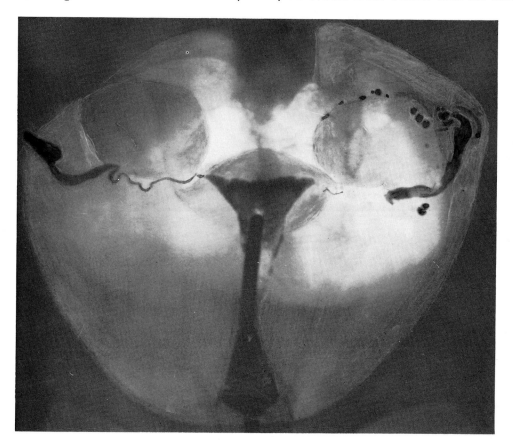

RECORD OF BASAL BODY TEMPERATURES

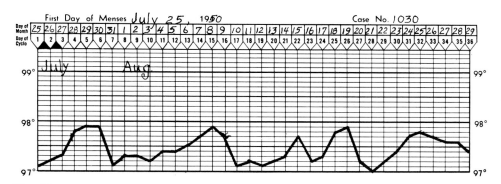

Fig. 6-2. Polycystic ovaries (Stein-Leventhal syndrome). Combined gynecography. Basal body temperature chart indicates anovulatory cycle. (From Williams, W. W.: Sterility; the diagnostic survey of the infertile couple, Springfield, Mass., 1953, the author.)

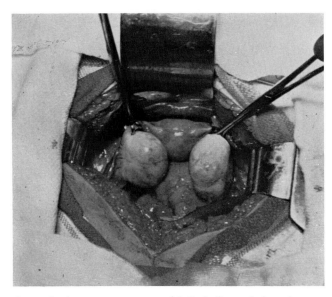

Fig. 6-3. Polycystic ovaries in a young woman with Stein-Leventhal syndrome.

Leventhal syndrome with selected substrates and found excessive androgen production in the ovarian tissue. Similar enlarged polycystic ovaries associated with disease of the adrenal cortex do not have the same capacity for increased androgen production. Successful therapy depends upon accurate diagnosis, and this is often quite difficult.

In both types of disorder, hormone studies are consistent with those in anovulatory cycles; the basal body temperature curve is monophasic, cervical mucus displays arborization with no significant change during the cycle, and the endometrium is nonsecretory in type. The excretion of estrogen is within normal limits. Gonadotropic hormone determination, performed in the usual manner without separation of FSH and LH, is within normal limits. Unfortunately, LH determinations are not generally available, but Ingersoll and McArthur found frequent and erratic bursts of LH excretion in women with the Stein-Leventhal syndrome. Most authorities believe that this is because of the prolonged absence of progesterone and that it is not the basic cause of the disorder. The 17-ketosteroid values are normal or slightly elevated.

The diagnosis of polycystic ovary syndrome is suspected in young women who develop oligomenorrhea, particularly if infertility is a problem. Obesity and hirsutism may or may not be associated. The finding of bilaterally enlarged ovaries, either on pelvic examination, gynecography (x-ray examination of the pelvis after injection of carbon dioxide), laparoscopy, or culdoscopy confirms the diagnosis. (Figs. 6-2 and 6-3). An ACTH-stimulating test resulting in a twofold or threefold increase in the 17-ketosteroid or oxycorticosteroid excretion would point to an adrenal origin. Finally, examination of androgen conjugates as described by Baulieu and co-workers will distinguish between primary and secondary polycystic ovarian disease, but this is still a highly specialized test. The condition may be differentiated from an adrenogenital syndrome by the mild degree of virilism and the normal 17-ketosteroids and from primary or early secondary ovarian failure in which FSH is elevated, ovaries are not enlarged, and hirsutism is not an associated finding.

Ovarian wedge resection with removal of a sufficient number of androgen-producing cells is effective therapy in the primary ovarian disorder, but it does not reverse the process if the ovarian changes are secondary to adrenal hyperactivity. In the latter disorder, suppressive therapy with oral cortisone is indicated.

Medical management with clomiphene citrate is of particular value in a patient desirous of pregnancy. The success of the

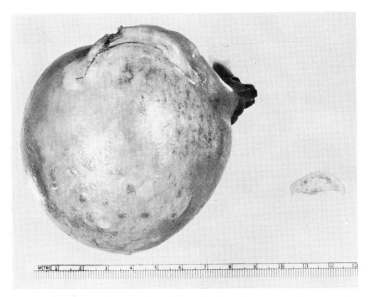

Fig. 6-4. Arrhenoblastoma and resected wedge of the other normal ovary in a 22-year-old patient. Chief complaints were amenorrhea and hirsutism. After the operation menstrual periods became regular and pregnancy ensued.

drug in inducing ovulation appears to be greater in individuals showing high rather than low unopposed estrogen effects prior to therapy. Unfortunately, "carry-over" effect in succeeding cycles is infrequent, thus limiting its usefulness when conception is not the objective of treatment.

Ovarian neoplasms. Ovarian neoplasms rarely cause amenorrhea, but they must be considered in the differential diagnosis. *Arrhenoblastoma* is the most important of the so-called masculinizing tumors of the ovary, all of which can cause amenorrhea. *Adrenal rest tumors of the ovary* are rare lesions that produce a syndrome similar to that seen in arrhenoblastoma. The tumor is usually of small size and is made up of tissue resembling adrenal cortex. *Masculinizing hilus cell tumor* is an exceedingly rare growth arising from the hilus cells of the ovary, which are probably the homologues of the Leydig cells of the testis. Therefore, these tumors, although rather small in size, produce distinct virilization. *Germinoma* is a rare ovarian tumor that originates from undifferentiated gonadal cells and may be responsible for amenorrhea in young women. The tumor is hormonally inert, however, and usually does not produce masculinizing symptoms.

Thyroid gland. The thyroid gland is not directly concerned with menstruation, but ovarian function often is disturbed in women with either hypothyroidism or hyperthyroidism. Amenorrhea may be associated with either mild or severe hypothyroidism and occasionally may be a symptom of Graves' disease.

Adrenal gland. Amenorrhea and signs of masculinization may be produced by hyperplasia, benign adenomas, or malignant tumors of the adrenal cortex. Apart from amenorrhea, which is common to each, more specific clinical syndromes and laboratory findings reflect involvement of different components of the adrenal cortex. Thus Cushing's syndrome is characterized by excessive production of the major glucocorticoid, cortisol, whereas congenital adrenal hyperplasia is characterized by excessive production of adrenal androgens. Adrenal neoplasms may produce either substance, or the typical features of each may overlap. Furthermore, adrenal hyperactivity may be secondary to excessive pituitary ACTH secretion. The most useful tests for differential diagnosis of these disorders include measurement of the 17-ketosteroids and 17-hydroxycorticoids, utilizing the cortisone or dexamethasone suppression tests and the ACTH stimulation test. X-ray examination of the skull and neurologic tests, as discussed under pituitary adenoma, may be definitive in localization of a central nervous system lesion, and intravenous pyelography and presacral air insufflation may demonstrate an adrenal tumor.

Amenorrhea caused by adrenal insufficiency (Addison's disease). Amenorrhea is usually a late symptom of Addison's disease and is either caused by the extreme debility or by the diminished activity of the anterior lobe of the pituitary gland—a condition often present in such cases.

CONSTITUTIONAL FACTORS

The pituitary gland and ovary are quite sensitive to deviations from normal function of the general body processes. Almost any disease with which there is a disturbance of metabolism and nutrition may be associated with amenorrhea. This is most often seen in wasting diseases such as tuberculosis and diabetes but may also occur in obesity during periods of increasing weight. The depression of ovarian function in the more serious wasting diseases is probably mediated through the hypothalamic-pituitary controls. The mechanism by which amenorrhea is pro-

duced in obese patients is not clearly understood, but it is a well-established clinical fact that such patients frequently resume normal menstruation after appropriate diet and weight reduction.

PSYCHOGENIC FACTORS

Although we cannot directly trace the pathways by which emotional and psychic stimuli affect the menstrual cycle in the female, there is ample evidence that the autonomic nervous system, the hypothalamus, and even higher cerebral centers exert a distinct influence on this function. Thus mental disorders, fears, anxieties, and psychic trauma may alter the secretion of gonadotropic hormone and disrupt the normal sexual cycle. The most striking example of the intimate relationship between the psyche and the soma is a condition known as *pseudocyesis.* This condition, which usually occurs in emotionally unstable women who are infertile and who have an intense desire for pregnancy, is discussed in Chapter 17.

Anorexia nervosa, too, is a psychogenically induced condition in which amenorrhea

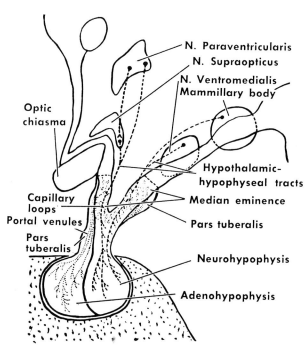

Fig. 6-5. Diagram representing median sagittal section of human hypothalamus and hypophysis. The dotted lines indicate only the hypothalamic-hypophyseal portal elements of the hypophyseal blood supply. (Redrawn from Cleghorn, R. A., and Graham, B. F.: Recent Progr. Hormone Res. 4:323, 1949.)

is an early and prominent symptom. The malady theoretically is brought on by a prolonged, serious emotional conflict that causes a depression of the secretory activity of the anterior pituitary gland. This results in symptoms not unlike Sheehan's syndrome, with which it is often confused. The antecedent histories of the two conditions, however, are quite dissimilar. Anorexia nervosa usually affects adolescent girls or young women with severe neurotic tendencies, whereas Sheehan's syndrome usually follows severe postpartum hemorrhage, shock, or sepsis.

■ Diagnosis

Often the physician may establish the cause of a particular patient's amenorrhea after taking a brief history, making a pelvic examination, or performing a simple laboratory procedure. On the other hand the etiology of the symptom may be so obscure as to defy the most careful investigation. Usually a complete history, physical examination, and indicated laboratory studies will serve to identify possible physiologic, anatomic, or constitutional factors that might be responsible for the amenorrhea.

The history is not complete if it fails to include details of early psychosexual development, sexual experiences, and the patient's adjustment to these and other problems of her emotional life. The physician should obtain information regarding the patient's early childhood and her attitude toward parents, siblings, husband, and other important members of her family. These facts may be helpful in ascribing a psychogenic cause for amenorrhea.

A thorough physical examination, including inspection of the genitals and palpation of the pelvic organs, will enable the physician to detect gross anatomic abnormalities as well as deviations in somatic growth and genital development. Endocrine stigmas such as abnormal hirsutism, deposition of body fat, and enlargement of the clitoris are significant physical findings in the clinical evaluation of amenorrhea.

In order to investigate the endocrine factors involved in the production of amenorrhea, endometrial biopsy, examination of vaginal smears and cervical mucus, and hormone assay will usually indicate whether the ovary or the pituitary gland is primarily involved.

Diagnostic survey. Following is a list of investigative procedures that will serve as a guide in the study of the more serious and persistent cases of amenorrhea:

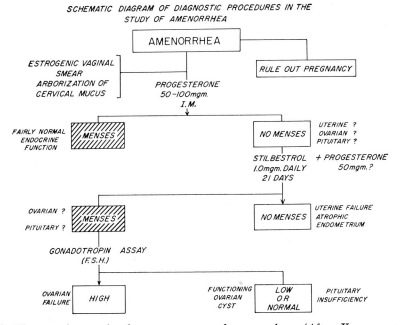

Fig. 6-6. Therapeutic test in the management of amenorrhea. (After Kupperman, H. S., Blatt, M. H. G., Wiesbader, H., and Studdiford, W. E.: Obstet. Gynec. **1:**650, 1953.)

1. Complete history
2. Complete physical examination
3. Complete blood count
4. Urinalysis
5. Buccal smear for sex chromatin (chromosomal number and karyotype as indicated)
6. Serum cholesterol test
7. Protein-bound iodine test
8. Basal metabolic rate determination
9. Sugar tolerance tests
10. Examination of vaginal smears
11. Examination of cervical mucus
12. Basal body temperature charts
13. Endometrial biopsy
14. Visual field examination
15. X-ray examination of skull
16. X-ray examination of chest
17. Pregnancy tests
18. Determination of urinary gonadotropins
19. Determination of urinary 17-ketosteroids, pregnanetriol, and 11-ketopregnanetriol
20. Psychiatric evaluation

From a practical standpoint, if no gross pathologic or anatomic lesions are evident or suspected and if pregnancy has been ruled out, the physician may employ the following clinical tests to determine the cause of the amenorrhea prior to the performance of the more extensive investigative procedures.

If bleeding can be induced by the injection of 50 to 100 mg. of progesterone, it may be assumed that the amenorrhea is not caused by any serious derangement of either the pituitary, ovary, or uterus. This would indicate that the patient probably manufactures sufficient *gonadotropins* to stimulate a fairly adequate ovary to secrete enough *estrogen* to "prime" a *responsive endometrium*. **Note:** A favorable response to a single injection of progesterone may usually be predicted if the examination of the cervical

mucus and vaginal smear shows evidence of good estrogen effect.

If bleeding does not occur, it may be assumed that the amenorrhea is caused by either failure of the ovary to secrete estrogen or by an atrophic, unresponsive endometrium. To rule out an endometrial factor, estrogen in the form of stilbestrol, 1 mg., or 17-ethinyl estradiol, 0.1 mg., is given daily for 21 days. If withdrawal bleeding does not occur within 5 to 7 days after this treatment, it may be assumed that the endometrium is unresponsive. To prove this assumption the physician should repeat the estrogen therapy and on the twenty-second day perform an endometrial biopsy. If no endometrium is present or if it should be reported as atrophic, the diagnosis of an unresponsive endometrium may be made. If bleeding does take place after withdrawal of estrogen, however, we have reasonable evidence that the patient has an adequate endometrium and that the amenorrhea is caused by either ovarian or pituitary dysfunction.

To differentiate these two causes for the amenorrhea it is necessary to perform a bioassay of urinary gonadotropins. A high titer of these hormones indicates deficient ovarian function (agenesis, aplasia, or hypofunction); absence or low levels of gonadotropins indicate pituitary hypofunction.

Hormone values. The hormone patterns in amenorrhea are given in Table 4.

■ Treatment

If the cause of the amenorrhea can be established, the physician can decide whether effective treatment is feasible or even neces-

Table 4. Hormone patterns

Etiology	FSH	Estrogen	17-Ketosteroids
Pituitary hypofunction	Low	Low	Low
Ovarian hypofunction	High	Low	Normal
Functioning cysts ovary (hyperhormonal)	Normal	High	?
Stein-Leventhal syndrome	Low	Low	Normal
Arrhenoblastoma	Low	Low	High
Adrenocortical hyperplasia			High
Adrenocortical adenoma			Very high
Chiari-Frommel syndrome	Low	Low	Normal
Hypothalamic disorders	Normal or low	Low	Normal
Pseudocyesis	Low	Normal	?
Pregnancy	Measurements unsatisfactory	High	Slight increase

sary. Patients with serious anatomic malformations or absence of important pelvic structures obviously cannot be helped, and when the amenorrhea results from a physiologic cause, no active therapy is indicated.

CONSTITUTIONAL THERAPY

Patients who are suffering from a clinical disease such as tuberculosis or diabetes require specific therapy for that condition. However, most patients with amenorrhea will be benefited by measures directed toward the improvement of their general health and well-being. One of the first considerations is adequate nutrition. The diet should be high in protein and vitamin values and relatively low in carbohydrates and fats. When obesity is associated with amenorrhea, the caloric intake should be reduced. Regular exercise in the outdoors is most advisable.

PSYCHOTHERAPY

Psychotherapy plays an important role in the management of all types of amenorrhea, but it is particularly applicable to those that are psychogenic in origin. A variable amount of anxiety and emotional tension is present in all women whose menstruation is unduly delayed. The anxiety may either be the cause of the amenorrhea or be caused by it. In either case a sympathetic and understanding attitude on the part of the physician, as it relates to the patient's emotional and sexual behavior, will accomplish a great deal toward relieving the amenorrhea and the anxiety. Every physician who attempts to treat these problems should provide the young woman with the opportunity to ventilate her feelings and fantasies regarding menstruation and her attitude toward sexuality and childbearing. This may enable the physician to clear up any misconceptions that the patient may have had on these subjects. Sympathetic encouragement, a factual explanation of the purpose and mechanism of menstruation, as well as a realistic approach to the patient's sexual problems are basic elements in the superficial psychotherapy of amenorrhea. Most patients suffering from the milder forms of psychogenic amenorrhea will readily respond to this type of therapy or will make an adequate adjustment to the symptom once they understand that the failure to menstruate regularly implies no threat to their health and happiness.

HORMONE THERAPY

When amenorrhea is associated with infertility or with serious emotional disturbances, the reestablishing of a normal cycle by endocrine therapy is definitely indicated. The administration of hormones will usually produce a flow, but such bleeding is unaccompanied by ovulation and recurs only in response to repeated courses of hormone therapy. Psychologically these women feel very much relieved by the reappearance of the flow, even though the basic problem of ovulation is not being solved. Occasionally in mild cases of secondary amenorrhea of short duration (less than 1 year), substitution therapy may result in the restoration of spontaneous ovulatory cycles. Hormone replacement is of particular value in cases of primary or early secondary ovarian failure, chiefly to prevent atrophy of the secondary sexual organs in young women but also for the relative value that estrogens appear to have in protecting against osteoporosis and atherosclerotic disease.

Thyroid. Hypometabolism is not a particularly common cause but when amenorrhea results from reduced thyroid activity, response to thyroid hormone replacement is dramatic. Triiodothyronine (T_3) has a more rapid onset and shorter duration of action, whereas tetraiodothyronine (T_4, thyroxine) may take weeks to reach maximum effects. Desiccated thyroid, which is a natural mixture of T_3 and T_4, is still a favored medication for maintaining a normal protein-bound iodine once a euthyroid state is achieved. Initial dosage is 30 to 60 mg. daily. The empiric use of thyroid substance, administration of thyroid to tolerance or in excess of the amounts required by the body, is not beneficial and may be detrimental because of the depression of pituitary tropic activity that it causes.

Progesterone. In instances of amenorrhea of very short duration with clinical evidence of adequate estrogen activity (arborization of cervical mucus and/or estrogenic vaginal smears), a single injection of 50 to 100 mg. of progesterone will result in bleeding within 7 to 10 days. The administration of progesterone will not induce a flow if the patient is pregnant or if the endometrium is unprimed by estrogen or already in the secretory phase.

Estrogen. The administration of estrogen in the form of diethylstilbestrol, 1 mg., or

17-ethinyl estradiol, 0.1 mg., daily for 21 days, will stimulate the endometrium to proliferation and will result in withdrawal bleeding 5 to 7 days after the last dose of hormone. This may be repeated for 3 months. This is a very simple and inexpensive method of treatment and occasionally will restore normal, cyclic bleeding. If this does not take place, another type of therapy should be employed.

Estrogen and progesterone. The addition of progesterone toward the end of the estrogen schedule just given improves the effectiveness of the estrogen therapy. Buccal tablets of progesterone, 10 mg. twice daily, or synthetic Provera orally, 10 mg. daily, for the last 10 days of the treatment schedule or 50 to 100 mg. of progesterone by intramuscular injection at the end of the estrogen therapy will induce bleeding. A simplified method of producing withdrawal bleeding has been recommended by Zondek. This consists of a single injection of a combination of 10 mg. of estrone and 50 mg. of an aqueous suspension of progesterone. Withdrawal bleeding occurs within 7 to 10 days. This method has the advantage of simplicity and economy, but some patients complain of considerable pain at the site of the injection.

The long-acting progestational steroid 17-alpha-hydroxyprogesterone caproate, if administered in doses of 375 to 500 mg. (3 to 4 ml. of Delalutin) to patients whose endometria have been previously primed with estrogen, will induce a well-developed secretory response. Withdrawal bleeding will occur 10 to 17 days after a single injection. Withdrawal bleeding, anovulatory in nature, can be produced by the use of oral progestins administered from the fifth to the twentieth days of the cycle, but these agents induce neither normal endometrial growth nor normal cyclic stimulation—inhibition of pituitary activity. It is therefore important that true cyclic therapy be used when estrogen deficiency is part of the problem.

Whenever estrogen-progesterone cyclic therapy is employed, the treatment should be continued over a period of 3 to 4 months. Basal body temperature charts and examination of vaginal smears will help in the clinical evaluation of treatment. If cyclic bleeding recurs and if a biphasic basal body temperature curve persists after cessation of treatment, it is an indication that normal ovarian function has been restored.

Cortisone. Cortisone is of value in the treatment of patients with amenorrhea secondary to adrenal cortical hyperplasia. Theoretically in these patients the anterior pituitary gland secretes excessive quantities of adrenocorticotropic hormone, which stimulates the adrenal cortex to increased output, primarily of androgenic steroids. This produces the virilism and also depresses the gonadotropic function of the anterior pituitary. Cortisone or hydrocortisone inhibits ACTH production, and the overstimulation of the adrenal cortex is arrested. With the resulting drop in secretion of adrenal androgens, the pituitary gonadotropic function is resumed, the ovary is stimulated to cyclic activity, and menstruation is reestablished. The usual dose of cortisone in these cases is 25 mg. orally given daily and continued for 2 to 3 months or longer if necessary.

Clomiphene citrate. Clomiphene citrate, which is a nonsteroid compound, is an analogue of the estrogen chlorotrianisene (TACE). It is of greatest value in patients with low pituitary gonadotropic secretion and anovulation, which often result in menstrual irregularity, amenorrhea, or oligomenorrhea. The drug causes an increase in both FSH and LH, either by direct action upon the hypothalamus with a secondary increase in ovarian hormones or primarily upon the ovary in stimulating estrogen synthesis at the preestradiol phase. It is ineffectual in the absence of endogenous estrogen, as in Turner's syndrome, but has been effective in the treatment of the Chiari-Frommel syndrome.

Menotropins (Pergonal). Human menopausal gonadotropin (menotropins), extracted from menopausal urine, has been successful in correcting amenorrhea and including ovulation even in women with 24-hour urine values for estrogens below 10 μg., the level below which clomiphene therapy has been less effectual. Dosage of menotropins is adjusted to increase the urinary estrogen to between 30 and 60 μg./24 hr., at which time cervical mucus shows approximately 3 plus arborization pattern. Human chorionic gonadotropin (HCG), 5,000 I.U., is administered daily for 3 days thereafter. Both clomiphene and menotropins may overstimulate the ovaries, giving rise to multiple births, considerable ovarian enlargement, and ascites. These effects occur more readily with menotropins, but this may be because of the greater difficulty of adjusting the dosage to the individual need.

SURGERY

Surgery is essential and generally curative in cases of obstruction of menstrual flow such as imperforate hymen, cervical stenosis, and traumatic uterine adhesions. When there is definite evidence of pathologic changes in the ovaries such as tumors or cysts, operative procedures may remove the cause of the amenorrhea. Stein reported his experience of 25 years with wedge resection of polycystic ovaries. Of 93 patients with amenorrhea so treated, 59 subsequently became pregnant, and a considerable number of the remainder of the group had been experiencing regular cyclic bleeding over long periods of time.

References

Asherman, J. G.: The myth of tubal and endometrial transplantation, J. Obstet. Gynaec. Brit. Comm. 67:228, 1960.

Baulieu, E. E., Mauvais-Jarvis, P., and Corpechot, C.: Steroid studies in a case of Stein-Leventhal syndrome with hirsutism, J. Clin. Endocr. 23: 374, 1963.

Bergman, P.: Amenorrhea of uterine etiology, Obstet. Gynec. 2:454, 1953.

Bongiovanni, A. M., and Root, A. W.: The adrenogenital syndrome, New Eng. J. Med. 268:1283, 1342, 1391, 1963.

Cleghorn, R. A., and Graham, B. F.: Manifestations of altered autonomic and humoral function in psychoneuroses, Recent Progr. Hormone Res. 4:323, 1949.

Cronin, T. J.: The influence of lactation upon ovulation, Lancet 2:422, 1968.

Fluhmann, C. F.: The management of menstrual disorders, Philadelphia, 1956, W. B. Saunders Co.

Fried, P. H., Rakoff, A. E., Schopbach, R. R., and Kaplan, A. J.: Pseudocyesis; psychosomatic study in gynecology, J.A.M.A. 145:1329, 1951.

Haskins, A. L., Moszkowski, E. F., and Cohen, H.: Chiari-Frommel syndrome; medroxyprogesterone acetate therapy, Amer. J. Obstet. Gynec. 88: 667, 1964.

Ingersoll, F. M., and McArthur, J. W.: Longitudinal studies of gonadotropin excretion in the Stein-Leventhal syndrome, Amer. J. Obstet. Gynec. 77:795, 1959.

Jayle, M. F., Scholler, R., Mauvais-Jarvis, P., and Metay, S.: Excrétion des stéroids chez des femmes présentant un virilisme pilaire associe à des troubles du cycle menstruel, Acta Endocr. (Kobenhavn) 36:375, 1961.

Kaiser, I. H.: Pregnancy following clomiphene-induced ovulation in Chiari-Frommel syndrome, Amer. J. Obstet. Gynec. 87:149, 1963.

Kase, N.: Steroid synthesis in abnormal ovaries. III. Polycystic ovaries, Amer. J. Obstet. Gynec. 90:1268, 1964.

Keettel, W. C., and Bradbury, J. T.: Premature ovarian failure, permanent and temporary, Amer. J. Obstet. Gynec. 89:83, 1964.

Kinch, R. A. H., Plunkett, E. R., Smout, M. S., and Carr, D. H.: Primary ovarian failure; a clinicopathological and cytogenetic study, Amer. J. Obstet. Gynec. 91:630, 1965.

Kupperman, H. S., Blatt, M. H. G., Wiesbader, H., and Studdiford, W. E.: Progesterone in menstrual disturbances; its diagnostic value in amenorrhea, Obstet. Gynec. 1:650, 1953.

Lloyd, C. W.: The hypothalamus and anterior pituitary in obstetrics and gynecology, Clin. Obstet. Gynec. 3:971, 1960.

Mahesh, V. B., Greenblatt, R. B., Aydar, C. K., and Roy, S.: Secretion of androgens by the polycystic ovary and its significance, Fertil. Steril. 13:513, 1962.

Mellinger, R. C., and Smith, R. W.: Effects of oral administration of estrogens on the 17-ketosteroid excretion of virilized women, J. Clin. Endocr. 21:931, 1961.

Miller, O. J.: The sex chromosome anomalies, Amer. J. Obstet. Gynec. 90:1078, 1964.

Philip, J., Sele, V., and Trolle, D.: Primary amenorrhea; a study of 101 cases, Fertil. Steril. 16:795, 1965.

Riley, G. M., and Evans, T. N.: Effects of clomiphene citrate on anovulatory ovarian function, Amer. J. Obstet. Gynec. 89:97, 1964.

Roger, J.: Menstrual disorders, New Eng. J. Med. 270:194, 356, 1964.

Sheehan, H. L.: Post-partum necrosis of the anterior pituitary, Irish J. Med. Sci. 6:241, 1948.

Stein, I. F.: Ultimate results of bilateral ovarian wedge resection; twenty-five years' follow-up, Int. J. Fertil. 1:333, 1956.

Stein, I. F., and Leventhal, M. L.: Amenorrhea associated with bilateral polycystic ovaries, Amer. J. Obstet. Gynec. 29:181, 1935.

Taymor, M. L., and Bernard, R.: Luteinizing hormone excretion in the polycystic ovary syndrome, Fertil. Steril. 13:501, 1962.

Taymor, M. L., Sturgis, S. H., Lieberman, B. L., and Goldstein, D. P.: Induction of ovulation with human postmenopausal gonadotropin, Fertil. Steril. 17:731, 1966.

Wallach, S., and Henneman, P. H.: Prolonged estrogen therapy in postmenopausal women, J.A.M.A. 171:1637, 1959.

Warner, R. E., and Mann, R. M.: Hematocolpos with imperforate hymen; report of five cases, Obstet. Gynec. 6:405, 1955.

Wilkins, L.: The diagnosis and treatment of endocrine disorders in childhood and adolescence, ed. 3, Springfield, Ill., 1966, Charles C Thomas, Publisher.

Zondek, B., Rozin, S., and Vesell, M.: Uterine bleeding induced by progesterone, Amer. J. Obstet. Gynec. 40:391, 1940.

7

Abnormal uterine bleeding

I. Complications of pregnancy
   A. Abortion
   B. Ectopic pregnancy
   C. Hydatidiform mole
   D. Chorioadenoma destruens
   E. Choriocarcinoma
   F. Placental polyp
II. Organic lesions
   A. Uterine myomata
   B. Malignant tumors of corpus uteri
   C. Malignant tumors of cervix
   D. Endometrial polyp
   E. Benign cervical disease
   F. Adenomyosis
   G. Endometriosis
   H. Salpingo-oophoritis
   I. Ovarian tumors
III. Constitutional diseases
   A. Acute infections
   B. Cardiovascular diseases
   C. Thrombocytopenia
   D. Hepatic cirrhosis
   E. Hypertension
   F. Lymphatic, hematopoietic, and reticular tumors
   G. Anticoagulant therapy
IV. Hormonal (dysfunctional) uterine bleeding
   A. Anovulatory cycles
   B. Endometrial hyperplasia
   C. "Irregular shedding"
   D. Functioning ovarian cysts
      1. Follicular
      2. Lutein
   E. Functioning ovarian tumors
      1. Granulosa cell
      2. Theca cell
   F. Estrogen therapy
V. Intrauterine contraceptive devices
VI. Psychogenic uterine bleeding
VII. Cryptogenic uterine bleeding

Irregular or excessive bleeding from the uterus is one of the most common symptoms the gynecologist is called upon to diagnose and treat. Abnormal bleeding may manifest itself by profuse, prolonged, or too frequent periodic flow or by bleeding between periods. Profuse and prolonged bleeding at the time of the period is called *hypermenorrhea,* or *menorrhagia;* too frequent bleeding is called *polymenorrhea;* bleeding between periods is usually *metrorrhagia.*

■ Etiology

Most abnormal bleeding results either from organic causes or from complications of pregnancy, but in a considerable number of instances no obvious cause can be found. A careful study usually discloses either a hormonal, constitutional, or psychogenic cause for the abnormal bleeding. Following is a classification of abnormal uterine bleeding:

COMPLICATIONS OF PREGNANCY

Abortion is by far the most common complication of pregnancy associated with bleeding. It should be considered as a possible reason for abnormal bleeding in any woman of childbearing age. Other less common causes are *ectopic pregnancy, trophoblastic diseases,* and *placental polyp,* all of which are discussed in other chapters.

ORGANIC LESIONS

Uterine myomata, particularly those of the submucous variety, are the genital tract lesions that most often cause abnormal bleeding in women who are not pregnant. Other entities include *benign cervical disease, carcinoma of the vagina, cervix, uterus, and ovaries, adenomyosis, endometriosis,* and *chronic salpingo-oophoritis* with extensive ovarian destruction. These are discussed in other chapters.

Endometrial polyps may cause intermenstrual staining and postmenopausal bleeding as well as menorrhagia and hypermenorrhea. Since polyps generally do not cause an appreciable enlargement of the uterus, they are frequently overlooked. A polyp may be missed during diagnostic currettage unless the physician suspects its presence and makes a special effort to detect it with polyp forceps. X-ray visualization of the uterine cavity (hysterogram) is a valuable aid in the diagnosis and localization of endometrial polyps.

CONSTITUTIONAL DISEASE

It would seem probable that a number of systemic diseases, particularly hypertension, would cause uterine bleeding. This is not the case. Constitutional diseases most likely to cause uterine bleeding are those that interfere with blood-clotting mechanism, such as purpura and leukemia.

DYSFUNCTIONAL UTERINE BLEEDING

The term *dysfunctional uterine bleeding* means hypermenorrhea and/or metrorrhagia caused by disturbances of the endocrine mechanism that controls normal menstruation. The term is virtually synonymous with anovulatory bleeding.

Incidence. Dysfunctional uterine bleeding may occur at any age between puberty and the menopause. It is encountered most frequently at the two extremes of menstrual life, when disturbances of ovarian function are most common. More than 50% of dysfunctional bleeding occurs in premenopausal women (aged 40 to 50 years); about 20% occurs in young girls during adolescence, and the remaining 30% is distributed among women in the reproductive period. Regularly menstruating women of childbearing age rarely develop dysfunctional uterine bleeding; however, it does occur in adult women who experience periods of oligomenorrhea and other menstrual irregularities.

Etiology. The underlying cause of dysfunctional uterine bleeding is still uncertain. This is not surprising, since we do not yet know the exact mechanism of normal menstrual bleeding. Most competent observers agree that, whatever the actual mechanism of dysfunctional bleeding may be, in most cases it is associated with failure of ovulation and a consequent hormonal imbalance.

Ovarian dysfunction may be caused by either a primary defect or pathologic lesion within the ovary itself, or it may be secondary to malfunction of other endocrine glands, notably the pituitary and thyroid. When the ovary is unresponsive, as is the case at the menarche or in the aging gland of the premenopausal women, follicles fail to rupture and become luteinized, despite adequate gonadotropic stimulation. If the ovaries are healthy and responsive, the failure to ovulate and luteinize may be a result of inadequate gonadotropin secretion. In either case the result is the same—absence of or faulty progesterone secretion. The follicle continues to secrete variable quantities of estrogen until the granulosa and theca cells surrounding its cavity are obliterated. This causes a drop in the estrogen level that results in irregular bleeding from the endometrium. Once such bleeding has begun, it may continue until sufficient estrogen is produced or administered to stimulate the endometrium to growth and regeneration.

Pathology of the endometrium. Dysfunctional bleeding is usually associated with a hyperplastic endometrium, but it may also occur from a normal proliferative, atrophic, or rarely a secretory structure. In the latter instance the bleeding is said to result from *irregular shedding*. This term relates to a prolonged shrinking, shedding, involution, and epithelization of the endometrium rather than the rapid disintegrative process during the normal cycle. The cause is probably the slow decrease in progesterone production with continuing irregular endometrial stimulation rather than the abrupt cessation of hormone secretion preceding normal menstruation. With the latter all endometrial stimulation ceases and disintegration occurs. Endometrial regeneration under the stimulus of estrogen alone limits normal menstruation to a few days. With irregular shedding the flow may continue for as long as 10 days before enough estrogen is produced to stimulate cell growth.

Hyperplastic endometrium may appear thickened and polypoid, or it may be rather normal in appearance. Microscopically the typical picture is that of benign cystic hyperplasia (Swiss cheese appearance) (Fig. 7-1). There is great disparity in the size and shape of the glands, the epithelium is cuboid or cylindric with deeply stained nuclei, and usually there is no evidence of secretion. The

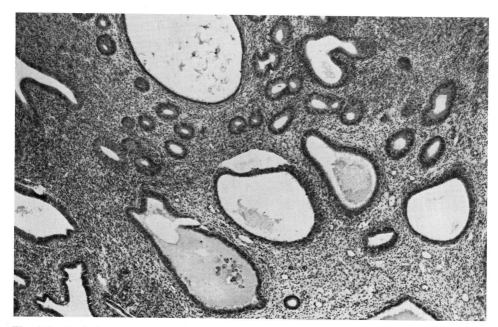

Fig. 7-1. Cystic hyperplasia. Note the nonsecretory character of the glands and great variation in their size, resembling the holes in Swiss cheese. (×60.)

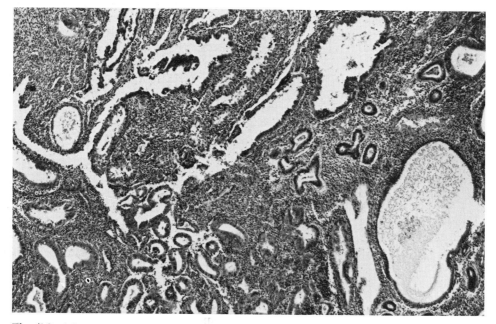

Fig. 7-2. Adenomatous hyperplasia. Glands are closely packed and back to back as a result of extraluminal budding. Intraluminal budding is also present. (×60.)

stroma is dense and hyperplastic. This is the usual picture; however, in a small percentage of patients a greatly proliferative, adenomatous pattern, closely resembling adenocarcinoma, is seen (Fig. 7-2).

Pathology of the ovary. Grossly, the ovary may show a single, large follicular cyst or a group of smaller follicles but no evidence of a corpus luteum. Microscopically, the absence of corpora lutea is confirmed. The follicles are lined by intact, functioning granulosa cells and contain follicular fluid rich in estrogen.

Symptoms. The flow in dysfunctional bleeding is usually painless because dysmenorrhea characteristcially occurs only during ovulatory cycles. The abnormality may be either hypermenorrhea or metrorrhagia. The bleeding may vary from minimal, persistent staining to severe hemorrhage. Occasionally periods of amenorrhea of 2 to 3 months precede the bleeding episode.

PSYCHOGENIC UTERINE BLEEDING

It has been known for many years that psychic trauma may result in profuse bleeding from the uterus. There have been many instances of prolonged, irregular bleeding with no evident cause, other than emotional factors, that were relieved by psychotherapy. The exact mechanism for the production of this type of bleeding is poorly understood. The following theories have been advanced to explain uterine bleeding on a psychogenic basis:

1. Emotional stimulation, either conscious or unconscious, can influence the hypothalamus and alter the secretion of gonadotropic hormones. Thus a primary, psychogenic mechanism could induce hormanal or *dysfunctional* bleeding.
2. The emotions also may exert a direct effect on the uterine blood vessels and thus cause bleeding. Markee has shown that fright will cause bleeding in endometrial transplants in the eye of the monkey.
3. The autonomic nervous system exerts control over the myometrium and may conceivably be a factor in some cases of functional uterine bleeding.

The diagnosis of uterine bleeding caused by psychogenic factors may be made only after the presence of an organic lesion or constitutional disease has been ruled out in a patient who is known to be suffering from an emotional disturbance brought on by a definite conflict in her life situation.

CRYPTOGENIC UTERINE BLEEDING

Despite the most exhaustive and careful studies, the physician encounters an occasional case of uterine bleeding whose cause escapes detection. Fortunately this is a rare occurrence.

■ Diagnosis of abnormal bleeding

Our aim in all instances of uterine bleeding is to determine the cause of the prolonged, excessive, or irregular flow.

DIAGNOSIS DURING ADOLESCENCE

In adolescent girls, abnormal bleeding is almost always caused by a disturbance of ovarian function. However, the possibility of an organic lesion, pregnancy, or even malignancy should be kept in mind if the symptom persists. A careful history and pelvic examination may suffice to rule out these conditions, but in cases of severe or prolonged bleeding, complete study including dilatation and curettage may be necessary to determine the cause of the hemorrhage.

History. A carefully taken history may indicate the presence of constitutional, nutritional, or psychogenic factors.

Physical examination. A complete examination should be made with special emphasis for evidence of cardiovascular disease, obesity, or endocrine stigmata. Vaginal or rectal examination should be performed to determine the presence of pelvic pathology. If the pelvic structures cannot be felt readily, examination under general anesthesia is indicated.

Laboratory studies. A complete blood count should be made to ascertain the degree of anemia and to determine the possibility of infection or leukemia. A platelet count should always be performed to rule out thrombocytopenia. Thyroid function should be evaluated by appropriate tests.

Dilatation and curettage. Dilatation and curettage is rarely necessary for the diagnosis of uterine bleeding in the adolescent, but it may be indicated in severe cases.

DIAGNOSIS IN THE CHILDBEARING PERIOD

In mature women, complications of pregnancy, pelvic infections, adenomyosis,

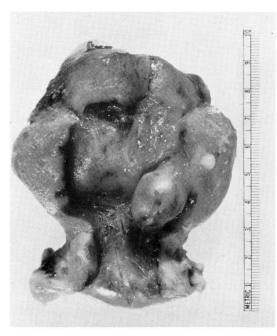

and uterine neoplasms are the most likely causes for irregular bleeding. These conditions, as well as constitutional factors, are to be carefully excluded before the diagnosis of *dysfunctional* bleeding is considered. *The diagnosis of dysfunctional bleeding should be made only after the elimination of all local and constitutional causes and in the presence of definite evidence of hormonal dysfunction, such as anovulatory cycles or endometrial hyperplasia.*

History. A carefully taken history is very helpful in making a differential diagnosis. Data relating to the age of onset, regularity, rhythmicity, and amount of flow during the first few years of menstruation are quite relevant. Is the bleeding intermenstrual staining? Is it a profuse flow at the time of the period? Or is the menstrual phase remarkably prolonged? Is it bright red or dark brown in color? Does it occur after coitus or the taking of a douche? Was the onset of the irregular bleeding preceded by a period of amenorrhea, a known pregnancy, or infection? Have there been similar

Fig. 7-3. Pedunculated submucous myoma. Uterus is normal size. Diagnosis is made by hysterogram (see Fig. 7-4).

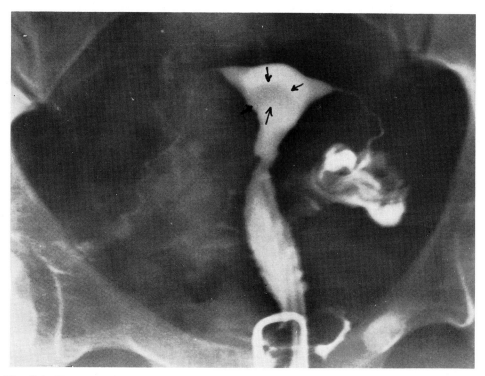

Fig. 7-4. Hysterogram showing submucous myoma. Uterine cavity is normal but has filling defect. Two previous curettages failed to disclose tumor.

episodes of bleeding in the past, and if so, how were they managed? Does the patient suffer from any known constitutional disease? Has there been any hormone therapy?

Physical examination. A complete general physical and pelvic examination should be performed.

Laboratory studies. Laboratory studies should include tests for endocrinologic evaluation, complete blood count including platelet count, and studies of thyroid function.

Hysterography. Hysterography is an often-neglected but valuable aid in the diagnosis of uterine bleeding. Endometrial polyps, submucous myomas, adenomyosis, carcinoma of the endometrium, and adnexal lesions may be visualized by this procedure.

Ovulation studies. The usual tests for evidence of ovulation should be carried out. Determination of pregnanediol in the urine may be helpful in estimating corpus luteum function, but microscopic examination of the endometrium is much more reliable.

Cervical biopsy with dilatation and curettage. Dilatation and curettage with cervical biopsy may provide important information concerning the cause of the abnormal bleeding. Whenever possible, curettage should be performed premenstrually, if the cycle is reasonably regular, to determine if ovulation has occurred.

DIAGNOSIS AT THE CLIMACTERIC

Dysfunctional bleeding occurs frequently in the premenopausal and menopausal age groups, but uterine neoplasms, both benign and malignant, also occur commonly and must be ruled out before a diagnosis of dysfunctional bleeding is made. In addition to the other studies, cytologic examination and cervical biopsy with a diagnostic curettage are mandatory.

DIAGNOSIS IN THE POSTMENOPAUSAL PERIOD

A malignant tumor somewhere in the genital tract must be considered first as a cause for bleeding after the menopause, no matter how small the amount. Benign lesions, notably atrophic vaginitis and cervical polyps, can cause postmenopausal bleeding, but they must not be accepted as the cause without complete investigation. Dilatation and curettage and cervical biopsy are essential in the study of postmenopausal bleeding.

An adnexal mass must be considered as potentially malignant until exploratory laparotomy is performed.

Although endometrial hyperplasia may result from the effect of small amounts of estrogen secreted either by an aging ovary or by the adrenal cortex, it often is produced by the administration of estrogens to relieve symptoms of the climacteric or to treat arthritides and osteoporosis. Prior to widespread use of estrogens for relief of menopausal symptoms, bleeding in menopausal women was most often caused by malignancy of the genital tract. Today prolonged administration of estrogen has assumed a major role as a cause for postmenopausal bleeding. This often creates a real dilemma. Is the bleeding caused by a pelvic neoplasm, or is it a manifestation of excessive estrogen therapy? Under these circumstances a careful search for an organic cause for the bleeding is mandatory.

■ Treatment of dysfunctional bleeding

The aims of treatment of dysfunctional bleeding should be to eliminate local or constitutional disease, to arrest hemorrhage, and to prevent recurrence of bleeding. In general, the type of therapy employed depends primarily on age of the patient and secondarily on severity of the bleeding.

The average amount of storage iron in young healthy women is only 250 mg., whereas in men it is 820 mg. The difference is a result of the iron deficit that occurs during pregnancies and because of iron loss during menstruation. A few episodes of excessive bleeding can deplete the iron stores entirely; unless iron is replaced, the hematocrit will fall progressively. For some reason abnormal bleeding may persist until anemia is corrected. Most women, even those whose menstrual flow is normal, should take iron regularly; it is particularly important in those who are bleeding abnormally.

TREATMENT OF ADOLESCENT GIRLS

Endocrine therapy. Since dysfunctional bleeding occurs because of irregular or abnormal hormonal stimulation of the endometrium, it can usually be controlled by endocrine therapy. Estrogen alone, progesterone alone, combinations of the two, and other steroid hormones have all been used with varying degrees of success. It is not possible to correct every case of dysfunctional bleeding, but the results should be better if one attempts to mimic the hormone pattern of the normal menstrual cycle.

Normal menstruation is preceded by a preovulatory period of endometrial proliferation resulting from the increasing concentration of estrogen. Estrogen production continues after ovulation, and the endometrial glands and stroma undergo secretory changes because of the effect of progesterone. If the ovum is not fertilized, the corpus luteum regresses and the stimulating effects of estrogen and progesterone on the endometrium are withdrawn. As a consequence, the secretory endometrial pattern regresses, arterioles are disrupted, and a menstrual period occurs.

As a general rule actively stimulated, growing endometrium does not bleed; bleeding only occurs when hormonal stimulation, principally that from estrogen administration, is withdrawn. The therapeutic programs for dysfunctional bleeding are based upon this principle.

Estrogens. Dysfunctional bleeding can usually be brought under control with the use of estrogen. Bleeding episodes occur with falling estrogen concentrations; exogenous estrogen, in adequate dosage, stimulates endometrial growth, and bleeding stops. This can sometimes be accomplished by the intravenous injection of 20 mg. of conjugated estrogen (Premarin), bleeding usually decreases after the first injection, but it may be necessary to repeat administration in 6 to 12 hours to stop the flow completely. Norethindrone (Norlutin), 5 mg., or norethindrone acetate (Norlutate), 2.5 mg., daily by mouth for 3 weeks will prevent recurrence by maintaining endometrial stimulation.

Estrogen alone is physiologically inadequate for the treatment of dysfunctional bleeding. The therapeutic aim is to establish a balanced estrogen-progesterone endometrial effect. Estrogen should be used alone, therefore, only for the initial control of profuse bleeding.

Dysfunctional bleeding of hemorrhagic proportions can usually be brought under control in 1 to 3 days by using Deluteval 2X, which is a mixture of hydroxyprogesterone

caproate, 250 mg., and estradiol valerate, 5 mg./ml. Two milliliters of this long acting progestational combination will induce a completely mature secretory endometrium with decidual reaction.

Progesterone. Progesterone, when given in the usual dosage, has little effect on endometrium that has not been stimulated with estrogen, and it has no hemostatic action. If 25 to 50 mg. of progesterone is given intramuscularly to a women with anovulatory dysfunctional bleeding, the endometrium will undergo a secretory change like that after ovulation in the normal menstrual cycle. Also, as during the normal cycle, the endometrium will slough, bleed, and be discharged as the progesterone concentration diminishes. This is known as a "medical curettage" because after this occurs, bleeding usually ceases while the endometrium proliferates once more under the stimulus of ovarian estrogen.

The periodic injection of progesterone in women with dysfunctional bleeding may produce regular cyclic flow. This can be accomplished with a single intramuscular injection of 25 to 50 mg. of progesterone in oil or a long-acting preparation, such as hydroxyprogesterone caproate (Delalutin), 250 mg. The latter preparation is somewhat less satisfactory than regular progesterone. It is metabolized and excreted slowly, hence the endometrial effect diminishes slowly and bleeding may be delayed and prolonged when compared to that after the rapid withdrawal of regular progesterone.

Estrogen and progesterone. The usual "cyclic therapy" for women with dysfunctional bleeding consists of the administration of estrogen alone for 2 weeks and then estrogen and progesterone for another week. This produces first a proliferation and then a secretory change in the endometrium, followed by bleeding a few days after hormone therapy is discontinued. Presumably the sequence of estrogen followed by estrogen and progesterone encourages the anterior pituitary to function as it does during the normal cycle. Since both the preparations and the dosages differ from the normal ovarian hormones, the pituitary effect may not be important. On about the fifth day after the first day of bleeding the medications are restarted.

Although this regimen has been reasonably successful, it is time consuming, expensive, and generally unnecessary. This program has to a great extent been replaced by the use of oral contraceptive agents, which contain estrogen as mestranol or ethinyl estradiol in combination with a variety of progestogens (depending on the commercial preparation used). These compounds have a progestogen-estrogen ratio that varies from 20:1 to 200:1, again, contingent upon the brand. Anterior pituitary function is inhibited by these drugs, hence the ovaries are quiescent; the endometrial changes result from direct stimulation by the medication. One tablet is taken daily for 21 days, and withdrawal bleeding occurs within a few days. The 21-day treatment cycle is resumed on the fifth day after bleeding begins.

The mechanism by which these drugs control bleeding probably is different from that with the usual estrogen-progesterone sequence. Women who are using oral contraceptive agents usually experience a considerable reduction in menstrual flow; some do not bleed at all. This probably occurs because these preparations do not produce a normal secretory response in the endometrium. Rather, the stroma is thin and dense and the glands are small and relatively sparse.

Cyclic therapy, whatever the type, is continued for about 6 months, after which it is stopped. Many women will have a normal menstrual cycle without medication, but in others the abnormal bleeding pattern recurs promptly. In the latter condition the treatment can be resumed and continued as long as necessary.

Androgens. Uterine dysfunctional bleeding can usually be checked by using aqueous testosterone, 100 mg., intramuscularly. Occasionally in the most severe cases a second dose the following day will be necessary. Testosterone must be considered an emergency hormone and should not be used otherwise.

Thyroid substance. When there are symptoms, signs, or laboratory evidence of hypothyroidism, adequate doses of thyroid extract are very effective in the prevention of recurrent dysfunctional bleeding.

Dilatation and curettage. Dilatation and curettage is rarely necessary to control adolescent bleeding. It should only be resorted to in cases of acute, exsanguinating hemorrhage or when hemostasis cannot be achieved by medical treatment. After curettage a 6-month regimen of cyclic estrogen-progesterone or progesterone therapy should be instituted.

Psychotherapy. Superficial psychotherapy in the form of education in sexual behavior, reorientation in domestic and social activities, and a sympathetic and understanding hearing of the patient's complaints may be very helpful. Refractory cases of abnormal uterine bleeding in which deep emotional problems seem to be a factor should be referred to a psychiatrist.

TREATMENT DURING THE CHILDBEARING PERIOD

Dilatation and curettage is the primary therapeutic and diagnostic measure in the childbearing age group. This procedure not only provides a diagnosis and often a cure but also affords the opportunity to carry out a careful pelvic examination under anesthesia. Patients with menorrhagia or hypermenorrhea should be curetted a few days before the onset of a period to determine whether they are ovulating. When the bleeding is irregular or profuse, curettage may be performed at any time, disregarding the cycle. A narrow ring forceps should be inserted into the uterine cavity and an attempt made to snare a polyp that may have been missed by the curet.

Endocrine therapy. Hormone therapy, as outlined earlier, may be instituted after the dilatation and curettage.

Hysterectomy. It is seldom necessary to remove the uterus because of dysfunctional bleeding, but hysterectomy may be indicated if bleeding cannot be controlled with hormone therapy. Operation should also be considered as an alternative to long-term medical treatment for women who must take hormones continually to prevent recurrence of profuse bleeding.

Radiation. Radiation has no place in the therapy of benign uterine bleeding of women in the childbearing period.

TREATMENT AT THE CLIMACTERIC

The management of women at the climacteric is similar to that in the childbearing period except that hysterectomy is more readily employed. Endocrine therapy should not be started until malignancy has been eliminated as a cause. If bleeding is not controlled or if it should subsequently recur, hysterectomy should be resorted to.

Radiation. For many years radiation of the pelvis, either by roentgen ray or by intra-uterine radium, was considered an acceptable method of treatment for benign uterine bleeding in premenopausal and menopausal women. This was a simple and effective method, involving less risk, less hospitalization, and a shorter convalescence than hysterectomy. The use of radiation in the treatment of benign disease has fallen into disfavor. Peter Alexander points out that, "high doses [of radiation] given only to small areas of the body will produce tumors at the site of radiation usually after long periods." Carcinoma of the endometrium does occur more often in women who have been given radiation treatment to control abnormal bleeding during the climacteric and preclimateric periods of life. It is unclear whether the malignancy is induced by the treatment or represents a continuing change in unrecognized uterine pathology.

TREATMENT IN THE POSTMENOPAUSAL PERIOD

The management of irregular bleeding in the postmenopausal age group consists mainly in eliminating and treating organic pathology of the uterus and ovaries. Hormone therapy is not to be considered in the treatment of bleeding in postmenopausal women.

References

Alexander, P.: Atomic radiation and life, London, 1957, The Whitefriars Press, Ltd.

Board, J. A., and Borland, D. S.: Endometrial effects of mestranol-norethindrone sequential therapy for oral contraception, Obstet. Gynec. **24**:655, 1964.

Davids, A. M.: X-ray diagnosis of uterine pathology, Amer. J. Obstet. Gynec. **65**:1167, 1953.

Fluhmann, C. F.: The management of menstrual disorders, Philadelphia, 1956, W. B. Saunders Co.

Geist, S. H., and Matus, M.: Postmenopausal bleeding, Amer. J. Obstet. Gynec. **25**:388, 1933.

Holmstrom, E. G.: Functional uterine bleeding, J.A.M.A. **156**:580, 1954.

Holmstrom, E. G.: Progesterone treatment of anovulatory bleeding, Amer. J. Obstet. Gynec. **68**: 1321, 1954.

Israel, S. L.: Diagnosis and treatment of menstrual disorders and sterility, ed. 5, New York, 1967, Harper & Row, Publishers.

Jones, G. E. S., and TeLinde, R. W.: An evaluation of progesterone therapy in treatment of endometrial hyperplasia, Bull. Hopkins Hosp. **71**:282, 1942.

Karnaky, K. J.: Dysfunctional bleeding, J. Clin. Endocr. **3**:648, 1943.

Kroger, W. S., and Freed, S. C.: Psychosomatic gynecology, Philadelphia, 1951, W. B. Saunders Co.

McKelvey, J. L.: Irregular shedding of the endometrium, Amer. J. Obstet. Gynec. **60**:523, 1950.

Morris, J. M., and Scully, R. E.: Endocrine pathology of the ovary, St. Louis, 1958, The C. V. Mosby Co.

Paloucek, F. P., Randall, C. L., Graham, J. B., and Graham, S.: Cancer and its relation to abnormal vaginal bleeding and radiation, Obstet. Gynec. **21**:530, 1963.

Pritchard, J. A., and Mason, R. A.: Iron stores of normal adults and replenishment with oral iron therapy, J.A.M.A. **190**:119, 1964.

Riley, G. M.: Gynecologic endocrinology, New York, 1964, Harper & Row, Publishers.

block

8

Sexual responses of women, dysmenorrhea, and premenstrual tension

The physically mature woman may respond to sexual feelings in varying degrees. There is a normal spectrum of response; however, outside of this range symptoms may be produced.

■ Normal sexual response

A complete sexual response of a woman results in an orgasm, which physically is the fine involuntary contractions of the vagina and pelvic muscles. This orgastic response is dependent upon three closely integrated systems—the endocrinologic, the psychic, and the somatesthetic. The woman's satisfaction with intercourse is not as dependent on the climax as with the male. With inhibition of orgasm there is a tendency for the development of depressions, chronic fatigue, head-aches, pruritus vulvae, and other somatic symptoms such as chronic congestion.

Psychologically, the orgasm represents the woman's ability to relate well to the man and to accept her own feminine role in life.

ENDOCRINOLOGIC ROLE

There is evidence in the literature that in all mammals there are subcortical centers responsible for sexual activity. These areas are located in the hypothalamus and upper midbrain. In the lower order of mammals these areas are primarily activated by the gonadal hormones. This is why the female dog will accept the male when she is in so-called *heat*. In the human the higher cortical centers inhibit this hormonal influence so that the sexual response in the woman is independent of the ability to conceive.

Estrogen does exert a minimal effect upon the sexual desire of women, and its influence on the vaginal mucosa is important. Progesterone has a tranquilizing effect. The sexually unresponsive female is not affected by either massive doses of estrogen or progesterone. The libido of a responsive female may be increased with the administration of testosterone. This is probably brought about by an increase in the end organ (clitoris) sensitivity and without direct influence on the psyche. Hormonal therapy will not alleviate frigidity or dyspareunia except that caused by atrophic vaginitis.

PSYCHOLOGIC ROLE

The psychologic factors that are the essential preamble to the physiologic response of a climax in the woman are dependent upon her acceptance of the feminine role in herself. This role is determined by a complex interrelationship of social, cultural, familial, developmental, physiologic, and interpersonal factors. In the normal sexual act the woman must allow herself to be conquered by the male. This entails a masochistic surrender to the man. The desire to be conquered must be balanced by the need to be loved by a valuable person in order to evoke a normal response.

SOMATESTHETIC ROLE

When emotionally stimulated, a woman's whole body responds to a greater degree than does that of a male. These responses

87

are passive in nature. Her libido is stimulated by being looked at, by words of love, and particularly by touch. Specific areas of response are the skin, lips, mouth, breasts, abdomen, thighs, and genital region. As a result of the psychic physical sexual stimulation, the response of the pelvis is dilatation of the vascular tree with pelvic congestion. This results in the production of vaginal lubrication by the "sweating" of the engorged blood vessels around the vagina.

The gross anatomic reactions of the female have been divided into the following four phases by Masters: (1) excitement, (2) plateau, (3) orgasm, and (4) resolution. The skin, breast, clitoris, vagina, and uterus change during these phases.

There is no difference in the anatomic response of the pelvis in an orgasm, whether it be stimulated by manipulation of the breasts, clitoris, vagina, or even fantasy. The normal woman's sexual response is the sum total of psychic and physical stimulation that reaches a climax in an automatic reflex arc that produces multiple somatic responses. The more mature woman, with a wish to give and take, has a greater ability to achieve orgasm.

CHANGING ATTITUDES OF THE FEMALE

The twentieth century has brought a new attitude concerning sexuality in women. The artificial division of the behavior of women into the good woman (mother, asexual) and the bad woman (mistress, sexual partner) is being discarded. The emancipation of women has been both social and sexual. Most young women today seek sexual gratification before as well as after marriage.

This frequently begins in adolescence. These changes in female behavior have been aided by the advent of more effective contraceptive measures, freeing women of the responsibility of pregnancy and thus separating the pleasure of sexual response from the responsibility of the family structure.

CHANGING ATTITUDES TOWARD SEX

We are in a period of changing attitudes and practices in regard to sex. The woman's role has altered most dramatically. The concepts of modesty, chastity, and sexual inhibition have been under attack. The new ideal places the woman's position closer to that of the male. She is now allowed to show interest and desire. Virginity in some circles is considered a fault instead of a virtue. One factor causing this change is the development of safe, reliable contraceptives, which removes one of the main motivations for chastity: the fear of pregnancy.

The physician may be thrown into the middle of this conflict in values. The young girl seeking contraception and advice may also desire help with her internal conflicts or those with her parents. The main question is what reason is there for the young girl not to be sexually active. The pleasure in sex is obvious. The main practical danger can be removed. Why not indulge? The answer the physician can give beyond the moral religious ideal, is that sex can be more than a physical act. It is a reflection of and an enhancing factor to a deep commitment between two people. The physician can thus help the woman discover how she wishes to relate to men in a more meaningful manner.

Table 5. Anatomic sexual responses of the female

Phases	Skin	Breasts	Clitoris	Vagina
Excitement	Increased sensitivity	Nipple erection	Vasocongestion; tumescence	Expansion of inner two thirds
Plateau	Maculopapular flush	Increased breast size	Gland retraction	Vasocongestion in outer one third of vagina
Orgasm	No change	No change	No specific change	Involuntary contractions
Resolution	Perspiration	Loss of nipple erection	Loss of congestion and retraction	Loss of vasocongestion

■ Sexual problems of the female

The sexual symptoms that are the presenting complaints of women are dyspareunia and frigidity. It should be emphasized that these are symptoms of underlying conflicts and not a disease to be treated in themselves. Since most patients find sexual problems difficult to discuss, the physician should realize that no matter how the subject is presented, it is very important to the patient.

DYSPAREUNIA

Dyspareunia is the term that designates painful intercourse. This symptom may indicate local organic disease in the pelvis, or it may be secondary to psychologic conflicts.

Local causes. Any condition that obstructs the entrance of the vagina or narrows the vaginal tube may interfere with intercourse. This obstruction may be congenital or may be the result of faulty repair of an episiotomy. Inflammatory lesions of the lower genital tract may render the tissue so sensitive that coitus becomes either very painful or impossible. Less often, pelvic lesions such as salpingo-oophoritis, endometriosis, prolapsed ovaries, and retroversion of the uterus may be responsible for dyspareunia.

One of the most common causes of organic dyspareunia is a rigid hymen that interferes with intromission. Each coital attempt is thwarted by the narrow orifice and by the pain that the young woman experiences as a result of this. Usually the couple will seek medical advice early in their marital career, but it is not rare for women to allow this situation to continue for long periods of time.

We have encountered several instances of rigid, intact hymens in women who consulted us because of infertility of several years' duration and in a few women who presented themselves for prenatal care. None of these patients complained of dyspareunia. Actually they never really had normal intercourse. After the first few unsuccessful attempts to penetrate the obstructing membrane their husbands became discouraged and contented themselves with ejaculation outside the vagina.

These patients do present a local anatomic difficulty, but in most instances there is a psychologic mechanism operating as well. The pain experienced in the early attempts at intercourse is tolerated without much concern by the average, mature young woman. The fearful, anxious girl may react by tensing the muscles that surround the introitus of the vagina—a condition known as *vaginismus*. This spasmodic reaction almost completely closes the entrance of the vagina and thus makes intercourse virtually impossible. When examining such a woman, the physician usually will find tightening of the thigh muscles as well as spasm of the levator ani muscles.

The psychologic mechanism that is usually responsible for vaginismus is an inordinate fear of injury to the genitals, which may have been conditioned by experiences in childhood. Many guilt feelings about being sexual find expression in a tendency to overemphasize the pain.

Treatment. The dyspareunia caused by local inflammatory lesions, painful scars, or pelvic pathology is usually amenable to either medical or surgical correction. When the cause of difficulty is a thick, rigid hymen, gentle but forceful dilatation repeated at regular intervals by either the physician or the patient is preferable to the often-recommended incision or divulsion of the hymen under anesthesia. In the dilatation the patient does experience some discomfort and pain, but this is usually a valuable part of therapy. It demonstrates to the patient that she is quite capable of withstanding the discomfort produced by the insertion of a well-lubricated speculum or dilator, and therefore, the vagina should be able to admit her husband's penis, which is usually much smaller, without undue pain. It is important that the physician doing the dilatation be aware that this treatment will represent a defeat for the husband and that the wife may interpret it as symbolic of her husband's lack of masculinity.

Discussion with the husband regarding the technique of the sexual act should take place during the period of instrumental vaginal dilatation. Suggestions relating to the primary sex play and the use of lubricating jelly may be most helpful. A need for a gentle but firm approach on the part of the husband should be stressed. Communication between the couple is the key in solving many of these problems. There is usually a breakdown in this area because the mutual frustration has led to unexpressed anger. The couple may also have guilt about discussing sex or even desiring to enjoy it. They may be helped by reading and discussing together books relating to the subject.*

Ordinarily these measures will succeed in correcting the sexual difficulty, mostly because the accepting attitude of the physician relieves guilt and fears. In the more refractory patients intensive psychotherapy is definitely indicated. This therapy is directed toward helping the patient uncover unconscious fears and/or hostility relating to men.

FRIGIDITY

The woman who is unable to respond sexually with an orgasm is classified as being frigid. This symptom may be temporary or of long duration. It may be present in a minimal degree or severe in character. Many classifications have been proposed, but from a clinical standpoint Weiss and English's classification seems most appropriate: (1) occasional failure to obtain orgasm, (2) only occasional orgasm, (3) mild pleasure in intercourse but no orgasm, (4) vaginal anesthesia with no special aversion to coitus, (5) vaginal anesthesia with aversion to coitus, and (6) dyspareunia and vaginismus with marked aversion to coitus. Many apparently normal women fall into the second and third categories. They experience some degree of pleasure during the act but achieve orgasm only on occasion. Very few of these women ever complain or seek medical help for their sexual inadequacy. Most often they consult the physician for a somatic symptom such as pelvic pain or vaginal discharge and will disclose their coital problem only if questioned directly about their sex life. Women in the last three categories less often develop pelvic symptoms, but they may seek medical help because of their complaint. When these women become ill, it is usually a severe neurosis or psychosis that the physician will have to treat. Women in the first category will require only reassurance and support, and no extensive therapy is indicated.

Another method of examination of frigidity is in what area pleasure is blocked. This can be determined by the following

questions. Is there vaginal sensation or pleasure? Is there masturbation and/or only pleasure in clitoral stimulation? Does the patient primarily get pleasure in being held or touched? Is loving or giving pleasure the main goal? Is there sexual fantasy and pleasure in it?

Etiologic factors. The etiology of sexual frigidity may be somatic, environmental, coital, or psychogenic.

Somatic factors. Patients who experience pain at intercourse because of some genital lesion or abnormality can hardly be expected to look forward to the act with pleasurable anticipation. The obvious solution is to correct the lesion, whether it be an abnormal hymen, vaginitis, or a severely retroverted uterus.

Environmental factors. It is common knowledge that problems of everyday living may adversely affect the libido. A woman who is overworked, plagued by overdue household bills, or suffers from poor health is relatively uninterested in sex. An improvement in these factors often corrects this type of frigidity. A common, unhappy environmental situation is fear on the part of the couple of being overheard in the act of coitus. Young couples living with parents often are inhibited in their lovemaking by this circumstance; a similar situation is the presence of children in the parents' bedroom. The increase in desire for sex on vacations is because of an ability to put these influences aside. The daily fluctuation of love and anger between the couple is very influential.

Coital factors. Many women who have perfectly normal sexual desires and inclinations remain relatively frigid because of inadequate coital technique on the part of the husband. His failure to recognize his wife's needs for preliminary caresses and sex play accompanied by endearing expressions of love frequently accounts for her lack of interest or her actual distaste for coitus. It is hardly likely that a woman will enjoy the sexual act when it is performed under such circumstances. Women are, by nature, romantic, and as one patient expressed it, "We want to be made love to, not had intercourse with." Obviously serious sexual difficulties in the male such as impotence or premature ejaculation will be associated with apparent frigidity in the spouse. It is

---

*For example, Davis, M.: The sexual responsibility of women, New York, 1956, The Dial Press, Inc.

important to realize that a woman must take the pleasure in coitus—no mate can make her respond.

Psychogenic factors (conscious and unconscious). Conscious thoughts, feelings, and attitudes play a major role in some cases of frigidity. These interfere with the necessary excitement of anticipation that heightens a woman's sexual desire. A woman who resents her husband's preoccupation with his work or his recreational activities and interprets them as a seeming indifference to her may retaliate by sexual coolness. Some women will consciously remain passive during coitus because of a mistaken notion that conception is more likely to result if they actively participate and derive pleasure from the act. Others consider it unladylike to seem to enjoy intercourse.

Most women who are unable to enjoy intercourse and certainly those who have an aversion for it harbor some unconscious childhood sexual fantasy that they have inappropriately carried into adulthood. It may be the fear of injury, feelings of guilt, a continued attachment to the father, a disappointing relationship with a significant male figure, and/or hostility toward men. The woman may wish to express her hostility by defeating the man in his attempts to please her. She may be so afraid to lose control that she cannot contemplate the strong emotions felt during orgasm. Many women equate orgasm with loss of bowel control. Some women have a very maternal attitude toward men and approach intercourse with the idea of satisfying and pleasing the man. These women may never have an orgasm, but they will rarely complain. Extremely narcissistic people have difficulty experiencing an orgasm because they cannot identify with the pleasure of their partner.

Prophylaxis. A great deal may be accomplished by the enlightened physician in the prevention of this all too common disability, but the first and most important prerequisite for sexual adequacy in the adult female is a childhood atmosphere characterized by affection, understanding, and a sane and sensible attitude on the part of the parents toward the little girl's sexual curiosity and activity. Intimidation or punishment for childhood sexual activity such as masturbation and exposure of the genitals does much more harm than the acts themselves.

Adequate education at puberty that enlightens the girl in matters of menstruation, sexuality, and pregnancy without engendering fear of injury or disease is of considerable value. The calm accepting manner of the presenter is more important than the educational material. Unembarrassed explanations and preparation for the menarche should be made by the girl's mother. Careful premarital examination and a frank discussion between the couple and the physician regarding the techniques of coitus and family planning are most helpful in clearing up misunderstandings and in preventing sexual disharmony.

Treatment. Treatment of frigidity may range from rather simple to most difficult types of therapy, depending on the cause and the degree of the pathology. The first step is the taking of a history of the patient's sexual experiences. Once the physician has displayed a sincere interest in the woman's problem and has gained her confidence, he may obtain information concerning childhood experiences, parental attitudes toward her and her siblings, as well as an estimate of her husband as a satisfactory mate. As the physician listens to the patient's history, he should keep in mind that the problems in the patient's personality and interpersonal relations are reflected in the couple's sexual adjustment. If the sexual problem seems to result from some environmental, somatic, or coital factor, it is usually amenable to physical treatment and superficial psychotherapy in the form of reeducation, reorientation, and manipulation of the environment. Frank discussion with the husband separately and with the couple together often can help him to recognize his wife's needs and thus pave the way for a more satisfactory sexual adjustment through increased communication. On the other hand, prudishness on the part of the wife, as evidenced by aversion to so-called abnormal positions during intercourse or to certain types of sex play, may be overcome by the physician's tactful suggestion that there is nothing wrong in this type of experimentation if it culminates in normal coitus and mutual satisfaction.

Patients whose sexual problems seem to result from a deep-seated emotional conflict will require intensive psychotherapy, and they should be referred to a psychiatrist. It should be remembered in the management of these patients that the physician, whether he be the family physician, gynecologist, or psychiatrist, will usually be looked upon by the patient as a parental figure. The therapist's own feelings concerning sexuality then become an important part in the treating of such patients and in helping them to overcome this problem. The successful physician working in the area of frigidity will be a person the woman can trust with her feelings and one who will encourage her to mature sexually. In other words, he plays the role of a good father or mother.

Failure in the treatment of frigidity is usually caused by too much coldness on the part of the physician or too deep a degree of pathology in the woman, resulting in the patient's inability to give up her fears.

Drug therapy. Many drugs have been advocated in the treatment of frigidity, including the administration of alcoholic beverages at bedtime. These may at times achieve the desired effect, but at best such therapy is of only temporary benefit and may actually delay a more rational approach to the problem. At the present time there is no drug that has been proved to be an effective aphrodisiac.

■ Dysmenorrhea

Dysmenorrhea literally means painful menstruation; however, since most women experience some degree of discomfort or cramping during menstruation, clinically we reserve the term for those cases in which the pain is severe enough to limit the woman's normal activity or to require medical treatment for its relief. There are four clinical forms of dysmenorrhea: (1) pains similar to those of labor with discharge of blood clots, (2) pain occurring before the onset of menstruation caused by hyperemia and distention and subsiding after the flow has begun, (3) membranous dysmenorrhea, and (4) menstrual colic. The latter is the most frequent form of dysmenorrhea.

The symptom may result from a variety of causes, and depending on the mechanism responsible, it is said to be either *primary* or *secondary*. *Primary dysmenorrhea* is painful menstruation for which no pelvic pathology can be demonstrated. *Secondary dysmenorrhea* is caused by a definite pelvic lesion such as endometriosis, adenomyosis, or chronic pelvic inflammation. Whatever the cause of the dysmenorrhea, it has great significance for the woman because menstruation symbolizes her role in life and is the clock by which most of her life pattern can be established.

INCIDENCE

Several statistical studies to determine the frequency of dysmenorrhea among high school and college students, industrial workers, and other large groups of young women have not resulted in consistent estimates. The variations range from an incidence of as low as 3% to a high figure of 80%. The most acceptable study is one conducted among 1,606 healthy high school students; about 10% of these girls complained of pain severe enough to keep them home from school or to require absence from several classes during the school hours.

ETIOLOGY OF PRIMARY DYSMENORRHEA

The exact cause of primary dysmenorrhea is not known. Consequently there are numerous theories that attempt to account for the painful period. Normal uterine contractions in a nonpregnant woman are usually not painful. If for any reason the contractions are stronger than normal or if the woman's pain threshold is somewhat lowered, the increase in myometrial tone is perceived as a painful sensation by the sensorium. Factors that may predispose to forceful uterine contractions are obstructive, developmental, hormonal, allergic, and psychogenic.

Obstructive factor (acute anteflexion). Acute anteflexion, perhaps one of the oldest theories, was a commonly accepted concept of the mechanism of dysmenorrhea. Normally the adult uterus is in the position of slight anteflexion. If the angle between the corpus and the cervix becomes acute, it seems logical that this might impede the progress of menstrual blood and debris in their passage through the internal os and thus stimulate the myometrium to spasmodic contractions. Despite the reasonableness of this theory, clinical experience has shown that it applies to only a few patients with severe primary dysmenorrhea.

Retroversion, in a similar manner, may occasionally produce painful menstruation, but surgical innovation should not be performed unless the symptoms are relieved by pessary, which corrects the anatomic defect.

Developmental factors (hypoplasia of the uterus). Underdevelopment of the uterus at the time of puberty results in an abnormally small corpus with a relatively elongated cervix. Acute anteflexion is frequently associated with this abnormality. Theoretically the hypoplastic uterus, because of the paucity of muscle fibers and disproportionate amount of fibrous connective tissue, is incapable of normal, rhythmic contractions. Instead, its response to the stimulus of the menstrual flow is irregular, spasmodic, and painful. This is a rare cause of dysmenorrhea.

Hormonal factors. An "imbalance" in the normal estrogen-progesterone relationship during the luteal phase of the cycle has been advanced as a possible etiologic factor in the production of dysmenorrhea. The nature of the hormonal disharmony has not been clearly defined. As a matter of fact, one theory attributes dysmenorrhea to a deficiency of estrogen, as in instances of hypoplasia uteri, and another states that a relative excess of estrogen and lack of progesterone sensitizes the myometrium to overactivity. *Clinical experience has shown that anovulatory cycles, in which progesterone effect is absent, usually terminate with a painless flow, whereas dysmenorrhea is almost always associated with ovulation.*

Allergic factors. It is possible that in certain women allergens may so sensitize the myometrium as to produce spasm and uterine colic. The irritant may be certain foods, inhalants, or as has been suggested by some observers, the so-called menstrual toxin. There is some evidence that progesterone therapy can be helpful in relieving dysmenorrhea due to allergic factors.

Psychogenic factors. Fluhmann has very aptly stated that "whatever may be the cause of painful uterine contractions, a strong psychosomatic influence plays an important role in dysmenorrhea. There is usually a marked hypersensitivity to pain and, in many cases, there are evidences of personality disorders." The young girl who suffers from dysmenorrhea usually has some degree of emotional difficulty in the home, at school, or in her interpersonal relationships. She is very often shy and anxious. The adult woman who presents this symptom very often is resentful of the feminine role. Each succeeding period reminds her of the unpleasant fact that she is a woman, and this realization is painful. Her resentment may result from conflicts with her mother, since she represented femininity in her early life. These mothers have difficulty in preparing their daughters for sexuality and menstruation. To the average, healthy, well-balanced girl the "curse," the monthly "sickness," or the more euphemistic(?) "falling off the roof" are merely colloquial synonyms for menstruation, but to the neurotic, fearful, and often constitutionally inadequate youngster these terms suggest a threat of injury or illness to which she reacts accordingly. To summarize, it can be stated fairly that in the light of our present knowledge primary dysmenorrhea may be caused by a variety of developmental, hormonal, or constitutional factors in an individual who has been psychologically conditioned to this disorder.

PATHOLOGY

Most young women suffering from primary dysmenorrhea have perfectly normal pelvic viscera. The endometrium and ovaries usually display evidence of normal ovulatory, cyclic activity. In some cases of severe dysmenorrhea the presacral nerves have been found to be the seat of inflammatory or degenerative changes. This finding has not been consistently reported.

SYMPTOMS

There is usually a history of painful periods soon after the menses are well established. Periods during the first few months, or even years, after the menarche are often relatively painless, probably because of the predominance of anovulatory cycles. The pain is usually sharp, colicky, and centered over the lower abdomen, at times radiating to the back and thighs. Nausea, vomiting, headache, and nervous irritability often accompany the abdominal cramps and may be more distressing than the pain. Symptoms usually begin before the onset of the flow and persist for 12 to 24 hours, sometimes longer.

DIFFERENTIAL DIAGNOSIS

The first problem is to eliminate a local organic lesion as a possible cause of the painful period. This often may be accomplished by a careful history and thorough physical examination, but in rare instances hysterosalpingography and culdoscopy may be required to eliminate the possibility of endometrial polyps, cervical stenosis, myomas, endometriosis, or chronic salpingo-oophoritis as cause of the pain. Once these possible organic factors have been ruled out and the diagnosis of primary dysmenorrhea has been established, the aim is to ascertain the etiologic factor or factors responsible for the pain. This is usually a difficult task. It often involves a painstaking investigation of the patient's early childhood experiences, her present mode of living, and her attitudes toward menstruation, sexuality, and childbearing. It is important to ascertain how crippling the symptom is and how much emotional gain the patient is deriving from it. For example, does the whole household revolve around whether or not the mother is having menstrual cramps? Is the dysmenorrhea the locus for the expression of depression, anger, or a need to be dependent?

TREATMENT

The objective in the management of this condition is to remove the cause and thus prevent recurrence of the pain at succeeding periods. This ideal is seldom attained. Much, however, can be accomplished toward ameliorating the pain at the time of the period by constitutional therapy, hormone therapy, psychotherapy, drug therapy, or surgical treatment.

Constitutional therapy. An essential part of the treatment of dysmenorrhea is the elimination of systemic disease. Strict attention to matters of personal hygiene, exercise, adequate diet, and rest is of primary importance. Special exercising methods have been devised for the treatment of dysmenorrhea and have proved helpful in many cases.

Hormone therapy. The inhibition of ovulation by the administration of oral contraceptives will usually result in a painless menstrual period. Unfortunately this treatment has to be repeated during each succeeding cycle. The patient should be treated through the course of four cycles, after which the medication should be discontinued to observe the results.

Occasionally it is deemed advisable to postpone a menstrual flow because of an important school examination or social or athletic event that might coincide with the expected period. This can usually be accomplished by continuing administration of the oral contraceptive for a longer period of time.

Psychotherapy. The primary principle involved in the psychotherapy of the patient with dysmenorrhea is the sincere and sympathetic interest that the physician displays toward her as an individual, rather than as an interesting case. Unhurried discussion of the girl's everyday problems, particularly as they relate to her parents, teachers, siblings, and close relatives and friends, will encourage her to express her more intimate thoughts and feelings. Once the physician has gained the young woman's confidence and has become aware of her personal difficulties, a great deal can be accomplished by intelligent guidance of the patient and appropriate manipulation of her environment. In addition, affording relief of pain by appropriate hormone or drug therapy is in itself a psychotherapeutic agent and is often the first step in this method of treatment. As in all psychosomatic illnesses, the problem is not solely psychologic or somatic but, as the name implies, a combination of the two. Therapy therefore should be directed toward the patient's emotional problems as well as toward amelioration of her symptoms. The physician should be sympathetic yet firm. He must not minimize or ridicule the girl's symptoms; neither should he be too sympathetic and pamper the patient. Symptomatic relief should be afforded, but the young woman should be discouraged from going to bed and from avoiding social and school activities during her menses.

Kroger and Freed have reported remarkable cures in refractory cases of dysmenorrhea by means of hypnotherapy and hypnoanalysis. These are very specialized techniques and should be employed only by a therapist who has had adequate training in these methods.

Drug therapy. In almost every patient the symptoms of dysmenorrhea can be controlled by medication administered during the painful period.

Treatment of the symptoms. Many drugs have been recommended for the treatment of dysmenorrhea. Most women obtain adequate relief from a mild analgesic aspirin, whereas some require additional sedation or antispasmodic drugs. In severe cases ethoheptazine citrate plus aspirin (Zactirin) gives sufficient relief. Codeine is rarely if ever needed for dysmenorrhea, and its use should be discouraged along with alcohol, Demerol, and morphine. The danger of addiction is too real to be disregarded, and furthermore, patients whose pain requires such potent drugs are probably in need of deep psychotherapy or a surgical procedure to cure their dysmenorrhea.

Surgical treatment. If after adequate trial medical measures prove ineffective, surgery is the next consideration.

Presacral and ovarian neurectomy. The hypogastric plexus, which lies directly below the bifurcation of the aorta in a triangle formed by the common iliac vessels laterally and the sacral promontory inferiorly, contains sympathetic preganglionic nerve fibers along with afferent and somatic nerves. The simplest way to ensure removal of all the pertinent nerve tissue plus ganglia is to remove the retroperitoneal tissue over the sacral promontory down to the periosteum and lateral to the ureters and common iliac veins. In this fashion the uterus is deprived of all autonomic stimulation except that from the parasympathetic postganglionic fibers from S_2, S_3, and S_4. For obvious anatomic reasons these must not be sectioned. Although neurectomy is rarely necessary to relieve dysmenorrhea, it is highly successful if meticulous dissection is carried out.

Prognosis and summary. Most patients complaining of moderate menstrual pain will be relieved by careful attention to physical and mental hygiene and the administration of mild analgesic drugs.

Superficial psychotherapy in the form of reassurance, sex education, and a sympathetic interest, combined with hormone and drug therapy, should relieve most patients with moderately severe dysmenorrhea.

The pain from severe dysmenorrhea frequently may be controlled by the use of the newer progesterone agents. Rarely will surgery ever be necessary, although presacral neurectomy will give relief in the most intractable cases of dysmenorrhea.

Although marriage and pregnancy often exert a favorable hormonal and psycho-therapeutic effect, it is generally unwise to recommend these momentous ventures simply to cure a woman's menstrual cramps. Such a remedy may only serve to provide new and more serious emotional problems to an already overburdened personality.

■ Premenstrual tension

Female patients and their physicians have been aware for many years that menstruation is often ushered in by mildly disturbing systemic symptoms. In 1931 Frank described this syndrome and named it *premenstrual tension.* The chief characteristic of this symptom complex is its regular occurrence a few days prior to the onset of a menstrual flow.

Most women experience some premonitory symptoms for several days before the onset of menstruation, but usually they pay very little attention to them. An exaggeration of these manifestations sufficient to disturb the patient and to prompt her to seek relief occurs in about 10% to 20% of women, generally in the fourth decade of life. Rarely are the symptoms severe enough to incapacitate the patient. It is during the premenstrual phase and during menstruation that women are most likely to become emotionally disturbed, suicidal, or homicidal.

ETIOLOGY

The cause of premenstrual tension is unknown, but its cyclic nature and timing suggest a causal relationship with the ovarian hormones, estrogen and progesterone. The following theories and explanations of the pathogenesis of the various symptoms of premenstrual tension have been advanced: excess estrogen, excess estrogen and progesterone, avitaminosis, allergy, and a psychogenic factor.

Excess estrogen. Frank suggested that the underlying cause of the syndrome was a high level of estrogen in the blood because of an unusually high renal threshold for this hormone. Israel confirmed the findings of hyperestrogenemia, but he theorized that this resulted from inadequate utilization of the hormone because of a deficient corpus luteum function.

Excess estrogen and progesterone. Greenhill and Freed stated that the condition was caused by the retention of sodium brought on by excessive secretion of both ovarian steroids during the postovulatory phase. The sodium retention causes accumulation of fluid in the extracellular tissue spaces. Various symptoms develop, depending on the organs involved.

Avitaminosis. Biskind explained the high estrogen level on the basis of inadequate inactivation of the hormone by the liver because of a vitamin B deficiency.

Allergy. Zondek has advanced the theory that some patients become sensitized to their own steroid hormones and react with symptoms of premenstrual tension whenever the levels of estrogen or progesterone become abnormally high.

Psychogenic factor. Emotional factors per se probably do not initiate symptoms of premenstrual tension, but the condition is encountered more often and the symptoms are more distressing in the "high-strung," anxious woman. Most of the clinical evidence supports the view that premenstrual tension is usually associated with sodium ion and water retention and is most likely to occur in women with neurotic tendencies.

SYMPTOMS

Headache, nervous irritability, insommia, and crying spells are the most common symptoms of premenstrual tension. Many women complain of backache, lower abdominal pain, and tender, painful breasts. Symptoms appear about 10 days to a week prior to the expected menstrual period, gradually increase in intensity, and usually are gone once the flow is well established. A weight gain of 3 to 5 pounds during the premenstrual phase is a common finding. Generalized edema and oliguria frequently occur. Rapid loss of weight and marked diuresis usually follow the onset of menstruation.

TREATMENT

Since water retention and a neurotic predisposition are the most common manifestations of premenstrual tension, therapy should be directed toward their correction.

Dehydration. A number of diuretic agents are suitable for dehydration programs. Most of these drugs are thiazides, which as a group may cause electrolyte imbalance from prolonged or too vigorous administration. We have found trichlormethiazide (Naqua), 4 mg., or bendroflumethiazide (Naturetin), 5 mg., once daily to be quite satisfactory.

The short intervals of cyclic treatment necessary to eliminate premenstrual tension should not create an electrolyte disturbance. A tranqulizing agent, meprobamate, 200 mg., combined with hydrochlorothiazide (Cyclex), 25 mg., administered once or twice a day during the troublesome phase, generally affords prompt relief from the premenstrual tension complex.

Psychotherapy. The patient should be informed as to the known causes of the symptoms. She should be assured that it is not an unusual or serious condition and can, as a rule, be relieved. Most women who have had a relative degree of premenstrual tension are depressed. The reason for this depression is anger over their discomfort and the guilt that they feel because of their behavior within the family. The husband often can be helpful by not being too sympathetic and increasing the woman's guilt, but rather he should be firm in a gentle way. Adjustment of environmental conditions in the home and in the patient's interpersonal relationships may help to reduce tension. Women suffering from other neurotic symptoms may require more intensive psychotherapy.

Hormone therapy. The administration of the steroid hormones, which has been recommended by some authors, seems to us to be an illogical approach to the problem of premenstrual tension. Firstly, there is no real evidence that steroid therapy is indicated, and secondly, dehydration therapy, which is quite effective, is much less expensive and less likely to produce undesirable effects.

Vitamin B therapy. Biskind recommended the administration of vitamin B complex on the assumption that the excess estrogen, said to be the precipitating factor in the production of symptoms, was caused by a deficiency of vitamin B. A small percentage of patients who suffer from premenstrual tension associated with poor nutrition do benefit from an improvement in diet and supplementary vitamin therapy.

Sedatives and tranquilizers. In some patients, particularly in those who do not show signs of great fluid retention, the administration of mild sedatives or mood-ameliorating drugs, such as Compazine, 5 to 10 mg., meprobamate, 200 to 400 mg., or Trilafon, 4 to 5 mg., may be sufficient therapy.

References

Burger, E., and Kroger, W. S.: Dynamic significance of vaginal lubrication to frigidity, Western J. Surg. 61:711, 1963.

Cotte, G.: Resection of presacral nerve in treatment of obstinate dysmenorrhea, Amer. J. Obstet. Gynec. 33:1034, 1937.

Davis, M.: The sexual responsibility of women, New York, 1956, The Dial Press, Inc.

Deutsch, J.: Psychology of women, vol. 1, New York, 1944, Grune & Stratton, Inc.

Doyle, J. B.: Paracervical uterine denervation by transection of cervical plexus for relief of dysmenorrhea, Amer. J. Obstet. Gynec. 70:1, 1955.

Haman, J. O.: Pain threshold in dysmenorrhea, Amer. J. Obstet. Gynec. 47:686, 1944.

Hoffman, J. W.: Effect of gynecological surgery on the sexual reaction, Amer. J. Obstet. Gynec. 59:915, 1959.

Kinsey, A. C., et al.: Sexual behavior in the human female, Philadelphia, 1953, W. B. Saunders Co.

Kroger, W. S.: Psychosomatic obstetrics, gynecology and endocrinology, Springfield, Ill., 1962, Charles C Thomas, Publisher.

Kroger, W. S., and Freed, S. C.: Psychosomatic gynecology, Philadelphia, 1951, W. B. Saunders Co.

Mann, E. C.: Clinical obstetrics and gynecology, New York, 1960, Paul B. Hoeber, Inc., Medical Book Department of Harper & Row, Publishers.

Masters, W. H.: The sexual response cycle of the human female. I. Gross anatomic considerations, Western J. Surg. 68:57, 1960.

Masters, W. H., and Johnson, V. E.: The human female anatomy of sexual response, Minnesota Med. 43:31, 1960.

Ruderford, R. M., et al.: Frigidity and psychosomatic obstetrics and gynecology and endocrinology, Philadelphia, 1953, W. B. Saunders Co.

Simmons, S. C.: Dyspareunia following vaginal repair, J. Obstet. Gynec. 7:476, 1963.

Solomon, P.: Love, a clinical definition, New Eng. J. Med. 252:345, 1955.

Sturgis, S. H.: The use of stilbestrol in relief of essential dysmenorrhea, New Eng. J. Med. 226:371, 1942.

Waxenberg, S. E., Drellich, M., and Sutherland, H.: The role of hormones in human behavior, J. Clin. Endocr. 19:193, 1959.

Weiss, E., and English, O. S.: Psychosomatic medicine, Philadelphia, 1949, W. B. Saunders Co.

Yalom, I. D., Lunde, D. T., Maas, R. H., and Hamburg, D. A.: "Postpartum blues" syndrome; a description and related variables, Arch. Gen. Psychiat. 18:16, 1968.

9

Endometriosis

ovary as follows: "We were astonished to find areas which were an exact prototype of the uterine glands and interglandular tissue. The whole formed an exact reproduction of a portion of the uterine mucous membrane and muscle."* Significant advances in our knowledge of endometriosis have come from Sampson, Meigs, Cashman, and Scott, although the literature on the subject is voluminous.

About 5% of all women seen in the practice of obstetrics and gynecology have endometriosis in some diagnosable form. It is probably the most common lesion seen at pelvic laparotomy in the white female, often being a surprise finding of no clinical significance. Endometriosis occurs between the life phases of puberty and the menopause. The usual age at which symptoms occur is between 25 and 35 years; so it is largely a problem of the reproductive years.

■ Etiology

Iwanoff (1898) was the first to suggest that the endometrium-like pelvic-peritoneal tumors were caused by metaplasia of the mesothelium or serosal layer of the uterus. This *serosal theory* or *metaplasia factor,* which was further popularized by Robert Meyer in 1919, is based on the fact that all epithelia of the female genital system are derived from the coelomic epithelium of the urogenital folds, which in turn comes from the primitive peritoneum. Many undeveloped peritoneal cells remain in the adult, and to these Meyer ascribed differentiating potentials that could make them the anlage of endometriosis. He believed that the typical lesions developed in response to an inflammatory reaction. Novak accepted the Iwanoff-Meyer metaplasia theory but believed that an unknown endocrine factor rather than inflammation initiated the late differentiation.

Meigs advanced a theory of etiology on which we have been able to build a conservative therapeutic plan. He noted that endometriosis was common in private patients who married late and among whom contraceptive practices were widespread. By contrast, endometriosis was unusual in ward patients in whom marriages took place earl-

Endometriosis may be defined as an abnormal growth of endometrial tissue outside the uterine cavity. If the endometriosis is confined to the myometrium, it is referred to as *internal endometriosis,* or *adenomyosis.* Involvement of all other pelvic structures and remote areas is called *external endometriosis.* A circumscribed tumor mass containing endometrial glands and stroma within the uterine wall is spoken of as an *adenomyoma.*

The earliest description of this lesion was given in 1860 by von Rokitansky while writing about adenomyomas. Apparently little attention was given this work until 1895 when von Recklinghausen aroused new interest in the entity while attempting to show that these tumors came from wolffian duct rests. A year later Cullen began making vast contributions to the subject of adenomyoma. The first early description of ovarian endometriosis was given in 1899 by Russell, who recorded his microscopic study of an affected

*From Russell, W. W.: Aberrant portions of the mullerian duct found in the ovary, Bull. Hopkins Hosp. **10:**8, 1899.

ier and contraceptive practices were almost nonexistent. He theorized that the interruption of the rhythmic changes in aberrant endometrium by repeated early pregnancies must be beneficial and conversely that prolonged periodic menstruation without interruption favored the development of endometriosis. Scott and Wharton succeeded in making experimental endometriosis in monkeys grow and bleed by the cyclic administration of progesterone after estrogen priming. They believe that progesterone withdrawal is the most important factor in the process.

Sampson's scholarly papers on the subject of endometriosis led some to the belief that his theory of etiology was probably the correct one. He suggested that endometriosis was caused by the growth of endometrial fragments regurgitated from the uterus through the tubes. The Sampson theory is supported by the work of Ridley and Edwards. These investigators, by using endometrial fragments collected from menstrual blood, were able to make them grow when injected into the abdominal wall. The Sampson theory, although attractively simple, does not explain many of the endometriosis lesions encountered.

Halban proposed the lymphatic dissemination theory: that endometriun entered the lymphatic vessels at the time of menstruation and was disseminated about the pelvis. Although somewhat uncommon, ureteral obstruction from retroperitoneal endometriosis gives substance to Halban's theory.

■ Pathology

Gross. The gross appearance of endometriosis is variable, depending on the stage of the disease and the length of time it has existed. Minimal lesions are of little clinical importance and appear as bluish red spots scattered over the peritoneal covering of the pelvic viscera. With more advanced lesions, the rectum, cul-de-sac, uterosacral ligaments, tubes, ovaries, and broad ligaments are

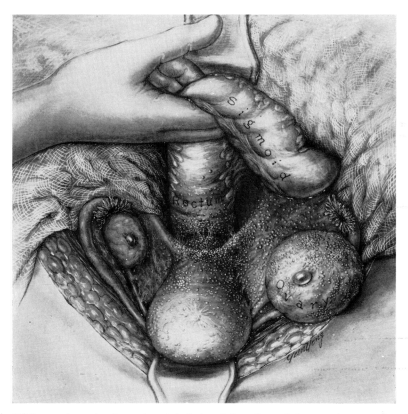

Fig. 9-1. Diffuse yet moderate endometriosis involving the cul-de-sac, uterosacral and broad ligaments, ovary, and corpus uteri.

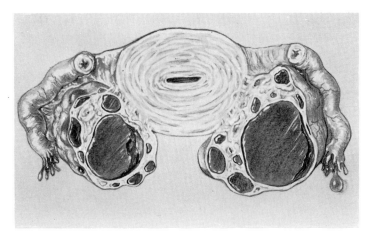

Fig. 9-2. Cross section showing the uterus in the center with bilateral ovarian endometrial cysts adherent to the uterus, the posterior leaves of the broad ligament, and tubes.

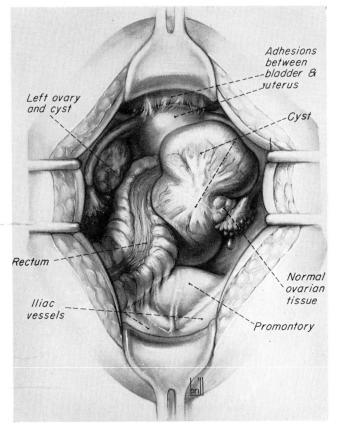

Fig. 9-3. Advanced endometriosis with previous rupture of the endometrial cyst on the right. Note adhesions and areas of normal-appearing ovarian tissue.

matted together. To some degree the retroperitoneal space is involved in all advanced lesions. Unlike tissue response from other irritants, endometriosis creates a fibrinocollagenous tissue reaction; ligneous adhesions result. The agglutinated surfaces of the structures are rough, granular, and brown in appearance, the glistening peritoneal covering having been destroyed. As the dissection is carried out, thick brown fluid escapes into the operative field. This fluid, which actually is old blood, may form collections in any plane of the adherent viscera or within the various organs themselves, notably the ovaries. Ovarian involvement varies from small cystic collections to a single loculated structure 10 cm. or more in diameter. The common practice of referring to endometrial cysts of the ovary as "chocolate cysts" is inaccurate. For instance, old blood may form a hematoma in an ovarian follicle and present a similar picture, but the nonpathologic entity of follicle hematoma is not to be confused with nor treated as endometriosis. *Every collection of old blood in an ovary is not endometriosis.*

The rectosigmoid and urinary tract may be involved in endometriosis lesions. Occasionally an implant may be found in one of these structures without evidence of endometriosis elsewhere in the pelvis. Rarely, the vagina, cervix, episiotomy scars, laparotomy scars, umbilicus, round ligaments, lungs, and extremities are sites of endometrial implants. Wherever the lesion is found, its behavior is essentially the same.

Microscopic. The microscopic like the gross appearance is subject to much variation. Classically one should find tissue resembling endometrial glands and stroma. In some instances endometriosis undergoes cyclic changes like those of the uterine endometrium, but this is not the rule, and a constant proliferative pattern in the aberrant glands is more to be expected.

Sometimes it may be difficult for the pathologist to recognize endometrial glands or even stroma, since degeneration is common and there may be nothing more than hemosiderin deposits to suggest the diagnosis. Whenever endometriosis is removed, the surgeon should mark the specific area he wishes studied. This will aid the pathologist in obtaining representative sections and will more often permit microscopic verification of the clinical diagnosis.

■ Symptoms

Pain. Lower abdominal and pelvic pain in some form is the most common symptom

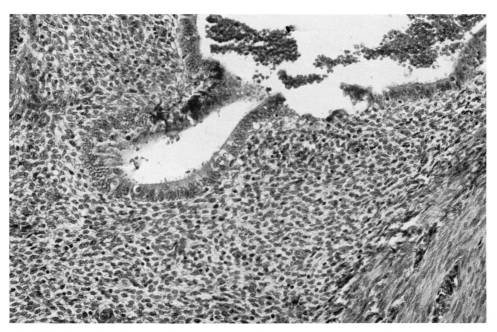

Fig. 9-4. Internal endometriosis or adenomyosis demonstrating the early secretory phase. Cyclic changes in endometriosis are a variable feature.

of endometriosis. Since some of the aberrant endometrium demonstrates cyclic changes, it obviously bleeds at menstruation, and the blood is contained within the involved organ or affected tissue, distending it and the surrounding peritoneum. As one would expect then, *dysmenorrhea* is a common symptom, but dysmenorrhea in women with endometriosis is not always a result of the disease. Menstrual pain associated with endometriosis is generally severe and steady rather than cramplike. In the far-advanced cases the pain may last throughout the period. Whenever dysmenorrhea is caused by endometriosis, there usually is considerable involvement of the uterosacral ligaments, the cul-de-sac, and the myometrium (adenomyosis). Ovarian endometriosis alone or an uncomplicated endometrial cyst of the ovary does not usually cause pain. *Rectal tenesmus* is common and severe at the time of the period if there is considerable involvement in the cul-de-sac and uterosacral ligaments. This same area of involvement will frequently cause *dyspareunia*. Advanced cases of endometriosis create the impression of a "frozen" pelvis, and as such may cause steady pelvic pain. *The disturbing features of endometriosis are that all degrees of involvement are encountered without a single symptom and that severe dysmenorrhea often occurs in women with minimal endometriosis.*

Intermittent crampy, colicky pain may occur with advanced endometriosis of the lower bowel. This suggests partial obstruction and may produce more symptoms at the time of the period.

Abnormal bleeding. Abnormal uterine bleeding may occur in women with endometriosis. In advanced lesions enough ovarian tissue may be destroyed to interfere with function, but in most instances adenomyosis (internal endometriosis) without ovarian involvement is found by the pathologist.

■ Differential diagnosis

Pelvic inflammation. The most common entity to be confused with endometriosis is pelvic inflammatory disease. The symptoms of both conditions are similar, and at times bimanual rectovaginal examination is of little help in differentiating the two diseases. The history is often helpful; when inflammatory disease is present, the patient may relate an episode of acute urethritis and/or cervici-

tis followed by the typical symptoms of extension upward to the tubes. There is nothing in the history of endometriosis to parallel these data. In both conditions the tubes and ovaries tend to become adherent to the posterior leaves of the broad ligaments and the rectosigmoid, and it is here that their resemblance is greatest. With inflammatory disease, however, the masses are relatively smooth when compared to the beaded, fixed, tender uterosacral ligaments and the irregular cul-de-sac obliterated by endometriosis.

Ovarian carcinoma. A cul-de-sac obliterated and bulging with endometriosis may on occasion resemble ovarian carcinoma. The patient's history may be helpful. Endometriosis usually causes pain and examination is painful, whereas ovarian carcinoma is devoid of symptoms until very far advanced and is not tender. A laparotomy may be necessary to differentiate these two conditions.

Benign ovarian neoplasms. An endometrial cyst of the ovary without other pelvic involvement cannot be distinguished from a primary benign ovarian neoplasm on pelvic examination. Laparotomy should usually be performed.

Other carcinoma. Endometriosis of the cervix, vagina, and vulva resembles early squamous cell carcinoma upon casual inspection. The raised, red, friable areas that bleed so easily to the touch make the physician strongly suspect malignancy. A punch biopsy is the quickest and easiest way to make the correct diagnosis.

Urinary tract lesions. Urinary tract endometriosis is suggested in women with cyclic or intermittent hematuria. Whereas intrinsic bladder lesions are easily seen, ureteral involvement can best be demonstrated by pyelography. Hydronephrosis from ureteral compression may progress to complete loss of kidney function.

Bowel lesions. Endometriosis of the bowel usually is visualized on x-ray examination as an extraluminal growth. At times it may even be annular. Rarely will the lesion be seen within the lumen so that a biopsy may be taken.

■ Treatment

A conservative approach to the treatment of endometriosis is imperative, since it is a nonneoplastic entity affecting women in the reproductive years. If the physician will keep in mind Meigs's clinical observations along with Scott and Wharton's progesterone withdrawal concept, he has the framework of a conservative therapeutic plan for endometriosis.

Pregnancy. A married patient should be advised to become pregnant when endometriosis is diagnosed. Physiologic amenorrhea often causes a truly remarkable regression in aberrant endometrium. In many patients it may be difficult to palpate the lesion after the first trimester of pregnancy. At full term the cul-de-sac and other areas previously so deeply involved will present white, soft, puckered clusters of peritoneum. This same appearance is often noted in the postmenopausal pelvis.

In severe cases of endometriosis that have been quiescent during pregnancy, symptoms and palpable nodules may recur as early as the second postpartum period. A second pregnancy has proved to be most helpful in delaying a recurrence of symptoms; many patients will remain symptom free for months, whereas in others the pains recur promptly.

Desirable as pregnancy is in the treatment of endometriosis, not all women with the disease are able to conceive. Endometriosis is a common cause of infertility. Why this is true is not entirely clear because most women with endometriosis have normal patent tubes and ovulate at reasonable intervals. If endometriosis itself is a factor in sterility, it must be on the basis of immobilization of the tubes and ovaries.

Oral contraceptive drugs. The advent of 19-norsteroids has added an extraordinary dimension to the treatment and prevention of endometriosis. Acting through hypothalamic-pituitary suppression, estrogen in these estrogen-progesterone combinations produces anovulation. High doses bring about amenorrhea. 19-Norsteroids have been so successful that generally no other therapy is necessary in the average case. With these preparations it is unnecessary to produce amenorrhea to control symptoms. Various progestogen combinations may be continued indefinitely, depending on age, desire for additional pregnancies, and total clinical response.

After an extended period of progestogen use a few women will develop irregular and/or profuse uterine bleeding, which is usually due to adenomyosis. After the usual diagnostic studies hysterectomy is the treatment of choice. No amount of 19-norsteroid

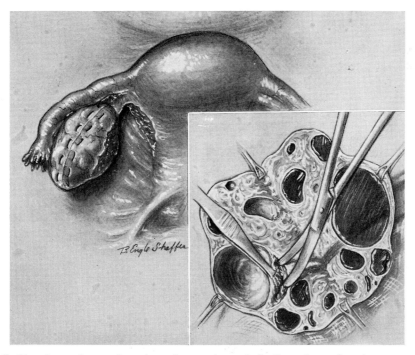

Fig. 9-5. Bisection and resection of ovarian endometriosis. Enough ovarian tissue to maintain normal function can almost always be salvaged.

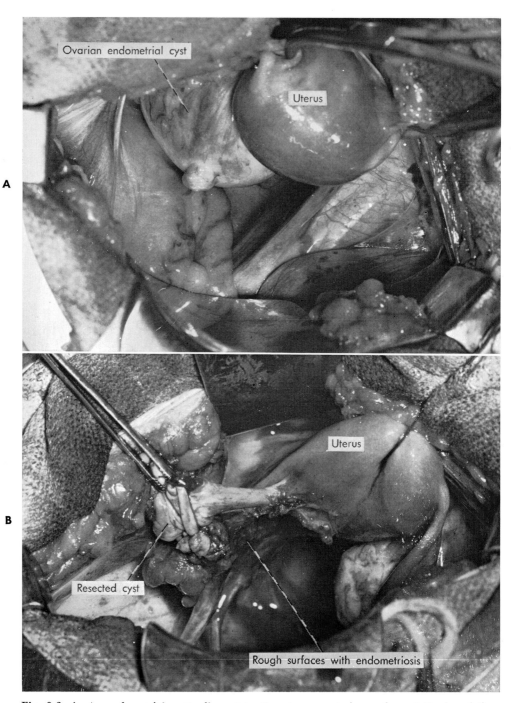

Fig. 9-6. A, An endometrial cyst adherent to the uterus, posterior surface of the broad ligament, and the cul-de-sac. **B,** The same ovary after resection. Note the substantial amount of
ovarian tissue remaining. Induced anovulation will resolve the implants on the broad ligament
and cul-de-sac.

or other endocrine manipulation will help control the bleeding in such cases.

Surgical treatment. We do not regard endometriosis as an entity requiring primary surgical therapy. Massive excisions and resections, not unlike those for a pelvic malignancy, are generally unjustified. Although superficial endometrial implants on pelvic viscera are frequently cauterized, there is no need to invite adhesions by this overzealous therapy when response to pregnancy or induced anovulation by decidual transformation, necrobiosis and absorption is so rewarding. Extirpation of any organ for endometriosis in young nulliparous women is seldom necessary. This applies particularly to the ovary.

Surgical exploration must be carried out in patients with endometriosis who have bilateral or unilateral ovarian enlargement greater than 5 cm. in diameter, because it is impossible to differentiate ovarian endometriosis from true neoplasms by physical examination. Treatment of ovarian endometriosis is different from that of true tumors of the ovary, for which cyst-oophorectomy is almost always necessary. Endometriomas of the ovary are dissected free from their adhesive beds and bisected at a point opposite the hilus. The cyst contents are evacuated and the cyst lining gently dissected away, leaving as much normal tissue as possible. Extensive alteration in ovarian function might be suspected from the great distortion when the ovary is enlarged many times by blood-filled cysts, but when the cysts are resected, there usually is enough normal tissue to maintain adequate function, even with ovulation and conception. In rare instances castration might be necessary but never without a trial of conservative measures first.

Cashman advised hysterectomy with conservation of the ovaries in women in the late childbearing years or in women with several children. This is a highly successful treatment, and again we have produced amenorrhea, this time permanently. All manner of endometriosis lesions left behind (from bowel endometriomas to ovarian endometrial cysts) usually atrophy, even though ovarian function continues. These effects are in keeping with Meigs's idea of interrupting rhythmic change in ovarian-uterine function and Scott's work on cyclic progesterone withdrawal.

Endometriosis of the rectosigmoid is encountered often enough to be considered as a possible cause for partial and complete bowel obstruction. Resection is not always necessary unless the lesion cannot be differentiated from carcinoma or unless obstruction is almost complete.

X-ray therapy. With any medical or surgical procedure there will be some failures in attaining a desired result. For example, a rectosigmoid endometrioma might not respond to hysterectomy, or a pregnancy might not improve a cul-de-sac endometriosis. If this happens and if the patient is truly miserable with the disease, she may be castrated by radiation. Knowing that we always have the radical plan of castration available, we apply the conservative measures with confidence. The need to castrate either by surgery or by radiation is *rare*.

References

Beecham, C. T.: Conservative surgery in endometriosis, Amer. J. Obstet. Gynec. **52**:707, 1946.

Beecham, C. T., and McCrea, L. E.: Endometriosis of the urinary tract, Urol. Survey **7**:2, 1957.

Cashman, B. Z.: Hysterectomy with preservation of ovarian tissue in the treatment of endometriosis, Amer. J. Obstet. Gynec. **49**:484, 1945.

Cullen, T. S.: Adenomyoma of the round ligament, Bull. Hopkins Hosp. **7**:112, 1896.

Halban, J.: Hysteroadenosis metastatica (die Lymphogene Genese der sog. Adeno-fibromatosis heterotopica), Wien. Klin. Wschr. **37**:1205, 1924.

Iwanoff, N. S.: Drusiges cystenhaltiges Uterusfibromyom kompliziera durch Sarcom und carcinoma, Mschr. Geburtsh. Gynaek. **7**:295, 1898.

Javert, C. T.: The spread of benign and malignant endometrium in the lymphatic system with a note on coexisting vascular involvement, Amer. J. Obstet. Gynec. **64**:780, 1952.

Kistner, R. W.: The use of steroidal substances in endometriosis, Clin. Pharmacol. Ther. **1**:525, 1960.

Kluver, H., and Bartelmez, A. W.: Endometriosis in rhesus monkey, Surg. Gynec. Obstet. **92**:650, 1951.

Kourides, I. A., and Kistner, R. W.: Three new synthetic progestins in the treatment of endometriosis, Obstet. Gynec. **31**:821, 1968.

Meigs, J. V.: Endometrial hematomas of the ovary, Boston Med. Surg. J. **187**:1, 1922.

Meigs, J. V.: Endometriosis—a possible etiological factor, Surg. Gynec. Obstet. **67**:253, 1938.

Meyer, R.: Ueben den Stand der Frage der Adenomyositis und Adenomyome im Allgemeinen, und inbesonders über Adenomyositis seroepithelialis, Zbl. Gynaek. **36**:745, 1919.

Novak, E.: The significance of uterine mucosa in the fallopian tube with a discussion of the origin of aberrant endometrium, Amer. J. Obstet. Gynec. **12:**484, 1926.

Prakash, S., Ulfelder, H., and Cohen, R. B.: Enzyme-histochemical observations on endometriosis, Amer. J. Obstet. Gynec. **91:**990, 1965.

von Recklinghausen, E.: Ueber Adenomyome des Uterus und der Tube, Wien. Klin. Wschr. **8:** 530, 1895.

Ridley, J. H., and Edwards, I. K.: Experimental endometriosis in the human, Amer. J. Obstet. Gynec. **76:**783, 1958.

von Rokitansky, C.: Ueber Uterusdrusennebildung im Uterus, Z. d. kaiserlich-königlichen Gesell. d. Aertze zu Wien, 1860.

Russell, W. W.: Aberrant portions of the mullerian duct found in the ovary, Bull. Hopkins Hosp. **10:**8, 1899.

Sampson, J. A.: Cysts of the ovary, Arch. Surg. **3:**245, 1921.

Scott, R. B., and Wharton, L. R.: The effect of estrone and progesterone on the growth of experimental endometriosis in rhesus monkeys, Amer. J. Obstet. Gynec. **74:**852, 1957.

10

Fertilization; development, physiology, and disorders of the placenta; fetal development

Successful human reproduction is dependent upon an integrated sequence of physiologic mechanisms that first of all assure normal maturation, fertilization, and growth of the ovum and then, as gestation advances, permit normal differentiation and adequate nutrition for the fetus.

■ Fertilization

Union of male and female elements of procreation must be preceded by *maturation* of the germ cells. In the sexually adult male spermatogenesis occurs continuously, whereas in the female oogenesis is cyclic. Under the influence of pituitary follicle-stimulating hormone (FSH) numerous follicles are stimulated during the first 10 days of the cycle. Growth is principally related to an increase in granulosa cells and the accumulation of estrogen-rich liquor folliculi. Usually only one follicle is destined to reach maturity at each cycle. Its rate of growth is greatly accelerated as the ripening follicle migrates to the surface of the ovary. At approximately the fourteenth day, when the levels of FSH and luteinizing hormone (LH) reach a critical level, rupture of the follicle occurs, and the ovum together with some of the surrounding granulosa cells and follicular fluid is discharged into the peritoneal cavity. Release of pressure allows the walls to collapse, and blood from the congested vessels of the theca fills the cavity. The point of rupture (blutpunkt) seals off. Theca cells and especially granulosa cells undergo luteinization, producing a yellow lipid-laden body, the mature corpus luteum.

Final preparation of the ovum for fertilization involves the unique process of *meiosis* (Fig. 10-1). In contrast to somatic cell division, or mitosis, wherein a complete diploid chromosomal set is passed to the daughter cell, gametogenesis results in reduction of the nuclear chromosomes to one half the number characteristic of the species. This is accomplished by two maturation divisions, the steps involved being of utmost importance to an understanding of human chromosomal anbormalities. Prior to the first division homologous chromosomes arrange in pairs (association), then in the first meiotic, or reduction, division they separate (disjunction) to form the first two daughter cells, each containing the haploid complement of 23 chromosomes. The second meiotic division, which is mitotic in type, results in a total of four haploid gametes.

Union of the ovum and the spermatozoon restores the normal diploid number with formation of the zygote, containing 44 autosomal chromosomes and 2 sex chromosomes; the zygote is female if the sex chromosomes are XX and male if they are XY (Fig. 10-2). Thus the genetic or nuclear sex is determined and fixed at fertilization, and the sex genes direct and control differentiation of the gonad and accessory structures, beginning about the sixth week of embryonic life. However, the external sex is not clearly apparent until about the sixteenth week. The physical appearance of sex may be influenced by a nonphysiologic hormonal environment to which the fetus is exposed. If gonadogenesis is normal, if the

107

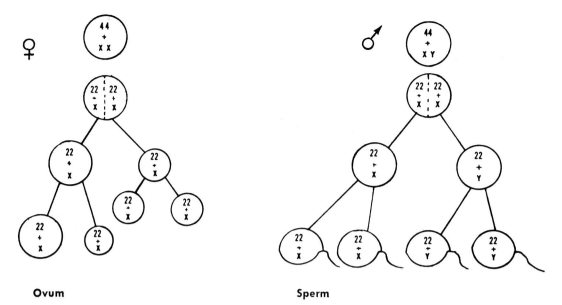

Fig. 10-1. Normal gametogenesis.

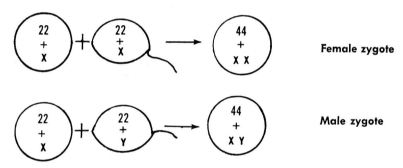

Fig. 10-2. Male and female zygote.

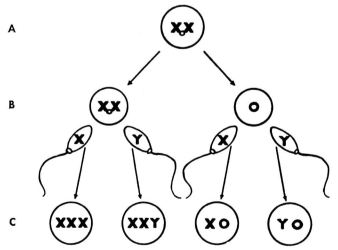

Fig. 10-3. Effects of nondisjunction during gametogenesis. **A,** Haploid daughter cell with two chromatids united by centromere. **B,** Nondisjunction. **C,** Four types of zygotes may be produced during fertilization. (From Eggen, R. R.: Amer. J. Clin. Path. **39:**10, 1963.)

fetal hormonal environment is appropriate, and if there is no interference from harmful physical factors or from exogenous hormonal influences, then the physical appearance of sex (phenotype) will be compatible with the chromosomal sex (genotype).

The genetic constitution may be altered in the process of gonadogenesis by nonassociation or by nondisjunction of chromosomes, resulting in defects that are often lethal if autosomes are involved—but there are exceptions. Nonlethal consequences are seen in developmental abnormalities that result from the number of chromosomes either exceeding or being less than normal (Fig. 10-3).

For many years the chromosomal num-

ber of man was thought to be 48. In 1956 Tjio and Levan made accurate chromosomal counts on cells prepared by culture of lung tissue obtained from aborted human embryos and established the chromosomal number of 46 in the human. Later in the same year Ford and Hamerton in England reported their studies of germ cells from human male testes. They demonstrated the formation of 23 chromosomal pairs in spermatocyte preparations and confirmed the chromosomal number of 46 (Fig. 10-4). The 22 autosomal pairs are similar in the female and the male, whereas the sex chromosomes differ in the two sexes (XX or XY, respectively).

The true genetic sex can be determined

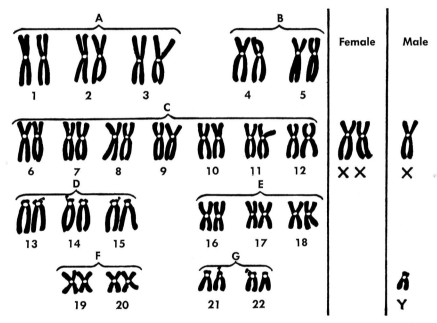

Fig. 10-4. Idiogram of human chromosomes—International System of Nomenclature (Denver). (From Eggen, R. R.: Amer. J. Clin. Path. **39:**10, 1963.)

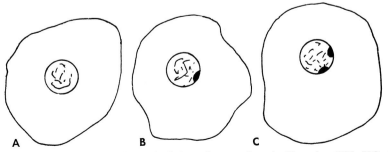

Fig. 10-5. Sex chromatin mass (Barr body) and examples. **A,** Negative XY, XO. **B,** Chromatin-1 positive XX, XXY. **C,** Chromatin-2 positive XXX, XXXY.

by cytologic examination of various somatic cells. The morphologic difference in the resting cell nuclei of the two sexes was first described by Barr and co-workers in 1950. A dense mass of chromatin known as the *sex chromatin mass,* or *Barr body* (Fig. 10-5), situated at the periphery of the nucleus just within the nuclear membrane is found in up to 90% of the somatic cell nuclei of normal females (chromatin positive) but is absent or is found in only about 1% to 3% of the nuclei of normal males (chromatin negative). The chromatin mass is derived from the female X chromosome. The number of Barr bodies found in each nucleus equals the number of X chromosomes minus one. Thus in normal females with an XX constitution one Barr body is seen. In females with Turner's syndrome, bearing the most characteristic XO pattern, and in normal males with an XY constitution the nuclear sex is chromatin negative. In Klinefelter's syndrome individuals with either an XXY or an XXXY constitution display a chromatin-one or a chromatin-two positive nuclear sex pattern, despite the fact that the phenotype is male.

Cells obtained by buccal smear are most commonly used for examination; occasionally skin or vaginal smears are taken. Polymorphonuclear leukocytes can also be used, in which case a characteristic mass or drumstick is found in normal females in about 3% of the neutrophils. However, this may appear as an accessory lobule, and differentiation is therefore more difficult.

Migration of the ovum. The precise mechanism by which the ovum gains access to the fallopian tube is unknown, although several factors conducive to its transport are demonstrable: (1) Peristaltic motions of the tube are influenced by hormone stimulation. The greatest amplitude and frequency of contractions are observed at the time of ovulation. (2) The ovary and its attached fimbria ovarica are drawn toward the uterus by contraction of the ovarian ligament. (3) Motion of the epithelial cilia lining the tube establishes a current that promotes migration of the ovum into and through the tube. Using culdoscopy for 4- to 5-hour periods, Doyle reported direct observation of ovulation in 3 patients. He noted elongation, edema, and congestion of the tube and spread of the fimbria over the supermedial aspect of the ovary. Trumpet-shaped cones of contraction developed at the fimbria at the rate of 6 per minute. Peristalsis continued to the isthmus, followed by a to-and-fro motion, and again peristalsis to the cornu. After a period of about 2 hours the tube slid down the ovary to the cul-de-sac. Suction developed in this location probably provides a means by which the tube on one side may pick up ova ruptured from either ovary.

Fertilization. The ovum is fertilized in the outer third of the tube within a short period of time, probably less than 24 hours, after ovulation. Viability of the ovum is somewhat less than that of sperm. The seminal fluid vehicle for transport is slightly alkaline, with a pH of 7.5. When the sperm are deposited in the vagina, they are placed in a hostile environment with a pH of 4.5. Although the buffering action of semen is to some extent capable of offsetting this difference, prompt migration is important to continued viability of sperm. The normal pH of cervical mucus is 7.5. Tyler suggests that the difference in vaginal and cervical pH is one of the factors that favor migration of the sperm into the cervical canal; cyclic variations in cervical secretion further enhance their passage. At the time of ovulation the mucus is thin, abundant, rich in glycogen, and most conducive for penetration.

Active sperm were shown by Brown to move at the rate of 2.7 mm. per minute and to reach the lateral portion of the tube within 65 to 75 minutes after ejaculation. Upon penetration of the vitelline membrane, male and female pronuclei, each with 23 chromosomes, unite to form the segmentation nucleus and restore the original 46 chromosomes. Repeated cell divisions result in the formation of a mulberry mass, the morula. The outer layer of cells secretes fluid that accumulates, forming the segmentation cavity. The mass at this time is called the blastodermic vesicle, or blastocyst. *Implantation* occurs at the blastocyst stage 6 or 7 days after ovulation. Formative cells crowded to one side represent the embryonic pole or inner cell mass. The single layer of cells surrounding the vesicle is the primitive trophoblast. There is much unresolved speculation regarding possible mechanisms in operation during implantation that may account for control of invasion on the one hand and prevention of immunologic rejection on the other. Just prior to attachment on the uterine endometrium, an aggregate of cells, the "syncytial knob," appears in the trophoblastic syncytium. These knobs are the portions of the trophoblast that penetrate the decidua. At the implantation site, fusion of maternal and fetal cells occurs temporarily. Behrman and others have speculated that such fusion of cytoplasmic and nuclear material may change the immunologic characteristics of maternal tissues and induce tolerance to fetal antigens rather than sensitization.

While these changes take place, the pregravid endometrium is prepared to provide for nidation and nutrition of the fertilized ovum. The decidua develops under the influence of increasing amounts of ovarian hormones, principally progesterone. The stroma is made up of characteristic large, polyhedral decidual cells, glands become thick and tortuous, and glycogen content is high. Vascularity is greatly increased. The epithelium of the endometrial cavity may play an active role in implantation. Fainstat and Chapman studied ultrastructure changes in the rat endometrial epithelium and found microvilli that serve as instruments for attachment of the ovum and, by increasing the free surface, facilitate the first direct metabolic interchange between maternal and fetal tissue during ova implantation. The number of these microvilli are increased as a result of the estrogen surge that occurs shortly before the attachment of the ovum to the epithelium.

The trophoblast secretes certain enzymes.

Proteolytic and cytolytic enzymes permit these cells to invade the prepared endometrium, destroying vessels, glands, and stroma locally. *Implantation bleeding* may occur. This is small in amount, is not associated with pain, and disappears within 1 or 2 days, when the aperture in the endometrium is sealed over. Decidua covering this portion of the ovum is the *decidua capsularis*, and that beneath the ovum is the *decidua basalis*. The remainder of the uterine cavity is lined by the *decidua vera*. During nidation trophoblastic cells provide nutrition for the embryo, first by destruction and absorption of decidua and later by absorption of substances from maternal blood.

■ Development and physiology of the placenta

The primitive *trophoblast* proliferates rapidly after implantation. Three layers appear, all of which are believed to be derived from this structure, which first develops as typical Langhans' cells. These in turn undergo differentiation into an outer syncytial layer and a thin layer of connective tissue called the mesoblast beneath the proliferating Langhans inner cell layer, the cytotrophoblast. The mesoblast provides, in effect, a supporting structure or central core of the villus and the site in which villous blood-forming elements and vascular structures make their appearance. The outer syncytial layer is far more complex than was formerly recognized. Detailed study by electron microscopy reveals the so-called brush border to be a profusion of microvilli projecting from the free surface of the syncytium and of

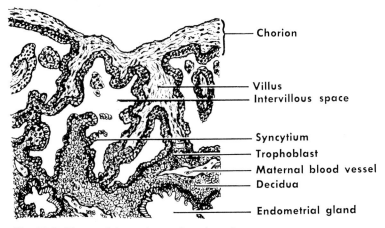

Fig. 10-6. Placental formation at 3 to 4 weeks.

Chorion

Villus
Intervillous space

Syncytium
Trophoblast
Maternal blood vessel
Decidua

Endometrial gland

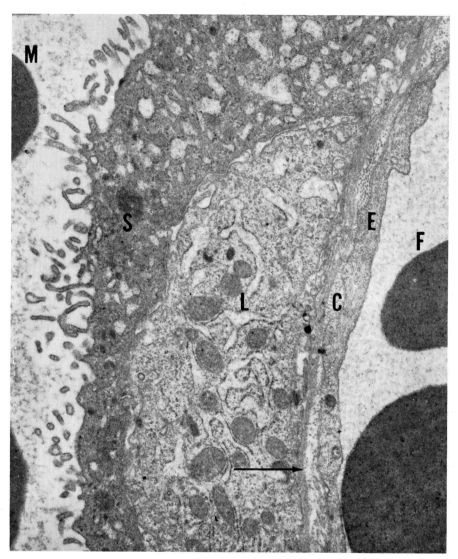

Fig. 10-7. Electron micrograph of villus of full-term human placenta. Both syncytiotrophoblast, **S**, with numerous microvilli, and Langhans' cell, **L**, persist throughout gestation. Arrow points to trophoblastic basement lamina. Connective tissue, **C**, is reduced to a minimum. The endothelium, **E**, of a capillary is seen. These placental elements separate maternal, **M**, from fetal, **F**, erythrocytes. (Glutaraldehyde and osmic acid. Araldite.) (×17,000.) (Courtesy Dr. Ralph M. Wynn.)

abundant highly developed structures—pinocytotic vesicles, lipoid droplets, and mitochondria, all providing structural evidence of secretory activity. Dempsey considers that this tissue is like a continuously streaming *ameboid mass* which is capable of actively engulfing substances, including maternal plasma, into the substance of the syncytium.

The fact that syncytial cells are rich in cytoplasmic ribonucleoproteins suggests that synthesis of proteins required by the growing embryo is one of the early functions of the trophoblast. Villee demonstrated that the early trophoblast has the *ability to synthesize glucose*. This function begins to decrease at about 12 weeks, when the fetal liver becomes capable of secreting glucose, and in late gestation placental synthesis disappears entirely. *Secretion of hormones* by the syncytiotrophoblast begins shortly after implan-

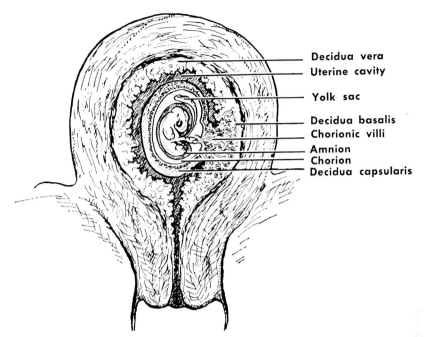

Decidua vera
Uterine cavity
Yolk sac
Decidua basalis
Chorionic villi
Amnion
Chorion
Decidua capsularis

Fig. 10-8. Diagram showing decidual, chorionic, and fetal growth at approximately 5 weeks.

tation, when chorionic gonadotropin appears, and later placental steroid hormones are secreted by cells of the syncytium.

During the first 2 or 3 weeks of gestation the chorionic villi are devoid of blood vessels. The villi project into the surrounding decidua and become filled with a core of mesoderm from the embryonal side. Islands of red blood cells develop in situ, and vascular channels appear. The villi in contact with the decidua basalis are exposed to a rich blood supply and multiply rapidly, becoming the *chorion frondosum,* or future placenta. Those in contact with the decidua capsularis become the atrophic *chorion laeve.*

Formation of the amnion occurs while the chorion develops. Two small cavities appear in the embryonic pole. The dorsal amniotic cavity is derived from ectoderm and the ventral yolk sac from entoderm. The amnion enlarges rapidly, causing disappearance of the extraembryonic coelom, and forces the body stalk, rudimentary blind allantois, vessels, and vitelline duct into a single pedicle, the beginning of the *umbilical cord.* The outer surface of the amnion applies itself to the inner aspect of the chorion. The two membranes are adherent but not fused.

IMMUNOLOGIC PROPERTIES OF THE PLACENTA

The placenta corresponds to a natural homograft in that it is a transplant of living tissue within the same species, yet it does not normally evoke the usual immune response reaction of homografts resulting in destruction and rejection of the graft. The explanation for its immunologic defense is not clear-cut. Theories have been proposed presuming the following: (1) antigenic immunity of the fetus, (2) depression of maternal immune response by increasing amounts of steroid hormones, (3) mechanical blockage or absorption of antigens by the fibrinoid layer, which separates trophoblasts and endometrial cells, and (4) the uterus as a "privileged site" for tissue graft. All of these theories discussed in detail by Behrman and Billingham have been vigorously explored and all can be contradicted. The most tenable explanation is found in the work of Simmons and Russell, who studied trophoblastic and embryonic implants in mice previously sensitized by skin grafts of the paternal type. Pure trophoblastic tissue failed to elicit the slightest cellular reaction in the host, whereas embryonic tissue was regularly destroyed by the sixth day. Thus syncytial and cytotrophoblastic cells appear to form an anatomic and immunologic buffer zone between the mother and the fetus and prevent immunologic destruction. The possibility that this protective mechanism is subject to failure and that certain cases of infertility or threatened abortion have an immunologic basis is the subject of a number of investigations.

CIRCULATION OF THE PLACENTA

By the fourteenth week the placenta is a discrete organ. Most of the villi lie free in

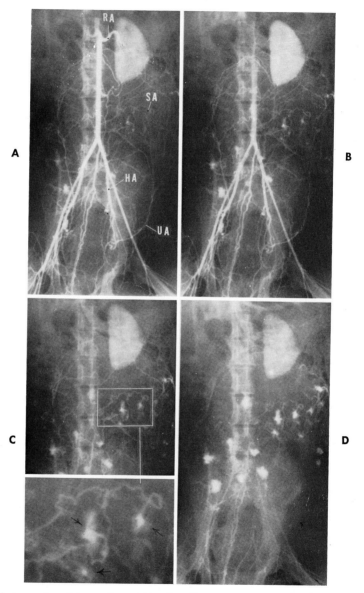

Fig. 10-9. Photographs of four of a series of radiograms made at 3½, 4, 5, and 6 seconds, respectively, after injection of a radiopaque dye into the right femoral artery of a monkey 111 days pregnant. The inset in **C** is a magnification (×4) of the area enclosed in the box. The arrows indicate spurts of dye into the intervillous space. **RA**, Renal artery; **SA**, spiral artery of endometrium; **HA**, hypogastric artery; **UA**, uterine artery. (From Ramsey, E. M., Corner, G. W., Jr., Donner, M. W., and Stran, H. M.: Proc. Nat. Acad. Sci. U.S.A. **46:**1003, 1960.)

maternal blood sinuses; anchoring villi are attached to the decidua basalis. At the point of anchorage a band of fibrin is deposited as a result of degeneration of fetal and decidual cells. This "fibrinous layer of Nitabuch" serves to resist overinvasion of maternal tissues by chorionic epithelium. This layer is absent in placenta accreta. *Circulation* of the blood through sinuses and intervillous spaces is dependent upon (1) maternal blood pressure with resultant gradient between arterial and venous channels and (2) uterine contractions. Ramsey and associates' work on placental circulation has clarified certain problems hitherto unexplained. These problems are concerned with (1) delivery of an arterial supply with suitable mixing throughout the entire organ, (2) an allowance of sufficient time for metabolic exchange, and (3) venous drainage through multiple channels, which Ramsey demonstrated in the various areas at the base of the placenta rather than via a single "marginal sinus," as proposed by Spanner. Ramsey contends that "marginal lakes" are actually the peripheral portion of the intervillous space lying within the placenta and that the course of the marginal lakes is discontinuous. This arrangement permits segmental "trapping" of blood when intervillous pressure is higher than that in endometrial veins and permits drainage when pressure is lower.

According to Ramsey, arterial blood enters the placenta from the endometrial arteries under a head of pressure. The incoming stream is driven up in a fountain-like jet toward the chorionic plate. The villi act as baffles, mixing and slowing the stream. The force is gradually spent, and eventually the blood that has dispersed laterally falls back on multiple orifices in the basal plate, which connects with maternal veins. Further fall in pressure in the intervillous space results in drainage through the endometrial veins. The circulatory process is enhanced by myometrial contractions. The authors demonstrated these events convincingly by radioangiographic study of the circulation in the placenta of the rhesus monkey (Fig. 10-9).

Krantz agrees that the villi by their presence act as a baffle and by their pulsations resulting from fetal cardiac action are of great importance in mixing the blood. He adds another factor, contraction of longitudinal smooth muscle of the villi, which he believes provides in effect a "peripheral heart." He suggests that contraction of these fibers brings maternal and fetal surfaces in closer approximation and thus serves a dual purpose: first, in assisting evacuation of the intervillous space and, second, in producing a "milking action" on the fetal side that enhances blood flow through the umbilical vein.

Normally there is no direct connection between maternal and fetal circulations.

TRANSFER MECHANISMS

Oxygen and substances for nutrition of the fetus must pass from the intervillous spaces through the surface epithelium of the villus, its thin stroma, and the endothelium of its capillary. Carbon dioxide and waste products from the fetus are transferred in reverse order. Damaged villi do occasionally break off into the maternal lakes and allow the escape of small amounts of fetal blood into the maternal circulation. Smith and associates, using Cr^{51}-tagged maternal erythrocytes, demonstrated passage of these cells to the cord blood of the newborn infants in 13 out of 18 instances. The rate of transfer averaged 0.3 ml. in 13 hours. The authors suggest that small leaks in the barrier are responsible and that these are common occurrences. Certain cases of Rh sensitization in which incompatible blood has never been given the mother and instances of ABO isoimmunization are related to this phenomenon.

Fetal growth is considerably greater than that of the placenta from the twelfth or fourteenth week to term. The placenta accommodates to greater demands (1) by increasing the surface area of the villi through arborization and (2) by thinning of the villus covering. Langhans' cells become thinned out but do not disappear. Wislocki and Dempsey have shown that many of these cells persist and continue to function throughout pregnancy; however, reduction in their number and in the size of the cells that persist leaves, in effect, a single layer of syncytial cells, thus increasing permeability.

Numerous factors, many of which are yet unknown, influence the *rate* of transfer of substances across the placental barrier. Materials of small molecular size such as electrolytes, water, uric acid, creatine, and creatinine can but do not always pass by simple diffusion. Many drugs, notably narcotics, barbiturates, general anesthetics, sulfonamides, and antibiotics, pass readily. Yet in spite of its obvious influence, the *size of the molecule* is not necessarily the determining factor in movement of materials in either direction. For example, the aldohexoses (glucose, mannose, and galactose) cross the placenta more readily than the ketohexoses (fructose and sorbose). Page refers to the process of speeding up the transfer of certain molecules such as glucose as *facilitated diffusion.* He considers this a form of *active transfer,* carried out by carrier molecules oscillating between the boundaries of the cell. In addition, the placenta achieves active transfer of a far more complex nature by the use of *enzymatic processes* requiring expenditure of energy. In some instances large molecules are broken down by enzymatic action before passage to the fetus, and in others enzyme transport is accomplished against the concentration gradient without alteration of the molecule. Histidine is an example of rapid active transfer of amino acid to the fetus. Fats, on the contrary, do not normally cross the placenta as such. Popjak, using radioactive fatty acids and fats, demonstrated that fats are broken down into fatty acids before passage and are resynthesized by the fetal liver. The passage without structural change of certain antibodies of higher molecular weight as diphtheria or tetanus antitoxin is not readily explained by any of the mechanisms mentioned. Visualization of the ameboid motion of syncytial cells has made tenable the concept of "droplet transfer," or *pinocytosis.* By this means intact macromolecules may be transferred slowly across the membrane.

A great deal remains to be learned in regard to *selective activity* in placental transfer. It is evident that the various mechanisms operate in accordance with the particular demands of the fetus, but the placenta may act as governor. For example, after removal of the fetus, Bothwell and co-workers demonstrated that the intact placenta continues to extract iron from the maternal circulation at approximately the same rate as it did beforehand. Furthermore, in the absence of the normal fetal destination the placenta proved capable of storing iron. Normally certain substances essential for fetal growth occur in higher concentration in the fetal than in the maternal circulation. These include calcium, inorganic phosphorus, free amino acid, nucleic acid, and ascorbic acid.

Bacteria do not normally cross the placenta. Thus the danger to the fetus of pneumonia in the mother is generally related to the degree of maternal anoxia rather than infection. Tuberculosis does not endanger the fetus in utero except when complicated by placenta tuberculoma that erodes into the fetal circulation. *Spirochaeta pallida* pass the placenta particularly after the seventeenth or eighteenth week when the cytotrophoblast is thinned out, but fortunately penicillin administered to the mother for treatment will also pass the barrier and provide fetal protection or treatment, depending upon whether or not the fetus is already infected. Placental transmission of certain viruses has engendered justifiable cause for concern. The virus of rubella crosses the placenta readily and may damage the fetus, especially if infection occurs before the tenth week of gestation. Measles, chickenpox, and poliomyelitis can be transmitted, although the incidence is low. The virus of cytomegalic inclusion disease may affect the fetus in the absence of discernible infection in the mother. These diseases are considered in more detail in Chapter 18.

PLACENTAL HORMONES

In addition to its function as an intrauterine organ of *respiration, nutrition,* and *excretion* for the growing fetus, the placenta functions as an *endocrine gland.* Maternal endocrine functions capable of providing a balance in the hypothalamic-pituitary-ovarian-endometrial axis to ensure ovulation and implantation are all-important in conception, but early in gestation, endocrine regulation is taken over by the fetus and its accessory endocrine organ—the placenta. The interrelationships of fetal, placental, and maternal compartments are extremely complex, but under normal conditions the conceptus maintains regulatory control of its own private hormonal environment. Abnormal conditions arising in any of the three compartments may jeopardize the fetus. The obstetrician encounters many situations in which assessment of the fetus at risk is mandatory. Under these circumstances, a clear

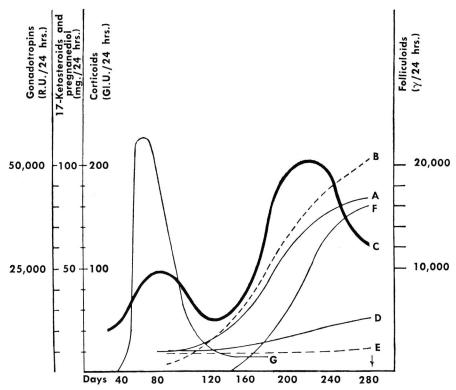

Fig. 10-10. Average values for excretion of various hormones during normal pregnancy. **A,** Pregnanediol; **B,** folliculoids; **C,** corticoids; **D** and **E,** 17-ketosteroids (depending upon method); **G,** gonadotropins. (After Venning; from Selye, H.: Textbook of endocrinology, Montreal, 1947, Acta, Inc.)

understanding of the physiologic and metabolic activities involved is of exceptional value.

The chief purpose of the dramatic changes in endocrine function during pregnancy is to maintain the gestation and to support the fetus in utero until the termination of the gestation period. Modern hormone assay techniques and methods for study of biosynthetic pathways and transfer mechanisms have evoked new concepts of endocrine activity. Several of these are of practical significance.

The classic hormone excretion curves (Fig. 10-10) still provide a valid overall view of alterations during normal gestation, although the excretion curves accepted as normal standards are clearly oversimplified. Normal ranges are variable, and day-to-day changes in excretion rates are found for all measurable hormones; some of them show more pronounced deviations than do others. Means of assessing the actual amounts of the various hormones secreted by (1) ma-

ternal endocrine glands, (2) placenta, and (3) fetal endocrine glands are limited. Degradation, inactivation, and other metabolic changes are carried out in maternal, placental, and fetal organs. Thus excretion rates of the steroids, for instance, represent the end result of many complex actions. Furthermore, increases in one hormone may cause changes in production and metabolism of another.

From a practical point of view the fetus and placenta should be regarded as a single functional unit with the uterus per se as an integral part of this unit.

Human chorionic gonadotropin. Human chorionic gonadotropin (HCG) provides the basis for biologic tests for pregnancy. The hormone is solely of placental origin. The precise site of production of HCG has recently become a controversial issue. The original investigators, Gey and others, grew what they considered to be cytotrophoblastic cells so successfully in tissue culture that they remained functional and produced measurable amounts of HCG. This evidence, and the fact that secretion of HCG is maximal when the cytotrophoblast is prolific and diminishes as this cell layer thins out, led to the belief that HCG is produced by Langhans' cells. Pierce and Midgley, using an immunohistochemical localization technique, found HCG only in the syncytiotrophoblast and could demonstrate none in the cytotrophoblast. It is likely that the syncytium plays an active role in production rather than simply storage and transport of this material. HCG is present in detectable amounts by about the eighth to tenth day after conception and reaches a peak in 50 to 60 days thereafter. During this time the hormone augments and prolongs corpus luteum function and thus maintains the endometrial bed.

HCG is a glycoprotein that in highly purified form exhibits an activity of 12,000 I.U./mg. One international unit represents the reaction produced by 0.1 mg. of a pure standard preparation. Ideally, sensitivity of laboratory test animals (immature rats) is attained when 1 I.U. just induces hyperemia in the rat ovaries. Then 1 I.U. equals 1 hyperemia unit. The kidney clears HCG at a fairly constant rate. Therefore clearance is not a limiting factor in excretion. Changes in urinary excretion determined over a sufficient period of time, that is, 24 hours, may reflect altered production, the direction and magnitude of which are approximately the same as the changes found in serial serum samples.

The hormone is found in all maternal tissues, blood, urine, cerebrospinal fluid, saliva, and vaginal secretions, as well as in placental tissue. Appreciable amounts are found in the amniotic fluid, but only trivial amounts in cord blood. The amount transferred to the fetus directly is not known, but since the fetus swallows amniotic fluid, differences in concentration suggest that the fetus is able to metabolize HCG and convert the hormone to compounds with little or no biologic activity.

Qualitative and quantitative assays. The immunoassay is exceedingly accurate in diagnosis of pregnancy and has all but replaced the bioassay as a straightforward pregnancy test. Bioassays are normally positive from the tenth day after conception until 1 to 3 days after delivery. Immunoassays are often positive by the eighth day after conception

and may remain positive for 8 days or longer after delivery. These differences may result from the fact that breakdown products of metabolism of HCG, which are biologically inactive, induce an immunologic response, or the differences may be because the standard HCG originally injected into rabbits in preparation of the antiserum used in the test is insufficiently pure to induce a totally specific response.

HCG titration test. Specialized immunotechniques have been developed for precise quantitative measurement of HCG in both serum and urine. The immunoassay of serum HCG by quantitative complement fixation devised by Lau and Jones and the radioimmunoassay, which detects levels of HCG in amounts as small as 0.06 I.U./ml., are examples. It is therefore possible to assess disturbed or abnormal pregnancies in the early months of gestation or to evaluate the course of hydatidiform mole or choriocarcinoma equally well and often more rapidly with one of the specific quantitative immunoassays as with a comparably precise bioassay method. Maintenance of a well-standardized rat colony is the first prerequisite of an accurate bioassay. The difficulties that this requirement poses have gradually overshadowed the virtues of the method.

Progesterone. Progesterone can be formed by all steroid-producing endocrine tissues: a small amount from the adrenal, much larger amounts from the corpus luteum of the ovary, the major production by the placental syncytial cells, and an undetermined amount by the fetal adrenals. In the human adrenal gland, progesterone is an intermediary in the biosynthesis of cortisone and aldosterone. It can also be converted to androgens by both adrenal and testes. In the ovary, progesterone can be converted to estrogens. See diagram at the top of the following page.

Functions. The functions of progesterone are chiefly the development and maintenance of the decidual bed. The work of Csapo suggests that it reduces excitability of the uterus, possibly by affecting membrane potentials of the myometrial fibers, particularly at the placental site. Csapo's theory is based on convincing evidence that the effects of the increasing amounts of progesterone transferred from these lipid-rich tissues to

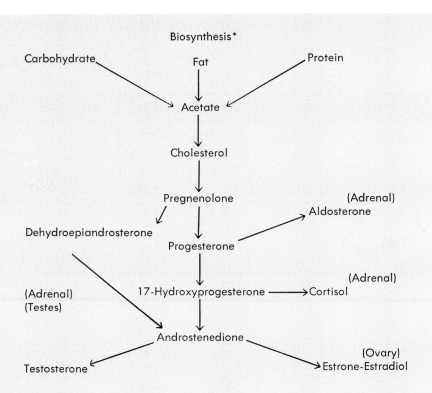

Biosynthesis*

*After Carey, H. M.: Modern trends in human reproductive physiology, Washington, D. C., 1963, Butterworth, Inc.

the adjacent myometrium provide a "progesterone block," which is the major factor preventing the uterus from emptying itself, despite increased distention throughout the course of pregnancy. It is his contention that the uterine volume (V) and progesterone (P) affect the uterus in opposite directions and that the ratio (V:P) is a basic regulatory parameter of the pregnant uterus. His extensive experimental and clinical studies performed in connection with intra-amniotic injection of hypertonic saline to induce labor and delivery strongly support this concept. The hormone appears to have some inhibitory effect on smooth muscle of the ureter, large bowel, and stomach, and it stimulates lobule-alveolar development of the breast.

Metabolism. In late pregnancy the placenta produces about 250 to 300 mg. of progesterone per day. Blood progesterone is metabolized rapidly chiefly in the liver but also in the tissue at its site of action, and a considerable amount disappears into depot fat. The turnover time is approximately 3 minutes. Thus the excretion of the metabolic end product, pregnanediol, excreted in the urine as a glucuronide conjugate, averages only about 10% to 20% of the progesterone produced. On an individual basis excretion rates of pregnanediol show a wide normal range. The mean value is about 50 mg./24 hr. near term (Fig. 10-11). Early pregnancy serial pregnanediol excretion rates have been used by Hamblin and others in prediction of the outcome of threatened abortion with some success. Its use in late pregnancy as an index of fetal well-being is limited. Consistently low levels may indicate chronic placental insufficiency, but sudden drops in pregnanediol excretion rates do not appear promptly enough to detect fetal jeopardy in time to initiate definitive measures. At the end of a 15-year investigation of pregnanediol excretion rates, Rawlings concluded that serial tests do not provide a confident basis for the prognosis of a pregnancy. Perhaps some metabolites other than pregnanediol would provide a better picture of progesterone production. In this connection Hytten's comment is appropriate: "It is

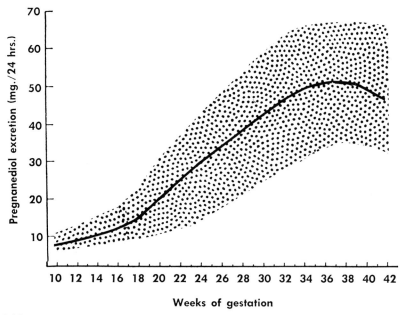

Fig. 10-11. Excretion of pregnanediol during normal pregnancy.

curious that so much research has been expended on polishing the technique for estimating pregnanediol and so little on discovering how faithfully it is likely to represent its parent hormone."

Estrogens. The amount of estrogens secreted in the third trimester is enormously increased over nonpregnant levels. Gestation levels drop precipitously after delivery or after intrauterine death of the fetus. The range of normal estrogen excretion rate is wide. Taken on an individual basis, the gestational increase in estrone and in estradiol is approximately a hundredfold, whereas the increase in estriol is a thousandfold as compared with individual nonpregnant values.

A comparison of mean values for 24-hour urinary estrogen secretion is given in Table 6.

Biosynthetic pathways of estrogens. New concepts of certain fetal and placental functions and new laboratory tools for assessing intrauterine fetal welfare have arisen as a result of recent studies of estrogen metabolism in gravid women. An understanding of the mechanisms involved is important in selection of the appropriate laboratory tests and for valid interpretation of results.

In normally menstruating women the ovary produces estrogens de novo princi-

pally, if not entirely, in the biologically active forms estradiol and estrone. Most of the estriol in nongravid women is derived from the peripheral metabolism of secreted estrone and estradiol. The following diagram of ovarian estrogen biosynthesis is based on the results of ovarian tissue incubation experiments performed by Smith and Ryan. Using radioactive substrates, these investigators obtained a yield of estrone plus estradiol amounting to 0.03% from acetate, 0.1% from cholesterol, 5.5% from progesterone, and 15% from androstenedione. (Note the increasing yield from intermediates closer on the pathway to the end product.)

The finding of these compounds in the incubation experiments indicates that any one or all of the biosynthetic pathways shown could be operative in human ovaries. Estradiol can be converted to estrone and vice versa, but estriol cannot be reconverted to either. Estradiol is by far the most biologically active, whereas estriol is biologically very weak. The biologic activity of estriol is approximately $\frac{1}{100}$ that of estrone and $\frac{1}{500}$ that of estradiol. It is obvious, therefore, that biologic assays of estrogens will not give the same answer as chemical assays. Since the bioassay results are determined to a great extent by the amount of

Table 6. Comparison of mean values for 24-hour urinary estrogen secretion*

Menstrual cycle	Estrone	Estradiol	Estriol	Total
Early proliferative (days 1 - 7)	0 - 7†	Trace	2 - 11	3 - 20
Ovulatory peak (days 10 - 16)	15 - 27	3 - 22	8 - 120	30 - 150
Postovulatory peak (days 20 - 26)	5 - 25	2 - 11	5 - 90	15 - 100
Pregnancy				
First trimester	To 200	To 70	To 500	
Second trimester	To 1000	To 300	To 10,000	
Third trimester	To 2000	To 1000	To 40,000	

*From Goldzieher, J. W.: Estrogens and progesterones. In Meigs, J. V., and Sturgis, S. H., editors: Progress in gynecology, vol. 4, New York, 1963, Grune & Stratton, Inc.
†All values are expressed in micrograms.

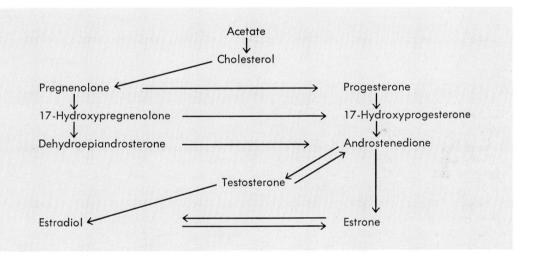

estradiol in the specimen, bioassay methods may be useful in certain endocrinopathies, but they are not applicable in assessing placental function.

Contrary to previous assumption, the placenta does not synthesize estrogen de novo to any significant degree. If placental tissue per se were capable of producing estrogens, high excretion might be expected in cases of hydatidiform mole, but such is not the case. Clearly the placenta is not autonomous in this regard. Instead, a viable placenta and an intact fetal circulation are necessary for continuous production of this steroid. When these two prerequisites exist, the placenta is highly efficient in conversion of steroid precursors to estrogens, mainly estriol. A much lower percentage of estriol is formed from conversion of estrone and estradiol in pregnant than in nonpregnant women. Most of the estriol of late pregnancy appears to be derived from primitive steroids such as pregnenolone and dehydroepiandrosterone. These precursors are produced by both the maternal and the fetal organisms, the fetal adrenal apparently playing a major role. This concept is supported by studies of pregnancies associated with an anencephalic fetus. Anencephaly is commonly associated with severe atrophy of the adrenal cortex involving the characteristic and ordinarily large fetal zone, which may disappear almost completely. Frandsen and Stakemann studied 15 cases of pregnancy associated with an anencephalic fetus and found critically low levels of estriol excretion in all but one. In the only exception the infant adrenals were of normal size and contained a well-developed fetal zone. Excretion of 17-ketosteroids, 17-ketogenic steroids, pregnanediol, and chorionic gonadotropin was normal. All fetuses were alive at the time of urine collection for assay. The placentas were normal, and there were no signs of a disturbed fetal circulation.

These investigators further demonstrated the important role played by the fetal adrenals by simultaneous injection of fetal adrenal tissue and placental tissue in castrate mice. Vaginal smears were obtained daily after injection of fetal adrenal tissue alone. Smears were negative in all tests. Negative results were also obtained after injection of placental tissue alone. But when both tissues were injected intraperitoneally or subcutaneously at the same time, positive vaginal smears were obtained in 12 of 15 cases. It was necessary to use living fetal adrenal and living placental tissues to obtain a positive response. The foregoing clinical and laboratory data point to the fetal adrenals as the source of precursors, and to the placenta as the organ for their metabolism to estrogens.

The importance of an intact fetal circulation in estrogen production is illustrated by the experiments of Cassmer. Therapeutic interruptions carried out by the vaginal route at approximately 20 weeks' gestation were studied as follows: The umbilical cord was brought through the cervix, ligated, and sectioned. Fetus and placenta were allowed to remain in situ for 3 days. Within 24 hours estriol values dropped more than 70% below previous levels. Progesterone values dropped only 20%, and chorionic gonadotropic titers remained the same. Perfusion of the placenta with maternal blood for up to 3 hours could almost restore preoperative estrogen levels, suggesting that the blood

perfused contained sufficient precursors to maintain estrogen production at least for the duration of the experiment.

The fetus actively conjugates estrogens, mainly as sulfates and, to a far lesser extent, as glucosiduronates. This ability is acquired at an early stage—usually by 16 weeks' gestation. Sulfurylation can be performed by many fetal organs: liver, lungs, gastrointestinal tract, skin. Through conjugation, biologically active compounds are converted to relatively weak compounds. The efficiency of this action suggests that it may be an important step for fetal defense against excessive estrogenization.

Some of the most precise studies of estrogen metabolism in pregnancy have come from Diczfalusy's laboratory at the Karolinska Institute in Stockholm. The results of in situ perfusion studies using various radioisotopes may be summarized as follows: The primitive steroids are produced mainly by the fetus, principally the fetal adrenal glands. The main precursor is dehydroepiandrosterone sulfate (DHAS). In the nonpregnant state most of the urinary estriol is derived from estrone and estradiol. During pregnancy the pathway exists within the fetoplacental unit for direct conversion of DHAS to estriol without estradiol as an intermediate. This involves the formation of 16-hydroxy-DHAS, which also takes places in the fetal adrenal. The placenta shows very little 16-hydroxylaing activity but strong enzymatic activity in the final conversion to estriol, the aromatization of ring A of the steroid nucleus. The conjugates are returned to the placenta and transferred to the maternal circulation, mainly as estriol. The estrogen is metabolized and conjugated in the maternal liver mainly as a glucosiduronate and is excreted largely in this form in the urine. The 24-hour urinary estriol values, therefore, can serve as an indication of fetoplacental function in the gravid woman whose hepatic and renal functions are within normal limits. Current studies in our laboratories suggest that renal clearance of estriol may be reduced in cases of maternal renal disease, and urinary values may be misleadingly low. In such cases estriol clearance determinations have proved useful.

One other aspect of estriol metabolism of clinical importance is the amount found in amniotic fluid in late pregnancy. Most of the free estriol returned to the fetus from the placenta is sulfurylated by various fetal organs, but a small amount is conjugated as the glucosiduronate, presumably by the fetal liver. Both the free and the sulfate forms clear the amniotic membrane rapidly, but the glucosiduronate accumulates. It is conceivable that compromise of fetal hepatic function, which occurs in erythroblastosis, for example, before fetal adrenal activity is affected, may be reflected in low amniotic fluid estriol values whereas maternal urinary estriol is still in the normal range. Behrman and co-workers found that values less than 100 μg./L. were consistently indicative of fetal jeopardy in cases of erythroblastosis.

The range of normal urinary excretion per 24 hours is quite wide, beginning with approximately 1 mg. at 18 to 20 weeks, gradually increasing to between 4 and 8 mg. at 28 to 30 weeks, and between 8 and 25 mg. or more at 38 to 42 weeks (Fig. 10-12). The curve for any given individual rises gradually to term and is roughly correlated with the fetal weight. Greene and Touchstone showed that when estriol output equals 12 mg./24 hr. or more, the fetal weight was 2,500 grams or more (P = 0.01). Daily fluctuations in estriol excretion values are common, but precipitous drops below 50% of previous peak values are warning signals. Fetal welfare is threatened when values in the range of 3 to 4 mg. are found in late pregnancy, and fetal death is almost inevitable if the daily excretion is below 2 mg.

Human placental lactogen. A growth hormonelike substance possessing lactogenic and luteotrophic properties, which like chorionic gonadotropin is synthesized solely by the placenta, was isolated in 1962 by Josimovich and Maclaren. This hormone, called "human placental lactogen" (HPL) by Josimovich and chorionic "growth hormone-prolactin" (CGP) by Kaplan and Grumbach, is a polypeptide and shows immunologic cross-reaction, although incomplete, with human pituitary growth hormone (HGH). Greater purification of these substances has proved that HPL can be distinguished from HGH, and its importance in normal pregnancy is only recently gaining recognition.

HPL is produced by the syncytiotropho-

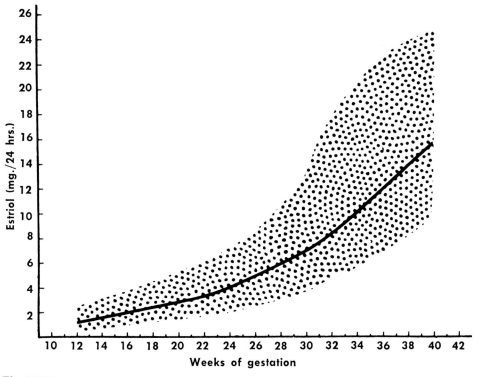

Fig. 10-12. Excretion of estriol during normal pregnancy.

blast and is transferred almost exclusively into the maternal circulation. Small but increasing amounts are transferred into the amniotic fluid, but negligible amounts are passed into the fetal circulation. The hormone is detectable in maternal serum or urine as early as the sixth week of gestation. Secretion increases progressively to term with serum values showing a tenfold or more increase in late pregnancy and prompt decrease after delivery. In contrast to the gestational increases in estriol or in diamine oxidase, production of HPL is not fully dependent upon the presence of a viable fetus. The hormone has been extracted from molar tissue as well as from the serum of patients with hydatidiform mole and choriocarcinoma. Serum levels have been found to be higher in healthy twin pregnancies than in singletons, but the weight of the placenta in single pregnancies, the birth weight of the infant, or the parity of the mother do not correlate well with the concentration of serum HPL at delivery. It is possible that placental function rather than placental weight is being measured. Nevertheless, the blood level curve for HPL during normal pregnancy appears to be sufficiently characteristic to indicate its potential use as an index of placental function and probably, therefore, of fetal health. Preliminary studies of Spellacy, Cohen, and Carlson demonstrated that the curve for serum HPL and 24-hour urinary estriol excretion rates showed parallel rises in normal cases and that the serum HPL level fell prior to fetal death in an abnormal pregnancy. The test deserves further study and may be of value in assessment of placental disorders in particular.

The appearance of a trophoblastic HPL early in pregnancy suggests that HPL may augment the luteotrophic effect of HCG and may be essential for full development of the corpus luteum of pregnancy. HPL shows no growth-promoting activity in itself, but it greatly increases the anabolic effects of HGH. This synergistic action is of importance in connection with nitrogen retention, essential for growth during pregnancy. New techniques have made possible critical studies of the growth hormonelike properties of HPL and its metabolic role in pregnancy. These have greatly enhanced understanding of protein, fat, and carbohydrate metabo-

lism during pregnancy, all of which show influences of growth hormone or growth hormonelike activity. The rate of secretion of HPL is very high and, according to Grumbach, far exceeds the excretion rate of any known human polypeptide hormone. During late pregnancy the concentration of HPL in the maternal circulation is approximately one thousandfold greater than that of HGH, but the HPL level in the fetal circulation is low (approximately $\frac{1}{300}$ that of the mother). In contrast the concentration of HGH is strikingly elevated in the fetal but not in the maternal circulation.

The concept that HPL plays a key role in maternal metabolic adjustments of pregnancy, as suggested by Grumbach and co-workers, is based upon these findings. Both HPL and HGH stimulate release of free fatty acids, the mobilization of fat stores thus providing an alternate pathway of metabolism. At the same time an elevated level of free fatty acids acts as a specific peripheral insulin antagonist and results in a compensatory exaggerated production of insulin. The utilization of fat stores as fuel through the concerted action of HPL and insulin would, in turn, increase maternal capacity for protein and glucose sparing. This hypothesis is particularly convincing in light of well-established biochemical changes characteristic of abnormalities in carbohydrate metabolism during pregnancy and is further discussed in Chapter 19.

Relaxin. The nonsteroid hormone relaxin appears in the blood of women early in pregnancy and increases gradually to term. Zarrow and co-workers found a serum level of 0.2 guinea pig units per milliliter at 7 weeks, a maximum of 2 guinea pig units per milliliter at term, and disappearance of this hormone within 24 hours post partum. For this reason it is thought possible that the placenta may be its source during pregnancy rather than the ovary, which is known to produce small amounts. Relaxation of the pelvic ligaments and connective tissues in various parts of the body may represent a relaxin effect per se or a synergistic action with progesterone.

Adrenocorticotropic hormone. The fact that corticosteroids are normally increased as pregnancy advances indicates an increased production of ACTH. Large quantities of ACTH have been repeatedly recovered from placental extracts, although there is some controversy as to whether the placenta acts as a repository for storage of ACTH or is the actual site of the increased gestational production.

Adrenal corticosteroid hormones. It is doubtful that the placenta synthesizes adrenal corticosteroids. Berliner and associates have demonstrated the presence of cortisol, cortisone, 11-dehydrocorticosterone, aldosterone, and several of their degradation products in placental extracts. Salhanick contends that the increased amounts of cortisone found in these placentas can be accounted for, first, by the volume of trapped blood present and, second, by the ability of the placenta to concentrate this hormone. His experiments in administration of radioactive cortisone to pregnant women revealed a placental concentration 2.2 times that in the peripheral blood. The increased binding capacity of plasma globulin during pregnancy probably accounts for the fact that the high levels of 17-hydroxycorticosteroids, which equal or exceed those normally found in Cushing's syndrome, do not produce symptoms of this disease. Sandberg and Slaunwhite demonstrated that the cortisol-binding protein transcortin is increased during pregnancy and after estrogen administration. Protein-bound cortisol appears to be biologically inactive. Aldosterone excretion begins to increase early in the second trimester and rises gradually to term.

Excretion of 17-ketosteroids shows only a slight rise during normal pregnancy. Venning found elevated values similar to those reported by several other investigators only when the method used was nonspecific and metabolites of progesterone were included in the final reading.

PLACENTAL ENZYMES

Considering the diversity of physiologic and metabolic functions required of the placenta for maintenance and development of the fetus, it is not surprising that a large number of enzymes should be demonstrated within its substance. Hagerman tabulates 64 of these catalytic agents whose presence within placental tissues have been established. Attempts have been made to correlate quantitative measurements of several enzymes in maternal plasma with normal and abnormal pregnancies.

Diamine oxidase (histaminase). Diamine oxidase (DAO) is an enzyme involved in the degradation of histamine and other diamines such as cadaverine and putrescine. Histamine is important in the metabolism of all growing tissues and is found in especially high concentration in fetal tissues. DAO is considered an adaptive enzyme produced by the mother in response to the increased production of the specific amine by the fetus. Southren and co-workers studied the relative DAO activity of fetal and maternal tissues and found maximal activity in the retroplacental decidua. No significant increase in maternal DAO is induced by trophoblastic tumors. Instead, the presence of a fetus is necessary to induce enzyme production. Measurable increases in DAO can be detected within 5 to 6 weeks after the last normal menstrual period, followed by a rapid rise to approximately 20 weeks, at which time levels tend to plateau and drop sharply within 2 to 4 days after delivery. The clinical use of DAO levels in following the course of pregnancy is evident in the extensive studies by Weingold and by Southren. Since the assay is economical and rapid, it is likely to gain more widespread use.

Oxytocinase (cystine-amino-peptidase). Oxytocinase activity increases between 50% and 100% during normal pregnancy. The source is presumed to be the syncytiotrophoblast. Babuna and Yenen contend that serial oxytocinase levels in the maternal serum accurately reflect the functional capacity of the placenta but that they are not useful in conditions where fetal jeopardy is due to fetal factors per se.

Alkaline phosphatase. Maternal serum alkaline phosphatase activity increases progressively during the last trimester of pregnancy. Both maternal and fetal sources contribute to the increase. The placental alkaline phosphatase is heat stable, whereas all other alkaline phosphatase is not. Thus the rising levels in maternal serum in late pregnancy represent placental function capacity, on the one hand, and the degree of mobilization of calcium from maternal bone, on the other. It does not appear to be sufficiently specific for clinical use at this time.

THE TERM PLACENTA

The *placenta at term* is a discoid organ, measuring 15 to 20 cm. by 2 to 3 cm. Its weight is roughly 500 grams, or about one sixth the weight of the infant at term except in patients with erythroblastosis or syphilis, in whom oversized placentas are characteristic. The maternal surface is divided by decidual septa into 15 or 20 cotyledons. The umbilical cord is usually inserted near the central portion of the smooth fetal surface. Fetal vessels are readily visible fanning out from the base of the cord. These diminish and disappear as they reach the periphery of the placenta.

The *umbilical cord* averages about 55 cm. in length. Cord measurements, however, may vary considerably in thickness as well as in length. Connective tissue with high water content (Wharton's jelly) surrounds the single umbilical vein and two arteries and facilitates desiccation after the cord is tied. The vessels are usually longer than the cord, become folded upon themselves, and give rise to false knots, which do not interfere with circulation.

Amniotic fluid. The volume of amniotic fluid usually averages about 50 ml. at 10 weeks' gestation, 200 ml. at 16 weeks' gestation, and approximately 1 L. at term. Water content is about 98%, and solids comprise 2%. Reaction is alkaline. Theories regarding its source include (1) secretion by amniotic epithelium, (2) transudation from maternal blood, (3) fetal urine, and (4) mixed origin. Recent experiments clearly demonstrate a mixed source. Chez, Smith, and Hutchinson performed direct catheterization of the monkey fetus in utero and confirmed the fact that the kidneys contribute significantly to the quantity of amniotic fluid. In the monkey fetus near term this amounts to 5 ml./kg./hr. Scoggin and co-workers, using an ingenious experimental model, demonstrated an exchange of water from mother to fetus and from amniotic fluid to maternal tissues across the placental site and the fetal membranes, respectively. According to their calculations the total body exchange across the amniochorion amounts to 25.5 moles per hour with a net flow of 100 ml./hr. from amniotic fluid to maternal circulation. The observations of Hutchinson and his colleagues indicate that the umbilical cord probably plays a very important role in the transfer of water from the amniotic sac, a fact not previously appreciated. It should be clear that the amniotic fluid is not a static medium but is continuously renewed. Vosburgh and associates, using radioactive sodium and deuterium oxide tracers, demonstrated a complete sodium exchange in 15 hours and water exchange in less than 3 hours.

Ultrastructure of the human amnion reveals the presence of an extensive system of canals and channels within the amniotic epithelium. Bourne and Lacy found that these channels communicate with lateral and basal vacuoles and with the extracellular space. It is a logical speculation that existence of this system is an important factor in the movement of amniotic fluid.

The rate of transfer of various substances, including drugs, is of practical importance in the management of the complications of pregnancy and in the conduct of labor and delivery of the infant. Apgar detected barbiturates in amniotic fluid, the placenta, and fetal organs within 15 minutes after intravenous injection in the mother. Since deglutition and respiration occur in utero from the fourth month on, amniotic fluid may afford an additional route for transmission of various substances to the fetus.

Constituents of amniotic fluid. Sampling of amniotic fluid has become one of the most important of diagnostic procedures for assessing the fetal status. Information regarding Rh isoimmunization, maturity, genetic disorders, and certain metabolic disturbances can now be obtained by cytologic and biochemical examination of the fluid at various stages of pregnancy.

Genetic information can be obtained from cells found in the amniotic fluid. Such studies are usually performed between the twelfth and fourteenth weeks of gestation. Prenatal sex determination can be made accurately and is useful in counseling regarding pregnancies in women who are heterozygous for sex-linked recessive disorders such as muscular dystrophy or hemophilia. Chromosomal aberrations involving the number and structure of chromosomes such as Down's syndrome have been detected as well as chromosomal breaks in fetal cells from mothers exposed to rubella and LSD. Biochemical studies of cultures derived from amniotic fluid containing cells allow pre-

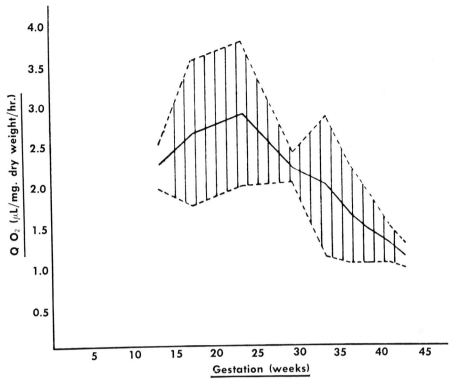

Fig. 10-13. Normal placental oxygen utilization. (From Tremblay, P. C.: Amer. J. Obstet. Gynec. **91**:600, 1965.)

natal diagnosis of an increasing number of hereditary metabolic disorders including cystic fibrosis, mucopolysaccharidosis, Marfan's syndrome, galactosemia, and Pompe's disease. The field of prenatal genetics, although newly born, is unquestionably a major medical advance.

Diagnosis of maturity. Creatinine concentration and fetal cells in amniotic fluid show changes with advancing pregnancy, and attempts are being made to determine which of these correlate most closely with fetal age. These studies are described in Chapter 17.

Placental oxygen utilization. During the first half of pregnancy the rate of oxygen uptake by the placenta is high, but according to Tremblay there is a gradual diminution in intrinsic placental metabolic activity from a high peak at about 25 weeks to more moderate levels at term as the fetus takes on more and more metabolic responsibility for itself (Fig. 10-13).

■ Disorders of the placenta

Variations in shape. The outline of the placenta may appear elongated or kidney shaped, or there may be two or three incompletely separated lobes. These lobes are termed *placenta bipartita* or *placenta tripartita*, respectively. Most of the atypical forms occur as a result of minor alterations in the blood supply or nutritional state of the decidua early in gestation, but they have no real clinical significance.

Placenta succenturiata. One or more accessory lobes may be found at variable distances from the main placenta. Vessels from the accessory lobe traverse the fetal membranes and continue over the surface of the placenta proper. During the third stage of labor these vessels may be torn and the succenturiate lobe retained within the uterus. Postpartum hemorrhage or infection may occur if the detached tissue is not recognized and removed. Diagnosis can be made if inspection of the fetal surface reveals an open vessel at the placental edge.

Placenta circumvallata. A white fibrous ring is occasionally visible on the fetal surface at a variable distance from the margin of the placenta. The ring is formed by a folding back of the amnion and of the

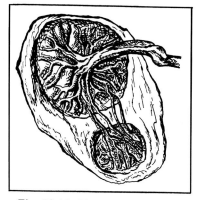

Fig. 10-14. Placenta succenturiata.

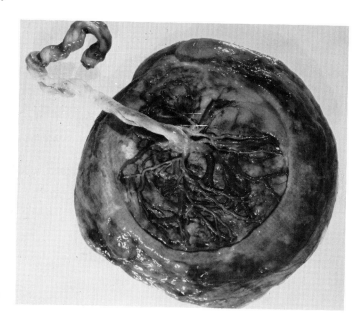

Fig. 10-15. Placenta circumvallata.

chorion upon itself, forming a double layer of fetal membranes at this site. This is presumed to occur when the early chorionic plate is relatively small. As the nutritional demands of the fetus increase, the limited decidua basalis is insufficient to meet the demand, and villi at the periphery grow out laterally into the decidua vera. The fetal vessels do not extend to the margin of the placenta but instead terminate at the ring. In other respects the placenta is normal.

The incidence of abortion early in pregnancy and bleeding late in pregnancy or during labor may be somewhat increased in association with this condition, but in most instances the course of pregnancy and the condition of the infant are unaffected.

Placenta membranacea. Occasionally the villi covering the decidua capsularis persist, continue to function, and form a large, thin, membranous placenta that entirely surrounds the fetal membranes. Its attachment therefore is not confined to one portion of the uterus but, instead, covers the surface completely. Separation or expulsion of a placenta membranacea during the third stage of labor may be incomplete, and consequently the danger of immediate or delayed postpartum hemorrhage is increased.

Placental infarcts. Avascular areas of varying size and consistency can be found in almost all placentas at term. Many of these are not true infarcts. White or yellowish

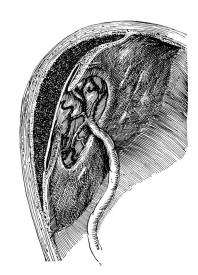

Fig. 10-16. Diagram of placenta circumvallata showing reduplication of chorionic plate and growth of villi beyond its margin.

nodules are commonly *fibrin deposits*, indicative of the aging process in the placenta. Zeek and Assali found evidence that small foci of degenerating trophoblasts initiate localized thrombosis of the surrounding maternal blood. Fine laminations of fibrin are laid down usually parallel to the chorionic plate. These were formerly designated as "white infarcts," but the term is misleading because the process is primarily degenerative

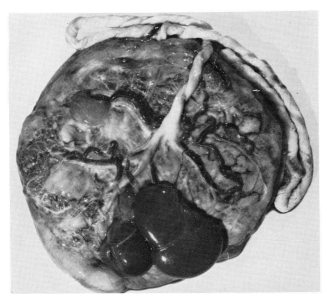

Fig. 10-17. Placental cyst.

rather than vascular. Fibrin deposition is rarely so extensive as to jeopardize the fetus.

True placental infarcts are localized areas of necrosis caused by obstruction of the nutritional blood supply. Since the placenta receives its nourishment through the maternal rather than the fetal circulation, infarction occurs only when the maternal side is interrupted. Upon cessation of the blood flow to a cotyledon, the intervillous spaces become ischemic, and the villi deprived of nutrition undergo necrosis. The lesion may appear pale, red, or grayish, depending upon its age.

Rupture of thin-walled or brittle vessels with extravasation of blood into the decidua and subsequent hematoma formation may also cause ischemic necrosis. The placenta becomes detached in the area of bleeding, and if separation is extensive, the fetus will die in utero. Although rupture of decidual vessels may occur without obvious cause, its occurrence is most common in patients with hypertension or chronic renal disease.

Calcification. Small areas of calcification are frequently found in the normal placenta. In some instances the entire maternal surface feels sandy upon palpation. Occasionally, firm white plaques are found in one or more regions. Like fibrin deposits, these are the result of degeneration of the villi, a late phase in the aging process of the placenta, and have no clinical significance.

Infection. Placental infection may occur in instances of prolonged rupture of the membranes with or without prolonged labor. An *amnionitis* develops first and may spread locally to the placenta. If the process extends through the chorionic vessels, general infection may develop in the fetus. Infection of the placenta is seldom primary, and infection resulting from a *maternal bacteremia* is relatively rare. *Syphilis* frequently involves the placenta, causing thickening and clubbing of the villi. The number of villous blood vessels is reduced because of endarteritic changes. Grossly the syphilitic placenta is large in relation to the weight of the infant and presents a greasy, yellowish surface with poorly defined cotyledons. Placental *tuberculosis* is exceedingly uncommon even when the disease in the mother is advanced.

Cysts. Cysts are frequently found on the fetal surface and arise from the chorionic membrane. They vary in size up to 5 or 6 cm. and are filled with yellowish or bloody fluid. Cysts found deep in the substance of the placenta usually represent advanced degenerative changes in areas of fibrin deposition or in old infarcts.

Tumors. Neoplasms of the placenta are unusual. Of those observed, chorioangioma is most common. DeCosta and co-workers found an associated hydramnios in one third of these cases.

■ Abnormalities of the cord

Variations in length of the cord between 35 and 70 cm. are normal, the average length being about 55 cm. Complete absence of the cord is sometimes observed in connection with defects in the fetal abdominal wall. A *short cord* may delay descent of the fetus during labor and result in detachment of the placenta or, rarely, rupture of the cord with traction. A *long cord* predisposes to prolapse or cord entanglement. Tightening of loops about the neck or body of the infant during descent may gradually impair circulation and cause asphyxia. *True knots* are found occasionally in the cord, but unless these become tightened, fetal circulation is unimpaired.

Variations in insertion of the cord. The umbilical cord is usually inserted eccentrically but nearer the central than the peripheral portion of the placenta. A marginal insertion, designated as *battledore placenta,* is relatively common and unimportant. On the other hand, *velamentous insertion* of the cord is potentially hazardous to the fetus. Vessels separate from the umbilical cord and traverse the membranes for a variable distance before reaching the placenta. Tearing or rupture of the vessels during labor may exsanguinate the infant. If the vessels course over the dilating cervix in bulging membranes *(vasa praevia),* pressure by the presenting part may cause fetal distress or asphyxia.

Vascular anomalies. The cord should be checked at delivery for the presence of one vein and two arteries. A single umbilical artery is found in slightly less than 1% of cases, but this abnormality is associated with a high incidence of congenital anomalies of the newborn as is the presence of intraplacental shunts and aneurysms. A specific type of arteriovenous shunt is seen occasionally in monozygotic twins; a fetoplacental transfusion syndrome is the result. The arterial donor twin is pale and dehydrated, whereas the venous recipient is plethoric, hypervolemic, and in greatest danger of cardiac overload.

■ Abnormalities of the amnion

Hydramnios. The accumulation of amniotic fluid in excess of 2,000 ml. is considered abnormal. Hydramnios usually develops gradually, but in rare instances acute hydramnios occurs, the uterus becoming remarkably distended within the course of a few days. The etiology remains obscure, although various factors associated with this condition are recognized. *Fetal anomalies,* particularly those of the central nervous system, are more frequent if hydramnios is present. The occurrence of anencephaly,

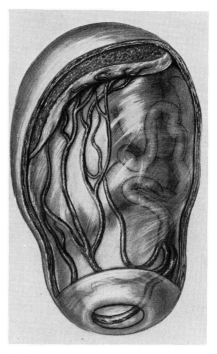

Fig. 10-19. Velamentous insertion of the cord with vasa praevia.

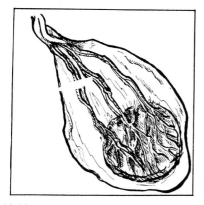

Fig. 10-18. Velamentous insertion of the cord.

spina bifida, duodenal atresia, or tracheo-esophageal fistula has led to the theory that an increased fetal output of fluid via the spinal fluid system or the urinary tract, or failure of the fetus to ingest fluid may cause hydramnios. This theory does not explain the increased incidence of hydramnios observed with *maternal diabetes* or *erythroblastosis.* An abnormality in placental transmission of fluids from the fetal circulation or an abnormally functioning amniotic membrane may be responsible.

Symptoms are more pronounced with acute than with chronic hydramnios. The patient suffers from pain due to overdistention of the uterus and abdominal wall, edema of the lower extremities, and severe dyspnea. The accumulation may be so rapid and so enormous that prompt evacuation is necessary to prevent maternal death.

Hydramnios should be suspected if the uterus appears larger than normal for the duration of pregnancy or if the fetal parts and fetal heart tones are indistinct. The condition must be differentiated from multiple pregnancy. Diagnosis can be made with certainty by x-ray examination, while at the same time certain fetal deformities involving the skull and skeletal part may be detected. Further information can be obtained by amniography. This technique includes amniocentesis with removal of 25 ml. of amniotic fluid under sterile conditions and insertion of 15 ml. or with severe hydramnios, 25 to 30 ml. of contrast media such as Renographin 60 or Hypaque 75. These dye solutions are hypertonic and may initiate labor. The inclination to use large amounts of dye to compensate for the excessive amounts of fluid should be rejected. The fetus swallows and concentrates the dye in the gastrointestinal tract. The roentgenogram should be delayed and taken 1 to 2 hours after instillation of contrast material, when concentration in the gastrointestinal tract can provide information regarding gastrointestinal atresia or other soft tissue abnormalities. This type of examination is also of great value in determining placental site, uterine deformities or tumors, intrauterine fetal death, and hydatidiform mole in addition to clear-cut information regarding the degree of hydramnios.

Medical treatment of hydramnios is generally ineffectual. The patient with chronic hydramnios and only mild symptoms should be kept as comfortable as possible with rest, low-salt diet, and diuretics and should be permitted to go into labor spontaneously. Since contractions are sometimes of poor quality because of overdistention of the uterus, progress in labor may be slow, and the incidence of postpartum hemorrhage is increased because of atony. Amniotomy becomes necessary if symptoms are progressive or severe. The cervix is usually effaced because of pressure. Rupture of the membrane should be carried out under aseptic conditions, and attempt should be made to drain the fluid slowly. Free or rapid flow may encourage prolapse of the cord or a fetal part, and sudden reduction in size of the uterus may cause placental separation.

Removal of fluid by transabdominal aspiration or insertion of polyethylene tubing into the uterus has met with little success, since the fluid reaccumulates or labor ensues shortly thereafter.

Hydramnios developing in Rh-sensitized mothers or in patients with diabetes offers an unfavorable prognosis for fetal survival. If the gestation period is sufficiently advanced, delivery is often advisable, and preparations should be made for special care of the infant.

Oligohydramnios. Marked deficiency or absence of amniotic fluid is exceedingly rare. The etiology is unknown, but when present the condition is generally associated with fetal urinary tract anomalies. Potter describes 49 cases of fetal renal agenesis from the Chicago Lying-In Hospital, and in none could the presence of any amniotic fluid be documented.

Relative diminution in the amount of amniotic fluid is sometimes noted late in pregnancy in connection with postmaturity.

■ Fetal development

From fertilization until organogenesis is largely completed, about the eighth week, the conceptus is designated as the *embryo,* after which time it is called the *fetus.* The significant features of the various developmental stages are shown in Table 7.

The rate of fetal growth is proportionately more rapid in the early months of pregnancy. According to *Haase's rule* the length of the fetus in centimeters equals the square of the lunar month during the first

Table 7. Principal embryonal and fetal characteristics at various developmental stages

Gestation period	Length (crown to heel)	Weight	Characteristics
3 weeks			Beginning of gastrointestinal tract followed by cardiac development; appearance of limb buds
4 weeks	1 cm.		Anlage for all organs present
12 weeks	9 cm.	15 grams	Fingers and toes visible; appearance of centers of ossification in most bones
16 weeks	16 cm.	110 grams	Sex revealed by external genitals; appearance of respiratory movements and swallowing reflexes; meconium present
20 weeks	25 cm.	300 grams	Fetal movements detectable
24 weeks	30 cm.	630 grams	Skin less transparent; fine lanugo over body
28 weeks	35 cm.	1,045 grams	Fetus viable although survival rate low
36 weeks	45 cm.	2,500 grams	Appearance of ossification center in distal femoral epiphysis

5 months. In the last 5 months the length is equal to five times the lunar month of pregnancy. Thus:

At end of third lunar month $3 \times 3 = 9$ cm.
fetal length
At end of sixth lunar month $6 \times 5 = 30$ cm.
fetal length
At term $10 \times 5 = 50$ cm.
fetal length

Despite obvious difficulties in obtaining precise crown-heel measurements, the length of the fetus usually provides a more reliable index of gestation period than does the weight. The importance of a more accurate estimate of fetal maturity is underscored by follow-up studies of "small for date" babies, "low birth weight infants," or intrauterine growth retardation problems. The common causes are intrauterine malnutrition or fetal maldevelopment. Comparison of the newborn measurements with those of standard fetal growth charts such as that developed by Lubchenco and co-workers should be routine nursery practice.

The *infant at term* measures 20 inches (50 cm.) and weighs about 7 pounds (3,175 grams). Very little lanugo remains except over the shoulders. A variable amount of vernix caseosa covers the skin surfaces; this is a mixture of epithelial cells, lanugo, and the secretion of the sebaceous glands. Characteristic features of the fetal head including suture lines, fontanels, and diameters are of obstetric importance. The sutures and fontanels that serve as useful landmarks are the

long *sagittal suture,* which separates the two parietal bones, and the *lambdoid suture* between the posterior edge of the parietal bones and the occipital bone. The triangular-shaped space at the intersection of these two lines is the *posterior fontanel.* The *frontal suture* separates the frontal bones from each other, and the *coronal suture* separates the anterior edge of the parietal bones from the frontal bones. The large *anterior fontanel* is the diamond-shaped space at the junction of the sagittal, coronal, and frontal sutures.

Fetal circulation. Initially the developing ovum derives nutrition from its own large cytoplasmic mass and then from the decidua by activity of the trophoblastic cells. The vitelline circulation is functional in the third and fourth weeks and temporarily provides nourishment for the embryo from the yolk sac. Thereafter connection is made between vessels developing in the chorion and those growing out from the fetus through the body stalk to establish the fetal-placental circulation.

Oxygen and nutrient substances pass from the maternal blood through the villi and are transported through small venules to the single umbilical vein. This divides at the liver edge. One branch empties into the portal vein, circulates through the liver, and enters the inferior vena cava through the hepatic vein. The larger portion passes directly to the inferior vena cava as the ductus venosus. In the right atrium oxygen-laden blood coming via the inferior vena cava

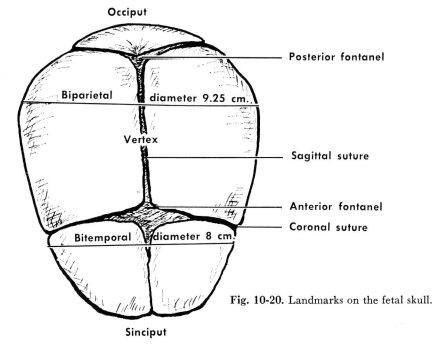

Fig. 10-20. Landmarks on the fetal skull.

passes for the most part through the foramen ovale into the left atrium. That blood from the head region delivered via the superior vena cava is low in oxygen and tends to pass in a direct stream into the right ventricle. Since the lungs are not functioning, most of this oxygen-low blood entering the pulmonary artery passes through the ductus arteriosus into the aorta and is mixed with blood of higher oxygen content pumped from the left side of the heart. In the fetus the internal iliac or hypogastric arteries send out large branches on either side, which traverse the lower abdominal wall to the umbilicus and continue through the cord as the paired umbilical arteries. Deoxygenated blood is thus transported back to the placenta.

Circulatory changes at birth. As soon as respirations begin and the cord is clamped, circulatory changes occur. (1) The *ductus arteriosus* closes as the lungs begin to function. A large volume of blood is pumped by the right ventricle into the previously collapsed pulmonary arteries, thus reducing pressure within the lumen. The ductus arteriosus becomes occluded and forms the *ligamentum arteriosum*. (2) The *foramen ovale* closes as a result of increased tension in the left atrium and concomitant reduction in the right atrium. This is because of the increased volume of blood returned from the

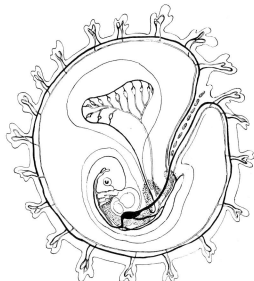

Fig. 10-21. Schematic drawing of vitelline and chorionic circulations.

lungs as respirations are established and the diminished quantity of blood to the inferior vena cava when the umbilical cord is tied. (3) The functionless umbilical vein becomes the *ligamentum teres*. (4) The ductus venosus closes and forms the *ligamentum venosum*. (5) The obliterated umbilical arteries become the *hypogastric* or *lateral umbilical ligaments*.

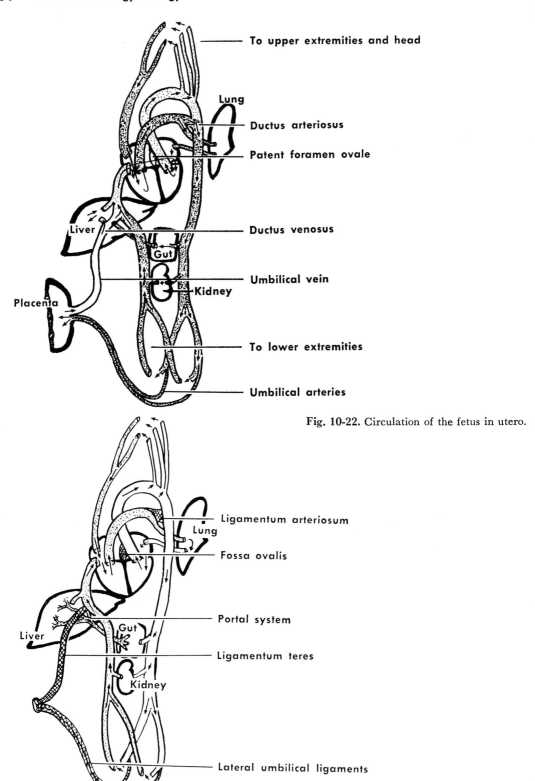

To upper extremities and head

Lung

Ductus arteriosus

Patent foramen ovale

Liver

Ductus venosus

Gut

Umbilical vein

Kidney

Placenta

To lower extremities

Umbilical arteries

Fig. 10-22. Circulation of the fetus in utero.

Ligamentum arteriosum

Lung

Fossa ovalis

Liver

Portal system

Gut

Ligamentum teres

Kidney

Lateral umbilical ligaments

Fig. 10-23. Circulatory changes in the infant after birth.

Fetal oxygenation. In the maternal circulation, arterial oxygen saturation is 96%, and venous oxygen saturation is 71%. Blood in the intervillous spaces is mixed, thus reducing the effective saturation.

In addition, oxygen diffuses through a wet membrane slowly. That oxygen passed to the fetus therefore provides only about 60% oxygen saturation. Fetal adaptation is effected by (1) high red cell count, (2) high hemoglobin values, and (3) differences in fetal hemoglobin as compared with the adult type. The oxygen dissociation curve of fetal blood is shifted to the left, and accordingly uptake of oxygen at low gas tension is enhanced. Studies of the oxygen and carbon dioxide pressure gradients across the placenta support the hypothesis that these gases are transferred by diffusion in accordance with differences in pressure on either side of the membrane. Although the human placental membrane is wet and consists of three layers (syncytium, stroma, and capillary endothelium), it behaves like the lung. Prystowsky and associates obtained intervillous-space blood and umbilical vein and artery blood at cesarean section for comparison. They found an average oxygen tension of 47 mm. Hg in the intervillous space, 30 mm. Hg in the umbilical vein, 18 mm. Hg in the umbilical artery, and an oxygen pressure difference of approximately 24 mm. Hg across the placenta. Carbon dioxide crosses the placenta more readily than oxygen and is found in higher concentration on the fetal than on the maternal side, with an average pressure gradient of 7 mm. Hg.

It is important to recognize that the fetus possesses compensatory mechanisms that increase the margin of safety in coping with temporary periods of hypoxia, but even these have limitations. Glucose breakdown is the major source of energy, which under normal conditions includes an aerobic as well as an anaerobic phase. If the fetus is deprived of oxygen, it has an alternate pathway, entirely anaerobic and much less efficient, to meet requirements. In the normal pathway for glucose oxidation a total of 38 high-energy phosphate bonds are produced (8 bonds in the anaerobic and 30 bonds in the aerobic phase). In the absence of oxygen, pyruvic acid is reduced to lactic acid, using 6 of the 8 high-energy phosphate bonds so

that the net result is only 2 instead of 38 energy sources. An increase in hydrogen ion concentration and a corresponding decrease in base is the final result. The fetal blood pH and base deficit therefore should indicate the severity of fetal hypoxia or distress, and this is the premise on which the Saling fetal scalp blood examination is based.

Fetal blood volume averages approximately 85 ml./kg., or about 300 ml. at term, blood pressure averages 80/40 mm. Hg, cardiac rate averages 120 to 140 beats per minute, and cardiac output averages 10 to 12 ml./100 grams per minute, which is about three times that of a normal adult.

■ Developmental anomalies

Normal growth and development of the fetus may be altered by a great variety of hereditary and environmental factors. These are outlined here and discussed elsewhere in the text. For a detailed description the reader may wish to refer to the comprehensive reviews of Hirschhorn and Cooper, Sohval, and Eggen.

It is important to realize the fact pointed out convincingly by Fraser that a minority of congenital malformations have a major environmental cause and a minority have a major genetic cause. Instead, complicated interactions between genetic predispositions and subtle factors in intrauterine environment form the basis for most. Furthermore, abnormal embryogenesis not only involves gross structural alterations in any of the systems undergoing sequential interrelated actions during development of the fetus, but it also involves functional derangements such as those reflected in inborn errors of metabolism or mental retardation.

Congenital defects may be classified on the basis of intrinsic factors, or genetic defects, and extrinsic factors. The latter may have a temporary effect on development or may cause genetic alterations of a hereditary nature.

INTRINSIC FACTORS

Chromosomal abnormalities include deviations from the normal chromosomal *number* of 46 (aneuploidy) and aberrations in chromosome *morphology*. Aneuploidy is caused by failure of the chromosomes to separate and divide equally in meiosis *(nondisjunction)*. *Monosomy* indicates the absence of one of a chromosome pair, for example, Turner's syndrome (45 XO), in which the total chromosomal number is reduced. *Trisomy* indicates a triple instead of a double dose of genetic material, for example, Klinefelter's and superfemale syndromes involving sex chromosomes (47 XXY and 47 XXX, respectively); there are trisomy syndromes involving autosomes with which multiple congenital anomalies and mental retardations are commonly associated. *Polysomy* refers to chromosomal numbers of 48 or more. These have been found to involve only the sex chromosomes. Presumably such marked deviations involving autosomes are lethal. *Mosaicism* is found in many of the syndromes associated with an abnormal chromosomal number. Adjacent cells from a given individual show different chromosomal counts; for example, patients with gonadal dysgenesis do not always show a chromosomal constitution of 45 XO. A variety of mosaics are now recognized in patients with this disorder, and these findings may modify the classic clinical picture to some degree (45 XO/46 XX), (45 XO/46 XX/47 XXX). Mosaicism involving autosomal abnormalities is seen in some cases of mongolism (46/47—trisomy-21).

Aberrations in chromosome morphology include the following: *Isochromosomes* represent genetic material that is split horizontally instead of vertically. The arms on either side of the centromere therefore are identical. If the short arm is lost, the functions carried on by the genes on the short arm are also lost. Certain cases of amenorrhea are believed to be due to this abnormality. *Translocation* indicates that a fragment of one chromosome is relocated on another (21/15—familial mongolism). This is apparently more common than *deletion,* in which a fragment of genetic material is lost during meiosis. This defect has been described only in connection with the sex chromosomes and may also be responsible for certain cases of amenorrhea.

Defective genes. Mutational alterations involving one or more genes result in defects that are transmissible to successive generations—either as a dominant or a recessive trait. Certain types of anatomic disorders with low but definite familial tendency belong in this group, for example, cleft palate, clubfoot, and congenital dislocation of the hip. A much larger group of functional disorders are caused by defective genes. Over 100 genetic biochemical derangements or inborn errors of metabolism have been described.

EXTRINSIC FACTORS

Extrinsic factors known to affect the development or the genetic makeup of the fetus or both include infection, particularly the viral and parasitic diseases (Chapter 18), radiation, chemicals such as drugs and hormones, and dietary deficiency, particularly those related to the vitamins.

Genetic effects of radiation. The Committee on Genetics of the Atomic Energy Commission recommends that no individual from conception to age 30 years be subjected to more than 10 r of x-ray radiation to the gonads. This does not include cosmic radiation, which amounts to approximately 4 r during this 30-year span.

1 r = 1 roentgen unit (a measurement based on ionization produced in air under standard conditions) = about 84 ergs per gram
1 mr = 1 milliroentgen, or 1/1,000 r
1 rad = amount of absorbed radiation per unit mass = about 100 ergs per gram

In the first few weeks of life serious anomalies may be produced by relatively low doses of radiation. A fetal exposure of 1 r is thought to be safe, but greater dosages are questionable. From day 18 through 38 after implantation, that is, from the beginning development of the neural groove and the neural components emanating from the neural axis including the developing central nervous system, radiosensitivity is maximal. Cells in the act of division, especially neuroblasts, are among the most sensitive of all cells to irradiation effects. Since their distribution at this stage is widespread, damage may vary from minor disturbances undetectable at birth to lethal injury. The dosage of irradiation incurred during diagnostic x-ray examinations is shown in Table 9 (Chapter 32). From a practical viewpoint, diagnostic x-rays should be kept at a minimum and deferred until after the first trimester whenever possible. On the other hand when essential for an immediate problem and when proper shielding and minimal numbers of films are used, this important aid should not be neglected. Fluoroscopic examinations and most radioisotopes should be avoided during pregnancy.

References

Apgar, V., and Papper, E. M.: Transmission of drugs across the placenta, Anesth. Analg. (Cleveland) **31:**309, 1952.

Assali, N. S., and Hamermesz, J.: Adrenocorticotropic substances from human placenta, Endocrinology **55:**561, 1954.

Babuna, C., and Yenen, E.: Enzymatic determination of placental function, Amer. J. Obstet. Gynec. **95:**925, 1966.

Barr, M. L.: Sex chromatin and phenotype in man, Science **130:**679, 1959.

Barr, M. L., Bartram, L. F., and Lindsay, H. A.: The morphology of the nerve cell nucleus according to sex, Anat. Rec. **107:**283, 1950.

Behrman, S. J., and Koren, Z.: Immunology of the conceptus. In Greenhill, J. P., editor: Year book of obstetrics and gynecology, 1967-68, Chicago, 1968, Year Book Medical Publishers, Inc.

Berliner, D. L., Jones, J. E., and Salhanick, H. A.: The isolation of adrenal-like steroids in human placenta, J. Biol. Chem. **223:**1043, 1956.

Billingham, R. E.: Transplantation immunity and the maternal-fetal relation, New Eng. J. Med. **270:**667, 720, 1964.

Blandau, R. J., and Rummery, R. E.: Observations on the movements of the living primordial germ cells of mouse and man, Anat. Rec. **148:**262, 1964.

Blechner, J. N., Stenger, V. G., Eitzman, D. V., and Prystowsky, H.: Effects of maternal metabolic acidosis on the human fetus and newborn infant, Amer. J. Obstet. Gynec. **100:**934, 1968.

Bourne, G. L., and Lacy, D.: Ultra-structure of human amnion and its possible relation to the circulation of amniotic fluid, Nature **186:**952, 1960.

Carey, H. M.: Modern trends in human reproductive physiology, Washington, D. C., 1963, Butterworth, Inc.

Cassmer, O.: Hormone production in the isolated human placenta, Acta Endocr. (supp. 45), 1959.

Chez, R. A., Smith, F. G., and Hutchinson, D. L.: Renal function in the intrauterine primate fetus, Amer. J. Obstet. Gynec. **90:**128, 1964.

Chinard, F. P., Danensino, V., Hartman, W. L., Huggett, A. S. G., Pauls, W., and Reynolds, S. R. M.: The transmission of hexoses across the placenta of the human and the rhesus monkey, J. Physiol. (London) **132:**289, 1956.

Csapo, A. I.: The termination of pregnancy by the intraamniotic injection of hypertonic saline, In Greenhill, J. P., editor: Year book of obstetrics and gynecology, 1966-67, Chicago, 1967, Year Book Medical Publishers, Inc.

Dancis, J., Lind, J., Oratz, M., Smolens, J., and Vara, P.: Placental transfer of proteins in human gestation, Amer. J. Obstet. Gynec. **82:**167, 1961.

Danforth, D. N., and Hull, R. W.: The microscopic anatomy of the fetal membranes with particular reference to the detailed structure of the amnion, Amer. J. Obstet. Gynec. **75:**536, 1958.

Davis, J.: Survey of research in gestation and the developmental sciences, Baltimore, 1960, The Williams & Wilkins Co.

Davis, M. E., and Potter, E. L.: Intrauterine respiration of the human fetus, J.A.M.A. **131:**1194, 1946.

DeCosta, E. J., Gerbie, A. B., Andresen, R. H., and Gallanis, T. C.: Placental tumors; hemangiomas with special reference to an associated clinical syndrome, Obstet. Gynec. **7:**249, 1956.

Denver Study Group: A proposed standard system of nomenclature of human mitotic chromosomes, Lancet **1:**1063, 1960.

Derom, R.: Anaerobic metabolism in the human fetus. II. The twin delivery, Amer. J. Obstet. Gynec. **92:**555, 1965.

Diczfalusy, E.: Endocrine functions of the human fetoplacental unit, Fed. Proc. **23:**791, 1964.

Doyle, J. B.: Direct observations of ovulation by culdoscopy, Fertil. Steril. **5:**105, 1954.

Eastman, N. J., Geiling, E. M. K., and DeLenoder, A. M.: Fetal blood studies. IV. The oxygen and carbon dioxide dissociation curves of fetal blood, Bull. Hopkins Hosp. **53:**246, 1933.

Eggen, R. R.: Cytogenetics; review of recent advances in a new field of clinical pathology, Amer. J. Clin. Path. **39:**3, 1963.

Fainstat, T., and Chapman, G. B.: Microvilli of endometrial epithelium in relation to ovo-implantation, Amer. J. Obstet. Gynec. **91:**852, 1965.

Federman, D. D.: Chromosome studies and disordered sex differentiation. In Meigs, J. V., and Sturgis, S. H., editors: Progress in gynecology, vol. 4, New York, 1963, Grune & Stratton, Inc.

Ford, C. E., and Hamerton, J. L.: The chromosomes of man, Nature **178:**1020, 1956.

Fraser, F. C.: Causes of congenital malformations in human beings, J. Chronic Dis. **10:**97, 1959.

Goldzieher, J. W.: Estrogens and progesterones. In Meigs, J. V., and Sturgis, S. H., editors: Progress in gynecology, vol. 4, New York, 1963, Grune & Stratton, Inc.

Greene, J. W., and Touchstone, J. C.: Urinary estriol as an index of placental function, Amer. J. Obstet. Gynec. **85:**1, 1963.

Grumbach, M. M., Kaplan, S. L., Sciarra, J. J., and Burr, I. M.: Chorionic growth hormone-prolactin (CGP); secretion, disposition, biologic activity in man, and postulated function as the "growth hormone" of the second half of pregnancy, In Sonenberg, M., editor: Conference on growth hormone, Ann. N. Y. Acad. Sci. **148:** 501, 1968.

Hagerman, D. D.: Enzymatic capabilities of the placenta. Symposia. Physiology of placenta, Fed. Proc. **23:**785, 1964.

Hendricks, C. H., Quilligan, E. J., Tyler, C. W., and Tucker, G. J.: Pressure relationships between the intervillous space and the amniotic fluid in human term pregnancy, Amer. J. Obstet. Gynec. **77:**1028, 1959.

Hertig, A. T., Rock, J., and Adams, E. C.: A description of 34 human ova within the first

17 days of development, Amer. J. Anat. **98:** 435, 1956.

Hutchinson, D. L., Gray, M. J., Plentl, A. A., Alvarez, H., Caldeyro-Barcia, R., Kaplan, B., and Lind, J.: The role of the fetus in the water exchange of the amniotic fluid of normal and hydramniotic patients, J. Clin. Invest. 38:971, 1959.

Hutchinson, D. L., Hunter, C. B., Neslen, E. D., and Plentl, A. A.: The exchange of water and electrolytes in the mechanism of amniotic fluid formation and the relationship to hydramnios, Surg. Gynec. Obstet. 100:391, 1955.

Hytten, F. E., and Leitch, I.: The physiology of human pregnancy, Philadelphia, 1963, F. A. Davis Co.

Jaffe, R. B., and Midgley, A. R., Jr.: Current status of human gonadotropin radioimmunoassay (review), Obstet. Gynec. Survey 24:200, 1969.

Jeffcoate, T. N. A., and Scott, J. S.: Polyhydramnois, Canad. Med. Ass. J. 80:77, 1959.

Josimovich, J. B., and Maclaren, J. A.: Presence in the human placenta and term serum of a highly lactogenic substance immunologically related to pituitary growth hormone, Endocrinology 71:209, 1962.

Jost, A.: Problems of fetal endocrinology; the gonadal and hypophyseal hormones, Rec. Progr. Hormone Res. 8:379, 1953.

Kaplan, S. L., and Grumbach, M. M.: Serum chorionic "growth hormone-prolactin" and serum pituitary growth hormone in mother and fetus at term, J. Clin. Endocr. 25:1370, 1965.

Klopfer, A.: The assessment of fetoplacental function by estriol assay, Obstet. Gynec. Survey 23: 813, 1968.

Krantz, K. E.: The anatomy and endocrinology of the human placenta. In Velardo, J. T.: Essentials of human reproduction, London, 1958, Oxford University Press.

Lanman, J. T., and Dinerstine, J.: The adrenotropic action of human pregnancy plasma, Endocrinology 64:494, 1959.

Lau, H. L., and Jones, G. S.: Immunoassay of serum human chorionic gonadotropin by quantitative complement fixation and its comparison with Delfs bioassay and two international standard preparations, Amer. J. Obstet. Gynec. 92:483, 1965.

Levine, B., and Wood, W.: Maternal serum alkaline phosphatase and placental function, Amer. J. Obstet. Gynec. 91:967, 1965.

Liley, A. W.: Amniotic fluid. In Carey, H. M., editor: Modern trends in human reproductive physiology, Washington, D. C., 1963, Butterworth, Inc.

Longo, L. D., Power, G. G., and Forster, R. E.: Respiratory function of the placenta as determined with carbon monoxide in sheep and dogs, J. Clin. Invest. 46:812, 1967.

Lubchenco, L. O., Hansman, C., Dressler, M., and Boyd, E.: Intrauterine growth as measured by liveborn birthweight; data from 24 to 42 weeks gestation, Pediatrics 32:793, 1963.

Marx, G. F., and Greene, N. M.: Lactate/pyruvate ratio of umbilical vein blood, Amer. J. Obstet. Gynec. 92:548, 1965.

McKay, D. G., Hertig, A. T., Adams, E. C., and Danziger, S.: Histochemical observations on the germ cells of human embryos, Anat. Rec. **117:** 201, 1953.

Nadler, H. L.: Prenatal detection of genetic defects, J. Pediat. 74:132, 1969.

Page, E. W.: Transfer of materials across the human placenta, Amer. J. Obstet. Gynec. 74:705, 1957.

Page, E. W., Glendening, M. B., Margolis, A., and Harper, H. A.: Transfer of D- and L-histidine across the human placenta, Amer. J. Obstet. Gynec. 73:589, 1957.

Pierce, G. B., Jr., and Midgley, A. R., Jr.: The origin and function of human syncytiotrophoblastic giant cells, Amer. J. Path. 43:153, 1963.

Pinkerton, J. H. M., McKay, D. G., Adams, E. C., and Hertig, A. T.: Development of the human ovary; a study using histochemical technics, Obstet. Gynec. 18:152, 1961.

Plotz, E. J.: Endocrine activities of the placenta, Clin. Obstet. Gynec. 8:580, 1965.

Potter, E. L.: Pathology of the fetus and infant, ed. 2, Chicago, 1961, Year Book Medical Publishers, Inc.

Prystowsky, H., Hellegers, A., and Bruns, P.: Fetal blood studies. XV. The carbon dioxide concentration gradient between fetal and maternal blood of humans, Amer. J. Obstet. Gynec. 81:372, 1961.

Prystowsky, H., Hellegers, A., and Bruns, P.: Fetal blood studies. XVIII. Supplementary observations on the oxygen pressure gradient between the maternal and fetal bloods of humans, Surg. Gynec. Obstet. 110:495, 1960.

Ramsey, E. M., Corner, G. W., Jr., Donner, M. W., and Stran, H. M.: Radio-angiographic studies of circulation in maternal placenta of the rhesus monkey; preliminary report, Proc. Nat. Acad. Sci. U.S.A. 46:1003, 1960.

Ramsey, E. M., Corner, G. W., Jr., Long, W. N., and Stran, H. M.: Studies of amniotic fluid and intervillous space pressures in the rhesus monkey, Amer. J. Obstet. Gynec. 77:1016, 1959.

Ratner, A., Dhariwal, A. P. S., and McCann, S. M.: Hypothalamic factors in gonadotropic hormone regulation, Clin. Obstet. Gynec. 10: 106, 1967.

Rawlings, W. J.: Pregnanediol excretion and placental insufficiency, Fertil. Steril. 16:323, 1965.

Salhanick, H. A.: Hormones in pregnancy, Clin. Obstet. Gynec. 3:295, 1960.

Scoggin, W. A., Harbert, G. M., Jr., Anslow, W. P., Jr., Riet, B. V., and McGaughey, H. S.: Fetomaternal exchange of water at term, Amer. J. Obstet. Gynec. 90:7, 1964.

Simmons, R. L., and Russell, P. S.: The immunologic problem of pregnancy, Amer. J. Obstet. Gynec. 85:583, 1963.

Smith, K., Duhring, J. L., Greene, J. W., Jr., Rochlin, D. B., and Blakemore, W. S.: Transfer of maternal erythrocytes across the human placenta, Obstet. Gynec. 18:673, 1961.

Smith, O. W., and Ryan, K. J.: Estrogens in the

human ovary, Amer. J. Obstet. Gynec. **84:**141, 1962.

Sobrero, A. J.: Sperm migration in the female genital tract. In Hartman, C. G., editor: Mechanisms concerned with conception, New York, 1963, Pergamon Press, Inc., p. 173.

Sohval, A. R.: Recent progress in human chromosome analysis and its relation to the sex chromatin, Amer. J. Med. **31:**397, 1961.

Southren, A. L., Kobayashi, Y., Brenner, P., and Weingold, A. B.: Diamine oxidase activity in human maternal and fetal plasma and tissues at parturition, J. Appl. Physiol. **20:**1048, 1965.

Spanner, R.: Mütterlicher und kindlicher Kreislauf der menschlichen Placenta und seine Strombahnen, Z. Anat. **105:**163, 1935.

Spellacy, W. N., Carlson, K. L., and Birk, S. A.: Human placental lactogen levels as a variable of placental weight and infant weight, Amer. J. Obstet. Gynec. **95:**118, 1966.

Spellacy, W. N., Cohen, W. D., and Carlson, K. L.: Human placental lactogen levels as a measure of placental function, Amer. J. Obstet. Gynec. **97:**560, 1967.

Streeter, G. L.: Weight, sitting height, head size, foot length and menstrual age of the human embryo, Contrib. Embryol. **9:**143, 1920.

Thompson, H. E., Holmes, J. H., Gottesfeld, K. R., and Taylor, E. S.: Fetal development as determined by ultrasonic pulse echo techniques, Amer. J. Obstet. Gynec. **92:**14, 1965.

Tremblay, P. C., Sybulski, S., and Maughan, C. B.: Role of the placenta in fetal malnutrition, Amer. J. Obstet. Gynec. **91:**597, 1965.

Turner, C. D.: Special mechanisms in anomalies of sex differentiation, Amer. J. Obstet. Gynec. **90:**1208, 1964.

Tyler, E. T.: Physiological and chemical aspects of conception, J.A.M.A. **153:**1351, 1954.

Velardo, J. T.: Essentials of human reproduction, London, 1958, Oxford University Press.

Venning, E.: Adrenal function in pregnancy, Endocrinology **39:**203, 1946.

Villee, C. A.: Metabolism of human placenta in vitro, J. Biol. Chem. **205:**113, 1953.

Villee, C. A.: Regulation of blood glucose in the human fetus, J. Appl. Physiol. **5:**437, 1953.

Vosburgh, G. J., Flexner, L. B., Cowie, D. B., Hellman, L. M., Proctor, N. K., and Wilde, W. S.: The rate of renewal in women of the water and sodium of the amniotic fluid as determined by tracer techniques, Amer. J. Obstet. Gynec. **56:**1156, 1948.

Weingold, A. B.: Enzymatic indices of fetal environment, Clin. Obstet. Gynec. **11:**1081, 1968.

Wislocki, G. B., and Bennett, H. S.: Histology and cytology of the human and monkey placenta with special reference to the trophoblast, Amer. J. Anat. **73:**335, 1943.

Wislocki, G. B., and Dempsey, E. W.: Histochemical age changes in normal and pathologic placental villi (hydatidiform mole, eclampsia), Endocrinology **38:**90, 1946.

Wynn, R. M., and Davies, J.: Comparative electron microscopy of the hemochorial placenta, Amer. J. Obstet. Gynec. **91:**533, 1965.

Zarrow, M. X., Holmstrom, E. G., and Salhanick, H. A.: The concentration of relaxin in the blood serum and other tissues of women during pregnancy, J. Clin. Endocr. **15:**22, 1955.

Zondek, B.: Hormonal diagnosis of placental dysfunction leading to fetal death, Clin. Obstet. Gynec. **3:**1083, 1960.

11

Infertility

From the beginning of recorded time the problem of the barren marriage has played a major role in the lives of human beings. Many ancient religious rites and social practices are specifically concerned with fertility and sterility. Magic potions and incantations are still utilized by primitive peoples to enhance the reproductive capacity of newly wed couples. Until a relatively short time ago little else could be done. During recent years our understanding of the reproductive process has increased to such an extent that many barren matings can be corrected. Yet in the United States today 1 marriage out of every 9 remains involuntarily barren. There is little doubt that the disappointment and sense of frustration associated with childlessness are often causes of marital discontent and much unhappiness.

Because of the prevalence and seriousness of this problem it deserves the interest of the general practitioner as well as of the spe-

cialist, since it is the family physician who is most often the first one to learn of the couple's difficulty and therefore is in the best position to give proper advice and guidance.

■ Definitions

Infertility can be diagnosed whenever a woman who desires children has not been able to conceive during a period of 1 year of unprotected intercourse. More than one half of normal couples will achieve a pregnancy within 3 months after discontinuing contraceptive measures, and 90% will be successful within 1 year. At the end of 2 years only an additional 5% will have conceived. Infertility is considered to be *primary* if conception has never occurred; it is termed *secondary* if there has been at least one pregnancy prior to the present difficulty. *Absolute infertility* or *true sterility* implies a situation in which conception is impossible and in which the causative factor is irremediable. *Relative infertility* is produced by various factors that may hinder or delay conception; these are often correctable.

■ Essential factors in fertility

Normal fertility is dependent upon many factors in both the male and the female.

Male. The male must produce a sufficient number of normal, motile spermatozoa that can enter the urethra through patent pathways in order to be ejaculated.

Male and female. The sperm must be deposited in the female in such a way that they reach and penetrate the cervical secretion and ascend through the uterus to the tube at the time in the cycle appropriate for fertilization of the ovum.

Female. The female must produce a normal, fertilizable ovum that must enter the fallopian tube within a period of a few hours and become fertilized. The resulting conceptus must move into the uterus and implant in an adequately prepared endometrium and there undergo normal development.

If any one of these essential processes is defective or impeded, infertility may result.

■ Etiology of infertility

Until recently the inability of a woman to conceive was considered to be solely her problem. Although the wife is still the one who first consults the doctor, it is now fairly well recognized that the husband may either be responsible for or contribute to her infertility. Reported studies indicate that in 30% to 40% of infertile marriages a male factor is either the sole cause of the failure to conceive or is an important contributing cause.

Faulty spermatogenesis and insemination. Faulty spermatogenesis may result from a number of congenital or acquired causes, which include those related to embryonic development, to abnormal endocrine function, and to environmental factors. Men with *gonadal dysgenesis* (Klinefelter's syndrome) and similar abnormalities in testicular development produce no sperm, even though the Leydig cells may be normal. *Endocrine abnormalities* include primary hypogonadism, as well as hypogonadism that is secondary to hypopituitarism and thyroid or adrenal gland dysfunction. *Infections,* particularly the suppurative orchitis accompanying mumps, will destroy the epithelium of the seminiferous tubules. Tuberculous orchitis, although uncommon, has the same effect. Spermatogenesis is often temporarily reduced after acute febrile illness, even though there is no actual involvement of the testis. *High temperatures,* and *disturbed circulation* from cryptorchidism, varicocele, hydrocele, and following herniorrhaphy may alter testicular function. *Radiation* and *direct trauma* may also disturb spermatogenesis. *Nutritional deficiencies* represent a minor cause of testicular malfunction because a change occurs only when depletion is advanced.

Murphy and Torrano diagnosed azoospermia in 8% of males in 3,620 childless marriages; in 34.4% the counts were less than 20 million per cubic millimeter. Azoospermia was found in less than 1% of normal college students, and in only 18% were counts below 20 million per cubic millimeter found.

The number of sperm in the ejaculate is definitely decreased with *frequent coitus.* This is usually of little significance in the normally fertile male, but if spermatogenesis is already reduced, it may never reach an optimum level unless coitus is restricted. On the other hand, the fertile period may be missed consistently with infrequent intercourse, which sometimes is the sole cause of failure to conceive.

Faulty sperm transmission because of obstructive postinflammatory scarring of the epididymis, vas, or urethra may occasionally interfere with insemination. If the penis is abnormally short, buried in fat, or malformed, emission may take place outside of the vagina; premature ejaculation may produce the same result.

In the female, dyspareunia, vaginismus, developmental anomalies, or an intact hymen may prevent intromission and normal deposition of the ejaculate. The practice of taking a douche or getting out of bed immediately after coitus may result in loss of the ejaculate.

Vaginal and cervical infections may alter the pH of the vaginal secretions and interfere with sperm motility. Normally the vaginal secretion is mildly acid in reaction with a pH of 4 to 5, whereas that of the seminal fluid is about 8. If the vaginal secretions are normal, sperm survival is good; but if because of chronic cervicitis or vaginal trichomoniasis they become less acid or even alkaline in reaction, the pH after ejaculation may be too high for normal sperm motility.

The cervical factor. Abnormalities of structure or of function of the cervix, which are present in 15% to 20% of infertile women, may play an important part in infertility. *Obstructive lesions of the cervix* such as large polyps, pedunculated fibroids, congenital atresia, or atresia following repeated cauterization or conization may interfere with ascent of the sperm. *Alterations in the cervical mucus,* either from endocervicitis or from hormonal deficiency, may also interfere with conception. Certain *bacteria* are lethal to sperm, but it is *chemical* and *physical alterations in cervical mucus* that more often impair fertility. Under the influence of estrogen from the developing follicle the cervical glands become progressively more active during the first 2 weeks of the cycle. At the end of menstruation the mucus is thick, viscid, and opaque, and the spinnbarkheit (ability to be drawn into long threads) is limited. The mucus is cellular, and ferning is slight or absent. As ovulation approaches and the peak of estrogen production is reached, the secretion is copious in amount (in some women it is actually annoying). The mucus is thin and clear and can be drawn into threads 10 to 15 cm.

long. Few cells can be seen, but ferning is pronounced. This type of mucus permits maximum sperm survival and penetration and is essential for normal fertility. Abnormalities in cervical mucus other than those caused by infection usually mirror defective ovarian hormone production.

The uterine factor. Malformations, malpositions, and tumors of the uterus do not often interfere with conception, but they may occasionally be a factor in faulty nidation and early abortion. Infertility often is attributed to an "infantile uterus," but this is usually secondary to a hormonal deficiency that is the primary factor in the difficulty. A movable retrodisplacement of the uterus is not ordinarily responsible for the failure to conceive. Submucous myomas may obstruct the uterine ends of the tube and thus prevent fertilization or may distort the uterine cavity and interfere with nidation.

The tubal factor. Partial or complete occlusion of the fallopian tubes is an important etiologic factor in infertility. It is encountered in about 30% of all women who fail to conceive. Tubal obstruction usually results from the destructive effect of pathogenic microorganisms on the mucosal surface. Although gonorrheal salpingitis is an important cause of obstruction, it is not the only one. Bacteria regularly ascend from the infected uterine cavities of women who have aborted or have had a normal delivery and may produce a destructive endosalpingitis. Uterine fibroids or cornual adenomyosis may distort and occlude the uterine ends of the tubes. The tubes also may be kinked by adhesions after appendicitis and other infections or by areas of pelvic endometriosis. Not infrequently intermittent obstruction occurs because of spasm of the uterine ends of the tubes.

Endocrine factors. The development of normal ova, their periodic extrusion from the follicle, and the cyclic secretion of adequate quantities of estrogen and progesterone are essential for normal fertility. This sequence of events occurs when the hypothalamus stimulates the anterior lobe of the pituitary to produce normal amounts of gonadotropin and when the ovary is responsive to this stimulation. Abnormal function of these glands, or of the thyroid or adrenal glands, can result in anovulation and infertility. The endocrine dysfunctions most often associated with female infertility are: (1) dysfunctional uterine bleeding and other disorders associated with ovulatory failure, (2) amenorrhea of any etiology, (3) inadequate progesterone production, (4) hypothyroidism and hyperthyroidism, (5) disorders of the adrenal glands, particularly the adrenogenital syndrome, and (6) tumors and dysfunctions of the anterior lobe of the pituitary gland. These factors are discussed in detail elsewhere.

Miscellaneous organic factors. Chronic infections, debilitating diseases, and severe nutritional deficiencies may alter the function of both male and female gonads and thus reduce fertility. Advancing age also may play a role; in women the fertility level reaches a peak at about 20 to 25 years of age and then slowly declines, reaching a low level after 40 years of age. Anovulatory cycles are quite common in the premenopausal period.

Emotional factors. It has long been recognized that impotence, premature ejaculation, vaginismus, and dyspareunia are usually a result of psychologic disturbances. More recently our attention has been directed to the possibility of psychogenically induced tubal spasm, inimical cervical secretion, and anovulatory cycles. The functionally infertile woman consciously verbalizes a wish for a child but unconsciously rejects pregnancy, childbirth, and motherhood. She has grave conflicts over femininity, being in hostile, dependent bondage to a mother image or aggressively imitating the male role. Mixtures of these attitudes are present in most persons, with one usually predominating. The patient is often unhappy in genital sexuality, and her menstrual function is often disturbed.

Immunologic factors. Investigation concerning the immunologic aspects of infertility are of relatively recent origin, but they have produced interesting results. Currently available evidence suggests that infertility may occur as a result of ABO incompatibilities and of the production of sperm-agglutinating antibodies both in men and in women. Further study is necessary before the place of these factors in infertility can be evaluated.

■ Investigation of the infertile couple

The investigation of the infertility must be conducted systematically, according to a planned program. Since multiple factors are so frequently found to be operating, the study of both partners should be carried out in its entirety, even though conditions that obviously would impair fertility are detected early in the investigation. Both husband and wife must be interested in the solution of their problem. The plan of study and the time and expense involved should be explained to them during the first interview in order to ensure full cooperation and to avoid future misunderstandings. The American Society for the Study of Sterility has recommended the diagnostic survey discussed in steps 1 to 5 for the evaluation of the barren marriage.

STEP 1—A COMPLETE HISTORY AND PHYSICAL EXAMINATION OF BOTH HUSBAND AND WIFE

After an initial interview with both partners, separate appointments are made for the examination of each individual.

History. The form on p. 145 is useful in obtaining important information concerning the history of each partner.

Physical examination. A complete general physical examination should be performed on each partner. Evidence of endocrine stigmas such as abnormalities of body configuration or of distribution of fat and hair may suggest a cause for the infertility.

Examination of the female. A systematic pelvic examination that includes careful inspection and palpation of the structures throughout the entire length of the genital tract ordinarily will indicate the residua of infections or abnormalities in development and growth that may prevent conception.

Enlarged Bartholin's glands suggest an old quiescent infection unless they are tender to palpation and pus can be expressed from their ducts, in which event a more acute process is probably present. Infection in the urethra or in Skene's glands is indicated if pus can be milked from the meatus by pressure on the urethra through the vagina. An intact hymen is an important although infrequent cause of infertility.

The normally developed and stimulated vagina is pink, distensible, and soft, and the mucosa retains the normal, rugous pattern. Inadequate estrogen stimulation can be suspected if the mucosa is smooth, thin, and pale or if the cervix is short and flush with the vaginal vault. Vaginitis is easily recognized by the inflammatory reaction and the discharge that accompanies it. The cause of the inflammation can usually be determined by the examination of a fresh, unstained saline suspension of the discharge for motile trichomonads and by culture for *Candida* and other organisms.

The cervix should be palpated and, in addition, carefully inspected for the presence of an obvious lesion through a vaginal speculum with a good light. Thick mucopurulent secretion exuding from the canal indicates infection, whereas clear, mucoid discharge, particularly if thin and watery, is more normal. The pH of the cervical secretions can be determined with Nitrazine paper.

If the uterus is retrodisplaced, it is important to know whether it is freely movable or fixed in the cul-de-sac by adhesions from old inflammatory disease or endometriosis. It also is important to determine whether the cavity of the uterus is larger or smaller than usual and, when possible, whether the usual adult ratio of one third cervix to two thirds uterine cavity exists. The depth of the cervicouterine canal, usually 6 to 7.5 cm., is measured by carefully passing a sound through the cervix and into the uterus until it meets the resistance of the fundus.

The adnexal areas and the parametria are palpated in an effort to detect abnormal tenderness or enlargement from inflammation, endometriosis, or tumors. The posterior surface of the uterus, the uterosacral ligaments, and the cul-de-sac can be palpated more accurately through the rectum than through the vagina.

Examination of the male. Complete physical examination, with a detailed study of the genital organs, of the male member of an infertile couple is essential. One should look particularly for evidence of endocrinopathy, developmental anomalies of the penis, testicular atrophy, varicocele, and for infection in the prostate, seminal vesicles, and urethra.

Laboratory studies. The following laboratory procedures are generally indicated: urinalysis, complete blood count, serologic test for syphilis, determination of blood type and of the Rh factor, and evaluation of thyroid function.

STEP 2—EVALUATION OF THE SEMEN

The semen examination is one of the most important parts of the infertility study since the male is often at least partially responsible for failure to achieve pregnancy. The simple microscopic examination of a drop of semen is utterly inadequate for accurate evaluation of fertility, and in order to assess the male factor properly, complete semen analysis and a study of the effect of the cervical secretions upon sperm survival must be made. A single analysis, particularly if it indicates lowered fertility, is inconclusive because the sperm count varies from day to day and is dependent upon emotional and physical, as well as sexual, activity. Previously performed sperm counts, particularly if the details of the analysis are unavailable, must be repeated, since they may not represent the current status of the male partner.

Semen analysis. The specimen should be collected by ejaculation into a clean, wide-mouthed, screw-top glass or porcelain jar after coitus interruptus or masturbation after a 5-day period of abstinence from intercourse. Catholic couples, who cannot use this method, can collect the semen in a plastic condom that has been punctured in several places. A rubber condom should never be used for the collection of semen because both the sheaths and the powder on them may be spermaticidal. The jar should be tightly capped and the specimen carefully transported to the laboratory within 1 hour of its emission. No particular precaution need be taken to control the temperature, except that excessive heat should be avoided.

The volume of the ejaculate varies from 2 to 5 ml., and the freshly collected semen is white, gelatinous, and semitransparent. It liquefies completely in 15 to 30 minutes, and the examination should be delayed until liquefaction has occurred.

The following method of determining the *total number of sperm* and the percentage of active forms is that described by Farris. Well-mixed, liquefied semen is drawn up to the 0.5 ml. mark of an ordinary white blood cell counting pipet and is diluted to 1:20 by filling the pipet to the upper mark with freshly prepared Locke's solution. After shak-

ing for 30 seconds the first 2 drops of solution are discarded, and the counting chamber of a Spencer Bright Line hemacytometer is flooded with the diluted serum. All the sperm in 5 groups of 16 small squares in the red field are counted. The addition of 6 zeros to this figure gives the total number of sperm per milliliter of semen. This first calculation should be checked by a similar count made in a different group of 5 large squares.

The *percentage of motile sperm* is of more importance than the total count and can be obtained easily. The number of active sperm per milliliter of semen is calculated by adding 6 zeros to the number of motile forms in 5 blocks of squares. This figure, divided by the total number of sperm per milliliter and multiplied by 100, gives the percentage of active forms in the specimen.

$$\frac{\text{Active sperm per ml.}}{\text{Total sperm per ml.}} \times 100 = \% \text{ active forms}$$

MacLeod believes that it is pointless to determine the *duration of activity* in semen because seminal plasma is not a physiologic environment for spermatozoa. Immediately after ejaculation the spermatozoa leave the plasma and enter the cervical mucus, through which they must pass to reach the tube. It is far more logical to study their activity in cervical secretions than in the semen.

The *speed of motility* can be checked by determining the time required for a spermatozoon to cross one of the small squares of the counting chamber. The normal spermatozoon crosses the square in 1 second or less, whereas the sluggishly moving forms may require 2 seconds or more to traverse the same distance.

Sperm morphology. The normal spermatozoon has an oval, flattened head, measuring 5 by 2.5 μ and containing the nucleus with the male contribution of chromosomes. The neck is 0.5 μ in length and lies between the head and the middle piece, which is a spiral filament coiled about a 4 μ length of axial thread. The tapering tail, which provides the motile power, is about 45 μ in length. The detailed structure of the sperm can be studied in a stained semen preparation and the number of abnormal forms calculated. Many staining techniques have been described, but most of them are too complicated for clinical use. Gram's or Wright's stain will usually suffice.

INFERTILITY HISTORY—WIFE

Age: Race: Religion:

Occupation:

Years of marriage: Previous marriage?

Duration of involuntary infertility:

Past history	*Present history*

1. Medical
    Tuberculosis
    Venereal disease
    Endometriosis
    Tumors
    Menstrual irregularities
2. Surgical
    Pelvic operations
    Appendectomy
3. Obstetrics
    Full-term deliveries—complications
    Abortions or premature delivery
    Previous infertility evaluation
	1. General
	    Habits
	    Diet
	    Work and health status
	    Menstrual
	2. Sexual
	    Frequency of coitus
	    Postcoital practices
	    Libido
	    Orgasm capacity
	    Position during and after coitus
	3. Personal
	    Motivation for childbearing
	    Attitude toward husband
	    What sort of man is he?
	    Relationship with parents, in-laws,
	      siblings, etc.

INFERTILITY HISTORY—HUSBAND

Age: Race: Religion:

Occupation:

Years of marriage: Previous marriage?

Past history

1. Medical
    Tuberculosis
    Venereal infection
    Mumps orchitis
    Varicocele
2. Surgical
    Herniorrhaphy
    Hydrocele
    Orchiopexy
    Injury to genitals

Present history

1. General
    Diet
    Habits
    Work and health status

2. Sexual
    Frequency of coitus and technique
      used
    Premature ejaculation
    Adequacy of erection
    Timing of coitus
3. Personal
    Motivation for childbearing
    Attitude toward wife
    What sort of woman is she?
    Relationship with parents, in-laws,
      siblings, fellow workers, boss
    Economic status
    What is his ambition?

Fertility standards. The standards for normal male fertility as determined by semen analysis have undergone considerable revision in recent years. Most authorities now agree on the following criteria for a normal range:

Volume	2 to 6 ml.
Count	20 to 200 million per milliliter
Motility	60% to 80% actively motile
Morphology	70% to 90% normally shaped

STEP 3—DETERMINATION OF TUBAL PATENCY

The usual tests for the study of tubal patency are dependent upon the injection of gas or a radiopaque substance through the cervicouterine canal and the tubes into the peritoneal cavity. If properly performed, the tests provide accurate information concerning tubal structure and function and should, unless contraindicated, be included as a part of every infertility study. They should never be performed in the presence of acute or subacute infections of the vagina, cervix, or tubes or during any episode of uterine bleeding since at that time the gas or the contrast medium may enter the open blood vessels. If pregnancy is suspected, tests for tubal patency ought to be delayed until the diagnosis can be definitely eliminated.

Patency tests are best performed 4 or 5 days after the end of a menstrual period. At this time there are no open vessels; the menstrual debris, which might be forced through the tubes and into the peritoneal cavity, has all been discharged; the tubal openings are not occluded by thick secretory endometrium, and there is little chance of pregnancy. Since the increased pressure may open minor tubal occlusions, insufflation shortly before ovulation may also aid in conception.

Uterotubal insufflation (Rubin's test). Rubin's test can be performed in the physician's office. Carbon dioxide under pressure is injected through a special cannula into the cervicouterine canal. If one or both tubes are open, the gas will pass into the peritoneal cavity, but if both tubes are occluded, this fails to occur. Air should never be used because deaths from embolism have occurred after its injection, but none has been reported with carbon dioxide. In addition it is more difficult to regulate the pressure and rate of flow of air, and abdominal and shoulder pains often persist for a day or two because the nitrogen is absorbed from the peritoneal cavity so slowly.

The necessary apparatus includes carbon

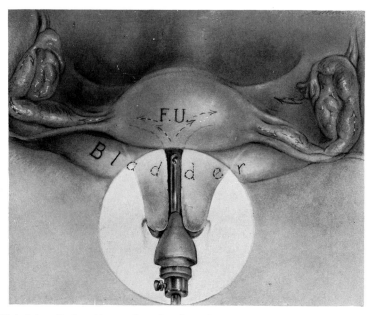

Fig. 11-1. Tubal insufflation. Front view showing dilatation of fallopian tubes. (From Willson, J. R.: Management of obstetric difficulties, ed. 6, St. Louis, 1961, The C. V. Mosby Co.)

dioxide gas under pressure and an easy means for controlling the volume of flow and the pressure as it passes through the cannula into the uterus. The inclusion of a kymograph to record the alterations in pressure will not only provide a permanent record but will demonstrate the minor changes caused by peristaltic activity in the tubes.

After having voided, the patient is examined in the lithotomy position to determine the position of the uterus and to be certain that no contraindications to insufflation are present. The cervix is exposed through a sterile bivalve speculum, and the anterior cervical lip is grasped with a tenaculum and pulled downward to straighten the uterine cavity, which is then sounded with a sterile sound. The cannula is inserted through the cervical canal, and the rubber tip is pressed tightly against the external os by combined downward traction on the tenaculum and upward pressure on the cannula to seal the opening. After a 2-minute interval to permit relaxation of tubal spasm, the valve is opened, and as the gas is allowed to enter the uterus, the pressure recorded by the manometer is observed. According to

Rubin the optimum flow rate is about 60 ml. per minute. This rate can be estimated fairly accurately without a flow meter because it takes about 30 seconds to raise the intrauterine pressure to 100 mm. Hg and about 1 minute to raise it to 200 mm. Hg. All tests should be performed with a standard rate of flow because variations may lead to misinterpretation of the results. The recorded pressure is determined by the rate of flow of the gas through the uterine cavity and the tubes, and the rate of flow is determined by the caliber of the tubes and their ability to expand. It is quite possible, therefore, to raise the recorded pressure well above 200 mm. Hg simply by increasing the flow rate, thereby simulating tubal obstruction.

In the normal test the pressure gradually rises to 80 to 100 mm. Hg and then falls as the gas passes through the tubes and into the peritoneal cavity. As the flow continues, the pressure oscillates between 40 and 80 mm. Hg as the normal peristalsis increases and decreases the resistance. After the test is completed and the patient sits up, she usually experiences pain in the shoulder be-

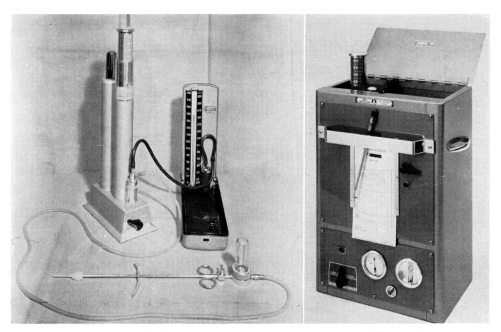

Fig. 11-2   Fig. 11-3

Fig. 11-2. Apparatus for insufflation of fallopian tubes (Rubin's test).
Fig. 11-3. Tubal insufflation apparatus with kymograph.

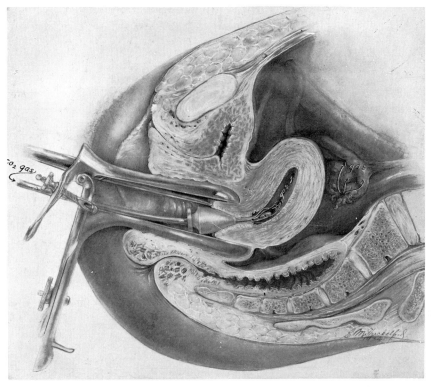

Fig. 11-4. Tubal insufflation. Sagittal section showing technique. Gas flows through intrauterine cannula and out through tubes, the cervix being closed by a rubber stopper. Resistance of tubes is measured by back pressure on the mercury gauge or is recorded by the kymograph. (From Willson, J. R.: Management of obstetric difficulties, ed. 6, St. Louis, 1961, The C. V. Mosby Co.)

cause of the subdiaphragmatic collection of the carbon dioxide. This occurs so regularly that if no pain is felt, occlusion of the tubes must be suspected even though the gas appeared to have passed through them at normal pressures.

If the tubes are blocked, the pressure rises sharply and continues to rise until the flow of gas is stopped or until the tube ruptures. The pressure will remain at a constant level after the flow ceases until the occluding cervical cannula is withdrawn. Since the gas cannot enter the peritoneal cavity, the patient feels no shoulder pain when she sits up.

Occasionally spasm at the uterine end of the normal tube may resemble organic occlusion, but ordinarily after an initial rise to 160 to 200 mm. Hg the pressure falls rapidly as the tube opens, and the remainder of the test appears normal. Spasm may be of emotional origin in part, but it may also be caused by pain. Drugs are not uniformly successful in relaxing spastic tubes, but a tranquilizer (meprobamate, 400 mg.) or an analgesic (Demerol, 50 to 75 mg.) given 1 hour before the test may help.

If the tubes are partially occluded, the initial pressure will be high; instead of the abrupt fall that is noted as the spasm relaxes, a more gradual decline is observed. The pressure rarely falls to a normal level, and tubal activity is decreased or absent. The amount of pressure required to force the gas through the tubes roughly indicates the degree of stenosis.

Since tubal occlusion can readily be differentiated from spasm at pressures less than 200 mm. Hg, an increase above this level rarely is indicated. Tubal occlusion should not be diagnosed, however, on the basis of a single study, even though the gas did not pass through them at a high pressure. Repeated attempts at the same sitting, as well as subsequent examinations and hysterosal-

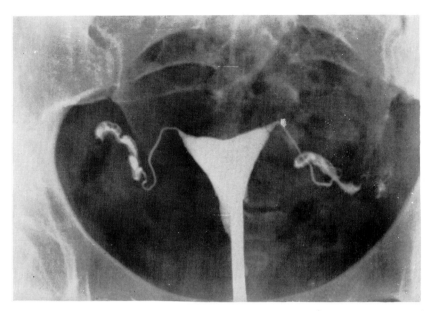

Fig. 11-5. Normal tubogram showing filling of tubes with radiopaque medium (see Fig. 11-6).

pingography are necessary to prove organic obstruction.

Hysterosalpingography. X-ray visualization of the uterine cavity and the tubal lumina is possible after the injection of radiopaque material into the upper genital tract. With this procedure the site of tubal obstruction can be located accurately, and valuable information concerning the presence of tubal abnormalities such as hydrosalpinx or fixation from adhesions is provided. It also is possible to demonstrate small submucous fibroids or other congenital or acquired defects that may be present in the uterine cavity. The contraindications are the same as those against uterotubal insufflation.

Hysterosalpingography is preferable to uterotubal insufflation in the study of infertility because it provides so much more information concerning the structure and function of the uterus and tubes. The only conclusion that can be drawn from a normal Rubin test is that at least one tube is patent.

The required apparatus consists of a bivalve speculum, a tenaculum, various cannulus of the same type as those used in the Rubin test, and a 10 ml. syringe, all of which must be sterilized. Both water-soluble and oil-soluble contrast media are available, and each provides satisfactory visualization of the uterine cavity and the tubes. The water-soluble media are preferable because they are absorbed from the peritoneal cavity rapidly and produce less local irritation than do the oily ones. In addition, fatal pulmonary embolisms have occurred after the unintentional injection of the latter into the uterine veins, but none has been reported with the water-soluble preparations.

The syringe containing the contrast material is attached to the cannula, and the air is displaced from the lumen by filling it with the media. The tip of the cannula is inserted into the cervical canal, and after a 2-minute wait 2 to 3 ml. of the media is injected. This is enough to fill the normal uterine cavity without distending it and may outline small irregularities that would be obscured by a larger amount. The first set of anteroposterior stereoscopic films is taken at this time. The rest of the contrast medium, which should distend the uterus and flow through the tubes, is then injected, but it may not be enough if the uterine cavity is unusually large or the tubes are distended. This will be obvious when the second set of stereoscopic films is examined. No test can be considered as satisfactory unless the uterus and tubes are distended to their maximum capacity or unless fluid spills from the ends of the tubes. Hysterosal-

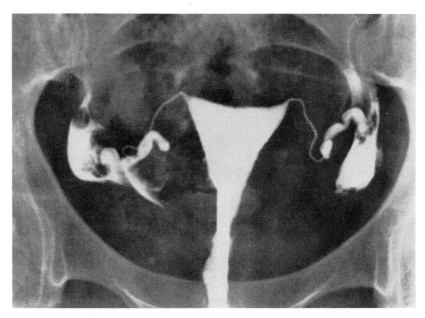

Fig. 11-6. Normal tubogram showing passage of radiopaque material through fimbriated ends of tubes and peritoneal "spill."

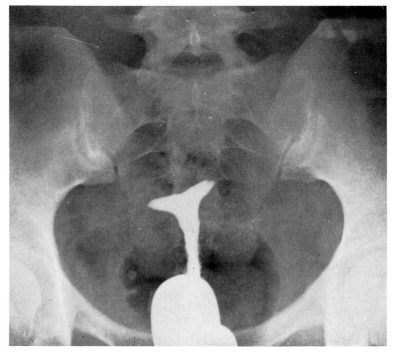

Fig. 11-7. Tubogram. Tubes occluded at cornual ends. (From Willson, J. R.: Management of obstetric difficulties, ed. 6, St. Louis, 1961, The C. V. Mosby Co.)

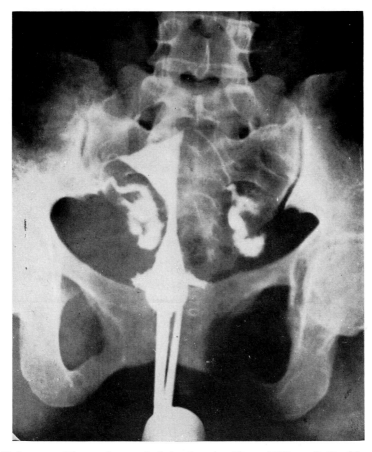

Fig. 11-8. Tubogram. Obstruction at fimbriated ends. (From Willson, J. R.: Management of obstetric difficulties, ed. 6, St. Louis, 1961, The C. V. Mosby Co.)

pingography can be controlled more precisely if the injection is made with the help of the fluoroscope; the use of an image intensifier will reduce the radiation hazard to a minimum.

Culdoscopy or laparoscopy. Direct observation of the passage of dye from the uterus through the fimbriated ends of the tubes is possible with the culdoscope or laparoscope and may be utilized for the determination of tubal patency by those experienced in the use of the instruments. An added advantage of this method is that it provides an opportunity for direct visualization of the pelvic structures, thus supplementing the other methods for evaluating normalcy.

STEP 4—DETERMINATION OF OVULATION

The production of normal ova and their expulsion from the ovary into the fallopian tube are the primary requirements for female fertility. The determination of the presence of this phenomenon and of the time of its occurrence is an important part of the investigation of all problems of infertility. The details of techniques, clinical application, and evaluation of the tests commonly employed for ovarian function are discussed in Chapter 2.

STEP 5—EVALUATION OF THE CERVICAL FACTOR

After normal fertility in the husband has been established by examination of the ejaculated semen, it becomes necessary to determine the effect of the vaginal and cervical secretions on the activity of the sperm. There is a period of only 24 to 72 hours in the entire menstrual cycle during which sperm can penetrate the cervical mucus. This occurs in the ovulatory phase of the cycle when the mucus is copious, thin, and watery and exhibits maximum spinnbarkheit and arborization.

The postcoital examination of cervical mucus (Sims-Huhner test) provides information concerning the number of spermatozoa that have entered the cervical canal and the percentage that retain their motility in the cervical mucus, but it gives no indication of the adequacy of the semen specimen. It is, therefore, not a substitute for semen analysis. It is essential that the postcoital test be performed when the secretions should be optimum for sperm penetration and survival; the day of ovulation is most appropriate.

The patient is instructed to report for examination 6 to 12 hours after coitus without having used a precoital lubricant or a postcoital douche. The cervix is exposed through an unlubricated speculum, and a specimen of mucus is obtained from the cervical canal with a uterine dressing forceps or a Palmer cervical mucus forceps. The material is examined for clarity, viscosity, and spinnbarkheit, and the pH is determined. The specimen is then spread on a clean glass slide and examined for the presence of sperm and, after it has dried, for aborization of the mucus.

Under normal conditions at least 10 to 15 active sperm can be seen in each high-power field. If sperm are present, but if none or only an occasional one is active, one can assume that the endocervical environment is unsuitable for their survival, if a previous semen analysis was normal.

Normal mucus at midcycle shows maximum spinnbarkheit and arborization. Inadequacies in these factors suggest either an estrogen deficiency or a defect in secretory activity of the cervical glands (*dysmucorrhea*).

■ Treatment of infertility

The treatment of infertility often begins with the first consultation, even though no specific therapy can be outlined until all the data obtained from the complete investigation of the couple have been analyzed and correlated. Not infrequently a woman may become pregnant soon after the initial visit or after the first tubal insufflation. Such a favorable outcome early in the investigation may be credited to the helpful hints regarding the technique and timing of coitus or to the correction of a minor abnormality.

However, it actually may be because of the psychotherapeutic effect of either the decision to deal with the problem actively or because of the positive transference reaction to the physician. In general the active treatment of infertility must be directed to the factors that the investigative procedures have indicated to be responsible for the failure to conceive.

Treatment of failure of insemination. Obvious abnormalities such as an intact hymen, developmental defects, or obesity should be corrected if possible. If failure in insemination occurs because of penile abnormalities, therapeutic insemination with the husband's semen should be considered. Inpotence, frigidity, vaginismus, and dyspareunia are seldom of organic origin, and psychotherapy usually is necessary for their correction. Faulty sexual techniques can be corrected by discussing the entire act with both partners and suggesting necessary modifications.

In order to be more certain that the semen remains in the posterior fornix and upper vagina, the woman should be instructed to maintain flexion of the thighs during and after intercourse, to remain supine for at least 30 minutes after the male ejaculation, and never to take a postcoital douche.

The time at which ovulation occurs can be estimated after the basal body temperatures have been recorded for three or more cycles. It is presumed that ovulation occurs as the temperature is falling or at the low point on the graph since the subsequent thermal rise is a result of progesterone production. If the length of the cycle is constant and if the fall in temperature occurs consistently at the same relative time, the fertile period can be calculated in advance each month without continuing the temperature recordings. The number of days between the low point preceding the thermal rise and the onset of menstruation is counted and subtracted from the date that menstruation presumably will begin. This will be the anticipated day of ovulation. Coitus during the period starting 2 days before and ending 2 days after ovulation is anticipated should cover minor deviations from the expected ovulatory pattern. If temperatures are being recorded, the couple should have intercourse on the day the temperature falls and the day after. Pregnancy sometimes occurs promptly after such a program is initiated, suggesting that the infertility was the result of consistent failure to deposit sperm at a time when ovulation was possible.

Frequency of intercourse should be drastically limited if the sperm count is low since emissions at 24-hour intervals greatly reduce the number of motile forms, thus further decreasing fertility. Ejaculation every other day affects the count less, and little change can be detected at 3-day intervals. The highly fertile male may become only relatively fertile after repeated ejaculations every 24 hours, but little change can be detected at the longer intervals. After a preliminary period of continence the subfertile male should time coitus to take place 2 days before the expected temperature fall, on the day of the fall, and 1 day afterward, in order that a maximum number of active sperm will be deposited during the period of greatest fertility.

Failure of spermatogenesis because of destructive testicular disease cannot be improved, and the inability to transport the sperm because of occlusions in the ductal system is difficult to correct. Reduced sperm counts can sometimes be improved by thyroid therapy if decreased thyroid function is the responsible factor, but other endocrine preparations are usually ineffectual in stimulating spermatogenesis.

Treatment of failure in ascent of sperm. Alterations in the pH of the vagina are not often responsible for inactivation of sperm unless the change in acidity is caused by vaginitis. If infection is present, it must be treated because the vaginal and cervical secretions are altered by the inflammatory response and may become lethal for the sperm. If all other factors have been eliminated and fertilization still does not occur, a precoital douche with 2 quarts of warm water and 2 tablespoonfuls of soda bicarbonate may be tried.

Cervical lesions should be eradicated and the cervix returned to as normal a state as possible. The treatment of benign disease of the cervix is discussed in Chapter 42.

Unusually viscous cervical mucus, which can interfere with the ascent of the sperm through the cervical canal, may be the result of a diminished production of estrogen because of defective ovarian function. The administration of 0.1 mg. of stilbestrol daily from the fifth to the fifteenth day of the cycle may decrease the viscosity of the cervical secretions, but if the primary defect lies in the ovary, pregnancy cannot be expected to occur. Large dosages of estrogenic substance early in the preovulatory phase may delay or even prevent ovulation.

Therapeutic insemination. Therapeutic, or artificial insemination refers to the artificial injection of semen into the cervical canal. It is termed *homologous* insemination if the husband's semen is used and *heterologous* insemination if the semen of a man other than the husband is utilized. Homologous insemination is indicated if the husband is normally fertile but is unable to ejaculate the semen over the cervix because of obesity or a penile defect or if a cervical abnormality appears to prevent the invasion of a sufficient number of sperm. Injection of the semen of a husband with oligospermia may sometimes initiate a pregnancy. Heterologous insemination is indicated if the husband's infertility has been proved to be irremediable. Neither type of insemination should be considered unless a complete study of the female partner proves her to be free from defects that might be partially responsible for the failure to conceive.

Insemination with the husband's semen presents no legal problem, but heterologous insemination involves a great many emotional, ethical, legal, and religious considerations. If the male partner is solely responsible for the failure to conceive, the couple can be offered only two choices, adoption or insemination, and the selection of the method must depend upon the wishes of both partners. Should there be a question in the mind of either as to the advisability of insemination, the physician should refuse to carry out the procedure. The decision must not be made at the initial discussion, but only after sufficient time has elapsed to make certain that it has been thoroughly thought through and discussed.

Therapeutic insemination must be timed to coincide with the ovulatory phase of the cycle. One can determine the appropriate time for insemination on the basis of several cycles of basal body temperatures and the daily examination of cervical mucus during the immediate preovulatory phase of the cycle. Insemination is usually carried out on the day before and the day after the estimated ovulation day.

Two highly fertile donors who have been continent for 5 days should be utilized during each series of insemination, and they must neither know who the barren couple is nor be known by them. Donors free from hereditary defects and clinical disease and with physical appearance and blood type similar to that of the infertile husband should be selected. Only Rh-negative donors should be used to inseminate Rh-negative women.

Treatment of uterine abnormalities. Changes in the position of the otherwise normal uterus rarely interfere with fertilization of the ovum, but if the uterus is retro-displaced, it should be replaced and maintained in the anterior position for several months with a properly fitting pessary while attempts at conception are continued. If pregnancy does occur, the pessary should be left in place until the end of the first trimester or until the uterus is large enough so that it cannot fall backward into the pelvis.

Uterine fibromyomas alone are seldom responsible for failure to conceive, and myomectomy seldom is indicated to improve fertility. This is particularly true if the tumors are small and of the subserous or intramural types. If myomas obstruct the cornual ends of both tubes, if the endometrial cavity is distorted by several submucous tumors that are associated with increased bleeding and that may interfere with nidation, or if a pedunculated, submucous fibroid is present, removal should be considered. Myomectomy alone is valueless if other causes of infertility remain uncorrected.

Although the incidence of infertility is increased in association with congenital or acquired structural defects in the uterus, such an abnormality alone is not always the factor that decreases fertility. Unless it can be clearly established that the defect is responsible for failure to conceive, its correction is unwarranted. A true infantile uterus ordinarily indicates a pronounced alteration in endocrine function and rarely occurs without evidence of underdevelopment in the breasts and in the other genital structures. Although most infantile uteri will grow when stimulated by estrogen, such therapy alone does not correct the underlying defect.

Treatment of tubal abnormalities. At-tempts to restore tubal patency by repeated uterotubal insufflation, the injection of oil-soluble contrast media, pelvic diathermy, administration of adrenal cortical substances, and other nonsurgical methods have been almost uniformly unsuccessful. The results from surgical procedures are better but far from spectacular. Pregnancy rates of 15% to 25% after tubal plastic procedures have been reported, but the incidence of pregnancy failure from abortion and tubal pregnancy is high. The main problem is that the tubes may not function normally, even though patency is reestablished, because of irreparable damage done to the muscle and mucosa by the condition responsible for the occlusion. The techniques of tubal reconstruction are delicate, and the best results are obtained when the operation is performed by skillful surgeons who are experienced in the surgical treatment of tubal obstruction.

Treatment of endocrine abnormalities in the female. Menstrual disorders such as amenorrhea and dysfunctional bleeding that are associated with endocrinopathic infertility are due mainly to disturbances of ovulation. Therapy in these situations is directed to the cause of the hormonal dysfunction, with the aim of regulating the menstrual function and effecting regular ovulatory cycles. These problems are discussed in detail in the chapters relating to menstruation and its abnormalities.

Improvement in general health and correction of malnutrition or obesity may favorably influence poor ovarian function. If there is evidence of *hypometabolism,* appropriate amounts of thyroid extract should be administered. The mechanism by which thyroid extract improves fertility is not known, and although it may prove effective in those patients whose thyroid function is reduced, it is of no value in women with normal metabolic activity.

Occasionally patients who menstruate and ovulate fairly regularly show clinical evidence of *inadequate progesterone effect.* This may be suspected if the basal body temperature chart shows a gradual instead of an abrupt ovulatory rise and is confirmed by the finding of an imperfect progestational endometrium on about the twenty-fifth day of the cycle. These patients may be given 25 mg. of progesterone intramuscularly every other day for 5 days beginning at midcycle, or oral Provera, 10 mg. daily for 10 days.

When the amenorrhea and infertility are found to be due to polycystic ovaries (Stein-Leventhal syndrome), the operation of *bilateral wedge resection* has given excellent results, but ovulation can often be induced with clomiphene.

Psychotherapy in infertility. A small percentage of patients show no organic or hormonal cause for infertility after careful investigation, and yet they fail to conceive. In a considerable number of these a psychogenic factor may be obvious, whereas in others the emotional conflict may be an unconscious one and most difficult to detect. Positive psychotherapy will come into play automatically if the physician can establish a good relationship with the couple. Unhurried consultations and a thorough and systematic investigation of their problems serve to inspire confidence. Instructions should be specific, but the physician must avoid unnecessary restrictions of sexual activity and prolonged basal temperature recordings.

As the investigation progresses, the physician should encourage the patient to vent her feelings regarding pregnancy, labor, and the rearing of children. The following simple questionnaire may be helpful in detecting the psychodynamics of the emotional conflict that may be interfering with the couple's reproductive potential:

1. Why do you want a baby? What does your inability to conceive mean to you?
2. What sort of woman was your mother? Would you rear your child the way your mother reared you?
3. What sort of man is your husband?
4. Would you rather work or keep house?
5. Do you want a boy or a girl? Why?
6. How many children would you like to have?

The answers to these questions must not be sought by direct interrogation or at one interview but should be obtained by cautious and gentle probing, ever mindful of the significant dynamic factors. Physicians who are unable or unwilling to carry out this type of management should refer the patient to a psychiatrist.

References

Behrman, S. J.: Artificial insemination, Fertil. Steril. **10:**248, 1959.

Behrman, S. J.: Agglutinins, antibodies, and immune reactions, Clin. Obstet. Gynec. **8:**91, 1965.

Behrman, S. J., and Kistner, R. W.: Progress in infertility, Boston, 1968, Little, Brown & Co.

Bos, C., and Cleghorn, R. A.: Psychogenic sterility, Fertil. Steril. **9:**84, 1958.

Buxton, C. L., and Southam, A. L.: Human infertility, New York, 1958, Paul B. Hoeber, Inc., Medical Book Department, Harper & Row, Publishers.

Cohen, M. R., Stein, I. F., and Kaye, B. M.: Spinnbarkheit, a characteristic of cervical mucus, Fertil. Steril. **3:**201, 1952.

Farris, E. J.: Human fertility and problems of the male, White Plains, N. Y., 1950, The Author's Press, Inc.

Ford, E. S. C., Forman, I., Willson, J. R., Char, W., Mixson, W. T., and Scholz, C.: A psychodynamic approach to the study of infertility, Fertil. Steril. **4:**456, 1953.

Forman, I.: Cervical mucus arborization; aid in ovulation timing, Obstet. Gynec. **8:**287, 1956.

Goldfarb, A. F., Morales, A., Rakoff, A. E., and Protos, P.: Critical review of clomiphene-related pregnancies, Obstet. Gynec. **31:**342, 1968.

MacLeod, J.: The semen examination, Clin. Obstet. Gynec. **8:**115, 1965.

Mastrioianni, L., Jr.: The diagnosis and timing of ovulation, Clin. Obstet. Gynec. **2:**797, 1959.

Morris, T. A., and Sturgis, S. H.: Practical aspects of psychosomatic sterility, Clin. Obstet. Gynec. **2:**890, 1959.

Murphy, D. P., and Torrano, E. F.: Male fertility in 3,620 childless couples, Fertil. Steril. **16:**337, 1965.

Rubin, I. C.: Uterotubal insufflation, St. Louis, 1947, The C. V. Mosby Co.

Stein, I. F., and Cohen, M. R.: Sperm survival at estimated ovulation time; prognosis and significance, Fertil. Steril. **1:**169, 1950.

Tompkins, P.: The use of basal body temperature graphs in determining the date of ovulation, J.A.M.A. **124:**698, 1944.

Weir, W. C., and Downs, T. D.: The optimal time for conception, Fertil. Steril. **19:**64, 1968.

12

Control of conception

There is little to indicate that uncomplicated pregnancy and delivery are harmful to normal women, but one cannot logically conclude from this that uncontrolled reproduction is desirable. The increasing social and economic demands, at both individual and community levels, make it essential that each couple reach a logical decision early in marriage concerning the number of children for which they can assume responsibility. Physicians, social agencies, or governments cannot tell normal couples how many children they can have, but each one can share in the responsibility of making effective and appropriate contraceptive methods available to those who want them.

It is estimated that more than 90% of all married couples in the United States either have used or intend to use some method for controlling fertility. About one fifth of all parous women wanted fewer children than they have, and as many as 75% of women registering in prenatal clinics have not planned their present pregnancies. How many unplanned pregnancies also are unwanted is not known.

Physicians, who should have the greatest interest in providing their own patients with adequate means of controlling fertility, have been apathetic. Many avoid the subject because they fear that they will become involved in troublesome legal or religious problems, because of a presumed moral issue, or because of their own religious backgrounds. A 1957 survey of physicians in various communities in the United States revealed interesting and startling information which suggests that many doctors, even obstetrician-gynecologists, attempt to avoid the whole subject of contraception completely. For example, over two thirds of the non-Catholic doctors surveyed thought that information concerning conception control should be provided *only* when requested by the patient. Of those who professed to do premarital counseling, only about one third brought up the subject of contraception often and almost half never mentioned it voluntarily; about half *never* initiated a discussion of contraception with women they had delivered. The situation has improved considerably in recent years, but there are still too many physicians who take too little responsibility for providing contraceptive counseling for their parents.

Every physician, particularly obstetrician-gynecologists, should feel responsible for providing contraceptive assistance for those of his patients who want it. He should always bring up the subject himself during premarital examinations, when he is consulted by young married couples, and after each delivery. If he chooses, for one reason or another, not to instruct the patient himself, he must refer her to another physician who will. Too often the patient will hesitate to ask about contraception, and if the doctor fails to mention the subject she will leave his office without having been instructed. The constant fear of pregnancy is a common cause for emotional illness and marital discord.

A perplexing problem, being encountered with increasing frequency, is the teenager who seeks contraceptive advice. We can anticipate meeting the situation more frequently in the future as young people mature, both physiologically and socially, at an earlier age and as sexual mores change. Each physician must make a definite decision as to how he is going to respond to such requests. The following are a few basic considerations that are essential to the problem:

1. It is illogical to respond with an unqualified "No" and to dismiss the girl without counseling. Some, particularly the younger girls, may be asking "Do I *have* to have intercourse" because they are confused by the pressures being put on them. Others who are already having intercourse will continue without protection and conceive.

2. It is unlikely that a girl who has been having intercourse regularly will stop simply because she is told it is "wrong." She already knows that, having been taught it by parents, teachers, minister, and friends. Her problem is that she already has made the decision for coitus and needs contraception.

3. An affirmative response to a request for contraception without exploring the relationship in some detail is also inadequate. Many girls who ask for contraceptive advice are really seeking help for the total problem. In fact the real reason for the request sometimes is that she has not yet had coitus and is being pressured to a point which she feels she must comply.

4. It is difficult to determine when to include the parents. It may be questionable for girls during their late teens who have what appears to be a good total relationship with a boy; this is particularly true if they plan eventually to marry. On the other hand, the parents of young girls who seek contraceptive advice must be involved. Before approaching the parents, however, one must learn all he can about the child and her need for contraception and be ready to support her in the solution of the problem.

There is no ready answer to teenage contraception. The solution is determined by the problem, which will never be clarified if the physician either complies with the request or denies it without exploring the situation.

There are many contraceptive methods, ranging from relatively simple forms to operative procedures that interrupt the continuity of the fallopian tubes or of the vas deferens. No single method is uniformly satisfactory, and the physician must be familiar with several types so that, after analyzing all the factors involved, he can select the one best suited for each individual couple.

In general, contraceptive methods can be divided into (1) physiologic, (2) chemical, (3) mechanical, (4) hormonal, and (5) surgical. All attempt to prevent the union of the sperm and ovum or to interfere with nidation. The protection rate for any contraceptive method can be calculated for its users as the number of pregnancies per hundred years of use by the following formula, which permits comparison of the methods:

$$\text{Pregnancy rate} = \frac{\text{Total number of conceptions} \times 1,200}{\text{Total months of exposure}}$$

PHYSIOLOGIC CONTRACEPTION

In physiologic contraception no chemical or mechanical device is used. The two methods are withdrawal and the calculation of the safe period.

Withdrawal. The penis is withdrawn from the vagina just before ejaculation occurs. This method does not afford maximum protection because fertilization can occur if live sperm are present in the seminal fluid that leaks from the urethra during coitus and if the withdrawal is not timed accurately, permitting at least part of the semen to discharge within the vagina. Repeated withdrawal before the female has reached her climax may well be responsible for emotional and marital disturbances. The pregnancy rate for withdrawal is about 16 per 100 years of use.

Rhythm (safe period). The human ovum probably survives no longer than 48 hours after it has been extruded from the ovary, and the life of the ejaculated sperm is little if any longer. If coitus is avoided during the *fertile period* (3 to 4 days before and after ovulation), unprotected intercourse during the *safe period* (the other days of the cycle) should not be productive of a pregnancy. Ovulation occurs fairly regularly about 14 days before the onset of menstruation, and the safe period can be calculated reasonably accurately in women whose cycles vary by no more than a day or two. Variations in the length of the menstrual cycles are ordinarily due to differences in the length of the preovulatory rather than the postovulatory phase; therefore in women with grossly irregular cycles the fertile period can be calculated only in retrospect.

If a patient with a regular cycle will avoid intercourse for 3 days before and 2 days after ovulation, she will not conceive unless she occasionally ovulates at an unusual time. The fertile period is determined after accurate recording of the number of days of each menstrual cycle during a period of 1 year. According to the Ogino formula the first unsafe day (beginning of the fertile period) can be determined by subtracting 18 days from the length of the shortest cycle and the last unsafe day by subtracting 11 days from the length of the longest cycle. For example, the fertile period for a woman with 25- to 35-day cycles would extend from the seventh to the twenty-fourth day of each cycle. It is quite obvious that few couples will abstain from coitus regularly during such long intervals.

Use of the safe period with its relatively narrow margin of safety is quite satisfactory for people who want more children, but it is not certain enough for those in whom pregnancy must for one reason or another be avoided. The pregnancy rate is about 34.5 per 100 years of use.

CHEMICAL CONTRACEPTION

The chemical methods of contraception consist of the deposition of a spermaticidal substance in the vagina before coitus. This material, usually a water-soluble jelly, coats the vaginal wall and the cervix and collects in the fornices, thus exposing the spermatozoa to its destructive action. It is reasonably reliable and offers more protection than the physiologic methods but less than a combination of the spermaticidal jelly and a contraceptive diaphragm. The pregnancy rate for jelly alone is about 20 per 100 years of use, but rates as low as 11 and as high as 39 per 100 years have been reported. Aerosol foams, which contain spermaticidal chemicals and which are used before coitus, offer about the same protection rate.

Other chemical methods include the use of various tablets, which may fail because they do not melt after they have been placed in the vagina, and postcoital douches, which offer almost no protection because the fluid cannot destroy the sperms that have already reached the cervical canal.

MECHANICAL CONTRACEPTION

Before oral contraceptives were developed, the most frequently prescribed method was a combination of an *occlusive vaginal diaphragm* and a *spermaticidal jelly*. It is necessary that the physician fit the diaphragm, instruct the patient in its use, and make certain, by having her return with the diaphragm in place after practicing using it at home, that she can insert it properly. For many women the insertion of a diaphragm is distasteful and too much trouble, but for those who use one regularly and properly they offer almost certain protection. The diaphragm must be inserted before intercourse and left in place at least 6 hours after ejaculation. The pregnancy rate is about 15 per 100 years of use.

The *condom* is a common form of mechanical contraceptive that offers good protection but has a number of disadvantages. It may break or slip off the penis and it dulls sensation. It provides better protection when used in conjunction with a vaginal spermaticidal jelly, and in fact this method is often prescribed at the premarital examination if it is impossible to fit a diaphragm. The pregnancy rate with the condom is about 15 per 100 years of use.

A more recent mechanical method is the use of *intrauterine devices,* small plastic or stainless steel coils, spirals, or rings that are inserted into the uterus and allowed to remain in place indefinitely. The prototype intrauterine device was the German silver Grafenberg ring, which was first used during the 1920's. The method was abandoned by most physicians because the rings caused ulceration of the uterine wall and infection.

In 1959 Oppenheimer reported on his use of a silkworm gut coil that effectively prevented conception with few ill effects. Since then several different devices have been developed and used successfully. These include the polyethylene Lippes loop, the Permaspiral and others, and the stainless steel Hall-Stone ring. These are inserted into the uterine cavity and allowed to remain in place. The patient often experiences intermenstrual spotting, increased menstruation, and cramping during the first month or two the ring is in place. After this she is unaware of its presence. There is no evidence to suggest that the device predisposes to uterine infection or to cancer. In about 10% of women the uterus repeatedly expels the device, and an additional 5% to 10% want the pessary removed for one reason or another. It provides a satisfactory method in about 80% of those in whom it is introduced. It is more suitable for multiparous than for nulliparous women.

The method by which intrauterine devices prevent pregnancy is not completely clear, but there are two possibilities. The ovum is transported through the tube to the uterus more rapidly when there is a foreign body in the uterus, thus the ovum may be fertilized in the tube, but it reaches the uterus before it is ready to implant and is cast off. There are local endometrial changes, consisting of stromal edema and an increase in the number of large thin-walled endometrial blood sinuses. Ovulation is not prevented. It seems certain that intrauterine devices interfere with implantation rather than cause repeated abortions. The pregnancy rate is about 3 per 100 years of use.

HORMONAL CONTRACEPTION

The ovarian hormones, estrogen and progesterone, when given in the proper dosage depress anterior pituitary function, thereby inhibiting the secretion of gonadotropic hormones and preventing ovulation. Large doses of progesterone, which is expensive, must be administered by injection to achieve this result, and estrogen, which costs less and can be taken orally, produces numerous side effects as well as irregular bleeding. The synthetic progestogens 17-alpha-ethinyl-19-nortestosterone (norethindrone) and 17-alpha-ethinyl-5,10 estraenolone (norethynodrel) combined with an estrogen act in the same manner and inhibit ovulation consistently. The amount of the estrogen-progestogen combination that is necessary to inhibit ovulation is much less than that contained in the early oral contraceptives. Most now contain less than 100 μg. of estrogen.

One tablet is taken each day for 21 days, starting on the fifth day of the menstrual cycle. The medication suppresses anterior pituitary secretion of gonadotropins, thereby inhibiting ovulation. It also has a direct stimulating effect on the endometrium so that from 1 to 4 days after the last tablet is taken the endometrium sloughs and bleeds as a result of hormonal withdrawal. The bleeding usually is less profuse than that of a normal period and may last only 2 or 3 days. Some women have no bleeding at all. The patient starts taking the medication again 7 days after she has taken the last pill, even though she does not bleed, and continues for another 21 days. This can be continued indefinitely.

The contraceptive effect is a combined result of ovulation inhibition, endometrial changes, and an alteration in cervical mucus. The glands are fairly widely scattered and remain straight throughout the cycle. Secretory activity can be detected in the gland cells after a few days of treatment, and it increases during the following few days, but by about the twentieth day the cells appear inactive. The stroma remains dense throughout, and a predecidual effect, which appears as early as the seventh day, does not often advance and usually disappears by about the middle of the cycle. The endometrium becomes quite thin after the patient has been on the medication for several months; this probably accounts for the reduced flow. The cervical mucus remains thick due to the effect of the progestogen, and it probably does not provide a suitable atmosphere for sperm survival as does the thin viscid mucus at ovulation.

Another type of oral contraceptive, the sequential, attempts to duplicate the hormone status during the normal cycle; estrogen alone is administered during the first 2 weeks and estrogen and progesterone during the third week. As might be anticipated, the endometrium responds differently and is more like that found normally. The change in cervical mucus also is more like that during the normal cycle. These factors may account for the slight decrease in protection against pregnancy as compared to the combined types.

In most women ovulation is resumed promptly, often during the first cycle, after the pills are discontinued. In an occasional instance women who have menstruated normally before taking the medication become amenorrheic when it is discontinued. The amenorrhea may be of short duration or it may last for months. It is probably caused by a depression of the hypothalamus rather than by a local effect on the endometrium because bleeding can be induced by the administration of estrogen. It is preferable not to prescribe estrogen or progesterone to induce bleeding because these substances merely serve to depress the hypothalamus even more and may delay recovery. Oral contraceptives have no effect on subsequent pregnancies.

Undesirable side effects are common but fortunately are transient, usually lasting for no more than 3 or 4 cycles. They include nausea, vomiting, breast engorgement, headache, vertigo, and fluid retention. The latter can usually be controlled by reducing sodium intake, but it is so distressing to some women that they will not continue taking the medication. Many women gain 6 to 10 pounds in weight while taking the medication and cannot lose it until they stop. If side effects do not disappear spontaneously, the physician should try another preparation because this may relieve them. Side effects are in part related to the amount of hormone since they are far less troublesome with low-dosage compounds.

The total incidence of "breakthrough" bleeding is about 8% to 10% but it occurs more often during the first few cycles than later. It also occurs more often when pills of smaller dosage are used. If the bleeding is slight and occurs only occasionally and particularly if it consists only of slight spotting during the last few days of pill ingestion, the physician should reassure the patient that it means nothing and attempt to convince her to ignore it. Some women must discontinue oral contraceptives because of irregular bleeding that can neither be controlled nor ignored.

Most of the complications are inconsequential when compared to the ease with which pregnancy can be prevented, but others may be more significant. Studies carried out under the auspices of the Committee on Safety of Drugs of Great Britain indicate that the estimated annual *death rates from thromboembolic disease* in women aged 20 to 34 years was 1.5 per 100,000 for users of oral contraceptives and 0.2 for nonusers. Comparable figures for women aged 35 to 44 years are 3.9 and 0.5. Studies in the United States support the concept that there is an increased risk of thromboembolism in oral contraceptive users. Changes in

blood coagulation factors have been found, but whether these are of importance in precipitating thrombosis is not known.

Women who become *jaundiced* during pregnancy because of cholestasis may respond in exactly the same manner to the administration of estrogen. *Hypertension* may be produced or augmented in certain women by oral contraceptives. These substances appear to have a *diabetogenic effect* similar to that of pregnancy, and glucose metabolism may be altered in some users. *Migraine* may be precipitated or become more severe in some women using these drugs.

Since there is still so much question concerning the physiologic effects of estrogen-progestogen combinations it seems wise to limit their use to perfectly normal healthy women who choose them over other methods after the risks have been described to them.

If contraceptive tablets are taken according to the recommended schedule, the incidence of unplanned pregnancy should be close to zero. If they are taken irregularly during the cycle, ovulation and fertilization may occur. With further improvements oral contraception will undoubtedly become the most widely used of all methods.

Ovulation can also be inhibited by injecting large doses of long-acting progestogens. This is still in an experimental stage, but it appears that pregnancy can be prevented by progesterone injections repeated at intervals of 3 to 6 months.

SURGICAL CONTRACEPTION

Termination of fertility by an operative procedure can be performed in both men and women. The most common reasons for surgical sterilization in women are chronic cardiovascular-renal disease, severe heart disease, advanced pulmonary tuberculosis, and diabetes mellitus. It may also be performed in conjunction with vaginal plastic operations and cesarean section; in the latter instance the physician may offer to sterilize a patient at the time of her third cesarean section if she and her husband wish, but he should not insist upon it. Elective sterilization also is appropriate for normal women who have completed their childbearing careers and who still have many years of fertility ahead. It may be particularly important if they cannot use an effective contraceptive method, and it may well be preferable to many years of using oral hormonal contraceptives.

The fallopian tubes can also be ligated in conjunction with other necessary abdominal operations or as a primary procedure. Puerperal sterilization is usually performed during the first 24 hours after delivery under local anesthesia.

The patient and her husband should understand that she will be unable to conceive after the operation but that she is being sterilized (termination of fertility) not castrated (removal of gonads). Although the law actually requires only the consent of the patient herself, both the husband and wife should usually give written permission for the procedure if the patient is married.

One must always consider the possible emotional effects of permanent elimination of procreative ability. It is not easy, even for a woman who wants no more children, to relinquish her ability to conceive. Men who are somewhat uncertain in their masculine roles may be impotent after vasectomy. These potential effects of sterilization must be explored before the operation is performed because even though each member of the couple may verbally agree, he may be unconsciously resisting.

FUTURE METHODS

The presently available methods for controlling conception leave much to be desired. With the exception of intrauterine devices and surgical procedures, each requires a considerable amount of motivation—particularly the taking of oral medication daily or the use of a physiologic or mechanical method consistently year after year. Many are able to do this, but it is unrealistic to expect it of primitive peoples and of most members of the lowest socioeconomic groups in the United States. The current research in immunologic methods, by which it will be possible to provide temporary immunity against spermatozoa, is promising, as are hormonal methods that require single injections at long periods of time. The ideal is a method that is completely effective and without danger but reversible and that requires no preparation for individual acts of coitus.

References

Calderone, M. S.: Manual of contraceptive practice, Baltimore, rev. ed., 1966, The Williams & Wilkins Co.

Dickinson, R. L.: Techniques of conception control, Baltimore, 1950, The Williams & Wilkins Co.

Goldzieher, J. W.: Future approaches to conception control, Pacif. Med. Surg. **73:**69, 1965.

Hartman, C. G.: Science and the safe period, Baltimore, 1962, The Williams & Wilkins Co.

Hellman, L. M.: The oral contraceptives in clinical practice, Family Planning Perspectives **1:**13, 1969.

Vessey, M. P., and Doll, R.: Investigations of relation between use of oral contraceptives and thromboembolic disease, Brit. Med. J. **2:**199, 1968.

Willson, J. R.: Intrauterine contraceptive devices; their effectiveness in controlling fertility and their effects on uterine tissues, Pacif. Med. Surg. **73:**44, 1965.

Willson, J. R., Ledger, W. J., Bollinger, C. C., and Andros, G. J.: The Margulies intrauterine contraceptive device; experience with 623 women, Amer. J. Obstet. Gynec. **92:**62, 1965.

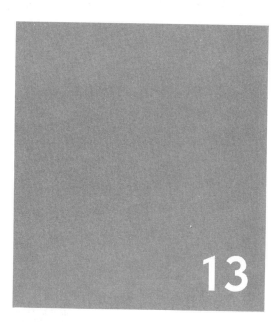

13

Spontaneous and induced abortion

Abortion is the termination of a pregnancy before the end of the twentieth week. Termination of pregnancy between the twenty-first and the end of the twenty-eighth week, when the infant, which weighs from 500 to 999 grams, theoretically can carry on an independent existence, is called *immature labor*. Abortions that occur accidentally because of some maternal or ovular defect are termed *spontaneous*, whereas those that are brought on intentionally are said to be *induced*, or *artificial*. An induced abortion is *legal* if performed by a physician in an approved hospital or other facility or *illegal* if performed by an individual or in a facility not approved by the law. Those abortions that are accompanied by infection are termed *septic*.

The incidence of abortion is difficult to estimate with accuracy because those that

are illegal do not come to the attention of the physician unless a complication develops, and many that occur spontaneously are accompanied by such minor symptoms that medical aid is deemed unnecessary. The incidence of spontaneous termination of early pregnancy has been estimated by various investigators as at least 10%. Taussig, however, has estimated that the total abortion rate in the United States is 43.4%, at least one half of which are induced.

■ Spontaneous abortion
ETIOLOGY

The causes of spontaneous abortion are multiple and include both fetal and maternal factors. A definite reason for a specific spontaneous abortion cannot always be established because a complete analysis of all causative factors is impossible. In most instances, however, the reason for the failure is temporary and does not interfere with the future childbearing capacity.

The possible etiologic factors in spontaneous abortion include the following:

I. Defective germ plasm
  A. Ovum
  B. Spermatozoon
II. Defective nidation
  A. Inadequate progestational endometrium
III. Maternal disease
  A. Severe acute infections
  B. Serious nutritional deficiencies
  C. Vitamin deficiencies (C and D)
  D. Chronic wasting disease (rare)
IV. Abnormalities of reproductive organs
  A. Laceration of the cervix
  B. Myomas of the uterus
  C. Congenital anomalies
  D. Displacements of the uterus
V. Physical trauma
  A. Severe external trauma (rare)
  B. Laparotomy (infrequent)
VI. Endocrine
  A. Chorionic gonadotropin deficiency
  B. Progesterone deficiency
  C. Thyroid deficiency
  D. Estrogen deficiency (?)
VII. Psychogenic
VIII. Blood group incompatibilities
  A. ABO
  B. Rh

Ovular factors. Defective growth of the ovum may include abnormalities in development and in implantation of the placenta as well as failure in the embryo itself. Mall was able to detect pathologic developmental changes in 48% of aborted embryos. Hertig, in a more recent study, reported a similar incidence. Recent observations suggest that many of the abortions of so-called blighted ova are actually a result of chromosomal aberrations. Thiede and Metcalfe found normal chromosome patterns in all but one of 37 specimens obtained by therapeutic abortion. In contrast, 24 of 54 chromosome preparations from 179 spontaneous abortions were cytogenetically abnormal, and 88% of blighted ova showed some type of genetic abnormality. Suzulman made similar observations. Singh and Carr studied tissue from 387 spontaneous abortions and found 168 embryos, 50 intact empty sacs, and 69 ruptured sacs. Sixteen of 95 embryos with normal chromosome patterns were structurally abnormal. Of 51 with abnormal chromosome patterns, an embryo or fetus was identified in 21. The karyotypes of these were XO (10), triploidy (5), D trisomy (3), 13 trisomy (1), G trisomy (1), and tetraploidy (1).

Late abortions are more often associated with defective placental implantations than with defects in the embryo. Nidation may take place in the lower uterine segment where decidual development and uterine circulation are inadequate to maintain the pregnancy. Abortion in patients with severe hypertensive cardiovascular disease may be in part caused by alterations in the circulation at the placental site secondary to the vascular abnormality.

Maternal factors. The maternal factors that may be responsible for abortion are many and include both local and systemic conditions.

Infections. Acute febrile illnesses may be responsible for death of the embryo and abortion, but tuberculosis and other chronic diseases usually do not disturb pregnancy. Syphilis rarely causes abortion because the spirochetes do not invade the fetal tissues until about the sixteenth week of pregnancy. Generalized peritonitis, appendiceal and pelvic abscesses, and other serious local infections often but not invariably cause abortion. The part played by undulant fever in human abortion has not as yet been clearly established, but it may well be a factor in certain instances of repeated pregnancy failure.

Nutritional deficiencies. A nutritional deficiency sufficient to cause pronounced loss of weight may interfere with both fertility and the maintenance of pregnancy, but the role of subclinical deficiencies is less clear. Vitamin E deficiencies are uncommon and play almost no part in failure of human reproduction. Some observers, notably Javert and Greenblatt, are of the opinion that vitamin C deficiency plays an important role in the etiology of early unintentional abortion. This has not been clearly substantiated.

Genital tract abnormalities. Cervical lacerations that extend through the internal os may be responsible for repeated late abortion and immature labor. As pregnancy advances, the support provided by the intact cervix is lacking; the membranes may rupture or labor may begin.

Developmental abnormalities of the uterus increase the abortion rate several fold if the abnormal structure cannot enlarge sufficiently to accommodate the growing fetus. The incidence of abortion in association with *uterine fibromyomas* also is increased, especially if multiple submucous tumors distort the uterine cavity and reduce the area in which normal placental implantation and growth can take place. Subserous and intramural tumors are less likely to interfere with the progression of the pregnancy.

The *position of the uterus* has little to do with abortion, except in the unusual instances in which a retrodisplaced uterus fails to rise out of the pelvis and becomes incarcerated beneath the promontory of the sacrum.

Endocrine disturbances. Endocrine disturbances undoubtedly play an important part in unintentional abortion, but an exact evaluation of the importance of hormonal deficiencies must await further information concerning the role of chromosomal abnormalities as well as progress in endocrinology.

If the ovum is fertilized, the corpus luteum continues to produce estrogen and progesterone rather than to regress as it does during the normal menstrual cycle. These hormones produce the decidual changes necessary for implantation and for maintaining the ovum during its early growth period. The trophoblastic cells soon begin to secrete estrogen and progesterone, as well as chorionic gonadotropins, and by the end of the sixth week probably supply enough of these hormones to support the pregnancy. Although the ovarian corpus luteum is maintained, it probably is not an important source of estrogen and progesterone. In many instances the ovary containing the corpus luteum has been removed during the first few weeks of pregnancy without disturbing embryonic development.

If the secretion of estrogen and progesterone by the corpus luteum is inadequate, the endometrium may be so poorly prepared for nidation and for support of the ovum that early abortion may result. Early regression of the corpus luteum before the placental production of hormones is adequate may allow the levels to fall below those necessary to maintain normal pregnancy. Or if the trophoblast fails to develop normally, it may be unable to secrete enough hormone to maintain the required level as the ovarian corpus luteum regresses. Hormonal function of the other endocrine glands (adrenal, thyroid, etc.) is important for normal gestation.

Physical trauma. Injury, even that associated with operative procedures on the uterus itself, does not regularly produce abortion. In many instances pregnancy has continued despite fractures or crushing injuries to the pelvic girdle. Although a minor bump or fall can almost always be remembered to have preceded an abortion, it seems highly unlikely that either is a responsible factor.

Emotional factors. Emotional stimuli, which do not need to be overt shocking experiences, may precipitate abortion, but their exact role has not as yet been established. Alterations in hormone secretion resulting from psychic stimuli are known to be responsible for variations in menstrual activity, and there is no reason to doubt that the same factors can operate during pregnancy. Normal placentation and placental function may be disturbed by abnormal vascular responses of the placental site, which also may be in part under emotional control.

Miscellaneous causes. Among the miscellaneous causes for abortion are many possible factors that are even less well understood than those already listed. In women with low fertility the same factors that interfere with impregnation may be responsible for the failure to maintain an environment suitable for fetal growth. The male factor in abortion has been inadequately explored, but it may account for some instances of pregnancy failure.

MECHANISM OF ABORTION

The immediate, precipitating cause of placental separation is necrosis of the decidua and hemorrhage caused by spasm of the spiral arterioles and the resultant patchy ischemia. Uterine contractions are then initiated, and the products of conception are expelled. In most instances fetal death, which may precede the clinical signs by several weeks, is the initial link in the chain of events terminating in abortion. After the stimulus of the growing embryo has been removed, the placental production of estrogen and progesterone gradually diminishes, allowing the regressive decidual changes to occur. Uterine activity normally is reduced during pregnancy, but as the steroid levels fall, the muscle becomes more irritable and eventually active contractions are initiated. These complete the placental separation and expel the ovum.

During the first 6 weeks after the onset of the last menstrual period the attachment of the fetus in the decidual lining is insecure, and in most instances the fetal sac and the decidua are extruded intact. During the next few weeks chorionic villi, which eventually will form the placenta, grow and invade the underlying decidua basalis at the area of the placental site, but until about the fourteenth week the placenta is not well formed. If abortion occurs during the period of placental differentiation, portions of the immature structure are torn from the uterine wall and expelled, but some chorionic tissue usually remains adherent.

CLINICAL STAGES AND TYPES OF ABORTION

As an abortion progresses, it advances through a series of fairly characteristic stages that can usually be recognized clinically. These are usually classified as *threatened, inevitable, incomplete* and *complete.* Abortions may also be *missed* or *habitual* (repeated).

Threatened abortion. The earliest stage that can be recognized clinically is spoken of as threatened abortion because the eventual outcome is uncertain and pregnancy may continue uneventfully. At some time during early pregnancy, usually after having missed one or two periods, the patient becomes aware of bleeding, which is slight and usually consists of the spotting of bright red blood or of dark brown discharge. She

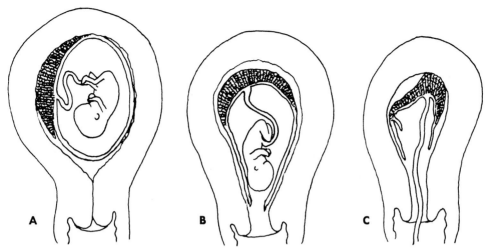

Fig. 13-1. A, Threatened abortion. The edge of the placenta has separated, but the cervix is closed. **B,** Inevitable abortion. The placenta has separated, the cervix is effaced and partially dilated, and the membranes may be ruptured. **C,** Incomplete abortion. The fetus and part of the placenta have been expelled.

may also experience some slight cramping pain. Usually the symptoms subside within a day or two and pregnancy continues, but in some patients both the pains and the amount of bleeding increase. No change is noted in the cervix during this stage.

Inevitable abortion. If the abortion progresses, the cramps become more severe, and as a result cervical effacement and dilatation occur. The bleeding increases and often is accompanied by the passage of clots, and the fetal membranes can be felt or seen bulging through the cervical opening before they rupture. The term *inevitable abortion* implies that the changes are irreversible and that any attempt to maintain pregnancy is useless.

Incomplete abortion. In the majority of spontaneous abortions varying amounts of placental tissue remain within the uterus either attached to the wall or free in the cavity. The patient usually reports the passage of some type of tissue, but she rarely observes the fetus because it has died and degenerated some time before the contractions began. The cramps are severe and the amount of bleeding may be sufficient to produce profound anemia, shock, and even death. The bleeding will continue until the remaining tissue has been removed or expelled because only then can the uterine muscle contract to compress the bleeding vessels and control the hemorrhage.

Complete abortion. A complete abortion is one in which the uterus empties itself completely of the fetus and its membranes and the decidual lining. This usually occurs only during the first 6 weeks and after the fourteenth week of pregnancy.

Missed abortion. Occasionally the products of conception are retained within the uterus long after the fetus has died. Because the interval between fetal death and expulsion in the usual abortion averages about 6 weeks, it has been suggested that the term *missed abortion* should not be applied unless the period of retention of the products has exceeded 8 weeks. The cause for this delay is unknown, but eventually spontaneous evacuation almost always occurs. The clinical picture of missed abortion is usually that of a threatened abortion which seems to have subsided spontaneously or after treatment. The amenorrhea persists, but in most patients brown vaginal discharge is noted intermittently. The subjective symptoms of normal pregnancy disappear, the breasts become smaller, uterine growth ceases, and eventually the size of the uterus diminishes. As placental activity ceases, the test for pregnancy becomes negative. The diagnosis of missed abortion can be made only after repeated examinations indicate regression of the uterine changes of pregnancy.

Habitual abortion. Although isolated in-

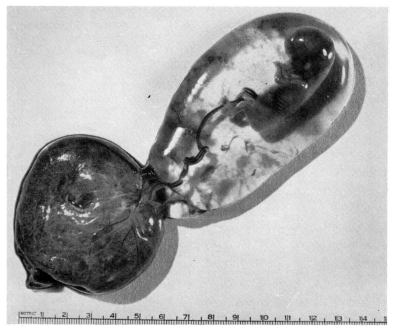

Fig. 13-2. Complete abortion. (From Willson, J. R.: Management of obstetric difficulties, ed. 6, St. Louis, 1961, The C. V. Mosby Co.)

stances of spontaneous abortion are fairly common and do not affect subsequent pregnancies, repeated abortions may be the result of a permanent maternal or paternal defect and are of greater significance. Since the reproductive capacity of women who have had one or two abortions is not reduced substantially, the term *habitual abortion* should be reserved for those patients who have lost three or more pregnancies consecutively.

TREATMENT OF ABORTION

Because the treatment of each of the various stages and types of abortion is different an accurate evaluation of the progress of uterine evacuation must be made before treatment can be planned. A properly performed pelvic examination does not adversely influence the course of the abortion and is necessary to establish the presence of a pregnancy, to eliminate tubal pregnancy as a cause of the symptoms, and to determine how far the process has advanced. Such examinations, which must be performed under aseptic conditions, should include gentle digital and visual examination of the cervix and bimanual palpation of the uterus and

of the adnexa. The degree of cervical effacement and dilatation can be determined by palpation, but the finger must not be inserted into the uterine cavity since pathogenic organisms may be carried directly to the placental site. All gloves, instruments, and materials used in the examination must be sterile, and the external genitals and the vaginal introitus must be thoroughly cleansed with green soap and water or with a hexachlorophene preparation.

Threatened abortion. In most instances the symptoms associated with the onset of abortion indicate that fetal death already has occurred and that the placental production of estrogen and progesterone has diminished to a point at which the pregnancy can no longer be maintained. Treatment started after the onset of the symptoms of a true abortion will not alter its course because irreversible changes already have taken place. In these patients the initial brown vaginal discharge resulting from decidual necrosis is soon followed by actual bleeding and uterine cramps that ultimately expel, completely or partially, the products of conception.

In other patients a small amount of bright

red bleeding begins a few days after a period is missed, when the ovum is actively invading the uterine epithelium. This is similar to implantation bleeding in monkeys, which is caused by the erosive action of the trophoblast on the vascular decidua. Later in pregnancy, bleeding may follow mechanical separation of the edge of the normally developing placenta. This type of bleeding usually is of short duration and does not recur, but occasionally it becomes progressively more severe, particularly if it is caused by separation of a placenta implanted in the lower segment. Benign lesions of the cervix such as polyps and cervicitis, as well as invasive cancer, may be a source of bright red bleeding. Such lesions can be detected by visual examination of the cervix.

Since the symptoms of abortion are the result of fetal death and the consequent reduced hormonel production, its progression cannot be prevented. Many women will want to go to bed because they have heard that bed rest is essential whenever bleeding occurs during pregnancy. Although this need not be discouraged, the physician should not make the patient feel it is essential because bed rest does no good and it may be impossible for a woman with small children for whom she is responsible. The physician also should not permit himself to be pressured into administering progesterone; the only effect it has on the course of the abortion is to delay evacuation of the uterus.

The bleeding associated with threatened abortion usually either ceases in 1 or 2 days or rapidly increases in amount as other symptoms appear, whereas that from cervical or vaginal lesions is more likely to continue unchanged from day to day. A complete, sterile vaginal examination therefore must be performed on any patient being treated for "threatened abortion" if the bleeding continues for a week in order that local lesions may be eliminated as a cause. The prognosis for continuation of the pregnancy is far better for those in whom bright red bleeding occurs initially than for those who first note brown discharge. Most of the latter proceed to rapid termination, regardless of the type of treatment.

Early bleeding that does not terminate in abortion has no effect upon fetal development. It is well to inform the patient specifically that the incidence of congenital anom-alies is not increased by threatened abortion.

Inevitable abortion. Since the diagnosis of inevitable abortion implies that irreversible progress toward uterine evacuation has already taken place, treatment should be directed toward reducing blood loss and pain. The administration of oxytocics is unnecessary because these substances do not hasten the process and serve only to increase the discomfort. In most instances uterine evacuation will be incomplete whether uterine stimulants are given or not, making surgical removal of the remaining tissue necessary. It is preferable, therefore, to empty the uterus mechanically as soon as a moderate amount of cervical dilatation has occurred or earlier in the event of profuse bleeding. Morphine sulfate, 0.010 to 0.016 Gm. ($\frac{1}{6}$ to $\frac{1}{4}$ gr.) or Demerol, 100 mg., will not retard the progress of the abortion and may be given as needed to relieve the pain.

Incomplete abortion. Placental tissue remaining in the uterus after a partial abortion should be removed because it often becomes infected and, in addition, may be responsible for continued and excessive bleeding. The majority of clinically recognized abortions occur between the sixth and the twelfth weeks of pregnancy, and since the passage of the products at this period is likely to be incomplete, a planned program for their management is important to keep complications at a minimum.

Patients with incomplete abortions are best treated in hospitals where facilities are available for evacuation of the uterus and where adequate amounts of compatible blood can be obtained rapidly for those who are bleeding excessively. The patient should be examined under aseptic conditions, and any placental tissue protruding through the cervical canal should be removed gently with sterile ring forceps because tissue in this location usually interferes with uterine contraction and with control of bleeding. The instrument must not be inserted into the uterine cavity in search of loose placental tissue because of the dangers of introducing infection and of injuring the uterine wall. If the patient is afebrile, if parametrial or uterine tenderness cannot be elicited, and if there is no evidence of previous instrumentation, early surgical evacuation of the uterus should be considered. If, however, physical signs suggest the presence of infection, the

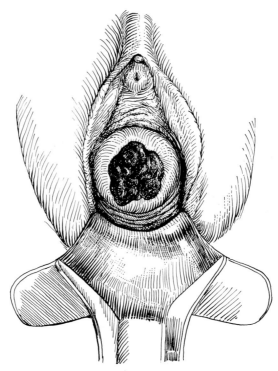

Fig. 13-3. Incomplete abortion. Appearance of secundines as they protrude from cervix. (From Titus, P.: Atlas of obstetric technic, St. Louis, 1949, The C. V. Mosby Co.)

operation should be delayed until the problem can be evaluated more completely unless bleeding is profuse.

Surgical evacuation of the uterus should be considered for most patients with early abortions even though the material that has been passed appears to represent the entire conceptus. Many who have had "complete" abortions between the sixth and the fourteenth weeks of pregnancy continue to bleed until the remaining placental tissue has been removed surgically. The procedure should be performed in the operating room under intravenous Pentothal sodium or local or inhalation anesthesia. Perforation of the soft and often retroflexed uterus can be avoided if caution is exercised during the manipulations.

Loose fragments of placental tissue can usually be removed by seizing them with ring or placental forceps and extracting them through the dilated cervix. In order to avoid grasping and tearing the uterine wall the instrument must be rotated slowly as the jaws are closing over a piece of tissue, and the downward traction should be slight at

first until it appears certain that the uterus has not been included in the bite. Fragments of placenta that remain adherent to the wall can be dislodged and removed with a large sharp curet.

Once the cavity is empty, the uterine muscle will contract and control the bleeding. A soft, boggy, bleeding uterus usually still contains placental tissue that may be lying free in the center of the cavity, and an effort must be made to locate and remove it. It is seldom necessary to pack the uterus to control bleeding if all the tissue has been evacuated, but the administration of Methergine, 0.2 mg. intravenously, will stimulate the muscle to contract. The blood loss in some patients with incomplete abortion is sufficient to require transfusion. If blood is necessary, its administration should be started before the uterus is evacuated, particularly if signs suggesting shock are evident.

Complete abortion. During the first 6 weeks after the onset of the last period nearly all abortions are complete and require no therapy. After the fourteenth week there

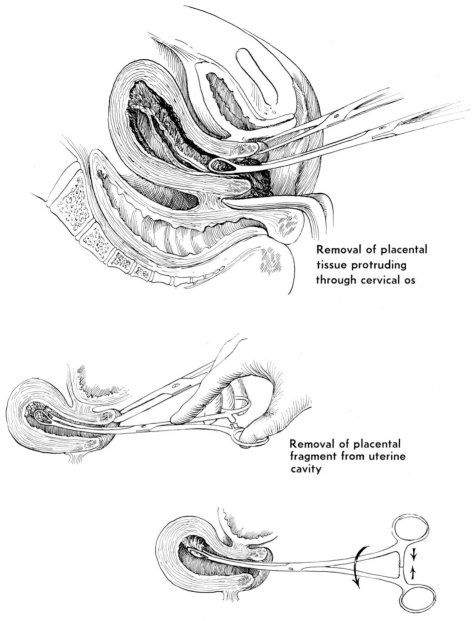

Removal of placental
tissue protruding
through cervical os

Removal of placental
fragment from uterine
cavity

Fig. 13-4. Use of ring forceps to remove placental tissue from cervix and uterus. (From Willson, J. R.: Management of obstetric difficulties, ed. 6, St. Louis, 1961, The C. V. Mosby Co.)

occasionally is a delay in delivery of the placenta following expulsion of the fetus, but in most instances it is passed intact and no further treatment is required.

Missed abortion. In the past, missed abortions were generally treated expectantly until the products were expelled spontaneously, after which the uterus was curetted. It is

possible to speed the process in carefully selected patients. Before any form of treatment is initiated the physician must be certain that he is dealing with a missed abortion and not with an altered growth pattern of a normal pregnancy. If the uterus becomes progressively smaller, if the physician no longer can hear fetal heart sounds that had been obvious, and if pregnancy tests are negative, the diagnosis is certain.

It may be possible to speed the process of evacuation by stimulating the uterus with a dilute oxytocin solution. Since the welfare of the infant need not be considered, the usual concentration of oxytocin can be increased considerably. In fact, Loudon uses as much as 100 units (10 ml.) in 500 ml. of fluid. If there is no response after 4 to 6 hours, the infusion should be stopped but should be repeated daily for 2 or 3 more days if necessary.

The uterus can also be evacuated by the intra-amniotic injection of hypertonic saline or glucose solutions. This technique is most appropriate when the uterine size is larger than that of a 14-week gestation. A 14- to 16-gauge needle is passed through the abdominal and uterine walls, and 100 to 200 ml. of 20% saline solution is injected into the amniotic cavity. It has been suggested that amniotic fluid be aspirated before the salt solution is injected, but this is not always possible because with missed abortion there may be little fluid within the sac. Contractions usually begin within a few hours, and in many instances the uterus evacuates itself within 24 hours without further stimulation. If the saline-induced contractions are irregular and ineffectual, the evacuation can be completed with intravenous dilute oxytocin solution.

Clotting defects caused by the development of hypofibrinogenemia may occur after prolonged retention of a dead fetus, particularly in Rh-negative women. This is not a problem during the first half of pregnancy.

Habitual abortion. The treatment of repeated abortion must be instituted prior to conception and is based upon the results of investigations of both the patient and her husband. The correction of physical abnormalities and of nutritional defects may be helpful, but often no definite cause is found by the usual methods of physical examination.

The following studies should be carried out between pregnancies: uterosalpingography to rule out congenital and other uterine abnormalities, glucose tolerance tests, serum cholesterol and protein-bound iodine determinations, serologic studies for Rh and ABO incompatibility, premenstrual endometrial biopsy, vitamin C estimation, tests for capillary fragility, and psychiatric evaluation when indicated. Karyotyping of both partners has been suggested because of the frequency with which abnormal chromosomal patterns are found in spontaneous abortions. Stenchever and co-workers, however, found only 1 patient with a chromosomal abnormality in 41 couples who were studied because of habitual abortions.

The administration of *thyroid substance* to either or both partners is indicated if the thyroid function is reduced.

Inadequacies in the production of ovarian hormones may be responsible for improper preparation of the endometrium and, when present, can sometimes be corrected by *endocrine therapy.* Stilbestrol, 0.1 mg., may be administered daily during the first half of the menstrual cycle. After ovulation this should be increased to 0.5 to 1 mg., and in addition, 30 to 50 mg. of progesterone should be added to reinforce the inadequate secretion of the natural hormone.

Surgical procedures are seldom required in the treatment of repeated abortion and should not be considered as long as any possible causes remain uncorrected. However, in an occasional carefully selected patient an operation may be effective. Removal of submucous fibromyomas may permit pregnancy to continue normally, but if the uterine cavity is symmetric and the tumors are of the subserous variety, myomectomy probably will not affect the outcome. The repair of congenital or acquired defects such as unification of a double uterus or an operation on an incompetent cervix may also permit pregnancy to continue normally.

Patients who have aborted three or more times, in whom no hormonal or organic causes can be demonstrated, and who manifest other symptoms of emotional instability may be benefited by a course of *preconceptual psychotherapy.* Since the psychic conflict that may be responsible for repeated abortion is usually on an unconscious level, these patients should be referred to a competent therapist or analyst for evaluation and treatment.

Active preventive treatment during pregnancy. When a patient who has aborted repeatedly again becomes pregnant, the active treatment to prevent another unfavorable outcome depends largely on the dominant etiologic factor involved. Obviously nothing can be done if defective germ cells are the cause of the abortion. But patients in whom a dietary deficiency, hormonal dysfunction, or psychogenic factors are responsible should be treated accordingly.

HORMONE THERAPY. Estrogen and progesterone, secreted first by the ovarian corpus luteum and later by trophoblastic cells, are essential for normal pregnancy. It is reasonable to assume, therefore, that a deficiency in the production of these hormones could be responsible for abortion. On the basis of this concept estrogen and progesterone, singly or in combination, have been employed over the years. Results, however, have been most discouraging because patients were treated without first establishing a definite hormonal insufficiency and because the dosages used were invariably totally inadequate to correct an existent deficiency.

If the physician could establish the presence of progesterone deficiency early in pregnancy and were able to supply an adequate dosage of exogenous progestational hormone, a favorable outcome might occur more often. Unfortunately, there are no reliable methods for diagnosing progesterone deficiency by readily applicable tests. Arborization of cervical mucus is inhibited by progesterone during the premenstrual phase of the normal cycle and during pregnancy. One can suspect progesterone deficiency if ferning is present during early pregnancy, but the reverse is not true. The fact that no ferning can be detected does not mean that progesterone production is normal because arborization is inhibited by amounts of progesterone far less than that found during normal pregnancy. The information derived from vaginal cytologic examinations is also inaccurate. McLennan and McLennan suggested that they might be able to predict progesterone deficiency and potential abortion by the karyopyknotic index of vaginal epithelial cells; those with few pyknotic cells were less likely to abort than those with greater numbers because progesterone inhibits the development of pyknotic cells. Further study did not substantiate this observation. The difficulty in correlating impaired hormone production and abortion should not be surprising; low levels may simply reflect abnormalities in the ovum or the trophoblast rather than impaired secretion with an otherwise perfectly normal pregnancy.

Although the administration of *progestogens* theoretically should reduce the possibility of abortion, practically it does not. Goldzieher studied 54 women who had aborted repeatedly with daily measurements of pregnanediol. Eighteen with pregnanediol excretions less than 5 mg. daily before the eighth week and less than 7 mg. daily before the fourteenth week of pregnancy and 13 with normal excretions were treated with medroxyprogesterone (Provera); 14 with low excretions and 9 with normal excretions served as controls, being treated with placebos. There was no difference in the abortion rate in the various groups; in fact 10 of the 13 placebo patients with the worst prognosis (no previous term pregnancy and subnormal pregnanediol excretions) had normal pregnancies.

Progesterone therapy is expensive and since its value is questionable it should be prescribed only for patients in whom there is a likely possibility of a deficiency. It also should be started as soon as there is a question of pregnancy, not after several weeks. The long-acting injectable preparations are likely to cause missed abortion if the pregnancy fails to survive, and some women will have prolonged periods of amenorrhea from the continuing effect of the progestogen after the uterus is emptied. It is preferable, therefore, to use an oral preparation such as Provera in doses of 10 mg. daily during the first trimester. There is no need to continue the drug any longer.

Some substances, notably Norlutin and Pranone, have adrogenic as well as progestogenic effects and are contraindicated during pregnancy because they can cause masculinization of female fetuses. Fortunately these changes affect only the external genitals, are not progressive, and can be corrected without difficulty. Nonadrenal pseudohermaphrodism may occasionally follow prolonged administration of progesterone, but this is so unusual that it should not deter its use when it is indicated.

THYROID. Hypothyroidism is not a common cause for abortion, but when there is evidence of hypometabolism, adequate dosage of thyroid during the preconceptual phase and continued during the gestational period may be of considerable value.

PSYCHOTHERAPY IN REPEATED ABORTION. Every woman who has aborted several times, especially if she has no living children, becomes anxious and fearful as soon as she realizes that she is pregnant once again. A sympathetic approach, interest, and patience on the part of the physician are potent factors in the ultimate successful outcome of every case of repeated abortion, no matter what the primary etiologic factor may be. It is not at all unreasonable to assume that good results obtained by various methods of hormonal, nutritional, and vitamin therapy may, in large part, be a result of the painstaking instructions, the frequent consultations, and the establishment of a good physician-patient relationship.

In the seriously disturbed patient, repeated abortion may be conditioned by unconscious desires and motivations to avoid pregnancy at all cost. These patients can be helped only by a prolonged period of treatment with an experienced therapist. Pregnancy should be attempted only after significant conflicts have been brought to consciousness, "worked through," and resolved. Therapy must be continued during pregnancy. Mann studied 160 women who had aborted repeatedly during previous pregnancies and found only 15 with demonstrable organic causes—13 with incompetency of the internal cervical os and 2 with bicornuate uteri. The remaining 145 women had psychiatric evaluation and therapy; 81% of this group completed pregnancy successfully.

Surgical treatment. The only surgical procedures that will help maintain a pregnancy already initiated are those directed toward closure of the *incompetent internal cervical os.* The characteristic history in patients with this abnormality is that they have had one or more successful pregnancies, that the uterus has been evacuated surgically after incomplete abortion, or that they have had dilatation and curettage performed. Each subsequent pregnancy terminates during the second trimester in a characteristic manner: The cervix effaces and dilates painlessly, the membranes rupture spontaneously, and labor begins.

The basic defect responsible for the repeated pregnancy loss is usually an injury in the area of the internal os. The stroma of the normal cervix is predominantly fibrous tissue, whereas that of the body of the uterus is almost entirely smooth muscle. During the second trimester of pregnancy the isthmus of the uterus expands and retracts, but the normal cervix remains relatively firm with its internal os closed. If the internal os has been injured, however, it may retract upward with the isthmus (effacement), and eventually the cervical canal will be obliterated, as it is when labor starts at term. The external os then dilates, permitting the membranes to pouch through into the vagina; they soon rupture, and labor starts. Although this does not often occur during the first pregnancy, it may. Roddick and associates attribute this to a congenital anomaly of cervical development in which most of the cervix is made up of muscle like that of the uterus rather than fibrous connective tissue.

Incompetence of the internal os may be suspected from the history and can be diagnosed by demonstrating the premature effacement and dilatation of the cervix. During pregnancy the cervix is inspected and palpated at weekly intervals, and the operation is performed when a change in its length is first detected. The diagnosis can also be made between pregnancies if a dressing forceps or a larger cervical dilator can be passed through the cervical canal without meeting resistance.

The cervix can be repaired before the patient conceives again by an operative procedure such as that described by Lash. The injured area is excised and the resultant surgical defect is closed. This operation does not decrease fertility and permits normal vaginal delivery. Incompetency that is first discovered during pregnancy is best treated by an operative procedure, such as that de-

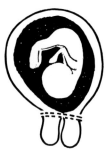

Fig. 13-5. Incompetent internal cervical os. Suture is in place.

scribed by Shirodkar and popularized in the United States by Barter and associates, with which the internal os is constricted by an encircling suture of Dacron, fascia, or silk. This suture is removed at term to permit the patient to deliver vaginally. It must also be removed at once if the membranes rupture or whenever labor starts.

The success rate with these procedures should approximate 80%; if nothing is done, almost all the pregnancies will terminate before the infant can exist independently. The results are poor if the repeated losses are due to factors other than the cervical defect; closing the cervix will not preserve the pregnancy.

■ Induced abortion

Most illegal abortions are performed because of unplanned pregnancies in married women as a way of regulating family size. Most of these unwanted pregnancies, subsequent abortions, and possible deaths could have been prevented had these women been given adequate instruction in contraception and pregnancy spacing. Control of conception should be discussed with each recently delivered woman. If she and her husband wish to make use of a method of birth control, the one most suitable for them should be provided.

The exact incidence of illegal termination of pregnancy is uncertain, but it has been estimated to account for from 4% to 20% of all abortions. The death rate after illegal abortion is far higher than that after spontaneous termination, because infection is more likely to occur and blood loss is greater. The instrument used to induce abortion is often unclean and may carry pathogenic organisms directly into the uterus, the bloodstream, or even into the peritoneal cavity if the uterus is perforated. The infection is similar to that after delivery at term but is far more serious because hemorrhage usually is more profuse, the organisms may be of a more lethal variety, and the patient may not seek treatment until the infection is advanced.

There is no reliable information concerning the frequency with which abortion is induced, but it is becoming progressively more important as a cause of maternal death. Over 50% of the maternal deaths in New York City follow induced abortion.

During the 5-year period from 1955 to 1959 there were 356 maternal deaths in the state of Michigan, 74 (21%) of which were due to illegally induced abortion. In the next 5-year period, 1960 to 1964, there were 321 maternal deaths, of which 120 (37%) were due to induced abortion. All could have been prevented by the use of an effective contraceptive method.

Most patients will deny having made any attempt to disturb the pregnancy, but during the examination suggestive evidence of manipulation can sometimes be detected. Tenaculum marks, fresh lacerations of the cervix or the vagina, and uterine perforations can be caused only by efforts to produce abortion since they do not develop spontaneously. The insertion of potassium permanganate tablets into the vagina and cervix is a popular, dangerous, and ineffectual method of inducing an abortion. The typical early lesion is a sharply punched-out vaginal ulcer covered by a black jellylike material. A number of deaths have been reported from hemorrhage, intravascular hemolysis, and hyperpotassemia, which occurred after the insertion of this drug.

An *infected abortion* is one with which there is clinical evidence of genital tract infection. The term is usually applied to abortions accompanied by fever and those in which the infection has spread to the parametrium or the peritoneum. Peritonitis may either be localized to the pelvic peritoneum or be diffuse, with accompanying ileus and abdominal distention. The parametritis may vary from severe, unilateral tenderness to fully developed cellulitis that fixes the uterus in an inflammatory mass. Pelvic examination is often unsatisfactory because of pain, but the cervix almost always is open, and thin, bloody discharge, placental tissue, or profuse bleeding usually is present. The patient appears gravely ill and dehydrated. The temperature is of a septic type with peaks of at least 103° to 104° F., and the pulse is rapid and thready.

The organisms most often responsible for serious postabortal infections are those of the *coli-aerogenes* group and anaerobic streptococci.

ACTIVE TREATMENT

The initial treatment of illegal abortion concerns itself primarily with evaluation of the general condition of the patient, the control of bleeding, the replacement of lost blood, and the initiation of necessary therapy directed toward combating the infection. A careful aseptic pelvic examination should be performed soon after the patient is admitted to the hospital to determine the extent of pelvic infection if it is present, to remove portions of the placenta that may be visible, and to obtain an intrauterine culture. All unnecessary manipulations must be avoided, and except for the insertion of the swab or the tube to obtain material for the culture, the uterine cavity must not be invaded. It is well to obtain a standing x-ray study of the abdomen and pelvis. Uterine rupture is suggested by the presence of air under the diaphragm, and foreign bodies that have been pushed through the uterus may be seen. In most communities the police are to be notified if there is any suspicion of nontherapeutic abortion.

Uninfected abortion. If the temperature is normal, if there is no evidence of infection outside the uterine cavity, and if the bleeding is slight, no immediate active treatment is necessary. If the hemoglobin is below 10 grams, compatible blood should be available as prophylaxis against a sudden, profuse hemorrhage. No antibiotic agents need be administered unless there is definite evidence of infection.

The uterus should usually be evacuated of the remaining placental tissue as soon as it is practical but certainly within 24 hours. Further delay in completing the abortion may serve only to increase the morbidity because the organisms proliferating in the placental tissue and the decidua have direct access to the blood vessels and thus may invade the parametrium rapidly. Early removal of the remaining placenta will eliminate this source of infection, and, in addition, will reduce the hazard from bleeding because as long as placental tissue remains in the uterus the possibility of hemorrhage exists.

Infected abortion. The early treatment of infected abortion is directed toward the control of infection unless the patient is bleeding heavily enough to endanger her life. Specific treatment should include morphine or Demerol to control pain, blood transfusions in a quantity sufficient to compensate for blood loss, enough 10% dextrose

to correct dehydration, and the administration of antimicrobial agents. Neither fluid nor food should be allowed by mouth, and constant suction should be instituted if the patient is vomiting. Ten million units of penicillin are added to the intravenous solution, and 0.5 Gm. of streptomycin is given intramuscularly. The streptomycin injection is repeated every 8 hours, and the daily intravenous dosage of penicillin is at least 50 million units. When the result of the uterine culture is available, it may be necessary to alter the treatment if an agent other than that already being administered is more effective against the responsible organism. Chloramphenicol may be given intravenously in doses of 500 mg. every 6 hours if the responsible bacteria are resistant to penicillin. Therapy should be continued for at least 48 hours after the uterus has been emptied.

The physician should usually delay surgical evacuation of the uterus until blood has been replaced, dehydration has been corrected, and high tissue levels of antimicrobial agents have been obtained. As soon as this has been accomplished, usually within 3 to 6 hours, the remaining placental tissue and decidua should be removed with a sharp curet. The curettage can be done under paracervical and pudendal block anesthesia, which adds little to the risk. Profuse bleeding accompanying incomplete abortion is usually caused by fragments of placenta that are only partially separated and are protruding through the cervical opening. The bleeding can usually be checked by removing the visible tissue with ring forceps. This is preferable to curettage before supportive treatment has been administered, but curettage should be done as soon as the general condition of the patient warrants it and whenever bleeding cannot be controlled by another method.

COMPLICATIONS OF INDUCED ABORTION

Most of the complications following induction of abortion are related to infection and blood loss. The majority of deaths are attributable to infection; the mortality from hemorrhage alone should be slight.

Bacterial shock. Endotoxin shock, thought to be caused by the release of a lipoprotein-carbohydrate complex from the cell walls of gram-negative bacilli, particularly those of the *coli-aerogenes* group, does not occur often but is one of the most lethal complications of septic abortion. The bacteria, which are introduced into the uterus during the manipulations to produce abortion, invade the uterine wall and enter the bloodstream. The toxin released from the lysed bacteria produces peripheral vasoconstriction, which is accompanied by reduced cardiac index, prolonged circulation time, hypotension, and tachycardia. The resultant reduced tissue perfusion becomes evident as urine secretion decreases or ceases completely. The hematocrit may be normal even though blood loss has been excessive because of hypovolemia, and the white blood cell count may be within the normal range even though it had been greatly elevated before signs of shock appeared.

The basic requirements for the successful treatment of septic shock include (1) the reduction of peripheral resistance, (2) the restoration of circulating blood volume, and (3) the treatment of infection.

A catheter is placed in the central venous pool and is attached to a three-way stopcock in order that *central venous pressures* can be measured periodically and *fluid* can be administered. If the central venous pressure is less than 10 cm. H₂O, an infusion of 5% dextrose is started and continued until the pressure is between 10 and 12 cm. H₂O. If the central venous pressure is below normal and the hematocrit is reduced, even to the lower limits of the normal range, *blood* should be given because the reading undoubtedly is distorted by the hypovolemia. In some patients correction of hypovolemia alone will restore normal tissue perfusion, which will be demonstrated by an *increase in urine volume.*

If oliguria or anuria persists, particularly if the central venous pressure is 10 to 12 cm. H₂O, one can assume that it is a result of peripheral vasospasm. It is essential that *peripheral resistance be reduced,* otherwise the venous pressure will continue to rise and the heart will decompensate. The medication that is most effective in accomplishing this is isoproterenol, which relaxes the peripheral arterioles (alphalytic action), constricts capacitance vessels, and stimulates cardiac action (betamimetic action). Isoproterenol is administered slowly intravenously (2.5 mg. in 500 ml. of 5% dex-

trose). The effect is determined by the urine volume and the central venous pressure, the former increasing and the latter decreasing as constriction is relieved. As the central venous pressure falls, more fluid must be infused to maintain an adequate circulating blood volume.

Corticosteroids aid in reducing peripheral resistance, stimulate cardiac action, and exert a protective effect on cell membranes that are damaged by the endotoxin and by ischemia. The equivalent of about 2 Gm. of cortisone should be administered every 24 hours. Hydrocortisone can be given intravenously; the synthetic substances, such as dexamethasone, appear to be as effective as the natural ones.

Permanent improvement cannot be expected until the infection is controlled; the two most important measures for accomplishing this are *removal of the infected placental tissue* and *prescription of appropriate antibiotic preparations.* Antibiotic therapy is similar to that recommended for septic abortions: penicillin, 50 million units or more, and chloramphenicol, 2 to 3 Gm. during each 24-hour period. These should be administered intravenously since little effect can be anticipated from intramuscular injection until circulatory failure has been corrected. The physician must consider the potassium administered with the large doses of penicillin in anuric patients. Kanamycin in doses of about 15 mg./kg. of body weight each 24 hours has also been recommended, but this cannot be continued in anuric or oliguric patients. Antibiotic therapy should be started as soon as the diagnosis of infected abortion is made; adjustments in dosage and preparation may be necessary when the responsible organism has been identified.

One of the most important parts of the treatment is to evacuate the uterus of the placental tissue from which the bacteria are disseminated into the bloodstream. Curettage, which should be performed early, even though the general condition of the patient seems hopeless, may mean the difference between death and survival. In an occasional patient with extensive myometrial involvement, hysterectomy may be necessary to eliminate the source of the infection.

Pelvic abscess. In some patients fever, pelvic pain, and signs of peritonitis persist despite antibiotic therapy and evacuation of

the uterus. This suggests advancing parametritis and pelvic cellulitis, which may
eventually end with pelvic abscess formation. Pelvic examination should be performed in such a patient every 3 or 4 days
in an attempt to detect the first evidence
of fluctuation in the area of cellulitis. Most
such abscesses eventually point into the
vagina and can be drained by posterior colpotomy. Some, however, extend upward between the leaves of the broad ligament until
they can be palpated above the pubis. These
must be drained through an abdominal incision, but they usually can be approached
without entering the peritoneal cavity.

Renal failure. Soap or other toxic materials injected into the uterus in an attempt
to produce abortion may enter the bloodstream, where they hemolyze red blood cells
and damage renal tubular cells. Bacteria or
their products may have the same effect on
the kidney. This is a highly lethal complication with a mortality of at least 75%. It
must therefore be recognized early in its
course. The treatment consists mainly of
fluid restriction to an amount with which
the patient will barely retain her weight,
or even lose a little from day to day, and
the maintenance of a reasonable electrolyte
balance. The greatest danger is from hyper-
kalemia. The diet should be high in carbohydrate and fat with a minimum of protein.
Dialysis may be required if anuria persists
and if the electrolyte levels are sufficiently
altered to constitute a threat to life. Hysterectomy often is necessary.

Ruptured uterus. Laparotomy should be
performed if uterine perforation is diagnosed
by x-ray examination or is thought to be a
possibility because of intraperitoneal bleeding or obvious local injury or if the uterus
is perforated during surgical evacuation of
the necrotic, infected contents. It usually is
necessary to remove the uterus. The bowel
should be inspected because it often is lacerated if the uterus is ruptured.

Thrombophlebitis. Puerperal infection
extends from its source in the uterine cavity
through the wall and into the parametrium
by progressive phlebitis and lymphangitis,
as well as by direct tissue involvement.
Thrombophlebitis eventually involves the
veins on the lateral pelvic walls, the ovarian
veins, and the vena cava. Septic emboli are
transported to distant parts of the body
where they set up secondary areas of infection, from which the patient may eventually
die even though the pelvic lesion clears.
When embolization continues in spite of
antibiotic and anticoagulant therapy, ovarian and vena caval ligation may be lifesaving.

■ Legal abortion

The term *legal abortion* refers to the termination of early pregnancy by a qualified
physician in an approved medical facility.

In past years termination of pregnancy
was considered only when it was perfectly
clear that the mother would die if she remained pregnant (therapeutic abortion).
Every effort was made to carry patients with
serious cardiovascular-renal disorders and
similar incurable processes through their
pregnancies, even though it seemed certain
that they could live only a few months.
Abortion was seldom considered in the interests of the fetus, even though one could
anticipate its being born with a lethal or
incapacitating condition, or for social reasons.
As newer methods for preventing and treating infections and for managing chronic
diseases were developed, the need for abortion as a lifesaving procedure diminished
and the incidence of therapeutic abortion
was reduced to about 1 in every 500 to 700
deliveries.

This situation prevailed until about 1960
when women and their physicians began to
express their concern over the moralistic
attitudes toward contraception and abortion
and their strict legal control. It became more
and more evident that the control of pregnancy should be a medical rather than a
legal problem. As a consequence, the indications were gradually expanded to permit
therapeutic abortion in the interest of the
mothers' physical and emotional health,
whenever there is a substantial risk of the
fetus developing abnormally, for example,
after rubella during early pregnancy, and
for social reasons such as pregnancy resulting
from rape or incest, those in unmarried
women, or those that would seriously disrupt
the stability of a family. By 1970 almost all
hospital abortions were being performed for
psychiatric or social rather than for medical
reasons.

Restrictive state laws are gradually being
changed and undoubtedly within the next

few years decisions concerning the termination of pregnancy can be made as are other medical decisions—upon the basis of individual need, not upon whether a legal loophole can be found.

INDICATIONS

When abortion becomes legal in all the states, it will be possible to divide the operations into those performed because of a systemic disorder that makes pregnancy hazardous *(medical indications)* and those performed for social or economic reasons *(nonmedical indications)*.

The *medical conditions* for which abortion is most often performed are discussed here. Other more unusual indications can be found in other parts of this book where each entity is considered.

Chronic hypertension or chronic nephritis. Therapeutic abortion is justified for women with chronic cardiovascular renal disease, particularly if there are degenerative vascular changes in the retinal vessels or if renal function is reduced. Under such circumstances the fetus has a limited chance of being born alive, and many of the mothers will die because the cardiovascular and renal functions cannot satisfy the increasing demands of advancing pregnancy.

Cancer. In patients with carcinoma of the uterus, ovaries, or lower bowel it often is necessary to remove the pregnant uterus as part of the treatment of the tumor. In some patients with cancer of the rectum or rectosigmoid, adequate removal is possible without disturbing the gravid uterus. Termination of pregnancy is justifiable for women who have recently been treated for carcinoma of the breast because the high levels of estrogen and progesterone may stimulate the growth of local and metastatic breast cancer.

Diabetes. Pregnancy should often be terminated in women with advanced or long-standing diabetes. This is particularly true if there is degenerative vascular disease or hypertension or if toxemia has developed in previous pregnancies.

Erythroblastosis fetalis. If infants have been severely affected and have died in previous pregnancies despite good treatment and if the father is homozygous Rh positive, termination can be considered. Abortion is more appropriate if the couple already has several living children than if it has none or only one, because intrauterine fetal transfusion, early delivery, and repeated exchange transfusions offer even the most seriously affected infant a reasonable chance of survival.

Heart disease. It is seldom necessary to terminate pregnancy because of heart disease if the patient can be treated properly. Termination can be considered for those who can neither obtain sufficient rest nor follow an acceptable program of treatment.

Pulmonary tuberculosis. Pulmonary tuberculosis is ordinarily not affected by pregnancy and can be treated as successfully in gravid as in nonpregnant women. Therapeutic abortions, however, should be considered for the patient who, because of family responsibilities, cannot treat her tuberculosis properly. Under such circumstances the additional responsibility of caring for a new baby full time may produce exacerbation of the infection.

Rubella. The indications for abortion in women who have contracted rubella are somewhat more clear cut than they have been in the past. Termination of pregnancy is certainly justifiable for those who have acquired German measles during the first 16 to 18 weeks after the onset of the last menstrual period. This is particularly true during epidemics when the fetal effects are more severe.

Other fetal indications. Termination of pregnancy can logically be considered whenever the fetus has little chance of developing normally or is destined to die at an early age from a lethal hereditary condition.

Psychiatric conditions. Therapeutic abortion for psychiatric conditions is justifiable when the pregnancy interferes with necessary psychotherapy, when there is a distinct possibility of suicide, or when the psychopathology of the patient and her family is severe enough to suggest that a baby reared in the atmosphere of the home would have a small chance for normal emotional development.

The *nonmedical* reasons for abortion cannot be described as precisely as the medical. They are primarily social or economic and the decision as to the advisability of terminating pregnancy will be one made individually by the woman and her physician.

PHYSICIAN RESPONSIBILITY

When abortion becomes legal in all the states there will be no need for "therapeutic abortion committees" or even for consultation except under unusual circumstances. The members of each hospital staff must develop the regulations under which the operations will be performed. It is not likely that every hospital will be required to permit physicians to perform abortions, and it is inconceivable that physicians will be required to do the operations, or that patients will be forced to accept termination of pregnancy against their wishes.

Physicians who choose to perform *nonmedical abortions* will make the decisions concerning the advisability of the procedure with individual patients. The request for the operation will always originate with the patient. One of the important responsibilities will be to recognize the occasional woman for whom termination of pregnancy may not be appropriate.

The responsibility of the physician in dealing with *medical abortions* is somewhat different. He must be able, with the help of appropriate consultants, to evaluate the severity of the systemic disease and to establish the potential risk of permitting the pregnancy to continue. He, therefore, must often advise termination. In many instances this is difficult because the patient wants the pregnancy, in direct contrast to those who request nonmedical abortion. The need for medical abortions can be kept at a minimum by prepregnancy examinations.

Complications are inevitable, but they can be kept at a minimum if the procedures are performed on carefully selected patients by skillful operators in properly equipped facilities. The complications most likely to occur during the operation itself are perforation of the uterus, hemorrhage, and anesthetic problems. Since these cannot be anticipated in advance it is desirable that abortions be performed in a hospital facility rather than in a doctor's office or in an outpatient operating area not a part of a hospital. Although women need not be admitted to a hospital for the procedure, it is essential that adequate facilities for treating major complications be immediately available.

At best, abortion is an unsatisfactory way of controlling reproduction. When effective contraceptive methods can be made available to every sexually active woman, the number seeking abortion will be substantially reduced.

TECHNIQUE

During the first trimester of pregnancy the uterus can usually be evacuated by dilatation of the cervix and removal of the products of conception with a standard curet or by suction curettage. After the fourteenth week the uterine cavity usually is so large that the products of conception cannot be removed safely through the artificially dilated cervix, and abdominal hysterotomy is more appropriate, particularly if sterilization as well as abortion is planned. The uterus can also be evacuated during the second trimester by injecting hypertonic saline solution into the amniotic sac as described for the treatment of missed abortion. This usually is preferable to an abdominal operation.

When pregnancy is terminated because of a chronic condition such as heart disease, diabetes, or essential hypertension, the patient should usually be sterilized because there is little hope that her condition will improve enough to permit pregnancy in the future. This is not true of abortions performed for other reasons.

■ Care of patients after abortion

Postabortal care depends upon the type of abortion, the amount of blood loss, and whether or not infection was present. The patient who has had an uncomplicated spontaneous abortion and little blood loss may be discharged a few hours after the uterus has been evacuated if she has recovered completely from the anesthetic. Those who have been more seriously ill should remain in the hospital for a longer time. Normal activity may be resumed whenever the patient feels able to carry out her usual duties. Involution usually is complete within 1 month, and menstruation begins 4 to 6 weeks after the abortion has occurred. Another pregnancy can be attempted, ordinarily, after the patient has had two or three normal menstrual periods. Before the patient is permitted to conceive, however, the physician must be certain that her return to normal is complete and that obvious factors that may have been responsible for the loss of the pregnancy have been corrected.

References

Adams, R. H., and Pritchard, J. A.: Bacterial shock in obstetrics and gynecology, Obstet. Gynec. **16:**387, 1960.

Barter, R. H., Dusabek, J. A., Riva, H. L., and Parks, J.: Surgical closure of the incompetent cervix during pregnancy, Amer. J. Obstet. Gynec. **75:**511, 1958.

Burge, E. S.: The relationship of threatened abortion to fetal anomalies, Amer. J. Obstet. Gynec. **61:**615, 1951.

Colvin, E. D., Bartholomew, R. A., and Grimes, W. H.: Salvage possibilities in threatened abortion, Amer. J. Obstet. Gynec. **59:**6, 1950.

Cosgrove, S. A., and Carter, P. A.: A consideration of therapeutic abortion, Amer. J. Obstet. Gynec. **48:**299, 1944.

Goldzieher, J. W.: Double-blind trial of progesterone in habitual abortion, J.A.M.A. **188:**651, 1964.

Greenblatt, R.: Habitual abortion; possible role of vitamin P, Obstet. Gynec. **2:**530, 1953.

Hertig, A. T., and Livingstone, R. G.: Spontaneous, threatened, and habitual abortion; its pathogenesis and treatment, New Eng. J. Med. **230:**797, 1944.

Hughes, E. C., Van Ness, A. W., and Lloyd, C. W.: The nutritional value of the endometrium for implantation and in habitual abortion, Amer. J. Obstet. Gynec. **59:**1292, 1950.

Javert, C. T.: Spontaneous and habitual abortion, New York, 1957, McGraw-Hill Book Co.

Kardos, G. G.: Isoproterenol in the treatment of shock due to bacteremia with gram-negative pathogens, New Eng. J. Med. **274:**868, 1966.

Lash, A. F.: Operations for habitual abortion, Clin. Obstet. Gynec. **2:**1083, 1959.

Lillehei, R. C., Dietzman, R. H., Movsas, S., and Bloch, J. H.: Treatment of septic shock, Mod. Med. **4:**321, 1967.

Loudon, J. D. O.: The use of high concentration I.V. drip in the management of missed abortion, J. Obstet. Gynaec. Brit. Comm. **66:**277, 1959.

McLennan, M. T., and McLennan, C. E.: Prediction of abortion from vaginal wall cytologic smears, Amer. J. Obstet. Gynec. **92:**620, 1965.

McLennan, M. T., and McLennan, C. E.: Failure of vaginal wall cytologic smears to predict abortion, Amer. J. Obstet. Gynec. **103:**228, 1969.

Mall, F. P., and Meyer, A. W.: Studies on abortions; survey of pathologic ova in Carnegie embryological collection, Contrib. Embryol. **12:**56, 1921.

Mann, E. C.: Habitual abortion, Amer. J. Obstet. Gynec. **77:**706, 1959.

Morris, J. A., Smith, R. W., and Assali, N. S.: Hemodynamic action of vasopressor and vasodepressor agents in endotoxin shock, Amer. J. Obstet. Gynec. **91:**491, 1965.

Reid, D. E.: Assessment and management of the seriously ill patient following abortion, J.A.M.A. **199:**141, 1967.

Roddick, J. W., Jr., Buckingham, J. C., and Danforth, D. N.: The muscular cervix—a cause of incompetency in pregnancy, Obstet. Gynec. **17:** 562, 1961.

Shirodkar, V. N.: A new method of operative treatment for habitual abortion in the second trimester of pregnancy, Antiseptic **52:**299, 1955.

Singh, R. P., and Carr, D. H.: Anatomic findings in human abortions of known chromosomal constitution, Obstet. Gynec. **29:**806, 1967.

Stenchever, M. A., Jarvis, J. A., and Macintyre, M. N.: Cytogenetics of habitual abortion, Obstet. Gynec. **32:**548, 1968.

Stevenson, L. B.: Maternal death and abortion, Michigan, 1955-1964, Mich. Med. **66:**287, 1967.

Studdiford, W. E., and Douglas, G. W.: Placental bacteremia; significant finding in septic abortion accompanied by vascular collapse, Amer. J. Obstet. Gynec. **71:**842, 1956.

Szulman, A. E.: Chromosomal aberrations in spontaneous human abortions, New Eng. J. Med. **272:**811, 1965.

Taussig, F. J.: Abortion: spontaneous and induced, St. Louis, 1936, The C. V. Mosby Co.

Thiede, H. A., and Metcalfe, S.: Chromosome aberrations in abortion, Mod. Med., June, 1967.

Wall, R. L., and Hertig, A. T.: Habitual abortion; a pathologic analysis of 100 cases, Amer. J. Obstet. Gynec. **56:**1127, 1948.

14

Ectopic pregnancy

An ectopic pregnancy is one that is implanted and develops outside of its normal habitat, the uterine cavity. It is sometimes referred to as an extrauterine pregnancy, but this term, strictly speaking, would not apply to the occasional cornual and interstitial pregnancies that are truly out of place but, nevertheless, are not outside of the uterus. An ovum may be fertilized and implanted at any point in its journey from the ovary to the uterine cavity.

■ Sites of implantation

The implantation sites of ectopic pregnancies in order of their frequency are:
1. Tubal (95% of all ectopic pregnancies)
   a. Ampullar
   b. Isthmic
   c. Interstitial
   d. Fimbrial
2. Abdominal

3. Ovarian
4. Interligamentary

Twins and even triplets have been found in one tube, and there are many reported instances of bilateral tubal pregnancies and of combined intrauterine and tubal gestations.

■ Incidence

In 1921 Schumann estimated that ectopic gestation occurred once in every 303 pregnancies. This ratio has gradually increased during the intervening years. Anderson states that the ratio of tubal pregnancy to total births in Baltimore during a 5-year period was 1:177 in white women and 1:120 in black women. He estimated the general incidence to be 1:190 in white women and 1:130 in black women. During a 14½-year period, ectopic pregnancy was diagnosed 591 times, and 46,062 women were delivered or treated for abortion in the Temple University Medical Center. The overall incidence therefore was 1 ectopic pregnancy to every 78 intrauterine pregnancies. The incidence in black patients was 1:60 intrauterine pregnancies and in white patients was 1:145.

■ Etiology

Except in the rare primary ovarian and possibly in some abdominal pregnancies, the ovum is fertilized in the outer one third of the fallopian tube. Under normal conditions it descends through the tube and enters the uterus at the blastocyst stage when active trophoblastic cells have developed. If its progress toward the uterus is delayed and if it survives, the trophoblast invades the tubal mucosa rather than the endometrium. The following conditions within or around the oviduct retard or prevent the passage of the fertilized ovum and are responsible for ectopic gestation.
1. Chronic gonorrheal or tuberculous salpingitis, which causes agglutination of folds of mucosa and narrowing of the lumen of the tube
2. Congenital tubal abnormalities, such as diverticula and atresia of the tube, which may distort the lumen
3. Peritubal adhesions, which may follow postabortal and puerperal infections or appendicitis and kink the tube
4. Tumors pressing against the tube
5. Previous plastic operations on the tube

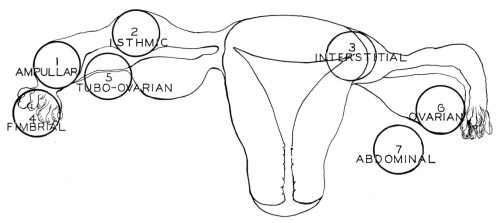

Fig. 14-1. Ectopic pregnancy. Diagram showing various sites of implantation, numbered in order of frequency of occurrence. (From Titus, P.: Atlas of obstetric technic, St. Louis, 1949, The C. V. Mosby Co.)

6. External migration of the fertilized ovum (An ovum produced in one ovary enters the fimbriated end of the opposite fallopian tube. If it has already been fertilized and the trophoblast has developed or if its transport through the tube is delayed until it is too large to enter the uterus, it may implant in the tubal mucosa.)
7. Ectopic endometrial implants in the fallopian tube
8. Tubal spasm or altered tubal peristalsis
9. Penicillin therapy of gonorrheal salpingitis, which may prevent sealing off of the fimbrial end of the tube but not the destructive changes in the mucosa

■ Pathologic anatomy

The process by which the fertilized ovum is implanted in the tube is similar to that in the uterus, but the tubal mucosa is a far less satisfactory implantation site than is the endometrium.

Implantation. Although decidual cells can usually be identified in tubal mucosa, the extensive decidual change that occurs in the endometrium is never seen. The fertilized ovum usually implants between two projecting mucosal folds, but it may become attached more superficially. As the trophoblastic cells proliferate, they erode through the mucosa and into the muscularis, destroying tissue and opening blood vessels as they invade. In the uterus the entire ovum is surrounded by decidua, but a true decidua capsularis cannot form in the tube. Instead, a *pseudocapsule* of muscle and connective tissue usually surrounds the ovum. The placenta, which is histologically identical to that in an intrauterine pregnancy, develops and continues to invade the surrounding tissues as it grows.

Uterine changes. The uterine endometrium is converted to decidua similar to that of normal pregnancy even though the ovum is implanted in the tube. In both instances the decidua develops in response to the stimulus of placental estrogen and progesterone. Decidual growth continues as long as the trophoblast is actively producing the gestational hormones, but when the placenta separates from the tubal wall or degenerates and can no longer function, the hormonal stimulation of the uterine endometrium is withdrawn and it degenerates and sloughs. The decidua usually is discharged in fragments, but occasionally an intact *decidual cast* of the uterus is extruded. The external bleeding that accompanies tubal pregnancy is due to decidual slough and indicates a failing placenta.

The size and consistency of the uterus change even though the pregnancy is in the tube. Both the cervix and the body of the uterus soften, and the corpus may enlarge to a size comparable to that of an intrauterine pregnancy of 6 or 8 weeks, but often it changes little. Uterine growth is caused by estrogen and progesterone.

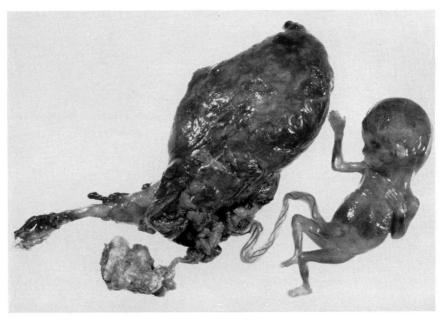

Fig. 14-2. Tubal abortion. Fetus is extruded through fimbriated end of tube, and placenta is in ampulla of tube.

■ Course and termination

The duration of tubal pregnancy and the eventual outcome are determined primarily by the area of the tube in which the pregnancy is situated.

Tubal abortion. If the ovum implants in the relatively large and distensible ampullary portion of the tube, the pregnancy will usually continue longer than it would in the narrow isthmus, but it almost always terminates 6 to 10 weeks after the onset of the last normal period. Local bleeding from trophoblastic invasion continues and increases, and eventually the hemorrhage separates the ovular sac completely or partially from the tubal wall. With complete separation, which usually occurs early, the entire sac may be extruded from the end of the tube, and unless a major vessel is injured the bleeding ceases. More characteristically, however, the process is prolonged. During an episode of active bleeding, which soon stops temporarily, only a portion of the placenta is detached, and the remainder continues to function. The blood escapes from the ostium into the peritoneal cavity, and a hematoma forms around the end of the tube in the cul-de-sac. After several similar episodes during which the

pelvic hematoma gradually increases in size, the ovum is completely separated from its attachment and is expelled into the peritoneal cavity *(tubal abortion)*. This process may continue over a period of 2 to 4 weeks, during which time the patient becomes progressively more anemic.

Tubal rupture. Trophoblastic cells proliferate and invade the isthmic and interstitial portions of the tube exactly as they do the ampulla. The tubal lumen in these areas is smaller and much less distensible than in the more distal portions, and rupture is inevitable as the chorionic tissue invades and weakens the wall and as blood accumulates. The placenta may grow directly through the tube, or the wall may become so thin and distended that it ruptures during examination or coitus or as the patient strains to defecate. Pregnancy in the isthmus usually terminates 6 to 8 weeks after the onset of the last period, but those that are implanted in the interstitial portion as it traverses the uterine wall characteristically continue for 14 to 16 weeks before rupturing.

The tube usually ruptures into the peritoneal cavity and its perforation is accompanied by sudden and profuse bleeding. Occasionally the implantation site is in the

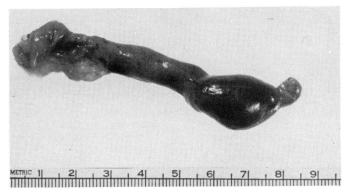

Fig. 14-3. Intact early isthmic pregnancy. The fimbriated end of the tube is at the left.

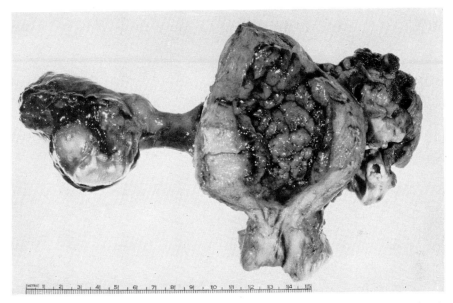

Fig. 14-4. Pregnancy in ampulla of right tube. Note the pronounced decidual reaction in the uterus and a chronic left tubo-ovarian abscess. (From Willson, J. R.: Management of obstetric difficulties, ed. 6, St. Louis, 1961, The C. V. Mosby Co.)

inferior wall, in which case the trophoblast erodes into the broad ligament.

Abdominal pregnancy. The fertilized ovum may implant directly on a peritoneal surface without entering the tube. This is *primary abdominal pregnancy* and must be rare. *Secondary abdominal pregnancy,* although it occurs only about once in 15,000 pregnancies, is more often encountered. An ovular sac that is suddenly and completely separated and extruded from the tube into the peritoneal cavity cannot possibly establish itself and grow. However, normal active trophoblastic tissue can implant on a peritoneal surface, grow, and function reasonably adequately. If the primary implantation site is just within the distal tubal opening, the developing placenta may grow through the ostium, attaching itself to the peritoneal covering of the pelvic viscera as it advances. If the embryo is properly nourished, the pregnancy will continue to develop, gradually extending out of the tube until the entire structure is in the abdominal cavity. An abdominal pregnancy may continue to term, but the infant usually dies before the fortieth week.

The placenta may also gradually erode

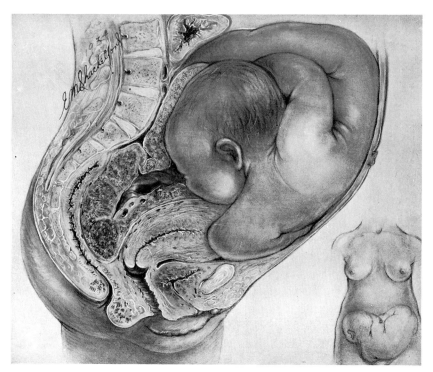

Fig. 14-5. Abdominal pregnancy near term. Placenta is attached over broad ligament, cul-de-sac, and anterior to sacrum. Delivery of living infant by laparotomy. (From Eisaman, J. R., and Ziegler, C. E.: J.A.M.A. **104:**2175, 1935.)

through the tubal wall into the broad ligament. A pregnancy that develops in this area is an *intraligamentous,* or *broad ligament pregnancy.* Although these are not strictly abdominal pregnancies, their course and termination are similar to those that grow in the peritoneal cavity.

Spontaneous regression. Many tubal pregnancies, probably more than become clinically obvious, must regress spontaneously. Either the ovum dies at an early stage or it implants so close to the tubal ostium that it is soon extruded. The woman may have a slight delay in menses and mild discomfort, but one does not usually suspect tubal pregnancy, much less make an accurate diagnosis.

■ Symptoms

The typical story of a *ruptured tubal pregnancy* is as follows: A woman who has had a rather long period of either primary or secondary infertility *misses a period;* she may experience some of the early subjective symptoms of pregnancy, but often does not. With-

in 2 to 4 weeks after the first missed period she will notice a small amount of *reddish* or *brownish vaginal discharge.* Preceding this spotting or coincident with it she may be aware of recurrent, sharp, *fleeting pain* in the lower abdomen, which is often described as a "stitch in the side." This symptom is so evanescent that it often escapes the patient's attention and is usually elicited only after close questioning. If the diagnosis is not made, the patient eventually experiences sudden, sharp abdominal pain, which is often severe enough to cause her to faint when the tube ruptures. She usually reacts from this primary shock, but if the intra-abdominal bleeding incident to the rupture continues, the symptoms of internal hemorrhage become progressively more severe, and the patient may lapse into profound shock.

Tubal abortion, which produces a less dramatic clinical picture than that just described, occurs more often than does tubal rupture, and its course is more prolonged. The pain, which is located in the lower abdomen and pelvis, is cramping and intermittent and may come in attacks lasting several hours. The episodes of pain are accompanied by visible uterine bleeding, the amount of which varies from spotting to a flow similar to that with impending abortion. The symptoms increase in severity as ovular separation progresses. The escaping intraperitoneal blood clots and forms a cul-de-sac hematoma, which enlarges with each episode of bleeding and which may press on the rectum, producing an urge to empty the bowel. The straining and increased intra-abdominal pressure that accompany the patient's attempts to evacuate the rectum may dislodge the ovum and produce the final episode of bleeding. The patient often faints at this time; in fact, sudden, severe abdominal pain and syncope during attempts to evacuate the rectum are so common with tubal pregnancy that the diagnosis must be considered whenever a patient describes these symptoms. *Shoulder top pain* may be present if there has been enough bleeding to permit blood to collect beneath the diaphragm.

The clinical course of *ovarian pregnancy* is similar to that of pregnancy in the tube, but it occurs rarely.

Abdominal pregnancy can be suspected in women who have experienced repeated episodes of pain and bleeding during the early weeks if abdominal discomfort, spotting, and digestive disturbances continue despite the fact that the pregnancy appears to be developing normally.

■ Physical signs

Pelvic examination ordinarily discloses the usual *signs of early pregnancy* such as cyanosis and softening of the cervix and uterine enlargement. The most important pelvic finding prior to tubal rupture or abortion is a *tender, sausage-shaped mass in one adnexal region*. Unfortunately this sign is not always present, and oftentimes, even though an adnexal mass has formed, it may not be felt because of the extreme pelvic tenderness and the patient's voluntary abdominal rigidity. *Unilateral pelvic tenderness* is a common finding, and pain in the affected side may be induced by either elevating the cervix or moving it from side to side. In patients who have developed a pelvic hematocele, *fullness or even bulging of the cul-de-sac* may be readily detected by vaginal or rectovaginal examination. *Signs of peritoneal*

irritation and of free fluid in the abdomen may be present if there has been profuse or prolonged bleeding within the peritoneal cavity. *Fever* is slight or absent except in persons with secondary infected pelvic hematocele; changes in *pulse rate* and *blood pressure* are dependent upon the amount of bleeding.

■ Laboratory findings

The *white blood cell count* may be normal or increased to about 15,000. The *hemoglobin* or *hematocrit* falls rapidly in cases of tubal rupture. The decrease is more gradual but progressive if moderate bleeding continues over a long period of time, as it does during tubal abortion.

The *pregnancy test* in tubal pregnancy may be helpful if interpreted in the light of physiologic principles upon which it is based and when its results are correlated with the pathologic physiology of ectopic gestation. The test generally will be positive if the embryo is living and the trophoblasts are in contact with the maternal circulation. It will be negative after death of the embryo or if there is interruption of the fetomaternal circulation. Thus it is quite possible that the pregnancy test will be negative with tubal pregnancy. A positive test, on the other hand, indicates only that the trophoblast is active and producing hormones; it is of little help in locating the implantation site.

■ Diagnosis

The diagnosis of an unruptured tubal pregnancy is not too difficult to make when classic symptoms and signs are present. Unfortunately symptoms are often atypical and the pelvic findings may be misleading. In general the diagnosis may be made with a considerable degree of accuracy if one has a high index of suspicion for this condition and by proper evaluation of the history. If the symptoms lead the physician to suspect the presence of a tubal pregnancy, all available diagnostic procedures must be employed to either prove or allay such a suspicion, even though the pelvic findings are not characteristic.

With *abdominal pregnancy* the uterus can often be felt as a mass separate from the extrauterine ovular sac. If uterine size remains the same while the other mass gradually enlarges, the diagnosis is more certain.

It is difficult to outline the structures precisely, however, and the uterus itself is often
interpreted as being an ovarian neoplasm
or a fibromyoma. Later in pregnancy the
fetus may be felt high in the abdomen and
in an abnormal position, which changes little
from week to week.

If fetal parts can be seen lying posterior
to the maternal lumbar spine in a lateral
x-ray projection of the abdomen, it is unlikely that the infant is in the uterus. A *hysterogram* will reveal a small uterine cavity
and an extrauterine fetus. The injection of
0.25 to 0.5 unit of *oxytocin* intravenously
will usually cause the uterine muscle to contract firmly, even though the pregnancy is
several weeks from term. With an extrauterine pregnancy the thick membrane surrounding the fetus, which may feel like
uterine wall and even look like it upon x-ray
examination, will not contract under the influence of an oxytocic agent.

SPECIAL STUDIES IN DIAGNOSIS OF ECTOPIC PREGNANCY

Diagnostic needle colpotomy. Intraperitoneal bleeding or a cul-de-sac hematoma can
be detected by *needle culdocentesis,* which
can be carried out in the clinic or ward examining room under local infiltration anesthesia. A 15-gauge needle is inserted through
the posterior fornix of the vagina about 1
cm. behind the point at which the vaginal
mucosa joins the cervix. If dark or bright
red blood flows freely through the needle,
the presence of intraperitoneal bleeding is
confirmed. If only a small amount of bright
red blood can be aspirated, the needle may
have perforated a blood vessel and should be
withdrawn and reinserted. Failure to obtain
blood does not rule out ectopic gestation
entirely; it only eliminates intraperitoneal
bleeding, which is not always evident in
early, unruptured tubal pregnancy.

Posterior colpotomy. If needle puncture
of the cul-de-sac is negative, the cul-de-sac
may be explored through a transverse incision in the vaginal mucosa and the peritoneum. This is preferable to an abdominal
exploratory operation because in the absence of an ectopic pregnancy the vaginal
incision can be closed and the patient can
be discharged from the hospital within 24
to 48 hours.

Culdoscopy. The insertion of a culdoscope into the cul-de-sac permits visualization of the pelvic viscera. This is a valuable
diagnostic tool in the hands of experienced
personnel, but it has certain disadvantages
and dangers. Culdoscopy is contraindicated
if there is a mass in the cul-de-sac or if acute
salpingo-oophoritis is suspected. It also is
contraindicated in patients with evidence of
excessive blood loss because the time involved
and the manipulations necessary for the examination may delay appropriate surgical
treatment.

Laparoscopy. Laparoscopy often is prefer-

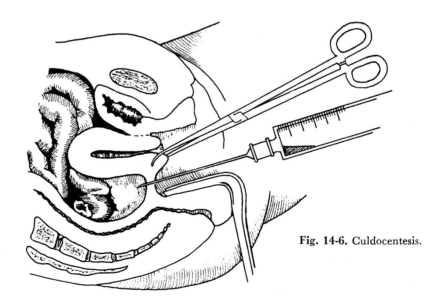

Fig. 14-6. Culdocentesis.

able to culdoscopy because the instrument is inserted through the abdominal wall rather than through the cul-de-sac and because it is performed with the patient in dorsal supine position. If laparotomy is necessary, there is no need to reposition the patient. Laparoscopy, like culdoscopy, is of greatest help in the diagnosis of ectopic pregnancy before the tube has ruptured.

Dilatation and curettage. Dilatation and curettage should be performed if vaginal bleeding has been profuse and prolonged. This affords an opportunity for careful pelvic examination under anesthesia and may rule out an ectopic pregnancy if placental tissue is obtained from the endometrial cavity. If the curettings grossly resemble normal endometrium, further investigation is indicated. If uterine bleeding has been scant and if there is a possibility of a threatened abortion of an intrauterine pregnancy, cul-de-sac puncture and exploration should be performed without invading the uterine cavity.

■ Differential diagnosis

Although it is usually possible to diagnose tubal pregnancy with reasonable accuracy, uterine abortion, salpingitis, appendicitis, and more rarely ruptured corpus luteum or follicular cysts may produce symptoms so similar that differentiation is difficult.

Threatened or incomplete abortion. The period of amenorrhea preceding the onset of symptoms usually is longer, the amount of vaginal bleeding is greater, the pain usually is less severe than in ectopic pregnancy and is in the midline and crampy in nature, and no adnexal mass and tenderness are present. When differentiation is difficult, the physician may have to resort to dilatation and curettage and colpotomy to establish a diagnosis.

Salpingitis. The symptoms accompanying acute tubal infection usually appear at the time of menstruation rather than after a period of amenorrhea, and the pain, tenderness, and palpable tubal enlargement usually are bilateral. The temperature ordinarily is quite high, and leukocytosis is much greater than with ectopic pregnancy. The pregnancy test is negative.

Appendicitis. There is usually a history of digestive disturbances such as nausea and vomiting, there is no amenorrhea or bleeding, and there is no adnexal mass unless an appendiceal abscess has developed. The pregnancy test is negative.

Corpus luteum cysts. The mass in corpus luteum cysts usually is larger and more globular than in ectopic pregnancy. It is also less painful and less tender. The pregnancy test usually is negative.

Ruptured graafian follicle with excessive bleeding. There is usually no amenorrhea associated with ruptured graafian follicle, and it occurs most often at midcycle, at the time of ovulation. The pregnancy test is negative.

■ Treatment

The treatment for tubal pregnancy consists of surgical removal of the involved tube and replacement of the blood lost as a result of the lesion. The patient with ruptured tubal pregnancy and massive intraperitoneal hemorrhage must be operated upon as soon as she can be transported to the hospital and the operating room can be prepared. If she is in deep shock, a surgical procedure without preliminary blood transfusion will increase the mortality. Consequently blood must be administered while the patient is being prepared and anesthetized, even though some of it will be lost through the bleeding vessels. Spinal anesthesia is contraindicated because of the bleeding and the shock, but the operation can be performed readily under general anesthesia with a high concentration of oxygen. A curare preparation may be utilized to produce relaxation of voluntary muscles, thereby reducing the amount of anesthetic agent needed.

The treatment of abdominal pregnancy is prompt operation with removal of the fetus. Except under unusual circumstances it is illogical to permit the pregnancy to continue to term because most of the infants are malformed and even those who are normal usually die relatively early in the pregnancy. Because the procedure usually is accompanied by excessive bleeding, particularly if an attempt is made to remove the placenta, the patient should be given blood preoperatively if she is anemic, and at least 2,000 ml. of compatible blood must be ready for immediate administration during the surgical procedure. The placental villi often penetrate the blood vessels of the omentum and mesentery, and because there is no cleavage plane as there is in the uterus, the placenta can be removed only by tearing or cutting through its vascular bed. Unless it can be separated easily by digital manipulation or unless it is already partially detached, it is preferable to permit the structure to remain in place after trimming the membranes and severing the cord close to its fetal surface.

■ Prognosis

If the diagnosis is made early, before rupture and severe bleeding occur, the operative results should be uniformly good, but if diagnosis and treatment are delayed or if blood replacement is inadequate, the number of deaths may be high. Statistical studies early in the present century showed a mortality of 10% to 15%, but more recent statistics indicate a reduction to somewhere between 1% and 1.5%. Leff reported a series of 266 tubal pregnancies without a death, and of 591 patients operated upon for ectopic gestation in the Temple University Hospital during a 14½-year period, only one died.

Because of the structural lesions responsible for the original tubal implantation, less than one half of the patients become pregnant after the first abnormal pregnancy, and of those who do about 10% have a recurrence in the remaining tube. Brey and his associates operated upon 241 women with ectopic pregnancies between 1955 and 1962. Of the 182 who responded to a questionnaire only 30% had intrauterine pregnancies after the tubal implantation and 7.9% had repeat ectopic gestations. These women frequently make a second diagnosis themselves because of the similarity of the symptoms to those of the first ectopic pregnancy.

References

Anderson, G. W.: The racial incidence and mortality of ectopic pregnancy, Amer. J. Obstet. Gynec. 61:312, 1951.

Brey, J., Schreiber, H., and Weinold, J.: Fertility after extrauterine pregnancies, Zbl. Gynaek. 86:825, 1964.

Clark, J. F. J., and Bourke, J.: Advanced ectopic pregnancy, Amer. J. Obstet. Gynec. 78:340, 1959.

Cross, J. B., Lester, W. M., and McCain, J. R.: The diagnosis and management of abdominal pregnancy with a review of nineteen cases, Amer. J. Obstet. Gynec. 62:203, 1951.

Daly, M. J.: Posterior colpotomy for the diagnosis and treatment of pelvic disease, Amer. J. Obstet. Gynec. 74:623, 1957.

Leff, B.: A thirty-seven year survey of ectopic pregnancy, Amer. J. Obstet. Gynec. 65:1313, 1953.

Schumann, E. A.: Extra-uterine pregnancy, New York, 1921, Appleton-Century.

Siddall, R. S.: The occurrence and significance of decidual changes of the endometrium in extra-uterine pregnancy, Amer. J. Obstet. Gynec. 31:420, 1936.

Weinberg, A., and Sherwin, A. S.: A new sign in roentgen diagnosis of advanced ectopic pregnancy, Obstet. Gynec. 7:99, 1956.

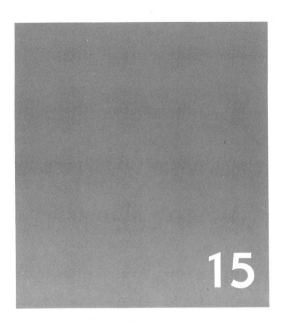

15

Trophoblastic disease: hydatidiform mole, invasive mole, and choriocarcinoma

Malignant diseases of trophoblastic tissue, although rare, are among the most lethal of all tumors arising in the reproductive organs. The trophoblastic lesions most often encountered are, in order of degree of malignancy, *hydatidiform mole, invasive mole,* and *choriocarcinoma.*

■ Hydatidiform mole

Hydatidiform mole is a term used to indicate a neoplastic proliferation of the trophoblast in which the terminal villi are transformed into vesicles filled with clear viscid material. Hydatidiform mole usually is benign, but at times it has malignant potentialities and precedes the development of choriocarcinoma.

Hydatidiform mole is an uncommon lesion in the United States, occurring about once in 2,000 to 2,500 pregnancies. It is much less rare in the Orient, where it is diagnosed once in 200 pregnancies in the Philippines and once in 82 pregnancies in Taiwan. Hertig believes that the usually quoted figures do not represent the true incidence because they disregard hydropic placental degeneration, which occurs so frequently with early spontaneous abortion.

Etiology. Hertig and Edmonds found pathologic ova in half of the spontaneously aborted specimens they examined. Early hydatidiform placental degeneration was present in two thirds of the specimens with abnormal ova. They suggest that the vesicles develop because of the absence of fetal circulation. The physiologic activity of the trophoblast continues, but the fluid accumulates and distends the villi because it cannot be removed by the embryo. The fact that a fetus is almost never found in conjunction with a well-developed hydatidiform mole suggests that this theory is a logical one.

Acosta-Sison suggested that the high incidence in Oriental women is related to dietary protein deficiency since the disease occurs much more often in poor than in well-to-do Filipinos. McCorriston, studying the incidence of trophoblastic disease in Honolulu, found that 54% of hydatidiform moles occurred in women of Japanese extraction, who make up 32% of the population, whereas Caucasians, who make up 30% of the population, contributed 11% of moles. Figures for other ethnic groups include Chinese, 6% of the population and 11% of moles; Filipinos, 11% of the population and 7% of the moles; and Hawaiian or part-Hawaiian 20% of the population and 11% of the moles. He suggests that diet probably plays an insignificant etiologic role because Hawaiians in Honolulu are far more likely to have inadequate diets than are the other racial groups.

Baggish and co-workers confirmed the observations of others that about 90% of hydatidiform moles have a female sex chromatin pattern. They suggest that two cell lines develop: one from the union of sperm and ovum and the other by endoreduplication of the second polocyte, which, of course, would be sex chromatin positive. Such an origin could account for the genesis of the mole, for the combination of mole and fetus, and for molar degeneration of the placenta.

Pathology. The whole placenta, or most of it, is converted into a mass of vesicles, which vary in size from a few millimeters to a maximum diameter of about 3 cm. The entire mass may be small, or it may enlarge the uterus to the size of a normal 24- to 26-week gestation. If a fetus can be identified, it is small and malformed, although occasionally a normal baby may be born at or near term with a considerable amount of the placenta having undergone hydatidiform degeneration.

The histologic pattern of a benign mole is characterized by trophoblastic proliferation, hydropic degeneration of the stroma, and the absence of blood vessels. The villous pattern is maintained, and there is neither anaplastic change nor epithelial penetration into the stroma or the myometrium.

Potentially malignant moles are characterized by more pronounced trophoblastic activity and anaplastic change. Attempts have been made to establish histologic criteria for estimating the degree of malignancy, but the most accurate method is still the clinical course.

The ovaries respond to the stimulation of the elevated levels of chorionic gonadotropic hormones by the development of *theca-lutein cysts,* which characteristically accompany hydatidiform mole. The cysts, which usually are bilateral, vary in size from those that barely enlarge the ovary to those 20 cm. or more in diameter. Definite ovarian enlargement is recognized clinically with a minority of hydatidiform moles, the change probably reflecting the stage of molar development and the amount of gonadotropin being produced. After the uterus is evacuated the ovaries gradually return to normal size as hormone levels decrease. The same change may occur during normal pregnancy.

Clinical course. After a period of amenorrhea, during which the patient considers herself to be pregnant, dark brown vaginal discharge appears. This may be followed rather rapidly by cramps and expulsion of the mole, or discharge and bleeding may continue intermittently for several weeks. Partial spontaneous evacuation, during which bleeding may be profuse, eventually occurs. These patients are usually diagnosed as having threatened abortion of normal pregnancy until the characteristic vesicles are passed.

All the symptoms of early pregnancy may be exaggerated in women with hydatidiform mole. Nausea and vomiting may begin earlier, be more severe, and last longer than during normal pregnancy. Severe preeclampsia may develop during the early part of the second trimester of a molar preg-

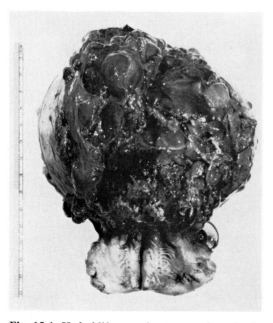

Fig. 15-1. Hydatidiform mole at approximately the hundredth day of pregnancy. Note the uneffaced, undilated cervix with deep molar penetration into myometrium. Patient is a 43-year-old primigravida.

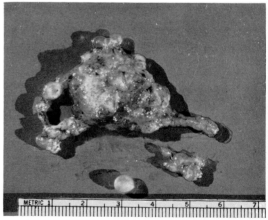

Fig. 15-2. Transitional mole found in a spontaneous abortion.

nancy; this is the only situation in which toxemia is diagnosed before the twenty-fourth week. Hypertension is most likely to occur when the uterus enlarges rapidly and is several times larger than might be expected for that stage of gestation.

Diagnosis. Most patients with moles are treated for threatened or inevitable abortion unless typical vesicles are passed. The correct diagnosis may first be made when the physician begins to evacuate the uterus. In about half these patients the uterus is larger than it should be for the calculated duration of pregnancy; in the rest its size is normal for the stage of pregnancy or smaller.

The uterus that is distended by a multicystic molar pregnancy feels firmer than does one containing a normal pregnancy; also, a fluid wave cannot be demonstrated. Between the sixteenth and twentieth weeks of normal pregnancy it is almost always possible to identify a living fetus by palpating its parts or hearing fetal heart sounds. Confirmatory evidence can be obtained by fetal electrocardiography, roentgen examination, or the use of ultrasound. None of these will give positive results with a molar pregnancy.

It may also be possible to differentiate hydatidiform mole from normal pregnancy by the use of *biologic tests for pregnancy* or, more accurately, by measuring *serum chorionic gonadotropin concentration*. The hyperplastic trophoblastic tissue secretes more gonadotropin than does a normal placenta; consequently, pregnancy tests are often positive even though the urine is diluted to 1:500 or more. During normal pregnancy positive tests cannot often be obtained with dilutions greater than 1:100, even during the period of maximum gonadotropin production.

A more precise evaluation can be made by measuring serum gonadotropin concentration. Even this may not be reliable because at the time of peak secretion during normal pregnancy, about the sixtieth day, the concentration may be in a range consistent with that of hydatidiform mole. According to Delfs the serum values rise during early normal pregnancy, reaching about 50,000 I.U. at 45 days and a maximum of as much as 600,000 I.U. at about the sixtieth day. The titer then decreases rapidly and is rarely above 20,000 I.U. after the

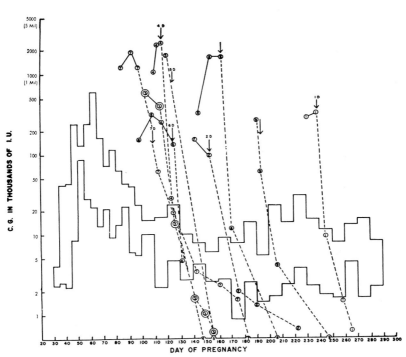

Fig. 15-3. Chorionic gonadotropin excretion during normal and molar pregnancy. (From Delfs, E.: Obstet. Gynec. **9:**3, 1957.)

hundredth day. The values for hydatidiform mole usually are higher than these, often reaching 1.5 to 2 million I.U., but they can also be low if the mole is regressing rather than growing.

It is evident that it would be hazardous to diagnose hydatidiform mole at the sixtieth day of pregnancy in a patient with a history suggesting threatened abortion and a uterus larger than anticipated simply on the basis of a serum gonadotropin concentration of 500,000 I.U. On the other hand, a similar concentration after the hundredth day undoubtedly would be significant.

Trophoblast hormonal secretion can be measured by radioimmunoassay techniques, which confirm the changes in chorionic gonadotropin production in molar pregnancies. They also offer an interesting differential diagnostic aid. The placenta during normal pregnancy secretes *human placental lactogen* (HPL) as well as *human chorionic gonadotropin* (HCG), but molar tissue is less able to produce the former. The values for HPL in molar pregnancy are ten to one-hundred times less than those expected at a comparable gestational age. The combination of a greatly elevated HCG and reduced HPL substantiates a clinical diagnosis of hydatidiform mole.

Amniography and *aortography* have been suggested as diagnostic measures, but they rarely are indicated. Uterine puncture or femoral vein catheterization and the subsequent x-ray exposure might prove to be disastrous if the pregnancy were normal.

Treatment. The uterus should be evacuated as soon as possible after the diagnosis is made. In most instances when bleeding begins during early pregnancy, the cervix has already effaced and is beginning to dilate, so the *tissue can be removed by suction curettage or with ring forceps and a sharp curet.* The former is preferable because the uterus can be evacuated rapidly with minimal blood loss. The uterus should be emptied as completely as is possible, but great care must be taken lest the thin, soft, uterine wall be perforated by the instruments. A repeat curettage after 48 to 72 hours is indicated if the uterus is large or if there is any possibility that some of the molar tissue may have been left. During the interval between operations, the uterus will have contracted, and a more vigorous curettage can

be performed with less likelihood of injuring the uterine wall.

If the uterus is larger than a 14- to 16-week gestation and the cervix is long and closed, *abdominal hysterotomy* is preferable to curettage. If the cervix is soft and effaced, an attempt can be made to induce labor with dilute intravenous oxytocin. If this is successful, the uterus should be curetted after the mole has been passed. If induction is unsuccessful or if the patient is bleeding profusely, hysterotomy should be performed. With the uterus open the cavity can be curetted under direct vision. The enlarged ovaries need not be removed since they will regress when the hormonal stimulus is withdrawn. Malignant potentialities of hydatidiform mole are greater in older than in young women. For this reason it is usually wise to perform *total abdominal hysterectomy* when a mole is diagnosed in multiparous women over the age of 35 years.

Follow-up examinations. Every patient treated for hydatidoform mole must be kept under observation until the physician can be certain that the patient does not have malignant trophoblastic disease. If the mole has been evacuated completely, uterine bleeding should cease within a week, and the uterus should return to its normal size within 4 to 6 weeks. If bleeding persists and involution is delayed, another curettage should be performed in an attempt to determine whether the cause is residual benign molar tissue or a chorionic malignancy.

A more precise method for detecting continuing trophoblastic activity is by the periodic measurement of gonadotropin concentration in the serum or urine. If the mole has been removed completely, the chorionic gonadotropin production will cease and the material will gradually be excreted. It usually has all disappeared from the serum within 4 to 6 weeks after removal of the mole. If active molar tissue remains or if a malignant trophoblastic lesion has developed, gonadotropin secretions will persist or increase, and the concentration actually may rise.

Delfs could still detect gonadotropin in 26 (21.8%) of 119 patients 60 days after evacuation of a mole. In 15 patients the concentration continued to regress and finally disappeared. The other 11 patients had either an invasive mole or a choriocarcinoma. The first measurement of serum gonadotropin should be made 2 weeks after evacuation of the uterus and subsequent ones at 2-week intervals until the physician can be certain that regression has occurred or that further treatment is required.

Brewer and co-workers observed 51 patients who had been treated for hydatidiform mole with HCG titers at 10-, 20-, 30-, 45-, and 60-day intervals and found persistently elevated titers in 15 women (29.4%) at day 60. The titers in 4 women had fallen slowly and were low at the sixtieth day; they became normal at 70, 90, 142, and 142 days without treatment. The titers in the other 11 women were either higher than anticipated, stable, or rising, each suggesting residual active trophoblastic disease. These patients were all treated with methotrexate. Brewer suggests that an evaluation of the need for treatment can be made on the basis of the titer at day 60 and the changes in titer between days 45 and 60. Treatment should be instituted if the titer between days 45 and 60 rises, if the titer between days 45 and 60 is steady but high, and if the titer between days 45 and 60 falls but is still greater than 2,000 I.U. at day 60.

After day 60 in those patients not treated the test should be repeated at monthly intervals for 3 more months and then every 2 or 3 months for 6 more months—a total of a year. A new pregnancy will confuse evaluation; consequently, an effective contraceptive technique should be used.

Pregnancy tests, as compared to gonadotropin titers, are inadequate for following patients who have been treated for hydatidiform mole or choriocarcinoma. The pregnancy test is significant only if it is positive because it is not sensitive enough to detect low concentrations of HCG. Presently available assay methods are sensitive enough to detect normal levels of pituitary gonadotropins, hence they must be used to evaluate the success of treatment of patients with trophoblastic tumors.

■ Malignant or invasive mole (chorioadenoma destruens)

Invasive mole is similar to hydatidiform mole, from which it arises, but its malignant potentials are much greater. It invades the myometrium, in some instances penetrating the uterine wall completely and extending into the broad ligament or the peritoneal cavity. In half or more of all cases, invasive mole metastasizes through the peripheral circulation to distant sites, most characteristically, the lung.

Pathology. The histologic pattern is similar to that of hydatidiform mole in that the

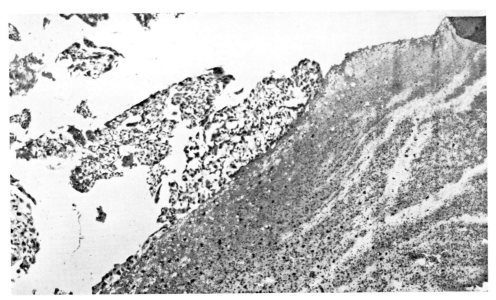

Fig. 15-4. Invasive mole. Note hemorrhage and necrosis as in choriocarcinoma and the villus (upper left corner). (×58.)

villous pattern is maintained, even in metastatic implants. The most important differences are the excessive trophoblastic proliferation and invasiveness. The degree of anaplasia is variable; in some patients the tissue looks completely benign, even though it has metastasized, whereas in others the cells are quite anaplastic. The preservation of the villous pattern serves to differentiate invasive mole from choriocarcinoma, which is so anaplastic that villi cannot form.

Clinical course and diagnosis. Bleeding may continue after the evacuation of a mole if the lesion is relatively superficial; there may be no blood loss if the trophoblast lies deep in the myometrium. The first evidence of the disorder may be cough or hemoptysis from metastatic lung lesions.

Invasive mole or choriocarcinoma can be suspected if the gonadotropin titers fail to regress or continue to rise after evacuation of a hydatidiform mole. When this occurs, repeat curettage is indicated. If the lesion is superficial, an exact diagnosis may be possible, but if it lies deep in the muscle, the curet will not reach it. A chest x-ray examination may reveal metastatic lesions if they are present.

The mortality from invasive mole is greater than that for benign mole, but much less than that for choriocarcinoma. Metastatic lesions may resolve spontaneously after removal of the primary lesion, and the primary lesion as well as the metastases usually respond well to chemotherapeutic agents. The main causes of death are hemorrhage, metastases, and infection.

Treatment will be discussed with that for choriocarcinoma.

■ Choriocarcinoma

Choriocarcinoma is a highly malignant trophoblastic tumor that may follow hydatidiform mole, abortion, or normal pregnancy. Although half to two thirds of choriocarcinomas are preceded by hydatidiform mole, less than 5% of the latter has malignant propensities. About 25% follows abortion, and a smaller percentage develops after delivery at term. There also have been patients in whom the malignant change occurred before delivery, and small foci of choriocarcinoma have been identified in otherwise normal term placentas.

Pathology. The tumor appears as an irregular or circumscribed hemorrhagic growth in the uterine wall. The ulcerating surface usually opens into the endometrial cavity, but on occasion the entire tumor is embedded in myometrium. It sometimes grows entirely through the uterus into the broad ligament or the peritoneal cavity. There may be dark red blood-filled metastases in the vagina or the vulva.

Masses of anaplastic syncytial and Langhans' cells invade the uterine wall, destroy-

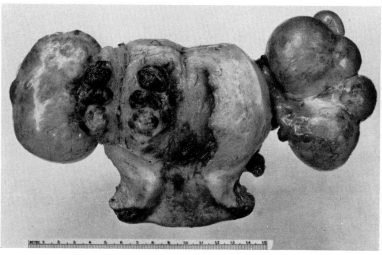

Fig. 15-5. Choriocarcinoma of uterine wall with multiple lutein cysts. (From Willson, J. R.: Management of obstetric difficulties, ed. 6, St. Louis, 1961, The C. V. Mosby Co.)

ing blood vessels and muscle tissue as they grow; consequently necrosis and hemorrhage are prominent in the histologic appearance. The cells proliferate in masses and sheets; villi cannot be recognized. The same pattern is retained in metastases.

Clinical course and diagnosis. Irregular bleeding continues after the passage of a hydatidiform mole or after abortion or delivery unless the growth is situated deep in the uterine wall. The bleeding usually increases in amount as more tissue is destroyed. Malignant tumor cells enter the circulation through the open blood vessels and are transported to the lungs, to the brain, or to other organs and soft tissues. The first evidence of an abnormality may be the appearance of symptoms caused by pulmonary or cerebral lesions or the discovery of a metastatic nodule in the vagina or vulva.

Choriocarcinoma must be suspected as a possible reason for continued bleeding after any pregnancy. A less serious lesion is more often the cause, but if each patient is studied by curettage, chest x-ray examination, and, when necessary, tests for gonadotropin, the diagnosis of malignant trophoblastic disease will be made as early as possible.

Curettage may be deceptive; if the tumor is situated deep in the myometrium, it cannot be reached with the curet. It may not even be possible to make an accurate histologic diagnosis from tissue curetted directly from a large ulcerating lesion because the material may contain only necrotic tissue from the surface.

The measurement of chorionic gonadotropin is the most important single diagnostic aid. Choriocarcinoma must be suspected whenever the concentration of this hormone remains high, or is increasing, and retained molar or placental tissue has been eliminated as its source. If the level remains elevated or continues to rise, the diagnosis is almost certain, and it is reinforced by the presence of characteristic lung lesions.

Treatment. Until recently, 80% to 85% of women with choriocarcinoma died within a year in spite of treatment. Total hysterectomy with bilateral salpingo-oophorectomy and resection of local metastases was the mainstay of treatment, but this was generally ineffective because by the time therapy was instituted the tumor had already metastasized widely.

The prognosis for choriocarcinoma has improved considerably as a result of the

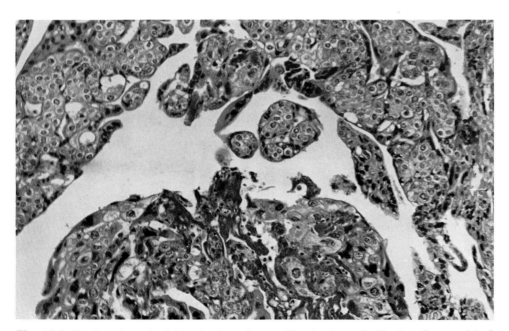

Fig. 15-6. Section through viable choriocarcinoma. Neoplastic trophoblastic cells are of both syncytial and Langhans type. There is no necrosis or hemorrhage in this field.

studies by Hertz and his associates on the use of methotrexate (4-amino-N^{10}-methyl-pteroylglutamic acid), which disrupts the metabolism of the actively growing trophoblastic cells. Methotrexate is a folic acid antagonist that inhibits the enzyme folic reductase, which is necessary for one of the steps in the synthesis of the nucleic acids. Hertz's most recent report concerns the treatment of 111 women with metastatic trophoblastic disease, 75 of whom had choriocarcinoma and the rest, other forms such as invasive mole. The remission rate in the patients with choriocarcinoma was 64% and for those with other malignant trophoblastic conditions, 75%. Most were treated with methotrexate alone, but in some, actinomycin D (formerly meractinomycin) was also administered.

The usual dosage of methotrexate for both choriocarcinoma and invasive mole is 25 mg. daily intramuscularly for 5 days, a total of 125 mg. This is repeated at intervals of 3 to 4 weeks for 5 courses or until chorionic gonadotropin can no longer be detected in the serum. In most patients, gonadotropin will disappear after the second or third course, but in others it persists. If the first 2 courses of methotrexate produce little change in gonadotropin concentration, actinomycin D may be added to the regimen. The dosage is 10 mg./kg. daily administered intravenously.

Some authorities recommend a triple-therapy regimen, which includes reduced dosages of methotrexate, actinomycin D, and Cytoxan or chlorambucil. The general effects of this form of treatment are much more pronounced than for methotrexate alone. Since almost all patients respond to the latter drug, it seems appropriate to use it for initial therapy, reserving the more drastic combinations for those who fail to respond.

Most women suffer toxic reactions, the principal ones being stomatitis, dermatitis, leukopenia caused by bone marrow depression, gastrointestinal ulceration, and alopecia, from the medications. As a consequence it is important that leukocyte, erythrocyte, reticulocyte, and platelet counts be made before treatment is started, daily during each course of therapy and weekly between courses. Chest x-ray examinations should be given at monthly intervals.

Chemotherapeutic agents have almost completely replaced surgical treatment of malignant trophoblastic disease. Not only was hysterectomy ineffective in the management of metastatic choriocarcinoma, but it eliminated all hope of future childbearing in young women. If the primary tumor and the metastases can be eradicated by drug therapy, there is no reason to remove the uterus. Menstruation will be normal and pregnancy can occur. There is no evidence to suggest that methotrexate affects the growth and development of the embryo during subsequent pregnancies.

In a few patients chemotherapeutic regimens are unsuccessful, either because the cells are unresponsive or because the drug fails to reach the primary tumor in the uterine wall. If the gonadotropin level does not fall after repeated courses of treatment, laparotomy must be considered. Primary invasive mole, and less frequently choriocarcinoma, can often be identified as a discrete, dark red hemorrhagic nodule in the uterine wall. If primary invasive mole can be completely resected, the metastatic implants will often regress spontaneously or they will respond to continued drug therapy. This is less likely to occur with choriocarcinoma. In young women if it is desirable to preserve the uterus for possible childbearing, it is quite possible to resect the myometrial lesion completely and to anticipate a remis-

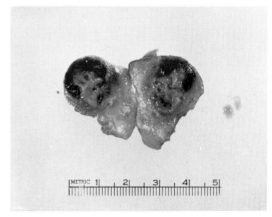

Fig. 15-7. Invasive mole lesion cut open. The dark clot is directly under the endometrial surface. Curettage had not touched the lesion. Note the depth to which the lesion has penetrated the myometrium.

sion with additional methotrexate therapy. Hysterectomy is preferable in multiparous women and those over age 35 years who usually are no longer interested in reproduction. Operation should be considered as being less adequate treatment than chemotherapy and should be used as part of the management of selected women rather than as primary treatment.

Follow-up examinations. Women who have been treated for invasive mole or choriocarcinoma should be checked at 1-month intervals for 1 year after the gonadotropin concentration has returned to normal. The essential studies are pelvic examination, chest x-ray examination, and a test for serum gonadotropin. The pulmonary lesions usually regress slowly and with successful treatment disappear completely.

After the first year the examinations are repeated at 4-month intervals. If there is no evidence of recurrence by the end of the second year, one can assume that the lesion has been eradicated.

References

Acosta-Sison, N.: Chorioadenoma destruens, Amer. J. Obstet. Gynec. 80:176, 1960.

Baggish, M. S., Woodruff, J. D., Tow, S. H., and Jones, H. W., Jr.: Sex chromatin pattern in hydatidiform mole, Amer. J. Obstet. Gynec. 102:362, 1968.

Brewer, J. I., Gerbie, A. B., Dolkart, R. E., Skom, J. H., Nagle, R. G., and Torok, E. E.: Chemotherapy in trophoblastic diseases, Amer. J. Obstet. Gynec. 90:566, 1964.

Brewer, J. I., Torok, E. E., Webster, A., and Dolkart, R. E.: Hydatidiform mole; a follow-up regimen for identification of invasive mole and choriocarcinoma and for selection of patients for treatment, Amer. J. Obstet. Gynec. 101:557, 1968.

Delfs, E.: Quantitative chorionic gonadotropin, Obstet. Gynec. 9:1, 1957.

Hertig, A. T., and Edmonds, H. W.: Genesis of hydatidiform mole, Arch. Path. 30:260, 1940.

Hertig, A. T., and Mansell, H.: Hydatidiform mole and choriocarcinoma, Washington, D. C., 1956, Armed Forces Institute of Pathology.

Hertz, R., Bergenstal, D. M., Lipsett, M. P., Price, E. B., and Hilbish, T. F.: Chemotherapy of choriocarcinoma and related trophoblastic tumors in women, J.A.M.A. 168:845, 1958.

McCorriston, C. C.: Racial incidence of hydatidiform mole, Amer. J. Obstet. Gynec. 101:377, 1968.

Mall, F. P., and Meyer, A. W.: Hydatidiform degeneration in uterine pregnancy, Contrib. Embryol. 12:203, 1921; cited by Hertig and Edmonds.

Sayena, B. N., Goldstein, D. R., Emerson, K., Jr., and Selenkow, H. A.: Serum placental lactogen levels in patients with molar pregnancy and trophoblastic tumors, Amer. J. Obstet. Gynec. 102:115, 1968.

Wilson, G., Colodny, S., and Weidner, W.: Comparison of amniography and angiography in diagnosis of hydatidiform mole, Radiology 87:1076, 1966.

Wilson, R. B., Hunter, J. S., Jr., and Dockerty, M. B.: Chorioadenoma destruens, Trans. Amer. Ass. Obstet. Gynec. 71:134, 1960.

Wilson, R. B., Beecham, C. T., and Symmonds, R. E.: Conservative surgical management of chorioadenoma destruens, Obstet. Gynec. 26:814, 1965.

Zondek, B.: Qualitative und quantitative Gewebsuntersuchung auf Hypophysenvorderlappenhormon nach Gewebsentgiftung. Bedeutung für die Diagnose des Chorionepithelioms, Zbl. Gynaek. 54:2307, 1930.

16

Physiology of normal pregnancy

Profound local and systemic changes in maternal physiology are initiated by conception and continued throughout pregnancy. After expulsion of the placenta many of these changes are rapidly reversed, although certain alterations, particularly those affecting the generative tract, are more gradual in their return to the nongravid state.

■ Genital changes

Uterus. The *size of the uterus* increases five or six times (from 7 by 5 by 3 cm. to 35 by 25 by 22 cm.), the *weight* undergoes a twentyfold increase (from 50 to 1,000 grams at term), and the capacity increases spectacularly one-thousandfold (from 4 to 4,000 ml.).

Uterine growth is caused largely by hypertrophy and to a lesser extent by hyperplasia of the muscle cells. In addition, an increase in the amount of elastic connective tissue adds considerably to the strength of the uterine wall, and a remarkable increase in the size and number of blood vessels provides the rapidly growing tissues with an adequate supply of oxygen and nutritive substances.

The initial stimulus to uterine hypertrophy is hormonal. Thus in the first 6 or 8 weeks the size of the uterus is similar in either intrauterine or extrauterine pregnancy. Enlargement thereafter is dependent upon intrauterine growth of the conceptus. Related uterine and fetal weights throughout gestation show that the greater part of the uterine weight is gained prior to the twentieth week, during which time the myometrial walls become progressively thicker. In the last half of pregnancy, when the fetal growth is accelerated, the myometrium is thinned out to accommodate the fetus (Fig. 16-1). Late in pregnancy, and particularly during labor, myometrial contractions with shortening of the muscle fibers cause progressive thickening of the upper uterine segment as the lower segment develops.

The *position* of the gravid uterus changes as gestation advances. Early, an exaggerated anteflexion is usual, and then as the uterus rises from the pelvis varying degrees of dextrorotation develop because the rectosigmoid occupies a relatively fixed position in the left posterior aspect of the pelvis.

Uterine blood flow in normal term pregnancy measured during cesarean section by Metcalfe and associates showed an average rate of blood flow of 500 ml./min. Oxygen consumption of the gravid uterus was calculated to be 25 ml./min. (5 ml./kg./min.) and the carbon dioxide production, 22 ml./min. On the basis of these determinations the average respiratory quotient of the uterus at term was found to be 0.91. A great deal more needs to be known regarding mechanisms regulating and influencing uterine blood flow throughout the course of pregnancy. Maternal arterial pressure and uterine contractions are only two such factors, but the most clearly recognized. Evidence for augmentation of uterine blood flow by biologically active estrogens, for alterations due to variations in blood gas tensions and chemical substances, and for a fine control superimposed by the autonomic nervous system are discussed in detail in a

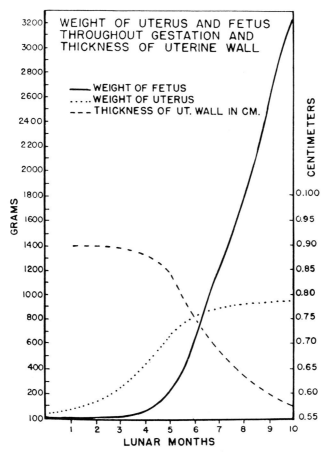

Fig. 16-1. This composite graph expresses certain weights and measurements. Note that around the twentieth week uterine growth diminishes; the myometrium therefore begins to thin, and the fetus begins to increase rapidly in weight. (From Gillespie, E. C.: Amer. J. Obstet. Gynec. **59:**949, 1950.)

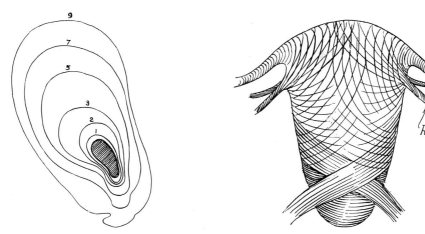

Fig. 16-2. Growth of the uterus during successive months of pregnancy.

Fig. 16-3. Diagram showing interwoven pattern of uterine muscle fibers.

recent review of mechanisms involved in uterine blood flow by Lewis. Elucidation of such mechanisms should have important applications in clinical practice.

Lower uterine segment. The body of the uterus is differentiated into an upper and a lower segment. The upper segment is the contractile portion, which undergoes brachystasis during labor; that is, the muscle fibers contract and then relax to a shorter length without change in tension. The wall in this portion of the uterus becomes thicker

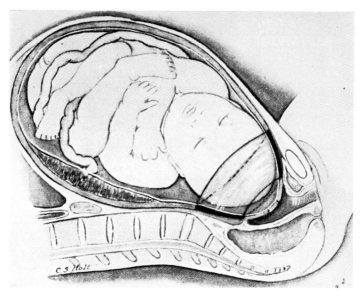

Fig. 16-4. Lower uterine segment early in labor. (From Danforth, D. N., and Ivy, A. C.: Amer. J. Obstet. Gynec. **57:**831, 1949.)

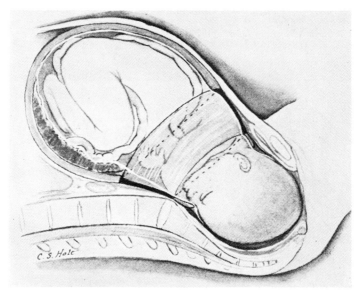

Fig. 16-5. Lower uterine segment in second stage of labor after circumferential dilatation and final elongation. (From Danforth, D. N., and Ivy, A. C.: Amer. J. Obstet. Gynec. **57:**831, 1949.)

during labor, whereas the lower uterine segment, which must undergo circumferential dilatation in order to permit passage of the presenting part, becomes thinned out and about 10 cm. in length. Danforth and Ivy have shown that the lower uterine segment takes its origin from the isthmic portion of the uterus (Figs. 16-4 and 16-5). Its lower border at the histologic internal os is recognizable by the transition from endometrial to endocervical cells at this point. The cervix below the histologic internal os is a fibrous structure. The upper border located at the level of the anatomic internal os is less definite. Early in pregnancy the isthmic portion between these two landmarks softens and lengthens. The softness noted upon compression of this area between the palpating fingers can be detected (Hegar's sign) at 6 to 8 weeks.

From the beginning of the second trimester until the last few weeks of pregnancy the isthmic portion hypertrophies and becomes incorporated or indistinguishable from the rest of the uterine muscle. Late in preg-

nancy, and most particularly during labor, the lower uterine segment becomes thinned out, and its upper pole is more clearly demarcated from the thick upper segment.

Uterine contractility. The uterus contracts irregularly throughout pregnancy. Caldeyro-Barcia and Poseiro have measured intrauterine pressures via a polyethylene tube introduced into the amniotic cavity. Uterine activity is measured in Montevideo units, that is, the intensity of the contractions in total mm. Hg per 10 minutes. From early pregnancy until 30 weeks' gestation, uterine activity is less than 20 Montevideo units. Irregular, painless contractions (Braxton Hicks contractions) increase gradually thereafter from about 30 to 80 Montevideo units as the cervix ripens. At the onset of labor intrauterine activity averages between 80 and 120 Montevideo units, and at peak activity near the end of labor, when the intensity is about 50 mm. Hg and the frequency 5 contractions per 10 minutes, an average of 250 Montevideo units is reached.

Cervix. Changes in the cervix are appar-

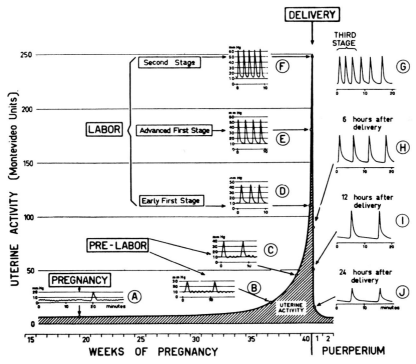

Fig. 16-6. The evolution of spontaneous uterine activity throughout the pregnancy cycle is illustrated by the striped area. Typical (schematic) tracings of uterine contractility at different stages of the cycle are shown. (From Caldeyro-Barcia, R., and Poseiro, J. J.: Ann. N. Y. Acad. Sci. **75:**813, 1959.)

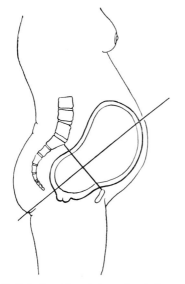

Fig. 16-7. Relationship of the axis of the pregnant uterus to the pelvic inlet.

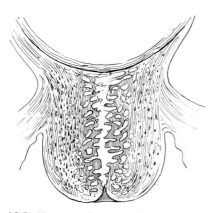

Fig. 16-8. Hypertrophy of cervical glands during pregnancy.

ent by the sixth week. Softening and congestion are the result of increased vascularity. The glands hypertrophy, mucous secretion is greatly increased, and the consistency is altered by steroid hormone activity. Inspissation of the water content of cervical mucus results in the formation of the thick mucous plug that acts as a barrier, protecting the conceptus against mechanical or bacterial invasion throughout the course of pregnancy. Progesterone effects overshadow the effects of increased estrogen production upon cervical mucus; hence the fern reac-

tion is negative when corpus luteum activity is sufficient to support a normal intrauterine pregnancy.

The cervical epithelium is far less responsive to the hormone stimulation of pregnancy than is the endometrium. The stromal cells show a decidual reaction in about one half of pregnant women, but aside from this change, the increased vascularity, and the edema, there are no alterations that can be considered characteristic or specific pregnancy effects. The squamous epithelium is often thicker, and the basal layer may be increased from one- up to four-cell strata. Growth of the endocervical epithelium is more pronounced, and squamous metaplasia is common. Frequently the columnar proliferation advances beyond the external os for a variable distance on the surface of the cervix. This so-called erosion is actually a *cervical ectropion* or *eversion* of the cervical canal. Its gross appearance may be indistinguishable from pathologic conditions of the cervix. Cytologic or histologic examination is necessary.

The most controversial problem concerns the interpretation of basal cell hyperactivity when this change is found in the gravid cervix. Carrow and Greene point out that all the types of epithelial abnormalities found in pregnant women have been found in nonpregnant women as well, and the subsequent behavior of basal cell hyperplasia depends upon whether or not the general architecture is maintained, whether mitoses are found in the lower layer only or in both lower and upper layers, and the type of nuclear changes. These authors and others present convincing evidence indicating that the diagnosis of any type of epithelial abnormality must be made on the basis of changes in the cellular characteristics, particularly those of the nuclei, irrespective of pregnancy.

Fallopian tubes and round ligaments. The *round ligaments* are hypertrophied and elongated. Since their relationship to the uterine fundus is retained, their position in late pregnancy is almost vertical. The round ligaments help to stabilize the uterus and tend to keep the heavy organ closer to the abdominal wall.

The *fallopian tubes* are also elongated and ultimately lie almost in line with the long axis of the uterus, but unlike the round ligaments their muscular coats are not hypertrophied.

Ovaries. Because of the increased vascularity, both ovaries become somewhat enlarged and elongated. The enlargement is more pronounced in the ovary containing the corpus luteum, which reaches its maximum development during the third month. Israel and associates studied the ovary at term in patients delivered by elective cesarean section. The patchy, reddened areas and elevated ridges seen so commonly on the surface of the ovary at cesarean section proved upon microscopic examination to be decidua-like reaction of the stroma and hyperplasia of the surface epithelium, respectively. These reactions are probably related to some hormone of chorionic origin, either chorionic gonadotropin or progesterone from the same source. Ovulation is suspended during pregnancy because of pituitary inhibition. The infundibulopelvic ligament is greatly enlarged during pregnancy, largely because of the great distention of the ovarian veins. Hodgkinson found that the capacity of the veins increases over sixty times. Such a vast change in diameter is possible because the ovarian veins are not confined within fascial sheaths as are the veins in the extremities. Compensatory hypertrophy of the smooth muscle of the vein media provides protection against spontaneous rupture.

Vagina. The vagina becomes deeply congested and cyanotic (Chadwick's sign) because of the greatly increased vascularity. In preparation for the great distention that the vagina must undergo during delivery, the mucosa thickens, the connective tissue becomes less dense, and the muscular coat hypertrophies to such an extent that the vault is considerably lengthened and the lower portion may protrude through the introitus, giving the appearance of a cystocele even in the primigravida. Secretions present in the vaginal vault during pregnancy have a highly acid pH (3.5 to 5.5) because of the increased glycogen content of the vaginal epithelium.

■ General maternal changes

Abdominal walls. Tension and stretching of the anterior abdominal wall and the tissues over the outer aspect of the thighs frequently cause certain changes in the col-lagen and elastic fibers of the deep layer of the skin, producing reddish, irregular lines, the *striae gravidarum*. Poidevin did microscopic studies of striae and found that collagen and elastic fibers lost their crisscross appearance and became thinned and straightened out longitudinally but not disrupted. He suggested that the effect is exerted upon the ground substance matrix, causing this substance to lose its adhesive quality and, further, suggested a relationship between adrenal cortical hyperactivity and the development of striae because of this and other similarities between Cushing's syndrome and normal pregnancy.

After delivery the discoloration gradually fades out, but the scarred lines do not disappear. In the latter part of pregnancy the rectus abdominis muscles are under considerable strain, and their tone is reduced. Wide separation of the muscles (*diastasis recti*) develops when the linea alba gives way to the stress and permits abdominal contents to protrude in the midline.

Breasts. The breasts become enlarged and sensitive by the eighth week of pregnancy. The primary areola deepens in color, and a more lightly pigmented secondary areola develops at the periphery. Sebaceous glands located in the primary areola undergo hypertrophy, forming the so-called *Montgomery's tubercles*. Colostrum may be expressed from the nipples after about the tenth week, but lactation is inhibited by the high estrogen-progesterone levels. Growth of the mammary apparatus is a direct response to hormone stimulation. Estrogen stimulates proliferation of the ducts; progesterone causes proliferation of lobule-alveolar tissue. Development is functionally complete by midpregnancy. As the breasts enlarge, the vascular supply is increased, engorged veins are frequently visible beneath the surface of the skin, and striae may appear over the outer aspects. After delivery, anterior pituitary *prolactin* stimulates synthesis and secretion of milk. Continued production and ejection of milk are under the control of the hypothalamus. The sucking reflex mediated through the hypothalamus results in the secretion of an oxytocin-like substance from the posterior pituitary, which in turn stimulates milk ejection.

Skin. Pigmentation of the skin in areas other than the breasts is a common finding.

The *linea nigra,* a brownish black streak down the midline of the abdomen, is especially prominent in brunettes. Occasionally pigmentation occurs in a characteristic distribution over the face, forming the "mask of pregnancy," or *chloasma,* which may persist for many months after delivery. The external genitals are similarly affected. Palmar erythema and spider nevi or telangiectases sometimes appear over the face and upper trunk and are believed to result from the increased concentration of estrogen.

■ Changes in the circulatory system

Vast alterations in hemodynamics occur as a result of (1) the increased metabolic demands of new tissue growth, (2) the expansion of vascular channels, particularly those of the generative tract, and (3) the increase in steroid hormones, which exert a positive effect upon sodium and water balance.

Blood. The *total blood volume* increases approximately 30%. The range is wide, and increases up to 50% are reported. Although the *red cell volume* and the *total hemoglobin* increase during pregnancy, the expansion of plasma volume is greater than that of the red cell mass. Caton and colleagues, using red cells tagged with radioactive iron, found an average increase in red cell mass of 495 ml. at term and calcu-

lated the concomitant whole blood rise at 1,800 ml. The disparity between the increase in fluid and cellular elements is reflected in the peripheral blood count as an apparent or dilution anemia, since both hemoglobin and hematocrit determinations are usually decreased in the third trimester as compared with the first. Cohen and Thompson showed that the average reduction in hematocrit was 15%, whereas the decrease in viscosity was 12% as a result of this dilution. True anemia is present if the hemoglobin is less than 12 grams, the red cell count less than 3.75 million and the hematocrit less than 35%.

The *plasma volume* begins to increase during the first trimester, reaching a peak approximately 40% above normal at 32 to 34 weeks. From this time until term there is a gradual reduction amounting to about 25% of the increase. During and immediately after the third stage of labor there is a sharp temporary rise in plasma volume, followed by a rapid drop toward the normal nonpregnant range, although the original level is not actually reached until 3 or 4 weeks post partum. On the contrary, the red cell mass continues to rise until the end of pregnancy, and, according to Lund, does not decline to its original level until the eighth postpartum week. Not all investigators agree that the decrease in plasma volume from the ninth to the tenth lunar

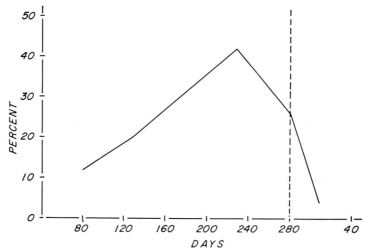

Fig. 16-9. Trend of plasma volume changes during normal pregnancy. (Based on data from Caton, W. L., Roby, C. C., Reid, D. E., and Gibson, J. G., II: Amer. J. Obstet. Gynec. **57:**471, 1949.)

month of pregnancy is of the magnitude described by Caton and his group. McLennan determined plasma volume by chromatographic extraction and spectrophotometric determination of Evans blue dye. In his series the total increase of plasma volume during the entire pregnancy was 40%. A diminution in plasma volume occurred in 17 of 23 pregnant women from the thirty-sixth week to term. Although the range varied widely from 790 ml. for the greatest drop to 20 ml. for the smallest drop, decreases greater than 200 ml. were unusual, and the mean value at term was not significantly below that at the thirty-sixth week. Lund and Donovan also found no evidence of a distinct peak in plasma volume during the last trimester nor any significant fall in the last 3 or 4 weeks of pregnancy. Furthermore, their studies show that almost all the increase in plasma volume occurs between the sixth and the twenty-fourth week of gestation. These findings parallel the curve of increases in cardiac output demonstrated by Kerr. Thus, maximal risk for the patient with heart disease is reached earlier in pregnancy than previously thought and persists throughout gestation.

Interstitial fluid volume expansion is less pronounced than the plasma volume rise during the first and second trimesters. The rate is accelerated in the latter part of pregnancy and continues until term, when the maximum increase of 40% or an average of 4,600 ml. (Caton) is reached. Return to original levels occurs gradually during a 6- to 8-week period after delivery.

The *bone marrow* is hyperplastic throughout pregnancy and remains so for about 2 months post partum. Gemzell and co-workers suggest that the increased hematopoiesis may be related to the rise in adrenal steroids, which occurs in the first half of pregnancy. Blood formation can be stimulated in mammals by administration of these substances. The white cells are increased as well as the erythrocytes. A *leukocytosis* in the range of 10,000 to 12,000 is normal in gravid women. Lowenstein and Bramlage studied the peripheral blood (Fig. 16-11) and performed bone marrow aspirations in 200 normal pregnant women throughout the three trimesters of pregnancy and the puerperium and in 30 non-pregnant women of childbearing age. In the pregnant group all cellular components were shown to increase progressively, becoming maximal in the third trimester. A curious finding was that normoblastic erythropoiesis with relative increase in nucleated red cells and granulopoiesis diminished during the first week post partum but did not return to nonpregnant normal values; activity increased again at the sixth postpartum week. These authors suggest

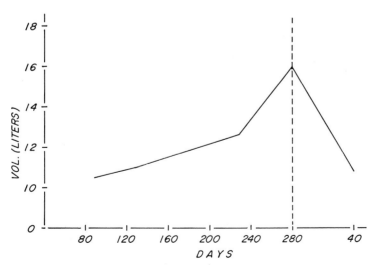

Fig 16-10. Trend of extravascular fluid volume changes during normal pregnancy. (Based on data from Caton, W. L., Roby, C. C., Reid, D. E., and Gibson, J. G., II: Amer. J. Obstet. Gynec. **57**:471, 1949.)

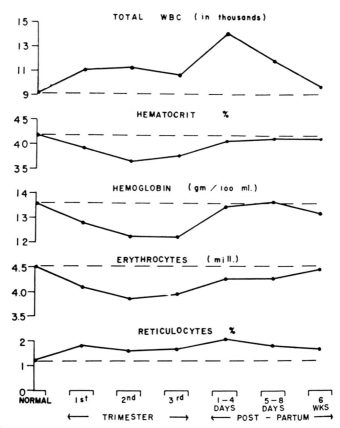

Fig 16-11. The peripheral blood of pregnant and nonpregnant women. (From Lowenstein, L., and Bramlage, C. A.: Blood **12**:261, 1957.)

that this late activity may be stimulated in response to postpartum decrease in total circulating hemoglobin and red cell mass.

Serum protein concentrations are approximately 1 to 1.5 grams per 100 ml. lower in pregnant than in nonpregnant women. It is not unusual to obtain values of 5.5 to 6 grams per 100 ml. The colloid osmotic pressure of the plasma is thereby reduced by about 20%. This is in part but not entirely a result of dilution. Miller and co-workers demonstrated a significant drop in the albumin fraction that is incompletely compensated by the rise in alpha and beta globulin. The albumin-globulin ratio is reduced from 1.5 to 0.8. Serial studies of plasma proteins determined by electrophoretic fractionation during the course of pregnancy and in the puerperium have been reported by Coryell and associates and by Mack. Their findings in normal mothers reveal a decrease in total plasma protein concentration amounting to 13% by the third

trimester. The albumin and gamma globulin concentration decreased progressively, but at the same time the alpha$_1$, alpha$_2$, beta fraction, and fibrinogen increased. The lipoproteins also increased. Of particular interest is the fact that these investigators found no significant increase in the concentration of total protein in the last weeks of pregnancy, which would be expected if there were a large decrease in plasma volume during this time. These studies support McLennan's contention that the diminution in plasma volume in late pregnancy is frequently an insignificant amount. *Fibrinogen* concentration increases progressively to term. Chemical values show an increase from 300 mg./100 ml. to over 400 mg./100 ml. Electrophoresis values are approximately 100 mg./100 ml. higher. *Urea* and *creatinine* are found in lower concentrations in the plasma during pregnancy because of the normal increase in renal filtration fraction.

Serum enzymes. During the prenatal pe-

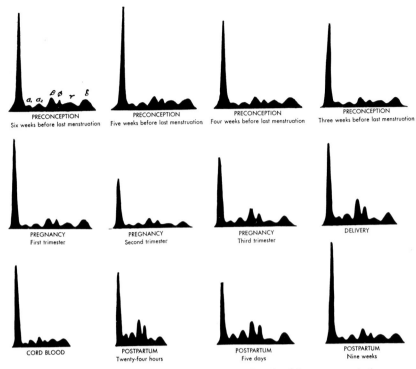

Fig. 16-12. Electrophoretic patterns of the plasma of a healthy woman before conception, during pregnancy, and during the puerperium and of the cord blood of her normal full-term infant at delivery. (From Mack, H. C.: Clin. Obstet. Gynec. 3:336, 1960.)

riod a profound change in the maternal serum enzymes is found in the increase in serum alkaline phosphatase (SAP). Individual variation is considerable, but Meade and Rosalki reported concentrations of SAP gradually increasing from approximately 2.2 Bodansky units in early pregnancy to a high of 20 Bodansky units or more at term. Serum glutamic oxaloacetic transaminase (SGOT) and serum glutamic pyruvic transaminase (SGPT) concentrations showed significantly increased activity only during labor.

Diamine oxidase (DAO) concentrations rise in an almost linear fashion from nonpregnancy values of 3 to 4 units beginning about the fifth week of gestation to the twentieth week when values exceed 500 units in normal pregnancy. Concentrations then fluctuate but tend to continue to increase more slowly to term. Weingold and Southern have employed serial determinations of DAO concentrations in maternal plasma extensively as an aid in diagnosis of pregnancy or prognosis in cases of threatened abortion during the first half of preg-

nancy and as an index of fetoplacental function in the latter half. DAO is an adaptive enzyme produced chiefly by maternal decidua, where its action in degradation of histamine produced by the fetus apparently provides necessary protection against transfer of histamine to the mother.

Serum cystine aminopeptidase (oxytocinase) is the primary oxytocin inactivating enzyme of pregnancy plasma. Babuna and Yenen demonstrated a sharp progressive rise in oxytocinase beginning at about 6 weeks' gestation to term in normal pregnancies. The enzyme appears to be mainly of placental origin, but it is of limited clinical value in assessing placental function and, more particularly, fetal welfare.

Heart. Serial orthodiagraphic tracings obtained at various stages of gestation reveal an actual alteration in position and apparent increase in size of the cardiac silhouette. The heart is rotated slightly anteriorly and displaced upward and to the left. Thus the area of dullness is increased, and the apical impulse may be located 1 to 1.5 cm. beyond the point of maximal impulse normally found in nonpregnant women. The factors responsible for these alterations are controversial, although recognized changes in the chest wall doubtless play an important role. The rib cage is flared out so that its circumference is increased at the base. The diaphragm is pushed up along with the rib cage, but it may or may not appear disproportionately elevated. The fact that the heart appears enlarged upon roentgen examination long before the uterus is large enough to push the abdominal contents upward raises the question as to whether or not the cardiac muscle undergoes some hypertrophy during pregnancy. If it does so, it is likely that the hypertrophy is in proportion to the increase in total body weight. It is quite possible that the increased blood volume is accompanied by slight cardiac dilatation.

In addition to the altered x-ray appearance of the heart, functional changes simulating organic heart disease in nonpregnant patients must be recognized and carefully evaluated. A soft systolic *murmur* at the base or over the precordium is demonstrable in over 50% of patients. *Extrasystoles* are common, and the *pulse rate* is slightly increased. There is a distinct change in heart rate immediately after delivery, when bradycardia is the rule. These findings and the frequent occurrence of dyspnea make the diagnosis of cardiac disease during pregnancy more difficult. Sodeman found a combination of signs and symptoms sufficient to suggest heart disease in 9.6 of 73 healthy gravid women.

Blood pressure. *Arterial blood pressure* does not increase in normal pregnancy. The level remains unchanged or may decrease during the second trimester and return to the normal range during the third trimester. Burwell found the maximal *pulse pressure* during the twenty-eighth to thirty-second week, at about the time of the maximal pulse rate. *Venous pressure* measured in the anticubital region remains constant and normal. Elevated venous pressure in the upper extremity is indicative of cardiac overload. Femoral venous pressure rises 10 to 15 cm. HO_2 above normal as a result of increasing pressure by the enlarging uterus upon the pelvic veins, a factor that contributes to the development of ankle edema and varicose veins.

Late in pregnancy, patients will sometimes complain of faintness in attempting to lie flat on their back, especially if the uterus is greatly enlarged. The syncope is attributed to the *vena cava syndrome.* When the heavy uterus falls back on the inferior vena cava, venous return to the heart is sufficiently impeded to cause a precipitous drop in blood pressure. The patient appears pale and apprehensive, but if she can change her position, which she usually does promptly, symptoms disappear almost immediately. This phenomenon is accentuated when the patient is unable to move about after anesthesia is administered. We have seen a few patients exhibit a profound drop in blood pressure after low-dosage spinal anesthesia given for cesarean section, although the level of anesthesia was no higher than the eighth or ninth thoracic segment. When pressure was exerted against the lateral abdominal wall, displacing the uterus to one side of the inferior vena cava, the blood pressure rose without any other aids. In such cases delivery should be carried out without delay. If initial hypotension is caused by this condition, there is no difficulty in maintaining blood pressure once the uterus is emptied.

Capillary permeability remains unchanged except with the increased hydrostatic pressure in the lower extremities.

Cardiac output. Increased tissue demands for oxygen may be met physiologically by (1) an increase in cardiac output of oxygenated blood or (2) an increased extraction of oxygen from blood at the capillary level. Measurements of cardiac output during pregnancy indicate that normally there is a rise, primarily in stroke volume, with the maximal increase being observed at about the twenty-eighth week, thereafter, most authors report a gradual decline until term. The heart rate follows the same general course but with a much lower increment of rise. In Adams' series the peak elevation in cardiac output occurred at 28 weeks and averaged 32% above nonpregnant levels. A steady decrease began thereafter and continued throughout the remainder of gestation until nonpregnant levels were reached by term. Immediately after delivery there was a second and sudden increase amounting to 29%. According to most authors it is during these periods, at about the twenty-eighth week and again immediately after delivery, that the patient with a diseased heart experiences the greatest cardiac strain. Kerr contends that most of the increase in cardiac output is established by the end of the first trimester and that this high level is maintained until term. Pressure measurements in the inferior vena cava by retrograde catheterization of the femoral vein indicate that compression or occlusion is consistently demonstrable in late pregnancy in the supine position. Measurements of cardiac output taken in this position showed diminution amounting to 10% to 25% of the peak output in the last stages of pregnancy. Serial studies of cardiac output performed in the lateral recumbent position show no significant reduction of output, and therefore ventricular work, in late pregnancy.

Since the overall increase in *oxygen consumption* is between 10 and 20% during pregnancy, it is evident that the heightened cardiac output exceeds this demand until the last trimester. Bader and associates found that the arteriovenous oxygen difference was reduced to 3.4 vol.% during the fourteenth to thirtieth weeks. This adjustment would appear to favor the margin of safety for fetal oxygenation. However, in the last trimester, when the cardiac output decreases, a larger percentage of oxygen must be removed at the uterine level, and the arteriovenous oxygen difference increases to values similar to or exceeding values found in nonpregnant women (4.4 vol.%).

The reason for the decrease in cardiac output in late pregnancy, if this change is actual and not related to the supine position, is not fully understood. The theory that the placenta acts as an arteriovenous shunt was proposed by Burwell in 1938 and has gained many followers. Pregnancy effects simulating an arteriovenous shunt are increased cardiac output, increased blood volume and accelerated pulse rate, slight decrease in arterial blood pressure, and increased venous pressure in the lower extremities. Those who concur with Burwell's concept point out that reduced cardiac output near term may be the result of partial closure of the shunt mechanism as part of the aging process of the placenta. The arguments against this hypothesis include the absence of true cardiac dilatation and the failure to discover fistulas upon microscopic examination. Other factors that may influence the changes in cardiac output are the alterations in plasma volume, increased metabolism, and the alterations in renal function. Of these, the sequence of change in renal plasma flow most nearly parallels those of the cardiac output with respect to the timing of maximal increases and the degree of fall that approximates normal nonpregnant levels in late pregnancy.

■ Changes in the respiratory system

Functional changes in the respiratory tract are demonstrable early in pregnancy, whereas anatomic alterations become evident later in gestation when intra-abdominal pressure is increased. The thoracic cage is pushed upward and widened out in its lower half, and the diaphragm is accordingly elevated, especially at the periphery. The central portion may appear flattened and its excursion reduced; hence breathing is more costal than abdominal. Cugell and co-workers demonstrated an increase in ventilation at rest as early as the first trimester.

The *vital capacity* remains unchanged or undergoes a slight increase. A decrease in vital capacity should always be considered significant. In gravidas with pulmonary or cardiac disease, particularly with mitral stenosis, reduced vital capacity is one of the earliest signs of impending failure.

Hyperventilation. The respiratory rate is slightly increased, and there is a rise in tidal volume. These changes may increase the margin of safety for the fetus. Hyperventilation lowers the carbon dioxide content of alveolar air, and in turn reduced carbon dioxide tension favors diffusion of carbon dioxide from fetal to maternal circulation.

■ Changes in the urinary system

Pregnancy exerts a profound influence upon the entire urinary tract. The outstanding effect is a dilatation of the *ureter* and *renal pelvis*. Crabtree demonstrated that the capacity of a dilated kidney pelvis and ureter increases from an original 10 or 15 ml. to 60 ml.

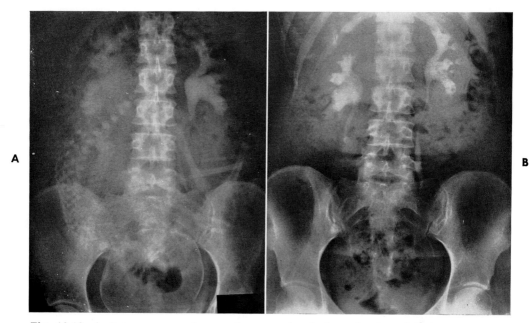

Fig. 16-13. A, Intravenous pyelogram demonstrating hydronephrosis and hydroureter at 34 weeks' gestation. **B,** Comparison at 6 weeks post partum.

Changes appear early and are progressive until the last month or two of pregnancy. The ureter is elongated as well as widened, and although it becomes curved and tortuous, actual kinking is rare. The flow of urine is reduced because ureteral peristalsis and tone are diminished. All of these alterations, especially those affecting ureteral function, are basically hormonal influences caused mainly by progesterone. During late pregnancy, pressure from the enlarged uterus may be a contributory factor. Dilatation is often considerably more pronounced in the right ureter than in the left, probably because of the cushioning effect of the rectosigmoid and the dextrorotation of the uterus. The muscular wall of the lower one third of the ureter undergoes hyperplasia similar to that involving most structures within the broad ligament. Reduction of the lumen at this level may also contribute to dilatation of the ureter above.

Renal function. Changes in renal function during normal pregnancy follow a recognized pattern, although the extent of the alteration may vary from one individual to another. Sims and Krantz did serial studies of para-aminohippurate (PAH) and inulin clearances that demonstrated the following: (1) *Effective renal plasma flow* increases approximately 25% during the first and second trimester and then falls to normal nonpregnant levels in the last trimester (600 ml./min.); (2) *glomerular filtration* increases by about 50% and remains in this range until the last 2 or 3 weeks of pregnancy, when the rate declines somewhat but does not fall to normal (125 ml./min.) until early in the puerperium; and (3) the *filtration fraction* is elevated throughout pregnancy, particularly in the third trimester, when renal plasma flow decreases while glomerular filtration remains elevated. Filtration fraction at this time is approximately 40% above control levels. The late pregnancy regression of renal blood flow and glomerular filtration may be related to position. Most studies have been carried out with the patient supine. Chesley, Sloane, and Wynn found that urine flow, PAH and inulin clearances, and sodium and chloride excretion were all depressed in the supine position as compared with the lateral position. Potassium excretion did not change. The fact that the lateral position is conducive to optimal function provides good reason for recommendation of programmed rest periods in this position in patients with borderline or diminishing renal function.

The alterations in renal function are most

probably the effect of increased maternal and chorionic hormonal secretions. Those hormones capable of increasing renal function include ACTH, antidiuretic hormone (ADH), aldosterone, cortisone, growth hormone, and thyroid hormone. The part played by each of these and by the increased plasma volume of pregnancy needs further study before the final answer can be given.

The known anatomic and physiologic changes in the kidney have important clinical implications. *Glycosuria* is common because of the increase in glomerular filtration, but before its occurrence can be assigned to a physiologic change a glucose tolerance test is indicated. *Amino acids* are excreted in larger amounts during pregnancy. This is particularly true of histidine, the glomerular filtration of which is raised by more than 50%, whereas tubular reabsorption appears to be partially inhibited. Blood concentrations of *urea, uric acid,* and *creatinine* are lowered as a result of increased clearance rates, but the clearance of *sodium* is not significantly altered in normal pregnancy. Renal *iodide clearance* is increased, and the plasma inorganic iodine level is reduced, which increases the physiologic demands on the thyroid.

Allowances must be made for changes in the genitourinary system in the interpretation of renal function tests. The results of the phenolsulfonphthalein (P.S.P.) test can be very misleading because the dye may be excreted normally, but dilatation of the renal pelvis and ureter and the relative stasis of this system may delay its arrival in the bladder. The test is better avoided during pregnancy. Concentration tests, when positive, are significant. If the urine does not show concentration, it may be related to the positive nitrogen balance, sodium retention, and low sodium intake, particularly if the salt has been restricted for a time before the test is performed. It should be performed in the late puerperium before a final diagnosis of failure of concentrating power is made.

The *bladder* is pulled up into the abdomen as the uterus enlarges. In the early weeks of gestation, pressure of the uterus upon the bladder, traction at the vesicle neck, and hyperemia of the trigone cause frequency of urination. The vascularity of the bladder is greatly increased, and upon cystoscopy engorged vessels or small varicosities are sometimes visible. Trauma late in pregnancy or during delivery may cause hemorrhage from these areas.

The hormonal influences responsible for dilatation of those structures of the urinary tract above the bladder exert a similar influence on the smooth muscle of the bladder. There is a decrease in bladder tone and a progressive increase in capacity of up to 1,300 to 1,500 ml. during pregnancy and in the postpartum period. Overdistention of the bladder in the postpartum period is a troublesome, often protracted complication of labor and delivery in which this physiologic reduction in tone plays an important role. Avoidance of overfilling in the immediate postpartum period is often preventive. However, when urinary retention occurs at this time, it must be differentiated from results of local trauma, perineal muscle spasm, and mechanical obstruction. Cholinergic drugs may be helpful in reversing physiologic atony but are of little value in treatment of any other of these causes.

■ Changes in the gastrointestinal tract

An alteration in the normal alkaline pH of the saliva toward the acid side is common in pregnancy. It is this change rather than withdrawal of calcium that predisposes to tooth decay. The quantity of saliva is frequently increased, sometimes excessively so (hyperptyalism), but the cause of the increased secretion is not yet known. In an occasional instance the gums become hypertrophied and spongy and tend to bleed easily. Ziskin and Nesse believe this is a hormonal effect, although vitamin C deficiency may contribute to the disturbance.

Gastric acidity is usually reduced, particularly in the first trimester, although the degree of hypochlorhydria is variable. Certain cases of otherwise unexplained severe anemia are occasionally related to an exaggerated gastric hypochlorhydria.

Gastric motility is somewhat diminished throughout pregnancy, and ultimately during labor the emptying time of the stomach is so slow that oral feedings are contraindicated from the onset. Nausea and vomiting of early pregnancy may well be influenced by these functional alterations.

Reduced peristaltic activity and diminished tone are evident in bowel function as well as in the stomach. Constipation, so common in pregnant women, usually results from these functional changes although the condition is undoubtedly aggravated by pressure of the uterus on the rectosigmoid early in pregnancy and again after lightening occurs near term.

During the last half of pregnancy the stomach is gradually pushed upward into the left dome of the diaphragm. Hormonal effects may cause relaxation or dilatation of the hiatus and predispose to the development of *hiatal hernia*. The condition is usually reversed after delivery. The cecum also undergoes a progressive upward displacement, beginning during the third month and continuing until term when the *appendix* is located out toward the right flank above the level of the iliac crest.

Gallbladder. Gallbladder emptying time is increased during pregnancy. Serum cholinesterase activity is reduced by about 25%. Relative biliary stasis and increased cholesterol levels may contribute to the formation of biliary calculi in gravid women. The ratio of women to men with calculous disease is approximately 4:1. In a large series reported by Glenn and Mc-Sherry, three fourths of the women with gallstones had been pregnant, and biliary tract symptoms usually were related to the gestation.

Liver. Measurements of hepatic function in human pregnancy are fragmentary and incomplete. Liver biopsies show no characteristic morphologic changes in normal mothers, but they tell us little regarding function. In some of the patients studied by Dieckmann and co-workers, direct bilirubin, urinary bilirubin, cephalin flocculation, and thymol turbidity were elevated, but these were exceptions.

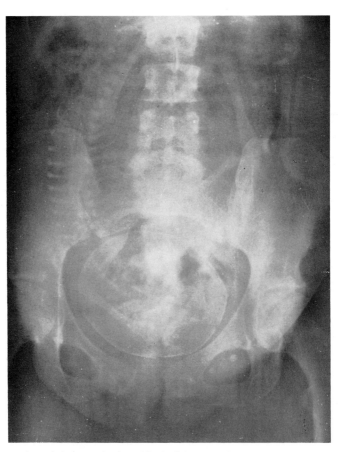

Fig. 16-14. Separation of the symphysis pubis during normal pregnancy.

■ Changes in the bones and joints

The sacroiliac synchondroses and symphysis pubis are widened and rendered movable beginning about the tenth or twelfth week of gestation. This alteration is believed to be almost entirely caused by the action of the hormone relaxin. Zarrow and associates demonstrated that blood concentrations of relaxin in pregnant women averaged 0.2 guinea pig unit per milliliter of serum at 7 to 10 weeks' gestation, with a maximum concentration of 2 guinea pig units per milliliter at 38 to 42 weeks.

Posture changes become evident as pregnancy advances. The upper spine is thrown backward to compensate for increased size of the abdomen. Disturbances arising from altered weight bearing and from relaxation of the pelvic articulations are discussed in Chapter 24.

■ Changes in the endocrine system

Thyroid. The thyroid gland is palpably enlarged in over 50% of persons during pregnancy. This is caused by a diffuse hyperplasia of glandular elements, new follicle formation, and increased vascularity. The actual change in secretory activity, however, is difficult to evaluate. An increase in basal metabolic rate is evident by the sixteenth week and rises 10% to 30% above the prepregnant rate during the third trimester. Since the basal metabolic rate measures total oxygen consumption rate, the growing fetal and maternal tissues logically increase the oxygen demand. Studies by Sandiford and Wheeler indicate that the elevation observed during pregnancy is proportional to this increased active protoplasmic mass. The increase in thyroid activity and in the size of the thyroid gland is more likely to represent compensatory changes because of the increased renal iodine clearance and resulting reduced plasma inorganic iodine level and the protein binding of thyroxin.

The increase in circulating thyroid hormone known to exist during pregnancy in euthyroid mothers thus appears paradoxical but may be related to alterations in serum proteins. Dowling and co-workers showed that thyroxin-binding protein (TBP) is increased during pregnancy and that the alpha globulin moiety of serum proteins is responsible for this increased ability to bind thyroxin. The same authors also demonstrated increases in TBP after the administration of estrogen. These findings are of particular interest since it is well recognized that during pregnancy (1) the alpha and beta globulins increase whereas the gamma globulins decline and (2) the estrogen level rises.

The best means of evaluating thyroid function during pregnancy is by determination of serum hormonal iodine. Direct and reasonably accurate measurements can be obtained by testing either for protein-bound iodine (PBI) or for butyl-extractable iodine (BEI). Heinemann and associates found a rise in the serum-precipitable iodine concentration as early as the third week after conception. Their normal pregnant values ranged between 6.2 and 11.2 μg./100 ml. As compared with normal nonpregnant values of 4 to 8 μg./100 ml. Protein-bound iodine concentrations fluctuate but do not continue to rise throughout pregnancy. They return to normal rapidly after delivery. Benson and co-workers find the BEI method more specific for thyroxin than the PBI method since chance contaminants are less likely to alter BEI values. A serum BEI concentration not lower than 6 μg. should be obtained in normal gestations. Values found in cord blood are only slightly lower but should **not** be less than 4.5 μg.

Evaluation of thyroid activity by radioactive iodine uptake is inadvisable during pregnancy since fetal thyroid follicles are differentiated by the fourth lunar month and may be damaged by I^{131}. Newer in vitro methods for measuring red cell or resin uptakes of radioactive triiodothyronine may be particularly helpful in evaluating thyroid function during pregnancy. Normal values for gravid women are 5% to 10% for red cell uptake and less than 21% for resin uptake. It should be noted that in these tests, values are lower in gravid than in nongravid women.

Parathyroid glands. The parathyroids undergo hypertrophy as the fetal demands for calcium increase. Although more parathormone is secreted at this time, many pregnant women show a relative deficiency or a predisposition to parathyroid tetany in late pregnancy. Chvostek's sign is frequently positive in the latter part of gestation.

Pituitary gland. The anterior lobe of the pituitary gland almost doubles in size during pregnancy. Increased secretory activity involves predominantly the growth hormone, although there is also evidence of increased secretion of lactogenic and luteinizing hormones with little change in the amount of follicle-stimulating hormone. Paschkis suggests that persistent headache in early pregnancy and the acromegalic-like changes in the skin and facial features may be related to enlargement of the anterior pituitary gland and increased activity of the growth hormone, respectively. In most cases these alterations return to normal after delivery.

The posterior lobe does not hypertrophy during pregnancy. The secretion of oxytocin and vasopressin-antidiuretic hormone is presumably increased. However, the measurements are made indirectly on the basis of increasing quantities of oxytocinase, which can be determined by electrophoresis.

Adrenal glands. Enlargement of the adrenal glands occurs progressively throughout the prenatal period because of *hyperplasia of the cortex.* A significant increase in corticosteroids can be detected in the first trimester, and according to Venning, a second higher peak reaching values similar to those found in patients with Cushing's disease normally occurs at about 200 days. The

peak in corticosteroid excretion corresponds with the period during which water retention is maximal. In Tobian's studies normal gravid women in the last trimester of pregnancy excreted twice the amount of corticosteroids as nongravid women; those with excessive edema excreted about 46% more corticosteroids than gravid women with no edema.

Not all the functions of the adrenal cortex are equally stimulated during pregnancy. Those corticosteroids that influence carbohydrate metabolism show the predominant and most universal rise, but at the same time binding protein (transcortin) is also increased as a result of the stimulus provided by increasing amounts of estrogen. As a consequence, significant amounts of otherwise excessive levels of corticosteroids are rendered biologically less active. An increase in aldosterone levels is noted by the fifteenth week of pregnancy. Values are in the range of 1,000 μg. per day during the last trimester. These high values are believed to be due to the high levels of progesterone produced in late pregnancy. Laidlaw and co-workers demonstrated a great increase in aldosterone secretion in nonpregnant subjects after the administration of progesterone, but it has not been clearly shown that circulating progesterone represents the major control mech-

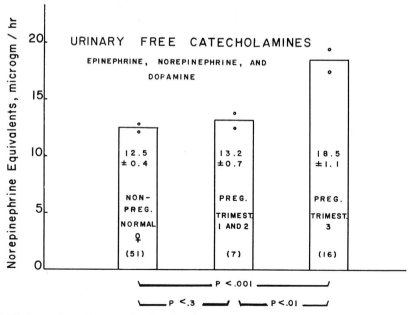

Fig. 16-15. Excretion of catecholamines in normal nongravid women of reproductive age and in normal gravid women. (Courtesy M. I. Oesterling.)

anism for aldosterone secretion in pregnancy. Lower levels of aldosterone found in association with severe toxemia of pregnancy as compared with normal pregnancy may be due to a fall in circulating progesterone of either placental or maternal adrenal origin. The 17-ketosteroids associated with androgenic activity are relatively unchanged or increase only slightly in the last trimester. *Adrenal medullary activity* is slightly increased in normal pregnancy. Oesterling and associates report mean values for urinary-free catecholamines expressed as norepinephrine equivalents in micrograms per hour as follows: 12.5 in normal nongravid women of reproductive age, 13.2 in normal gravid women during the first and second trimesters, and 18.5 in normal gravid women during the third trimester. Further increases in epinephrine secretion during the stress of labor might be expected. However, Israel and co-workers studied plasma epinephrine and norepinephrine during the third trimester, in labor, and post partum and found no significant change in either of the catecholamines. The mean plasma value of epinephrine was 0.1 μg./L. and of norepinephrine 1.5 μg./L.

■ Changes in metabolism

Protein metabolism. A positive nitrogen balance demonstrable early in gestation increases progressively through the third tri-mester when fetal requirements are greatest. Macy and Hunscher and other investigators have repeatedly shown an accumulation of nitrogen during pregnancy far beyond the needs of the conceptus. In Hunscher and associates' study the observed nitrogen accumulation during the last half of pregnancy totaled 446 grams. Net gain after delivery was 310 grams. A negative balance continues in the puerperium with blood loss, lactation, and involutional changes in the uterus and other maternal tissues. According to observations continued by Macy for 53 days post partum, a maternal nitrogen reserve still persisted at the end of the usual involutional period. Surplus protein is apparently stored in maternal viscera and other body tissues.

Another means of estimating protein alterations in pregnancy is by measuring total body water since this space and lean body mass are normally increased proportionately. Seitchik and Alper studied changes in body composition by measuring total body water (antipyrine) and extracellular water (mannitol). The expansion of both spaces paralleled one another, and the average increase was 40% for each. The gain in lean body mass of mother and fetus exceeded the maternal weight gain, and thus the authors contend that some solid (fat) must be lost or exchanged in favor of the increased active protoplasmic mass. They suggest that the

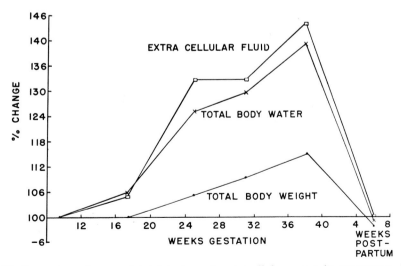

Fig. 16-16. Percentage change of total body and extracellular water in pregnancy. Average of 5 normal patients; 100% equals the average value found at initial study in early pregnancy. (From Seitchik, J., and Alper, C.: Amer. J. Obstet. Gynec. **71:**1165, 1956.)

excess nitrogen accumulation of pregnancy implies that synthesis of lean body mass must occur during pregnancy and that this is associated with the utilization of body fat stores. The process is reversed in the puerperium, when lean body tissue is lost and fat is apparently gained.

Carbohydrate metabolism. Reducing substances can be found in the urine at some time or other during pregnancy in about 30% of persons. In most instances the reducing substance is glucose. The presence of lactose in the urine is unusual except for the 2- or 3-week period preceding the onset of labor, although during the puerperium lactosuria is very common.

The renal threshold for glucose may be reduced from normal nonpregnant levels, which range between 150 to 200 mg./100 ml., to a range of 100 to 150 mg./100 ml. This is probably because of the increased glomerular filtration that normally occurs during pregnancy. Chesley states that renal tubular reabsorption of glucose may fail to increase proportionately. This phenomenon accounts for many cases of glycosuria and may contribute to the relatively low fasting level of blood sugar found in gravid women. In some instances, however, glycosuria during pregnancy will provide the first evidence of a diabetic state. Fasting blood sugar determination alone is not sufficient for diagnosis. Instead, a glucose tolerance test is essential for differentiation of physiologic and abnormal glycosuria of pregnancy.

In our opinion carbohydrate tolerance is not significantly reduced in normal pregnant women. A rise above 120 mg./100 ml. at the 2-hour period of the glucose tolerance test or a delay in return to normal beyond the 3-hour period indicates some disturbance in carbohydrate metabolism. These problems are discussed in detail in Chapter 19.

A maternal glucose sparing effect is noted in pregnancy that may be related to the demands of the fetus. Although there is an increased secretion of insulin during pregnancy, there is also an increased resistance to insulin by elevated free fatty acids and increased destruction of insulin by the placenta. The growth hormone per se is not appreciably increased, but its counterpart, chorionic growth hormone, prolactin, generally referred to as human placental lacto-

gen (HPL), is greatly increased and is probably responsible for the elevated free fatty acids and increased insulin resistance. Insulin resistance has been demonstrated by Burt and others on the basis of insulin tolerance tests and intravenous tolbutamide responses in normal women late in pregnancy. Increases in corticosteroids and thyroxin in normal gravid women may have some effect upon carbohydrate metabolism, but protein binding of these substances is sufficiently increased to suggest that the actual biologic activity of each is not much different in the pregnant than in the nonpregnant woman. Observations made by Bleicher, O'Sullivan, and Freinkel on normal gravid women late in pregnancy and repeated post partum indicate that the plasma insulin level after an overnight fast is higher ante partum than post partum and that the insulin response to an intravenous glucose load is greater in the same patients in the antepartum tests. Vallance-Owen and co-workers have shown that plasma antagonists are found in latent and overt diabetic women during pregnancy, but no such antagonists are detectable in the plasma of normal pregnant women.

Fat metabolism. Hyperlipemia is a normal prenatal finding. Most authors believe that the increase in blood lipids is related to the requirements of the fetus and to development of the mammary apparatus. The increased quantity of steroid hormones of pregnancy may be a factor. Estrogen is known to increase the production of the alpha globulins, including lipoproteins, and the glucocorticoids are known to increase serum cholesterol. The lipoproteins are significantly increased during pregnancy, particularly the beta lipoproteins. Neutral fats are approximately doubled. Gardner and Gainsborough found a progressive increase in free cholesterol until the thirtieth week of pregnancy. Ketonuria occurs more readily in pregnant than in nonpregnant women when carbohydrates are reduced or when dietary fat is increased.

The normal values for maternal and cord plasma glucose and nonesterified fatty acids (NEFA) have been established by Whaley, Zuspan, and Nelson in a group of rigidly controlled normal pregnancies. Maternal values average 92.9 mg./100 ml. for glucose and 881.8 mEq./L. for NEFA; umbilical cord values averaged 61.9 mg./100 ml. and

536.0 mEq./L., respectively. The differences in maternal to newborn ratios of glucose (1.3:1) and NEFA (1.7:1) suggest independent homeostasis in this biologic system. Because various metabolic diseases are known to influence blood glucose and NEFA levels, alterations in the ratio of these substances may provide a useful tool in investigation of these disorders.

Mineral metabolism. Demands for inorganic substances necessary for growth are increased sharply at about the fourth lunar month when the fetus begins to increase rapidly in weight. Materials used for blood and skeletal formation continue to increase progressively to term.

Calcium and phosphorus. Requirements for calcium and phosphorus are approximately doubled during pregnancy. These demands are satisfied by the daily intake of 1.5 grams of calcium and 2 grams of phosphorus. Total storage during the course of pregnancy is approximately 50 grams and 35 to 40 grams, respectively. Only about one half of these amounts are utilized by the fetus; the remainder is stored in maternal tissues. Ordinarily, serum calcium levels are unaltered. Since most of the fetal calcium deposition takes place in the latter part of pregnancy, relative deprivation or a deficiency in parathyroid function will cause a decrease in concentration of ionized calcium.

During pregnancy, calcium is more rapidly exchanged between the maternal circulation and bone. The bone therefore can be considered part of the metabolic calcium pool and can be drawn upon when calcium supplies are low. Osteomalacia, a condition in which softening and distortion of the long bones occurs due to excessive mobilization of calcium, is almost never seen in the United States. Dentin does not contribute to the metabolic pool and thus dental caries associated with pregnancy are not due to the removal of calcium from the teeth but to local changes in pH and oral bacteria flora.

Folic acid. Folates play an essential role in the metabolism of several amino acids and in the synthesis of nucleic acids. During pregnancy, rapid tissue growth of trophoblastic, maternal, and fetal origins creates an increased demand for folic acid. The undisputed example of maternal folic acid deficiency is seen in the development of megaloblastic anemia due specifically to inade-quacy of folate and not to vitamin B_{12} deficiency. Association of less severe depletion of folic acid with other obstetric complications has been suggested. These include spontaneous abortion, placental abruption, premature deliveries, toxemia of pregnancy, and fetal abnormalities.

The daily requirement of folic acid during pregnancy is about 300 to 500 μg. per day. Green vegetables, some fruits, liver, and kidney are the principal sources.

Iron. The demand for iron is increased, especially in the last trimester of pregnancy, because fetal absorption is far greater at that time. In addition, the hemoglobin mass continues to increase until term, and a small amount is necessary for other maternal tissues such as the uterus. Total body iron in the normal female ranges from 3.5 to 4 grams. Holly estimates a net loss of iron to the mother of approximately 400 mg. throughout pregnancy and delivery, or about one eighth of her total supply. Many women in apparently good nutritional state have less than the normal 1-gram amount of storage or available iron, and therefore iron supplements are necessary in most to avoid a nonanemic iron deficiency state or an obvious iron deficiency anemia.

Acid-base balance. Maternal plasma bicarbonate and total base are normally reduced during pregnancy. According to Kydd the values for total base averaged 146 mEq./L. in normal gravid women as compared with 154 mEq./L. in nonpregnant controls. At term the average carbon dioxide combining power value is about 45 vol.% as compared with the nonpregnant average of approximately 60 vol. % or plasma bicarbonate values of 22 to 25 mM./L., respectively. Since the blood pH /is unchanged, the alkali deficit is well compensated. The specific cause for this alteration remains unknown. It is probable that the normally increased ventilation effects the change, but whether the hyperventilation of pregnancy is of sufficient magnitude to reduce the carbon dioxide and induce the compensatory increase in renal excretion of sodium is as yet uncertain.

References
Aboul-Khair, S.: Iodine metabolism in pregnancy. In Hytten, F. E., and Leitch, I., editors: The physiology of human pregnancy, Philadelphia, 1963, F. A. Davis Co.

Adams, J. Q.: Cardiovascular physiology in normal pregnancy; studies with dye dilution technique, Amer. J. Obstet. Gynec. 67:741, 1954.

Assali, N. S., Douglass, R. A., Baird, W. W., Nicholson, D. B., and Suyemoto, R.: Measurement of uterine blood flow and uterine metabolism, Amer. J. Obstet. Gynec. 66:2‘8, 1953.

Babuna, C., and Yenen, E.: Enzymatic determination of placental function, Amer. J. Obstet. Gynec. 95:925, 1966.

Bader, R. A., Bader, M. E., Rose, D. F., and Braunwald, E.: Hemodynamics at rest and during exercise in normal pregnancy as studied by cardiac catheterization, J. Clin. Invest. 34:1524, 1955.

Bean, W. B.: Note on development of cutaneous arterial "spiders" and palmar erythema in persons with liver disease and their development following administration of estrogens, Amer. J. Med. Sci. 204:251, 1942.

Benson, R. C., Pickering, D. E., Kontaxis, N. E., and Fisher, D. A.: Thyroid function in pregnancy, Obstet. Gynec. 14:11, 1959.

Bleicher, S. J., O'Sullivan, J. B., and Freinkel, N.: Carbohydrate metabolism in pregnancy. V. The interrelationships of glucose, insulin and free fatty acids in late pregnancy and post partum, New Eng. J. Med. 271:866, 1964.

Burt, R. L.: Peripheral utilization of glucose in pregnancy. III. Insulin tolerance, Obstet. Gynec. 7:658, 1956.

Burt, R. L.: Reactivity of tolbutamide in normal pregnancy, Obstet. Gynec. 12:447, 1958.

Burwell, C. S.: Circulatory adjustments to pregnancy, Bull. Hopkins Hosp. 95:115, 1954.

Caldeyro-Barcia, R., and Poseiro, J. J.: Oxytocin and contractility of the pregnant human uterus, Ann. N. Y. Acad. Sci. 75:813, 1959.

Carrow, L. A., and Greene, R. R.: The epithelia of the pregnant cervix, Amer. J. Obstet. Gynec. 61:237, 1951.

Caton, W. L., Roby, C. C., Reid, D. E., Caswell, C. J., Maletskos, C. J., Fluharty, R. G., and Gibson, J. G., II: The circulating red cell volume and body hematocrit in normal pregnancy and the puerperium, Amer. J. Obstet. Gynec. 61:1207, 1951.

Caton, W. L., Roby, C. C., Reid, D. E., and Gibson, J. G., II: Plasma volume and extravascular fluid volume during pregnancy and the puerperium, Amer. J. Obstet. Gynec. 57:471, 1949.

Chesley, L. C.: Renal functional changes in normal pregnancy, Clin. Obstet. Gynec. 3:349, 1960.

Chesley, L. C., Sloan, D. M., and Wynn, R. M.: Effects of posture and angiotensin 2 upon renal function in pregnant women, Amer. J. Obstet. Gynec. 90:281, 1964.

Cibils, L. A., and Hendricks, C. H.: Normal labor in vertex presentation, Amer. J. Obstet. Gynec. 91:385, 1965.

Coryell, M. N., Beach, E. F., Robinson, A. R., Macy, I. G., and Mack, H. C.: Metabolism of women during the reproductive cycle. XVII. Changes in electrophoretic patterns of plasma proteins throughout the cycle and following delivery, J. Clin. Invest. 29:1559, 1950.

Crabtree, E. G.: Changes in the urinary tract in women; the result of normal pregnancy, New Eng. J. Med. 205:162, 1953.

Cugell, D. W., Frank, N. R., Gaensler, E. A., and Badger, T. L.: Pulmonary function in pregnancy. I. Serial observations in normal women, Amer. Rev. Tuberc. 67:568, 1953.

Danforth, D. N.: The fibrous nature of the human cervix and its relation to the isthmic segment in gravid and non-gravid uteri, Amer. J. Obstet. Gynec. 53:541, 1947.

Danforth, D. N., and Ivy, A. C.: The lower uterine segment; its derivation and physiologic behavior, Amer. J. Obstet. Gynec. 57:831, 1949.

de Alvarez, R. R., Gaiser, D. F., Simkins, D. M., Smith, E. K., and Bratvold, G. E.: Serial studies of serum lipids in normal human pregnancy, Amer. J. Obstet. Gynec. 77:743, 1959.

Dieckmann, W. J., Smitter, R. C., and Pottinger, S. M.: Liver function studies in normal and toxemic pregnancy, Surg. Gynec. Obstet. 92:598, 1951.

Dignam, W. J., Titus, P., and Assali, H. S.: Renal function in human pregnancy. I. Changes in glomerular filtration rate and renal plasma flow, Proc. Soc. Exp. Biol. Med. 97:512, 1958.

Dowling, J. T., Freinkel, N., and Ingbar, S. H.: Thyroxine-binding by sera of pregnant women, newborn infants and women with spontaneous abortion, J. Clin. Invest. 35:1263, 1956.

Engbring, N. H., and Engstrom, W. W.: Effects of estrogen and testosterone on circulating thyroid hormone, J. Clin. Endocr. 19:783, 1959.

Gemzell, C. A., Robbe, H., and Sjöstrand, T.: Blood volume and total amount of hemoglobin in normal pregnancy and the puerperium, Acta Obstet. Gynec. Scand. 33:289, 1954.

Gillespie, E. C.: Principles of uterine growth in pregnancy, Amer. J. Obstet. Gynec. 59:949, 1950.

Glenn, F., and McSherry, C. K.: Gallstones and pregnancy among 300 young women treated by cholecystectomy, Surg. Gynec. Obstet. 127:1067, 1968.

Gray, M. J., and Plentl, A. A.: Variations of sodium space and total exchangeable sodium, J. Clin. Invest. 33:3‘7, 1954.

Grumbach, M. M., Kaplan, S. L., Sciarra, J. J., and Burr, I. M.: Chorionic growth hormone-prolactin (CGP); secretion, disposition, biologic activity in man, and postulated function as the "growth hormone" of the second half of pregnancy. In Sonenberg, M., editor: Conference on growth hormone, Ann. N. Y. Acad. Sci. 148:501, 1968.

Gylling, T.: Renal hemodynamics and heart volume in normal pregnancy, Acta Obstet. Gynec. Scand. (supp. 5) 40:1, 1961.

Hamilton, H. F. H.: Cardiac output in normal pregnancy as determined by Cournand right heart catheterization technique, J. Obstet. Gynaec. Brit. Comm. 56:548, 1949.

Hamolsky, M. W., Stein, M., and Freedberg, A. S.: The thyroid hormone–plasma protein complex in man. II. New in vitro method for study of "uptake" of labelled hormonal components by human erythrocytes, J. Clin. Endocr. **17:**33, 1957.

Hayashi, T.: Uric acid and endogenous creatinine clearance studies in normal pregnancy and toxemias of pregnancy, Amer. J. Obstet. Gynec. **71:**859, 1956.

Heinemann, M., Johnson, C. E., and Man, E. B.: Serum precipitable iodine concentration during pregnancy, J. Clin. Invest. **27:**91, 1948.

Hendricks, C. H., Quilligan, E. J., Tyler, C. W., and Tucker, G. J.: Pressure relationships between the intervillous space and the amniotic fluid in human term pregnancy, Amer. J. Obstet. Gynec. **77:**1028, 1959.

Hibbard, B. M., and Hibbard, E. D.: Folate metabolism and reproduction, Brit. Med. Bull. **24:**10, 1968.

Hodgkinson, C. P.: Physiology of the ovarian veins during pregnancy, Obstet. Gynec. **1:**26, 1953.

Holly, R. G.: Dynamics of iron metabolism in pregnancy, Amer. J. Obstet. Gynec. **93:**370, 1965.

Israel, S. L., Rubenstone, A., and Meranze, D. R.: The ovary at term. I. Decidua-like reaction and surface cell proliferation, Obstet. Gynec. **3:**399, 1954.

Israel, S. L., Stroup, P. E., Seligson, H. T., and Seligson, D.: Epinephrine and norepinephrine in pregnancy and labor, Obstet. Gynec. **14:**68, 1959.

Kerr, M. G.: Cardiovascular dynamics in pregnancy and labour, Brit. Med. Bull. **24:**19, 1968.

Kydd, D. M.: Hydrogen ion concentration and acid-base equilibrium in normal pregnancy, J. Biol. Chem. **91:**63, 1931.

Laidlaw, J. C., Ruse, J. L., and Gornall, A. G.: The influence of estrogen and progesterone on aldosterone excretion, J. Clin. Endocr. **22:**161, 1962.

Langman, J., van Drunen, H., and Bouman, F.: Maternal protein metabolism and embryonic development in human beings, Amer. J. Obstet. Gynec. **77:**546, 1959.

Lewis, B. V.: Uterine blood flow, a review, Obstet. Gynec. Survey **24:**1211, 1969.

Lowenstein, L., and Bramlage, C. A.: The bone marrow in pregnancy and the puerperium, Blood **12:**261, 1957.

Lund, C. J.: Studies on the iron deficiency anemia of pregnancy, including plasma volume, total hemoglobin, erythrocyte protoporphyrin in treated and untreated normal and anemic patients, Amer. J. Obstet. Gynec. **62:**947, 1951.

Lund, C. J., and Donovan, J. C.: Blood volume during pregnancy; significance of plasma and red cell volumes, Amer. J. Obstet. Gynec. **98:**393, 1967.

Mack, H. C.: The plasma proteins, Clin. Obstet. Gynec. **3:**336, 1960.

Macy, I. G., and Hunscher, H. A.: Evaluation of maternal nitrogen and mineral needs during embryonic and fetal development, Amer. J. Obstet. Gynec. **27:**878, 1934.

McCall, M. L.: Cerebral blood flow and metabolism in toxemias of pregnancy, Surg. Gynec. Obstet. **89:**715, 1949.

McCartney, C. P., Pottinger, R. E., and Harrod, J. P., Jr.: Alterations in body composition during pregnancy, Amer. J. Obstet. Gynec. **77:**1038, 1959.

McLennan, C. E.: Antecubital and femoral venous pressure in normal and toxemic pregnancy, Amer. J. Obstet. Gynec. **45:**568, 1943.

McLennan, C. E., and Corey, D. L.: Plasma volume late in pregnancy, Amer. J. Obstet. Gynec. **59:**662, 1950.

Mattingly, R. F.: The physiology of the urinary tract in pregnancy. In Marcus, S. L., and Marcus, C. C., editors: Advances in obstetrics and gynecology, Baltimore, 1967, The Williams & Wilkins Co.

Meade, B. W., and Rosalki, S. B.: Serum enzyme activity in normal pregnancy and the newborn, J. Obstet. Gynaec. Brit. Comm. **70:**693, 1963.

Metcalfe, J., Romney, S. L., Ramsey, L. H., Reid, D. E., and Burwell, C. S.: Estimation of blood flow in normal human pregnancy at term, J. Clin. Invest. **34:**1632, 1955.

Miller, G. H., Jr., Davis, M. E., King, A. G., and Huggins, C. B.: Serum proteins in pregnancy, J. Lab. Clin. Med. **37:**538, 1951.

Mitchell, M. L., Harden, A. B., and O'Rourke, M. E.: In vitro resin sponge uptake of triiodothyronine I[131] from serum in thyroid disease and in pregnancy, J. Clin. Endocr. **20:**1474, 1960.

Oesterling, M. J., Tse, R. L., and Holmes, H. M.: Spectrophotometric determination of catecholamine excretion in the free and conjugated forms, Fed. Proc. **21:**192, 1962.

Page, E. W., Titus, M. A., Mohun, G., and Glendening, M. B.: The origin and distribution of oxytocinase, Amer. J. Obstet. Gynec. **82:**1090, 1961.

Paschkis, K. E.: Acromegaly and pregnancy, J. Clin. Endocr. **14:**32, 1954.

Poidevin, L. O. S.: Histopathology of striae gravidarum, J. Obstet. Gynaec. Brit. Comm. **66:**654, 1959.

Prowse, C. M., and Gaensler, E. A.: Respiratory and acid-base changes during pregnancy, Anesthesiology **26:**381, 1965.

Robbins, J., and Nelson, J.: Thyroxine binding by serum protein in pregnancy and in the newborn, J. Clin. Invest. **37:**153, 1958.

Romney, S. L., Merrill, J. P., and Reid, D. E.: Alterations in potassium metabolism, Amer. J. Obstet. Gynec. **68:**119, 1954.

Rose, D. J., Bader, M. E., Bader, R. A., and Brunwald, E.: Catheterization studies of cardiac hemodynamics in normal pregnant women with reference to left ventricular work, Amer. J. Obstet. Gynec. **72:**233, 1956.

Sandberg, A. A., and Slaunwhite, W. R., Jr.: Transcortin; a corticosteroid binding protein of plasma. II. Levels in various conditions and the effects of estrogens, J. Clin. Invest. **38:**1290, 1959.

Seitchik, J., and Alper, C.: The body compartments of normal pregnant, edematous pregnant, and pre-eclamptic women, Amer. J. Obstet. Gynec. 68:1540, 1954.

Seitchik, J., and Alper, C.: The estimation of changes in body composition in normal pregnancy by measurement of body water, Amer. J. Obstet. Gynec. 71:1165, 1956.

Sims, E. A. H., and Krantz, K. E.: Serial studies of renal function during pregnancy and the puerperium in normal women, J. Clin. Invest. 37:1764, 1958.

Sodeman, W. A.: Cardiac changes in pregnancy unrelated to the usual etiological types of heart disease, Amer. Heart J. 19:385, 1940.

Sterling, K., and Tabachnick, M.: Resin uptake of I[131] triiodothyronine as a test of thyroid function, J. Clin. Endocr. 21:456, 1961.

Stone, M. L.: Effects of the fetus on folic acid deficiency in pregnancy, Clin. Obstet. Gynec. 11:1143, 1968.

Tobian, L., Jr.: Cortical steroid excretion in edema of pregnancy, preeclampsia and essential hypertension, J. Clin. Endocr. 9:319, 1949.

Vallance-Owen, J., and Hurlock, B.: Estimation of plasma insulin by the rat diaphragm method, Lancet 1:68, 1954.

Vallance-Owen, J., and Lilley, M. D.: Insulin antagonism in the plasma of obese diabetics and prediabetics; preliminary communication, Lancet 1:806, 1961.

Venning, E. A.: Endocrine changes in normal pregnancy, Amer. J. Med. 19:721, 1955.

Watanabe, M., Meeker, C. I., Gray, M. J., Sims, E. A. H., and Solomon, S.: Secretion rate of aldosterone in normal pregnancy, J. Clin. Invest. 42:1619, 1963.

Weingold, A. B., and Southern, A. L.: Diamine oxidase as an index of the fetoplacental unit; clinical applications, Obstet. Gynec. 32:593, 1968.

Whaley, W. H., Zuspan, F. P., and Nelson, G. H.: Glucose and nonesterified fatty acid levels in maternal and cord plasma, Amer. J. Obstet. Gynec. 92:264, 1965.

Zarrow, M. X., Holmstrom, E. G., and Salhanick, H. A.: The concentration of relaxin in the blood serum and other tissues of women during pregnancy, J. Clin. Endocr. 15:22, 1955.

Ziskin, D. E., and Nesse, G. J.: Pregnancy gingivitis: history, classification, and etiology, Amer. J. Orthodont. 32:390, 1946.

17

Diagnosis and duration of pregnancy and prenatal care

Prenatal care can be defined as a program of examination, evaluation, observation, treatment, and education of pregnant women directed toward making pregnancy, labor, and delivery as normal and as safe as possible for mothers and their infants. Physical abnormalities and emotional disturbances that might alter the course of pregnancy can be detected and often corrected so that the mothers will approach the time for delivery in as perfect health as possible.

The current program of prenatal care, which was developed early in the twentieth century, was designed to help reduce maternal and infant deaths by giving the physician an opportunity to diagnose conditions such as preeclampsia-eclampsia soon after their onset rather than in their terminal stages. The effectiveness of a systematic prenatal care program is evidenced by the reduced mortality from such disorders. The general improvement of health of women in the United States has altered the emphasis on prenatal care somewhat. Since there is less need to concentrate on physical health, more emphasis can be placed on the individual patient's emotional responses to pregnancy. One of the most important objectives of prenatal care is to identify women who have unusual reactions to pregnancy and concentrate on supporting them in their areas of need.

There are still women with conditions that may constitute temporary or permanent contraindications to pregnancy. These can only be detected and treated effectively by *prepregnancy examination*. Every woman who is contemplating pregnancy should be examined completely before she attempts to conceive. At this time the physician should also attempt to evaluate her emotional reactions toward pregnancy and to initiate an educational program that may help her learn more about reproduction and her own responses to it.

Perkin has designed a method for assessing reproductive risk as a guide in establishing priorities for contraception (Table 8). Individual patients are scored in each of the factors that are known to be important in determining the outcome of pregnancy. This can be used quite appropriately for prepregnancy examinations as well as for determining the need for contraception.

Neither prepregnancy nor prenatal care can be expected to compensate for inferior care during labor and delivery. In order to achieve the lowest maternal and infant morbidity and mortality the physician must maintain careful supervision over the entire pregnancy and delivery. The best pregnancy care is not necessarily provided by the highly trained specialist who may be too busy to spend enough time with his patients to really know them and their problems, nor does the total number of office visits during the prenatal period determine the quality of the program. Good pregnancy care can and should be provided by family physicians who are willing to devote time to evaluation of prenatal patients and to the careful consideration of their problems and their pregnancies.

■ Initial examination

The patient should report for examination as soon as she is reasonably certain that

Table 8. Establishing priorities for contraceptive care*

Age	Under 17, over 34 (score 2) 17-19, 30-34 (score 1)	Maximum possible score	2
Parity	5 or more (score 2) 3 or 4 (score 1)		2
History	Previous relevant infant death, congenital defect, premature birth; obstetric complication, abortion; history of diabetes, cardiovascular, renal disease, or other medical condition increasing risk of pregnancy to mother or fetus	(score 1 for each to a maximum of 3)	3
Interval	Less than 24 months since termination of last pregnancy	(score 1)	1
Social	Medical indigency as defined by local standards Marital status—unmarried Maximum possible total score	(score 1) (score 1)	2 10

Interpretation

Score of 5 points or more	Highest risk group Contraceptive counseling by a physician should be considered mandatory Highest priority for follow-up
Score of 3-4 points	High priority Contraceptive counseling highly desirable Should receive periodic reevaluation of risk status
Score of less than 3	Contraceptive counseling should be available to patient

*From Perkin, G. W.: Assessment of reproductive risk in nonpregnant women, Amer. J. Obstet. Gynec. **101**:709, 1968.

she is pregnant, usually 2 or 3 weeks after she has missed a menstrual period. At the first visit a complete history is recorded; this includes a general medical and social review with particular reference to diseases or conditions in the patient or her family that might affect the course of pregnancy and a detailed analysis of gynecologic function. The date of onset and the duration of at least the last two periods are important. It is particularly important to determine specifically whether or not the last period was normal and came at the expected time. Many women report any bleeding, even spotting, as a "menstrual period" unless questioned in detail. The physician should inquire as to the duration of previous pregnancies at delivery, the length of labor, type of delivery, size, condition, and subsequent development of the infant, the occurrence of complications, and the patient's emotional reaction to the event. Previous pregnancy failures such as abortion, ectopic pregnancy, and stillbirths ought to be recorded also.

A general medical examination should be performed after the patient has been interviewed. The pelvic examination includes bimanual palpation of the structures and inspection of the external genitals, the vagina, and the cervix. Manual measurements of the bony pelvis are obtained during the initial pelvic examination unless the patient is unusually tense, in which event this part of the examination may be postponed until later in pregnancy.

Essential laboratory studies in the normal patient include determination of the hemoglobin or hematocrit, blood type, Rh and serologic reaction, and urine tests for protein and sugar and a screening cytologic examination of cervical secretions.

A *screening antibody test,* which is nonspecific in that it indicates the presence of any abnormal antibody not the precise type, should be run. If it is positive, further tests are necessary to identify the specific factor involved.

X-ray examination of the chest has revealed unsuspected pulmonary tuberculosis in from 1% to 3% of large groups of pregnant women. The advisability of routine chest x-ray examination has been questioned because the low incidence of important abnormalities detected might not justify the potential danger to the embryo. Chest x-ray examination should, without question, be a part of the prenatal examination for patient groups in whom the incidence of pulmonary tuberculosis is high, for individuals who have had previous infections, or if there is any question as to the presence of a disease process. The abdomen and pelvis must be properly protected.

It is unnecessary to *examine the urine sediment* in every prenatal patient, but when such an examination is indicated, it must be done on a clean voided specimen or one obtained by catheter to eliminate contamination by vaginal or vulvar secretions. Since about 7% of all pregnant women have asymptomatic bacteriuria and since most predelivery and postdelivery urinary tract infections occur in women with bacteriuria it is wise to obtain a urine culture some time after the eighteenth week in all pregnant women. This is particularly important in women who have had urinary tract infections.

After the examination has been completed and the diagnosis of pregnancy has been established, the findings are discussed with the patient. This portion of the interview should be unhurried and presented in words that she can understand easily. The physician first confirms the fact that she is pregnant if this is possible and indicates the date at which delivery can be expected. Unless there is some abnormality, she should be assured that her physical condition is satisfactory, that her pelvis is adequate, and that no complications are anticipated.

It has been customary to give a detailed description of what to expect during pregnancy, precise instructions concerning diet, general activities, what to do when labor starts, and numerous other directions at the time of the first visit and to believe that this needs be done only once. Unfortunately, patients ordinarily hear little of such monologues because they are so excited or disturbed by the confirmation of the pregnancy that they fail to listen. In addition it is impossible for most women to understand the full implication of pregnancy and to realize that they are going to have a baby, in contrast to being pregnant, until they actually can feel fetal activity. As a conse-

quence, it is preferable to discuss specific problems at appropriate times during the pregnancy when the patient has some interest in them and when they are applicable. It usually is helpful to have printed instructions to which the patient can refer.

■ Diagnosis of pregnancy

The diagnosis of pregnancy is made on the history of the *subjective symptoms,* which are the sensations experienced by the patient, and the detection of the *objective signs,* which are evident to the examiner. It may be difficult to establish an accurate diagnosis early, but the physician will make few mistakes if he uses all the available aids.

SUBJECTIVE SYMPTOMS

Amenorrhea. Although cessation of menstruation should always suggest the possibility of pregnancy, this symptom is not completely reliable. A few women bleed at irregular intervals throughout pregnancy because of some abnormality, and others may cease menstruating for reasons other than pregnancy. Regular cyclic bleeding cannot occur during pregnancy because ovarian function is suspended.

Morning nausea and vomiting. Morning nausea and vomiting usually appear a week or two after the period is missed and continue until about the tenth or twelfth week. They develop in one half or more of all pregnant women but may also occur in women who are not pregnant or even in the husbands of those who are.

Bladder disturbance. Frequency of urination is caused by pressure or tension on the bladder by the enlarging uterus.

Breasts. Enlargement, tingling, or actual discomfort in the breasts is the result of hormonal stimulation of alveolar and ductal structures. This may also occur premenstrually.

Quickening. Quickening is a term that indicates the perception of fetal motion by the mother. Multiparas first feel the infant in about 4 months and 4 days and primigravidas in about 4 months and 14 days after the first day of the last menstrual period. Women with pseudocyesis also experience "quickening." The first sensation is usually described as a slight fluttering or a feeling similar to gas passing through the bowel. As the fetus grows and becomes more active the

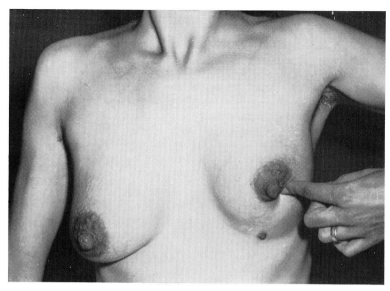

Fig. 17-1. Breast changes. Note the prominence of Montgomery's glands and the deep pigmentation of the nipples and areolae. An accessory nipple beneath the left breast is also pigmented.

stimulus becomes stronger and may even be painful.

OBJECTIVE SIGNS

Breasts. The breasts are firm and distended, and Montgomery's glands are prominent. The nipple and areola become darker and are surrounded by an area of increased pigmentation in the normal skin, the *secondary areola*. Colostrum can be expressed from the nipples, but it is not a reliable sign because it may also be produced in pseudocyesis and may be present in multiparas between pregnancies.

Genitals. The most remarkable changes take place in the genital organs.

Vagina. The vaginal mucosa becomes cyanotic and congested (Chadwick's sign). This may also be detected premenstrually or with increased local congestion from any cause.

Cervix. Softening in the tip of the cervix (Goodell's sign) can be detected soon after the onset of pregnancy. The entire cervix eventually is softened.

Uterine isthmus. The isthmus of the uterus is soft at 6 to 8 weeks and can be compressed between the fingers palpating the vagina and abdomen (Hegar's sign). Within a few weeks the entire cervix and

the corpus become much softer, and the difference can no longer be detected.

Uterus. The consistency and shape of the firm, pear-shaped nonpregnant uterus change as pregnancy advances. Soon after the fertilized ovum implants, a soft bulge can be detected in one half of the uterus, usually fairly high in the fundus, whereas the other side remains firm (Piskacek's sign). The softened area probably indicates the implantation site. As pregnancy advances, the uterus becomes globular and eventually it elongates.

The consistency of the uterus is soft and doughy rather than firm, and a definite increase in size can be detected by repeated examinations. Intermittent, painless uterine contractions (Braxton Hicks contractions) can sometimes be felt during the first trimester. Later they become stronger, and the patient may be aware of them.

Demonstration of the fetus. The fetal parts can usually be *palpated* by the sixteenth to eighteenth week of pregnancy unless the patient is too obese, the abdomen is tender, or there is an excessive amount of amniotic fluid (hydramnios). It may be possible to feel the fetus earlier by ballottement through the vagina. The examining fingers in the vagina push the anterior vaginal wall

Softening of the
isthmus
(Hegar's sign)

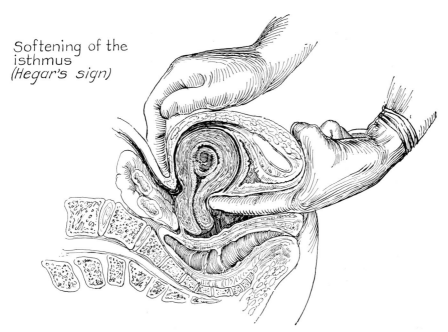

Fig. 17-2. Uterine changes in early pregnancy.

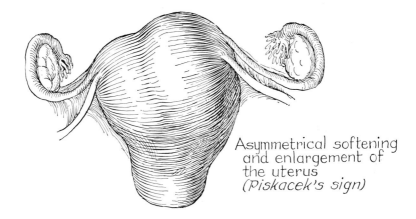

Asymmetrical softening
and enlargement of
the uterus
(Piskacek's sign)

and lower uterine segment sharply upward, and the fetus first rises and then falls back, bumping against the fingertips.

Fetal motion can usually be seen, felt, or heard by the physician after the eighteenth week. Quickening is subjective and therefore unreliable.

The *fetal heart tones* can be heard first with an ordinary stethoscope at about the eighteenth to twentieth week low in the midline. The normal rate varies from 120 to 160 beats per minute, and usually it is not difficult to differentiate them from the maternal pulse. The sounds may be obscured by obesity, hydramnios, or an unusual fetal position.

It is possible to detect fetal heart motion much earlier with ultrasonic equipment than to hear heart sounds with a stethoscope. The Doppler apparatus consists of a probe containing an ultrasound source, which emits a continuous signal, and an amplifier, which permits the examiner to hear the ultrasound waves that are reflected back from the beating fetal heart. With the Doppler apparatus one can detect the fetal heart quite consistently by the twelfth week and even earlier. Obesity, fluid, and other barriers do not alter the accuracy of the instrument.

The *fetal skeleton* can be detected by x-ray examination after some calcification has taken place. Under favorable conditions it may be seen at about 14 weeks and almost always after 16 to 18 weeks. X-ray studies at this stage of pregnancy are best avoided unless it is essential to attempt to demonstrate the presence of a fetus and no other method is available.

A *fetal electrocardiogram* is a certain indication of pregnancy. Although a positive tracing can sometimes be obtained early in the second trimester, the periods of highest accuracy are between 18 and 24 weeks and after the thirty-second week. A negative result during the periods of low accuracy cannot be accepted as proof that pregnancy does not exist.

Repeated examinations. Often the physician may suspect pregnancy from the history but be unable to confirm the diagnosis by pelvic examination because the patient has reported for examination too early. If she is reexamined 2 or 3 weeks later, the changes in size and consistency of the uterus will usually make the diagnosis obvious.

Pregnancy tests. The laboratory tests for pregnancy are based upon the production of chorionic gonadotropic hormones. Since similar hormones are produced by certain teratomas of the ovary and testes, choriocarcinoma, and hydatidiform mole, as well as by normal placenta, a positive test does

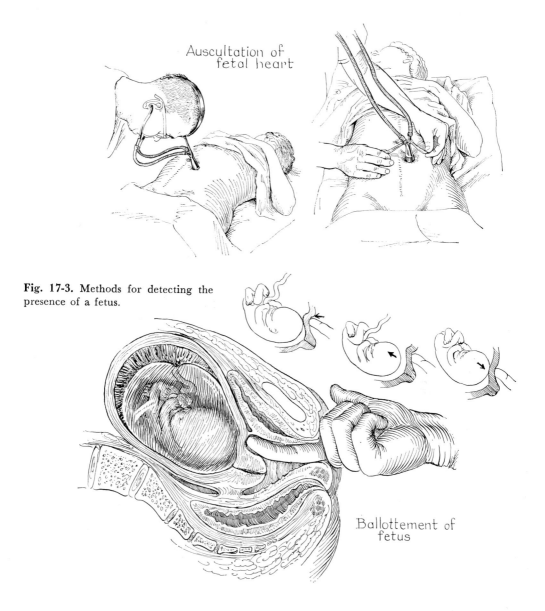

Fig. 17-3. Methods for detecting the presence of a fetus.

not necessarily indicate the presence of normal pregnancy. False positive tests are possible and false negative tests may be the result of running the test too early before sufficient hormone is being produced, dilute urine, the wrong urine, an unresponsive animal, an animal killed too soon, or the injection of an insufficient quantity of urine. These tests are seldom necessary and are not to be relied upon alone for the diagnosis of pregnancy.

POSITIVE DIAGNOSIS

A positive diagnosis of pregnancy can be made only if the fetus is identified by palpating its parts, palpating motion, hearing its heart, positive electrocardiogram, or demonstrating its skeleton by x-ray examination. This can seldom be accomplished during the first trimester of pregnancy.

DIFFERENTIAL DIAGNOSIS

Typical uterine changes must make the physician suspect pregnancy even though the patient denies the possibility. Repeated pelvic examination will clarify the problem because the size, shape, and consistency of the pregnant uterus will undergo the typical changes as pregnancy advances.

Cystic ovarian neoplasms situated either in the posterior cul-de-sac or in the anterior pelvis may simulate a pregnant uterus. Ovarian neoplasms alone do not often cause amenorrhea. They usually can be separated from the uterine fundus, and they do not increase in size as rapidly as the pregnant uterus.

Uterine fibromyomas, particularly a large single tumor situated in the fundus of the uterus, may be almost impossible to differentiate from a normal pregnancy. Uterine tumors do not cause amenorrhea, and since they grow slowly one can detect little or no change in the uterus by repeated examinations at intervals of 2 or 3 weeks.

Other disorders such as *hematometra* are uncommon and can usually be diagnosed by careful examination.

Pregnancy and fibromyomas or ovarian tumors often occur simultaneously. It is in situations of this sort that it may be necessary to use every possible diagnostic aid. Pregnancy must be considered in women who have missed one or more periods and in those whose periods have been normal but who are now bleeding irregularly, even though an ovarian cyst, a fibroid, or another obvious lesion is present. It is in such patients that pregnancy tests, x-ray examinations, fetal electrocardiograms, and similar studies are of greatest importance.

■ Pseudocyesis

Pseudopregnancy, during which the patient may experience all the subjective changes of normal pregnancy, such as nausea and vomiting, quickening, etc., is encountered occasionally. The menstrual flow may be reduced or completely absent, and the breasts may enlarge and become firm and may secrete colostrum. Abdominal enlargement may also occur, but it is caused by bowel distention or the deposition of fat in the subcutaneous tissue rather than by growth of the uterus.

Pseudocyesis may appear at any age but is more common in older women. It usually represents an emotional need for an infant in an attempt to maintain a failing marriage, to hold the husband's affection, to

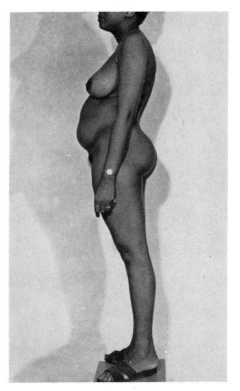

Fig. 17-4. Pseudocyesis. Note protrusion of abdomen, increased lordosis, and posture typical of pregnancy.

prove to herself that she can conceive, or for some other similar reason. The endocrine changes that accompany pseudocyesis—an increased production of pituitary luteotropic (lactogenic) principal, producing persistent luteinization of the ovaries—could produce the changes.

The diagnosis can be suspected if the physician cannot detect characteristic pregnancy changes in the pelvic organs and can be confirmed if the pregnancy test is negative or if the uterus does not enlarge progressively.

Because of the emotional factors involved it will do no good and in fact may be harmful simply to tell the patient that she is not pregnant. An attempt must be made to uncover the underlying emotional problem that makes pregnancy necessary to the individual. In some instances the patient should be interviewed several times before she is even told that she is not pregnant. Intensive psychotherapy may be necessary.

■ Signs of life or death of the fetus

During the first half of pregnancy the physician must usually rely upon progressive uterine enlargement to determine whether the fetus is alive, but during the second half the fetal heart tones can usually be heard, and fetal motion can be palpated or heard.

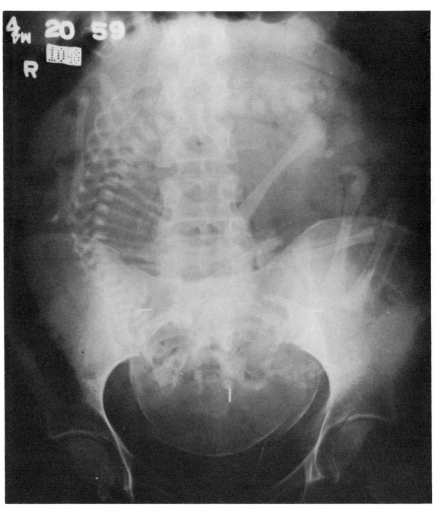

Fig. 17-5. Intrauterine fetal death near term. Note the overlapping skull bones, exaggerated flexion of spine, and collapsed rib cage.

If *fetal motion suddenly ceases* and cannot be detected by the mother or the physician and if the *fetal heart can no longer be heard,* the baby may have died. A *negative fetal electrocardiogram* in a patient in whom the test previously has been positive is a reliable indication of fetal death except during the period of low accuracy between 24 and 32 weeks. Occasionally the fetal heart cannot be heard with an ordinary stethoscope because the fetal chest wall is not in contact with the anterior uterine wall. Before assuming that the infant has died because the heart sounds are inaudible, the physician should check with the Doppler apparatus, which is far more accurate.

The physician can often confirm his suspicion of intrauterine fetal death by an appropriate *x-ray examination.* Such studies are of little help during the first half of pregnancy, but they become progressively more accurate as pregnancy advances. The usual x-ray evidences of fetal death—overlapping of the cranial bones before the onset of labor (Spalding's sign) and collapse of the spine and rib cage (Brakemann's sign)—occur because of softening of the interosseous tissues; consequently these signs will be absent for several days after the baby dies. One of the earliest of the x-ray signs of fetal death is the accumulation of gas in the heart and great vessels. This can usually be demonstrated in 3 or 4 days. The fetal fat line over the skull can be seen during the third trimester. After death the fat line is elevated from the skull bones by an accumulation of fluid.

The fetus begins to swallow amniotic fluid very early in pregnancy. If a contrast medium is injected into the amniotic sac it will enter the infant's gastrointestinal tract if the infant is alive; if it is dead, it will not swallow the fluid. This study is seldom necessary.

If the baby has died, *uterine growth ceases* or the size of the uterus may even regress, and when placental function is disturbed, the breasts become softer and smaller and the *pregnancy test becomes negative.* Estriol production also decreases when the baby dies, and the change can be detected by repeatedly determining the level of this estrogen fraction. A fall in estriol excretion may occur more rapidly than a reversal of pregnancy test because estriol production is a function of both fetus and placenta whereas the chorionic gonadotropins are produced entirely by the placenta. The placental cells may continue to survive and function for several weeks after the fetus dies.

■ Duration of pregnancy

The duration of pregnancy extends over an approximate period of 280 days from the first day of the last normal menstrual period or 268 days from fertilization. The duration of pregnancy therefore is about 40 weeks when calculated from the onset of the last period and 38 weeks when calculated from conception. Since the exact time of fertilization is problematic, whereas the day the last period began usually is obvious, the latter is most often used as a starting point. The thirteenth week of pregnancy, for example, means the thirteenth week after the first day of the last normal period rather than the thirteenth week after conception.

There is no accurate method for determining exactly when labor will begin, but the patient will want some day toward which to point, and this may be chosen by the following methods:

1. The date of the first day of the last normal menstrual period minus 3 months

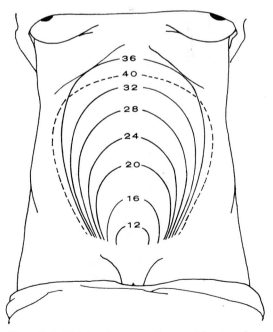

Fig. 17-6. Height of uterus above pubis at various weeks of pregnancy.

plus 7 days gives the day of expected delivery. Since the date of the last menstrual period often is unreliable and since the last period of bleeding recognized by the patient may or may not have been true menstruation, this date does not necessarily indicate the day delivery will occur, but it usually is within 2 weeks on either side.

2. Add 268 days to the day of ovulation as determined by basal temperature recordings or to the date of presumed fruitful coitus. The latter may well be inaccurate.

3. *Quickening* occurs 4 months and 4 days after the onset of the last menstruation in multiparas and 4 months and 14 days in primigravidas. This obviously is inaccurate, since some women feel the infant far earlier than others.

4. The *size of the fetus* is difficult to determine with accuracy and is at best only an approximation. The *size of the uterus* can be determined by measuring the height of the fundus above the pubis, but in pregnancies of comparable duration the measurement may be substantially different because of differences in thickness of the

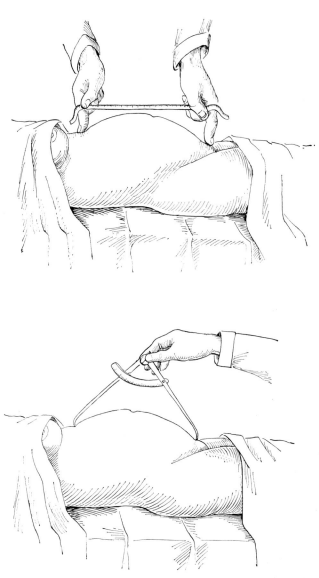

Fig. 17-7. Measurement of fundal height. An attempt should be made to measure the linear height rather than around the curve of the fundus.

abdominal wall, in the amount of amniotic fluid, and in fetal size. The duration of pregnancy may be approximated by the following calculation: The average height of the uterus above the pubis at term is 35 cm.; therefore, after the middle of pregnancy

$$\frac{height}{3.5} = \text{lunar months of pregnancy.}$$

Another method, which is based upon a measurement from the superior surface of the symphysis around the curve of the fundus to its top, can also be used. In the patient at term this arc averages 35 cm. if the presenting part is not yet engaged and 33 cm. if it is. Two sevenths of the length of the arc indicates the gestational age in lunar months. For example, if the arc measures 28 cm., the duration of pregnancy is 8 lunar months (32 weeks):

$$\frac{28 \text{ cm.} \times 2}{7} = 8 \text{ lunar months}$$

■ Fetal maturity

Unless he has a point of reference, such as the date of the last menstrual period or an isolated coitus, the physician may find it

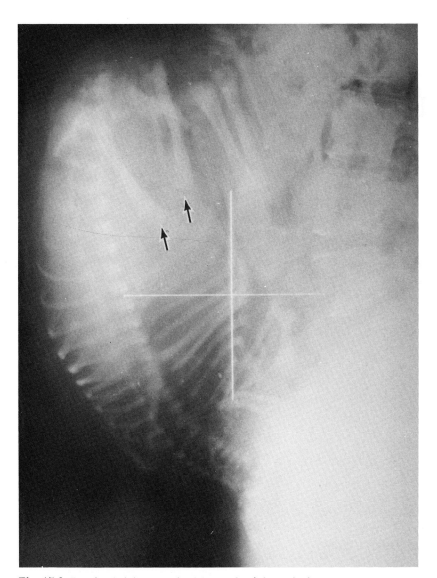

Fig. 17-8. Proximal tibial and distal femoral epiphyses in fetus near term.

difficult to determine when a patient is approaching term. The size of the uterus is helpful, but it is more important to determine, if possible, the age of the fetus. These problems are arising more often with increasing use of oral contraceptive agents: Ovulation and menstruation may occur irregularly for several cycles after discontinuing the pills, or amenorrhea may persist for months.

It is possible, however, by using all the available methods to arrive at a reasonable approximation of fetal age.

1. *X-ray examination.* It is difficult to measure body length and head diameters precisely unless the infant happens to be in a favorable position at the time of the examination, but it is possible to estimate fetal age by the appearance of ossification centers. The *distal femoral epiphysis* is present in 80% or more of infants at the thirty-sixth week of pregnancy and the *proximal tibial epiphysis* in 70% to 75% of infants at term. The demonstration of these ossification centers confirms the duration of pregnancy, but their absence does not eliminate the fact that the infant may be mature.

Well-developed *cortical bone* in the skull and long bones suggests that the infant is mature.

A well-developed *fetal fat line,* particularly when combined with good bony ossification and the presence of epiphyses, suggests a mature fetus.

2. *Ultrasound techniques* are also helpful in determining fetal size. The biparietal diameter of the fetal skull can be measured precisely by this method.

3. *Amniotic fluid* examination may be helpful in determining fetal age.

Fetal cells. Shed fetal cells, presumably from sebaceous glands, stain orange with Nile blue sulfate, whereas squamous cells stain blue. The number of orange-staining cells in amniotic fluid increases as the fetus matures and can be used as a rough determinant of fetal age. Bishop and Carson state that when the count of orange cells is less than 2%, the prematurity rate is 85%, but when more than 20% of the cells in amniotic fluid are of this type, the infant will weigh at least 2,500 grams.

Creatinine. The fetal kidneys become progressively more active as maturity advances. One evidence of improving renal function and of the increasing fetal muscle mass is the amniotic fluid creatinine concentration. The infant is presumed to be mature when amniotic fluid creatinine concentration is more than 2 mg./100 ml.

None of these studies of amniotic fluid is precise enough to justify acceptance without reinforcement by other examinations. They may provide supporting evidences of fetal development. All have the disadvantage of requiring amniocentesis.

■ Diet and weight gain

Weight gain. A total increase of about 18 to 20 pounds can be accounted for by the fetus (7½ pounds), placenta (1 to 1½ pounds), amniotic fluid (1 to 2 pounds), the increase in the size of the uterus (2 to 2½ pounds), and breasts (2 to 3 pounds), the increased blood volume (3 pounds), and the increased storage of extravascular fluid. If the patient gains this amount, she will usually return to her prepregnancy weight after delivery. Gains greater than this can be accounted for by the ingestion of a diet too high in calories, in which the patient increases her fat stores, or by an accumulation of fluid outside the vascular system. The former of these is responsible for many of the overweight women who find it difficult to lose the excess fat later and who repeat the same process with each subsequent pregnancy. Excessive storage of fluid is less likely to be a cause of obesity but has a more serious immediate significance because it is one of the warning signs that a toxemia of pregnancy may be developing. Excessive weight gain per se is not a cause of toxemia, but most women with preeclampsia do gain abnormally because of fluid retention.

Recent studies indicate that there is a definite relationship between weight gain and the outcome of pregnancy. Eastman and Jackson studied the records of 6,675 white women and 5,236 black women who were delivered of normal living single infants between the thirty-ninth and forty-second weeks of uncomplicated pregnancies. The mean weight gain for white women was 22.1 pounds and for black women 20.5 pounds. The mean birth weight of white infants was 3,395 grams, and progressive increases in maternal weight gains were accompanied by progressive increments in infant birth weights. The mean infant birth weights and maternal weight gains were as follows:

MATERNAL WEIGHT GAIN (pounds)	BIRTH WEIGHT (grams)
0 - 10	3,278
11 - 20	3,301
21 - 30	3,426
31 - 40	3,562
+41	3,636

An interesting finding is that the mean birth weights of 61 infants whose mothers had lost weight during pregnancy was 3,360 grams.

The incidence of babies weighing 2,500 grams or less decreased progressively from 4.4% if the mothers gained 0 to 10 pounds to 0.5% in 202 women who gained more than 41 pounds. Of the mothers who lost weight, 3.3% were delivered of low birth-weight infants.

The infants of black women followed a similar pattern but weighed less in each group than did the white babies.

Nyirjesy, Lonergan, and Kane, studying 12,569 primigravidas who were delivered at term, also noted progressively increasing infant weight and a decreasing incidence of low birth-weight babies with increasing maternal weight gains. They conclude that it is illogical to recommend that the mother gain excessively solely in an attempt to increase the size of the baby because she would have to gain about 50 pounds to increase the baby's weight by 1 pound.

The rate of gain ought to be fairly steady; during the first trimester little or no increase in weight is expected even though there is no nausea; hence during the last two thirds of pregnancy the average increase is about ¾ pound weekly. Sudden jumps in weight or gains over 2 pounds weekly are most likely caused by fluid retention.

Allowances must be made for the patient who is not at her normal weight at the beginning of pregnancy. For those who are underweight, gains greater than 18 to 20 pounds may be permitted if the physician can be certain that the increase is not caused by excess fluid retention. For the overweight individual a reduced caloric intake is permissible. The amount that the food intake is reduced depends upon how much above normal weight the patient is. Ideally, if she should weigh the same at delivery as she did at the time of conception, she can be expected to lose the 18 or 20 pounds accounted for by the products of conception and the physiologic changes of pregnancy and thus will be that much below her prepregnancy weight. If the weight decreases during the gestation period, the expected postdelivery weight will be the sum of the weight loss during pregnancy and the physiologic loss at delivery. If patients lose weight during pregnancy, it is essential that the reduced calorie diet contain all the ingredients necessary to meet the maternal and fetal nutritional requirements.

It is particularly important that the pregnancy diet contain an adequate amount of good quality protein because it is essential for fetal development and for maintenance of maternal health. Recent studies suggest that protein deficiencies during pregnancy may alter brain development. The brains of rats born of mothers who were maintained on a diet inadequate in protein were qualitatively and quantitatively inferior to the brains of rats whose mothers were well nourished before and during pregnancy. The brains of the experimental rats' offspring contained fewer neurons than did the controls, and each cell contained less protein.

Normal pregnancy diet. The normal pregnancy diet must supply the needs of both mother and infant during the pregnancy. Ingredients required by the infant and not supplied in the diet may be obtained at the expense of the mother's tissues, therefore they must be supplied by increasing the maternal intake. The following essential daily requirements are those suggested by the National Academy of Sciences –National Research Council:

Calories	200 over that recommended for age, weight, and height
Protein	65 grams
Calcium	1.4 to 1.7 grams
Iron	18 mg.
Vitamin A	5,000 I.U.
Vitamin D	400 I.U.

To provide these, each day's food intake should include the following:

Protein
Lean meat, fish, chicken—2 servings
Eggs—at least 1
Milk—1 quart; 10 tablespoonsful of dried skim milk powder provide an equivalent amount of protein
Additional protein—½ cup cottage cheese, additional meat or eggs

Vegetables
  Potato—1 serving
  Cooked vegetables (preferably colored such as carrots, spinach, greens, etc.)—2 servings
  Raw vegetables (cabbage, lettuce, carrots)—1 serving
Fruits
  Fresh fruit or fruit juice—2 servings, 1 of which should be tomatoes, oranges, or grapefruit
Bread and cereal
  Whole grain cereal (oatmeal, enriched grits, whole wheat cereal)—1 serving
  Bread—2 slices whole wheat or rye bread
Other foods
  Sugar—small amount as desired
  Butter or margarine—3 teaspoonsful
  Fluids—water or other nonfattening liquids may be taken in any quantity; 8 to 10 glasses daily are desirable
Supplements
  A multivitamin preparation and iron

Low-calorie pregnancy diet. The overweight woman can lose safely without affecting her own health or that of her infant if caloric reduction is accomplished by limiting the ingestion of fats and carbohydrates while an adequate intake of protein is maintained. A satisfactory pregnancy diet with a caloric content lower than 1,200 to 1,400 cannot be constructed. A multivitamin and an iron preparation must always be prescribed with a low-calorie diet.

The ingestion of 5 or 6 small feedings rather than 3 large ones will often decrease the sensation of hunger.

Each day's intake of food should include the following:

Protein
  Meat, chicken, fish—2 servings
  Milk—1 quart of skimmed milk or an equivalent amount of dried skim milk powder
  Eggs—at least 1 daily
  Cheese—½ cup cottage cheese or yellow cheese
Vegetables
  Two cups of any vegetables on the following list; one should be green, leafy type

Asparagus	Kale
Beets	Kohlrabi
Beet greens	Lettuce
Broccoli	Mushrooms
Brussels sprouts	Onions
Carrots	Pumpkin
Cabbage	Radishes
Cauliflower	Romaine
Celery	Rutabagas
Cucumbers	Sauerkraut
Dandelion greens	Squash
Eggplant	String beans
Endive	Swiss chard
Escarole	Tomato
Green peppers	Turnip
	Watercress

Fruits
  Three servings of unsweetened fruits in amounts suggested in the following list; one should be tomato or citrus fruit

Apples	1	small
Apricots	2	medium
Bananas	½	medium
Blackberries	½	cup
Blueberries	⅓	cup
Cantaloupe	¼	of 1 medium
Cherries	⅓	cup
Currants	⅓	cup
Gooseberries	½	cup
Grape juice	½	cup
Grapefruit	½	medium
Grapefruit juice	½	cup
Grapes	¼	cup
Huckleberries	⅓	cup
Oranges	1	medium
Peaches	1	medium
Pears	2	medium
Pineapple	1	cup cubed
Pineapple juice	½	cup
Plums	2	medium
Raspberries	⅓	cup
Strawberries	½	cup
Tomato juice	1	cup
Watermelon	¼	inch slice

Cereal
  Whole grain cereal—1 serving
  Whole wheat or rye bread—2 slices

The patient must be specifically instructed to eliminate the following foods from her diet:
  1. Fried foods, fat meat, and gravy
  2. Ice cream, cake, pie, cookies, candy, milk shakes, canned sweetened fruits, and soft drinks sweetened with sugar.
  3. Rice, macaroni, spaghetti, noodles, potatoes, and crackers
  4. Salad dressings or oils, olives, cream, and nuts

Before reducing calories in a woman of normal weight who is gaining excessively, the physician must make certain that she is not accumulating fluid. Another reason for unusual weight gain during pregnancy is that patients tend to become progressively less active as pregnancy advances but continue to ingest the same amount of food. Normal pregnant women who are gaining too rapidly should be ecouraged to exercise as well as reduce caloric intake.

Low-sodium pregnancy diet. A low-sodium diet may be prescribed for pregnant patients with chronic cardiovascular renal disease, preeclampsia, and edema, or if excessive weight gain is thought to be the result of fluid retention. Each day's food intake must provide the basic requirements for pregnancy and should be prepared without salt. Only fresh meats, fruits, and vegetables should be used. A multivitamin preparation and iron should also be prescribed. The dietary ingredients should be selected from the following list of low-sodium foods:

HIGH SODIUM

Meats
　All cured meats, brain, heart, kidney, clams, lobster, crab, haddock, shrimp

Starches
　Regular bread, "quick-cooking" cereals, potato chips, soda crackers, all dry cereals except those listed as "low sodium"

Fats
　Oleomargarine, peanut butter, bacon drippings

Vegetables
　Beets, beet greens, celery, dandelion greens, Swiss chard, kale, frozen peas, sauerkraut, spinach

Fruits
　Raisins, dried figs

Dairy products
　Regular milk, cheese, cream, sour cream, salted butter, ice cream

Desserts
　Cake, cookies, pie, sherbet, candy

Seasonings
　Baking powder, baking soda, bouillon cubes, catsup, celery salt, French dressing, garlic salt, mayonnaise, meat sauces, molasses, mustard, olives, pickles, relishes, salad dressing, brown sugar

LOW SODIUM

Meats
　Lean beef, lamb, liver, pork, veal, turkey, chicken

Starches
　Low-sodium bread, plain rice, hot cereals, corn, Puffed Rice, Puffed Wheat, Shredded Wheat, spaghetti, noodles, macaroni, lima beans, potatoes

Fats
　Lard, corn oil, olive oil, peanut oil, soybean oil, cottonseed oil

Vegetables
　Asparagus, broccoli, Brussels sprouts, cabbage, carrots, cauliflower, eggplant, endive, green beans, green pepper, lettuce, mushrooms, onions, parsnips, fresh peas, pumpkin, radishes, squash, tomatoes, turnips

Fruits
　Bananas, apples, fresh figs, oranges, cantaloupe, blueberries, blackberries, plums, raspberries, prunes, strawberries, rhubarb, cranberries, currants, grapefruit, apricots, dates, pears, cherries, gooseberries, peaches, tangerines, watermelon, pineapples

Dairy products
　Eggs, low-sodium milk, unsalted butter

Desserts
　Only homemade desserts prepared without salt

■ Prenatal instructions

In addition to advice concerning diet the patient must know what she is permitted to do and what she should avoid doing during her pregnancy. The normal individual does not need to alter her existence much because she is pregnant.

Exercise. The amount of exercise permitted is determined by the tolerance of the patient. Fresh air and activity are usually beneficial. Walking, golf, and swimming in clean water are permissible, but tennis, horseback riding, and cycling, although not necessarily too strenuous, should usually be avoided because of the possibility of injury. The multiparous woman with a house and several children to care for often will benefit more from rest than from exercise. Women who gain weight excessively should be encouraged to increase physical activity as well as reduce calories.

Travel. The only danger in travel for the normal patient is that she may abort or go into labor while away from home. Those who have aborted previously or who have abnormal pregnancies should not travel. Train, airplane, or automobile trips are permissible. The normal patient may drive her car or ride in buses or trolleys until term.

Intercourse. The normal patient may continue intercourse throughout pregnancy without fear of injury or introducing infection. The desire for intercourse may be reduced during pregnancy but returns after delivery.

Bathing. Tub or shower baths are permitted throughout pregnancy. As pregnancy advances, the patient must take care not to lose her balance as she climbs in and out of the tub.

Bladder. Pubococcygeus exercises, if performed daily, will aid in preventing postdelivery urinary incontinence.

Bowel. Constipation can ordinarily be corrected by prune juice, mineral oil, or milk of magnesia, 30 ml. once or twice daily.

Breast care. The breasts and nipples should be washed daily with soap and water. The nipples may be massaged and stretched with cocoa butter–lubricated fingers if the patient wishes, but this probably will not influence their response to nursing. The patient must be careful not to injure the nipples, particularly if they are inverted or abnormal.

Clothing. No special clothing is necessary, but all clothes should be loose and hang from the shoulders. *Circular garters* may promote the development of varicose veins. *Low-heeled shoes* increase stability and decrease backache. High heels rotate the body forward, thereby increasing the normal pregnancy lordosis and strain on the back muscles in order to balance the protuberant abdomen. A *maternity brassiere* that may be used after delivery should be worn if breast support is required. A *maternity girdle* is necessary only to control backache, pelvic pressure, or a pendulous abdomen.

Dental care. The teeth should be examined and any necessary repairs performed at least twice during pregnancy. Necessary extractions are permissible. Only local anesthesia should be used.

Alcohol. Alcohol may be used in moderation. Its caloric content and its effect on appetite must be considered in overweight women.

Tobacco. The babies of women who smoke heavily are smaller than those of non-smokers. According to Underwood and co-workers the mean birth weight of babies of 4,856 nonsmokers was 3,395 grams, that of women who smoked 1 to 10 cigarettes daily was 3,286 grams, that of women who smoked 11 to 30 cigarettes daily was 3,196 grams, and that of even heavier smokers was 3,182 grams. There was no difference in perinatal mortality rates.

Drugs. Peckham and King reported that drugs were prescribed during pregnancy for 92% of the women they surveyed and that 3.9% had been given 10 or more. It has long been known that fetal anomalies can be produced experimentally by the administration of certain drugs at appropriate times during embryonic development. Thalidomide, methotrexate, testosterone, and others are known to produce anomalous development of the human fetus, and many other presumably innocuous preparations may. As a general rule no drugs should be prescribed during the first trimester of normal pregnancy. Only medications that are essential to the health of the patient should be permitted.

■ Subsequent visits

Although the adequacy of care cannot be gauged by the number of visits to the doctor, frequent observation is necessary. For many years it has been customary to space prenatal visits at 3- to 4-week intervals during the first 28 weeks, at 2-week intervals between the twenty-eighth and thirty-sixth weeks, and then weekly until delivery. This schedule may be quite appropriate for the primigravida who has little responsibility at home, who will have many questions concerning the pregnancy, and who may need a considerable amount of support and reassurance. It usually is completely inappropriate for healthy multiparas whose previous pregnancies have been uncomplicated. These women have little to learn about the course of pregnancy, and their prenatal visits often are social calls rather than significant medical consultations. In contrast to the primigravida she and her obstetrician are well acquainted because they have managed several pregnancies together. If one can be assured after the first 2 or 3 visits that there are no abnormalities, the subsequent examinations can be scheduled at 6- to 8-week intervals until the twenty-eighth or thirtieth week, at 3- to 4-week intervals until the thirty-sixth week, and at 2-week intervals until delivery. Such a schedule is appropriate only if the patient is comfortable with it and understands that she can see the obstetrician whenever she thinks it necessary and that she must call at once if there is any question of an abnormality.

Women with proved or suspected abnormalities must be seen at much more frequent intervals. The spacing of the visits will be determined by the complication.

At each visit the following are done:

1. Weigh the patient and calculate not only the total gain but the gain since the last visit. Dietary adjustments if necessary are made at that time.

2. Record the blood pressure and compare it with the previous readings.

3. Examine a urine specimen for protein and sugar.

4. Question the patient regarding symptoms.

5. Suggest any change in treatment indicated by your findings.

Other examinations are unnecessary each time the patient is seen unless there is a reason for them. The pelvic examination may be repeated if the first was inconclusive, if any abnormality was encountered, or if pelvic symptoms appear.

Vaginal examinations may be done in the office at any time during normal pregnancy if the external genitals are cleansed with soap or an antiseptic solution and sterile gloves and instruments are used. *Abdominal examination* is unnecessary at each visit if the presence of a normal pregnancy has been proved and if fetal activity continues. The position of the fetus cannot be checked with accuracy until after the thirtieth week and is of little importance before this time. During the last few weeks, however, abdominal examinations will reveal not only the position but the degree of descent of the presenting part.

The *breasts* should be examined at least once during the last trimester of pregnancy. This provides a good opportunity to discuss breast-feeding. Determination of the *hematocrit or hemoglobin* should be repeated at about the thirty-fourth week.

Symptoms that appear during the prenatal period must be thoroughly investigated, making use of any physical or laboratory test that may be indicated.

It is during the return prenatal visits that the subjects often discussed only at the first examination are considered. For example, fetal growth may be discussed at the visit when the patient reports feeling fetal activity, the significance of edema if the patient is gaining excessively, the onset of labor during the last trimester, and anesthesia and delivery near term. Of course, throughout the pregnancy the obstetrician must try to learn all he can about the patient and her reactions to motherhood.

References

Apgar, V.: Drugs in pregnancy, J.A.M.A. **190:**104, 1964.

Bishop, E. H.: Estimation of fetal maturity by cytologic examination of amniotic fluid, Amer. J. Obstet. Gynec. **102:**654, 1968.

Bishop, P. A.: Radiologic studies of the gravid uterus, New York, 1965, Paul B. Hoeber, Inc., Medical Book Department, Harper & Row, Publishers.

Chadwick, J. R.: Value of the bluish coloration of the vaginal entrance as a sign of pregnancy, Trans. Amer. Gynec. Soc. **11:**399, 1887.

Eastman, N. J., and Jackson, E.: Weight relationships in pregnancy. I. The bearing of maternal weight and pre-pregnancy weight on birth weight in full-term pregnancies, Obstet. Gynec. Survey **23:**1003, 1968.

Fried, P. H., Rakoff, A. E., Schopbach, R. R., and Kaplan, A. J.: Pseudocyesis; psychosomatic study in gynecology, J.A.M.A. **145:**1329, 1951.

Hegar, A.: Diagnose der fruhesten Schwangerschaftsperiode, Deutsch. Med. Wschr. **21:**565, 1895.

Hicks, J. B.: On the contractions of the uterus throughout pregnancy; their physiologic effects and their value in the diagnosis of pregnancy, Trans. Obstet. Soc. London **13:**216, 1871.

Nyirjesy, I., Lonergan, W. M., and Kane, J. J.: Clinical significance of total weight gain in pregnancy, Obstet. Gynec. **32:**391, 1968.

Peckham, C. H., and King, R. W.: Study of intercurrent conditions observed during pregnancy, Amer. J. Obstet. Gynec. **87:**609, 1963.

Perkin, G. W.: Assessment of reproductive risk in nonpregnant women, Amer. J. Obstet. Gynec. **101:**709, 1968.

Pugh, W. E., and Fernandez, F. L.: Coitus in late pregnancy, Obstet. Gynec. **2:**636, 1953.

Seager, K. G.: The onset of labor in relation to the length of the menstrual cycle, J. Obstet. Gynaec. Brit. Comm. **60:**92, 1953.

Spalding, A. B.: A pathognomonic sign of intrauterine death, Surg. Gynec. Obstet. **34:**754, 1922.

Stewart, H. L., Jr.: Duration of pregnancy and postmaturity, J.A.M.A. **148:**1079, 1952.

Sunden, B.: On the diagnostic value of ultrasound in obstetrics and gynecology, Acta Obstet. Gynec. Scand. XLIII (supp. 6), 1964.

Thomson, J. L. G.: The differential diagnosis of Spalding's sign, Brit. J. Radiol. **23:**266, 1950.

Underwood, P. B., Kesler, K. F., O'Lane, J. M., and Callagan, D. A.: Parental smoking empirically related to pregnancy outcome, Obstet. Gynec. **29:**1, 1967.

Zamenhof, S., Van Marthens, E., and Margolis, F. L.: DNA (cell number) and protein in fetal brain; alteration by maternal dietary protein restriction, Science **160:**322, 1968.

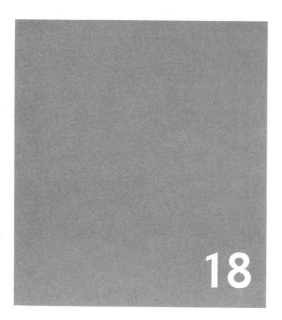

18

Infectious diseases during pregnancy

Pregnant women are susceptible to and can contract any of the infectious diseases as readily as nonpregnant women. In most instances infectious diseases neither affect the infant nor alter the course of pregnancy. There are, however, certain notable exceptions that are discussed in this chapter.

■ Acute infectious diseases

Upper respiratory disease. Pregnant women are somewhat more susceptible to the development of the common cold, and upper respiratory infections tend to last longer than in nonpregnant women. The usual symptomatic treatment can be administered.

Although there is no evidence to suggest that the usual viruses which presumably cause the common cold have a teratogenic effect, some viral diseases which are char-

acterized by respiratory symptoms may. Brown and Evans have found a significant increase in congenital heart lesions in the infants of mothers who had Coxsackie virus B, types 3 and 4 infections during pregnancy.

Pneumonia. Pneumonia is far less serious since the development of the antibiotic drugs than it was in the past, but when it does occur during pregnancy, it may prove fatal to the mother or her fetus. The bacteria most often responsible are pneumococcus, *Streptococcus hemolyticus, Staphylococcus aureus,* and *Klebsiella pneumoniae.* The choice of an antibiotic should be determined by the responsible organisms. Material should be obtained for culture before a decision is made, but treatment cannot be withheld until the results are available. If a Gram stain of the sputum reveals large numbers of gram-positive cocci, the infection probably will respond to adequate doses of penicillin or the broad-spectrum antibiotics. If the bacteria are mostly gram negative, penicillin probably will be ineffective.

Pneumococcus pneumonia will usually respond to 600,000 units of penicillin given every 3 or 4 hours or to chloramphenicol, 500 mg. every 6 hours for 24 hours and 250 mg. every 6 hours thereafter. For staphylococcus pneumonia the dosage of penicillin should be at least 10 million units daily combined with chloramphenicol as just decribed.

Since intrauterine death occurs as a result of anoxia as well as the infection, oxygen should be administered to the mother if she is cyanotic.

Influenza. During the 1918 influenza pandemic the total maternal mortality was 27% (50% in those who also developed pneumonia), and the infant mortality was 26% (52% if the mother also had pneumonia).

Chemotherapeutic agents have no effect upon the influenza virus, but they will reduce the severity of the complications.

Asian influenza. Gravid women appear to contract Asian influenza more frequently than do those who are not pregnant, and the infection is more severe. Fifty percent of the women of childbearing age who died of Asian influenza and its complications in Minnesota during the 1957 epidemic were pregnant, and the deaths accounted for 19% of the maternal mortality for that year. All had fulminating pneumonitis, many dying within 24 hours of the onset of symptoms. Treatment was ineffective. There was no evidence to suggest that the fetus was affected.

Measles (rubeola). Measles probably do not cause congenital defects, but they do increase the incidence of abortion and premature labor. The infant may be infected in utero and may even be born with a typical rash or develop it during the first few days of life.

Rubella (German measles). Gregg reported a high incidence of congenital defects in the eyes of infants whose mothers had contracted rubella during early pregnancy. Swan later calculated that 74.4% of infants would develop a congenital malformation if the maternal infection occurred during the first 4 months of pregnancy.

Siegel and Greenberg studied the effect of rubella on 180 women who were pregnant during epidemics of rubella and in 114 in whom the infection occurred sporadically. About one half of the patients who were infected during the first 8 weeks of pregnancy aborted, and about 20% aborted during the next 4 weeks. Only an occasional fetal death occurred after the first trimester. Of the infants whose mothers were infected during the first 8 weeks of pregnancy in epidemic years, 5 out of 16 were born with major congenital anomalies. None occurred after infections during the same period of pregnancy in nonepidemic years.

Rendle-Short, reporting on 200 women who had rubella during pregnancy, calculated the incidence of fetal anomalies to be 60% if the infection occurred between 1 and 4 weeks after the onset of the last menstrual period, 35% between 5 and 8 weeks, 15% between 9 and 12 weeks, and 7% between 13 and 16 weeks. Congenital heart lesions accounted for almost 50% of the defects if the infection occurred between the fifth and the eighth weeks. About 30% of the lesions involved the eyes. The rubella syndrome has also been observed in infants of mothers who had no clinical evidence of infection but who were pregnant during rubella epidemics.

It now appears that congenital defects alone are not the only result of intrauterine rubella. Early abortion, fetal death, and premature delivery rates are all significantly increased. Many babies whose mothers have had rubella during pregnancy are born alive with active infection, "the extended rubella syndrome," which is characterized by various combinations of purpura, thrombocytopenia, hepatosplenomegaly, jaundice, pneumonitis, encephalitis, and ocular and cardiac defects. Many of these babies die during the first few months of life, and those who survive longer may have active viral infection. The rubella virus has been cultured from affected infants as long as 18 months after birth. Such infants obviously are a potential source of infection for susceptible pregnant women.

Children of mothers who acquire rubella after the first trimester may also be affected. Hardy and co-workers studied 22 children of mothers who had rubella between the thirteenth and thirty-first weeks of pregnancy and found only 7 to be normal. Seven of the others have some degree of mental or motor retardation, 4 have cardiac murmurs, and others have findings typical of the extended rubella syndrome.

Therapeutic abortion is justifiable whenever unquestioned rubella is contracted during the first twenty weeks after the onset of the last menstrual period unless the woman and her husband are willing to accept the risk of the infant's being affected.

If the physician is to approve a request for termination, he must be certain that the patient actually had rubella. This may be difficult because the clinical course is much like that of several other viral infections. Serologic tests for rubella antibody have been developed and will soon be generally available. If maternal blood tested during the acute illness contains no antibody, but the level is high 2 weeks later, the physician can be certain of the diagnosis, and abortion can be considered if it is appropriate. If antibodies already are present or do not appear after the illness, the physician can conclude that the patient did not have rubella.

Gamma globulin has been given in an attempt to prevent infection after exposure or to modify the course of the disease. Its use often only obscures the issue because it may prevent only the rash without affecting the viremia and fetal involvement. Gamma globulin should not be given, even with definite exposure. If infection does not occur, nothing need be done; if rubella develops, abortion can be considered.

Rubella will undoubtedly become an unusual complication of pregnancy because an effective vaccine is now available and will eventually be used extensively. Sever and co-workers tested 500 pregnant women for rubella antibodies and found only 7.8% without it. A test for rubella antibody might well be included in the premarital or prepregnancy examination so that those who are not protected can be identified and immunized before they conceive.

Smallpox. Smallpox occurs only rarely. The infant can acquire the disease in utero. Pregnant women probably can be vaccinated without disturbing fetal development during the last half of pregnancy, but it is wise to avoid vaccination during early pregnancy because the resulting viremia could interfere with fetal tissue differentiation.

Chickenpox. The pregnant woman who develops chickenpox may be seriously ill with the disease and may die from the complications. The infant can be infected in utero. Fish reported 4 deaths, all from diffuse bilateral interstitial pneumonia.

Scarlet fever. The serious effects of scarlet fever can be reduced by the early administration of penicillin, but abortion occurs frequently. Because the infecting organism is a hemolytic streptococcus, infected women should not be treated or delivered in an obstetric unit.

Mumps. Hyatt found approximately a 15% incidence of abortion and fetal death and a similar incidence of congenital anomalies in the infants of 94 pregnant women with mumps (4 of his own patients and 90 collected from the literature). St. Geme, Noren, and Adams found positive mumps skin-test reactions in 13 of 14 children with primary endocardial fibroelastosis, but they were unable to detect a similar response when mumps-virus neutralizing antibody titers were measured. They conclude that there may be a relationship between intrauterine mumps-virus infection and endocardial fibroelastosis.

Whooping cough. Pertussis is rare in adults. If the mother has pertussis at the time she delivers, the child should be isolated from her until she is no longer infectious.

Typhoid fever. Typhoid fever is uncommon in the United States, but if it does occur, it can be treated with chloramphenicol, 500 mg. every 3 hours until the fever has subsided and then every 6 hours until the cultures are negative.

Cytomegalic inclusion body disease. Cytomegalic inclusion body disease is caused by a virus that is transmitted to the infant from a presumably well mother. It often is fatal. If the child does survive, it may be mentally retarded. The characteristic inclusion bodies are often best seen in microscopic sections of the kidney. The disease may also be diagnosed by finding the same structures in the urine.

Herpes simplex. Disseminated herpes simplex may develop in infants born of mothers with active genital herpetic lesions. The infant probably is infected by direct contact during delivery. The virus may also reach the infant in utero if the membranes are ruptured and possibly by transplacental transmission, even though the amniotic sac is intact. Nahmias, Josey, and Naib have suggested that if the mother develops primary or recurrent herpetic infection 3 weeks or more before delivery, the infant probably will have been immunized by antibodies which reached it through the placenta. In this event vaginal delivery might be appropriate. If the infection occurred less than 3 weeks before delivery, the infant would have no protection and undoubtedly would contract the infection during labor and delivery. In this event elective cesarean section in the interests of the baby would be justified unless the membranes already had ruptured.

Coxsackie virus disease. Sporadic cases of lethal Coxsackie virus disease in newborn infants have been described. The mother may have had only a mild respiratory infection, but as mentioned under the discussion of upper respiratory diseases, the infant might be in danger of developing a congenital heart lesion.

Toxoplasmosis. The protozoa causing toxoplasmosis can be transmitted to the fetus from a mother who shows no signs of the condition. The infant may die in utero or deliver prematurely; the death rate in premature infants is high. Most affected infants have chorioretinitis, and many have psychomotor retardation or cerebral calcification. Toxoplasmosis usually is not repeated in pregnancies after the birth of an affected infant.

■ Chronic infectious diseases

Pulmonary tuberculosis. Pulmonary tuberculosis complicates at least 2% of all pregnancies, but the frequency with which it is encountered varies with the type of patient. It is especially common in women of the poorest socioeconomic classes. It is important that the infection be diagnosed in order that the mother may be treated and that the infant as well as the mother's contacts can be protected.

Pregnancy has little effect upon pulmonary tuberculosis if the patient and her infection can be managed properly, but the outlook is different if the lesion is unrecognized and if the mother is not treated during pregnancy and after delivery.

The *maternal mortality* is determined primarily by the extent of the lesion rather than by the fact that the patient is pregnant. In those with minimal involvement the risk is slight; with advanced lesions the mortality may be 50% or more but is similar to the death rate in nongravid women with comparable lesions.

Diagnosis. Physical examination alone is inadequate for the detection of all cases of pulmonary tuberculosis, even though the lesion is active and relatively advanced. A chest x-ray examination should be included in the initial examination of prenatal patients in whom a high incidence of pulmonary tuberculosis can be anticipated.

Treatment. Ideally a chest x-ray examination should be given to all women who apply for prepregnancy evaluation. If there is a small, active tuberculous lesion, pregnancy should be delayed until it has been treated and is inactive. Those known to have pulmonary lesions ought also to be examined. If the lesion is small and inactive, the patient should be a reasonably good risk for pregnancy, provided that she can be treated adequately both during the period of gestation and after delivery. Women with advanced lesions should often be discouraged from ever becoming pregnant.

Treatment of the tuberculosis during pregnancy need not differ from that in nonpregnant individuals. Para-aminosalicylic acid, streptomycin, and isoniazid can be used safely, and as far as is known, none of these drugs has a deleterious effect on the infant. Collapse by pneumothorax or by thoracoplasty and lobectomy or pneumonectomy can be performed whenever it is necessary. In some instances, however, the pulmonary reserve is reduced to a dangerously low level in pregnant women in whom pneumonectomy has been performed.

Management during labor. There is no need to induce labor because of pulmonary tuberculosis, but certain precautions are necessary during labor and delivery.

SEDATION. Analgesics can be administered to relieve pain, but the patient should not be narcotized. Caudal or epidural analgesia can be used to advantage in relieving pain during labor.

DELIVERY. Low forceps delivery to eliminate the perineal phase of labor should be considered for many women with pulmonary tuberculosis. This will prevent the increased intrapulmonary pressure and possible dissemination of infection that may result from violent voluntary bearing-down efforts. If the patient is a multipara whose labor has progressed rapidly and who can be expected to deliver with one or two contractions, operative extraction is unnecessary. Difficult operative deliveries should be avoided whenever possible, and blood loss must be kept at a minimum.

The indications for cesarean section can be extended somewhat in women with pulmonary tuberculosis. Schaeffer reported a mortality of 33.3% in women with far-advanced lesions who were delivered by cesarean section; in another group with comparable lesions who were delivered vaginally the mortality was 63.1%. He suggests that abdominal delivery should be considered for almost all women with advanced pulmonary tuberculosis except multiparas whose previous labors have been short and normal. Cesarean section should be considered whenever labor is prolonged because of cephalopelvic disproportion or an abnormal mechanism and for unusual fetal positions, such as brow or face.

Therapeutic abortion. Schaeffer and Epstein found the death rate in 63 women who were aborted because of tuberculosis to be higher than that in 407 infected patients who were delivered at term. They conclude that therapeutic termination of pregnancy is rarely necessary. This certainly is true of women who can be treated adequately, particularly when the lesion is small and stationary, but there are circumstances under which abortion may be indicated. If a tuberculous woman with several children and a home to manage without help must add the burden of the complete care of a new baby to her responsibilities, the lesion is almost certain to advance or to be reactivated. If she can be hospitalized and treated and if her children can be cared for adequately, there is probably no justification for terminating the pregnancy on medical grounds, but usually facilities for the treatment of such a patient and for the care of her family are not available. Under such circumstances therapeutic abortion and tubal ligation are warranted. In a few other women with actively progressing fresh lesions that have not yet been treated or those with far-advanced or terminal disease, termination of early pregnancy may be considered.

Care of the infant. Tubercles are often found in the placenta, but intrauterine infection of infants of tuberculous mothers is unusual. In almost every instance the baby is infected by contact with the mother after delivery. Consequently the baby and the mother should be separated immediately after birth, and contact should be prohibited until it seems certain that the mother is not infectious. Nursing, of course, should be prohibited.

Bronchiectasis. Bronchiectasis is seldom encountered in association with pregnancy, but occasionally both may occur in the same patient. If a considerable amount of lung tissue is involved, pulmonary insufficiency may develop during late pregnancy and the patient may become dyspneic or even cyanotic. Postural drainage and chemotherapy and antibiotic therapy can be continued throughout pregnancy, but surgical procedures should be delayed until after delivery whenever possible. The management of labor and delivery is similar to that for patients with pulmonary tuberculosis.

Syphilis. Syphilis may be present in from 10% to 20% of women registering in prenatal clinics, but it is seldom encountered in private practice. In the past a large proportion of the total infant loss was caused by syphilis, but today severe intrauterine fetal infection is seldom encountered.

Pregnancy alters the course of early syphilis somewhat, probably because of the increased tissue vascularity. The primary lesion, which may be on the external genitals but which usually escapes notice because it is located in the vagina, often is large. Secondary skin lesions may not be obvious, but condylomas develop frequently.

The effect on the infant is determined in part by the age of the infection. If the syphilis has recently been acquired and is active, the child is almost certain to be affected and may die in utero or be born prematurely. If the infection is old and inactive, the infant may escape the disease completely. If the infection has been acquired shortly before delivery, the infant may be entirely normal unless it is inoculated from local primary or secondary lesions in the birth canal. In this event its initial blood serologic reaction may be negative, and evidences of infection may not appear for several weeks.

Syphilis rarely causes early abortion. The placenta is relatively impervious to spirochetes during the first half of pregnancy; consequently the fetus at this time is normal. Spirochetes have been recovered from fetal tissues during the fourth month, but they rarely can be found before the eighteenth week.

Diagnosis. Almost every case of syphilis, except those that are still in the seronegative phase, can be diagnosed by determining the blood serologic reaction. This should be part of every prenatal examination. The disease may be acquired during pregnancy; therefore, even though the screening test was negative, it should be repeated in high-risk patients during the final weeks.

Any open lesion of the genital tract during pregnancy should be studied by dark-field examination as well as by the usual bacterial cultures and biopsy.

Treatment. An adequate course of treatment started during the first half of pregnancy will afford almost complete protection for the infant. Regardless of the duration of pregnancy, however, treatment should be started as soon as the diagnosis is established. Even though the infant is already infected, its disease can be controlled and further damage prevented by treating the mother.

Most pregnant women with syphilis can be treated successfully with procaine penicillin G in oil with 2% aluminum monostearate. The first injection is 2.4 million units, and two subsequent ones of 1.2 million units each are given at intervals of 2 to 4 days for a total dosage of 4.8 million units. Aqueous penicillin, 600,000 units daily for a total dosage of 4.8 million units, or a single injection of benzathine penicillin G, 2.4 million units, may also be used successfully. The husband should also be examined and treated if he is infected.

The mother's serologic reaction may still be positive at delivery even though the infection has been eradicated. The baby's serologic reaction may also be positive at birth because the antibodies cross the placenta freely. The physician should not treat a newborn infant simply because of positive serologic reaction. If the test remains strongly positive for more than 3 or 4 weeks, if the titer remains constant or increases, or if there is unequivocal x-ray evidence of osteochondritis or periostitis in the infant, treatment should be started.

The baby should be isolated until it is proved to be free from infection. There is no reason why a mother with syphilis should not nurse her child; the organisms are not transmitted in the breast milk.

If syphilis has been treated with an adequate dosage of penicillin and if the infection has responded properly, retreatment during subsequent pregnancies is probably unnecessary. If the serologic reaction remains positive or if there is any suggestion of activity, a course of treatment should be advised during each subsequent pregnancy.

Malaria. Intrauterine infection of the fetus with malaria is rare because the parasites do not often cross the placenta. Quinine and other antimalarial drugs can be administered without hesitation to pregnant women.

References

Abramowitz, L. J.: Effect of Asian influenza on pregnancy, S. Afr. Med. J. 2:1155, 1958.
Alford, C. A., Neva, F. A., and Weller, T. H.: Virologic and serologic studies on human products of conception after maternal rubella, New Eng. J. Med. 271:1275, 1964.
Brown, G. C., and Evans, T. N.: Serologic evidence of Coxsackievirus etiology of congenital heart disease, J.A.M.A. 199:183, 1967.
Corner, G. W., Jr., and Nesbitt, R. E. L., Jr.:
Pregnancy and pulmonary resection, Amer. J. Obstet. Gynec. 68:903, 1954.
Dippel, A. L.: The relationship of congenital syphilis to abortion and miscarriage and the mechanisms of intrauterine protection, Amer. J. Obstet. Gynec. 47:369, 1944.
Fish, S. A.: Maternal death due to disseminated varicella, J.A.M.A. 173:978, 1960.
Forssner, H.: The relationship between pregnancy and tuberculosis, Acta Obstet. Gynec. Scand. 3:256, 1925.
Gregg, N. M.: Further observations on congenital defects in infants following maternal rubella, Trans. Ophthal. Soc. Aust. 4:119, 1946.
Hardy, J. B., Monif, G. R. G., and Sever, J. L.: Studies in congenital rubella, Baltimore 1964-65. II. Clinical and virologic, Bull. Hopkins Hosp. 118:97, 1966.
Hardy, J. B., McCracken, G. H., Gilkeson, M. R., and Sever, J. L.: Adverse fetal outcome following maternal rubella after the first trimester of pregnancy, J.A.M.A. 207:2414, 1969.
Hopwood, H. G.: Pneumonia in pregnancy, Obstet. Gynec. 25:875, 1965.
Hyatt, H. W.: Relationship of maternal mumps to congenital defects and fetal deaths, and to maternal morbidity and mortality, Amer. Pract. 12:359, 1961.
Nahmias, A. J., Josey, W. E., and Naib, Z. M.: Neonatal herpes simplex infection, J.A.M.A. 199:132, 1967.
Packer, A. D.: Influence of maternal measles (Morbilli) on unborn child, Med. J. Aust. 1:835, 1950.
Phillips, C. A., Melnick, J. L., Yow, M. D., Bayatpour, M., and Burkhardt, M.: Persistence of virus in infants with congenital rubella and in normal infants with a history of maternal rubella, J.A.M.A. 193:111, 1965.
Pineda, R. G., Desmond, M. M., Rudolph, A. J., Halleen, W., Rawls, W., and Ziai, M. H.: Impact of the 1964 rubella epidemic on a clinic population, Amer. J. Obstet. Gynec. 100:1139, 1968.
Plotkin, S. A.: Virologic assistance in the management of German measles during pregnancy, J.A.M.A. 194:105, 1964.
Rendle-Short, J.: Maternal rubella; the practical management of a case, Lancet 2:373, 1964.
Schaeffer, G.: Tuberculosis in obstetrics and gynecology, Boston, 1956, Little, Brown & Co.
Sever, J. L., Fuccillo, D. A., Gilkeson, M. R., Ley, A., and Traub, R.: Changing susceptibility to rubella, Obstet. Gynec. 32:365, 1968.
Siegel, M., and Greenberg, M.: Fetal death, malformation and prematurity after maternal rubella, New Eng. J. Med. 262:389, 1960.
St. Geme, J. W., Jr., Noren, G. R., and Adams, P., Jr.: Proposed embryopathic relation between mumps virus and primary endocardial fibroelastosis, New Eng. J. Med. 275:339, 1966.
Swan, C.: Rubella in pregnancy, an etiologic factor in congenital malformations, stillbirths, miscarriages, and abortions, J. Obstet. Gynaec. Brit. Comm. 56:591, 1949.

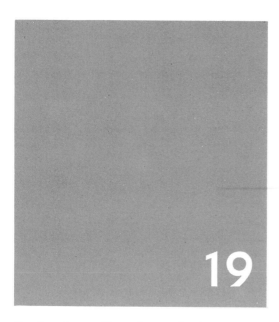

19

Endocrine disorders during pregnancy

Physiologic alterations in secretions of the endocrine glands are so essential to the reproductive process that even minor abnormalities in pituitary, ovarian, thyroid, placental, or other hormone production may seriously affect fertility, nidation, or the maintenance of pregnancy.

Diagnosis and management of endocrine disorders in pregnancy are often difficult. Fortunately, more precise methods are being made available for isolation of hormones, for quantitative determination of their circulatory levels, and for measurement of their urinary metabolites. Even so, it is increasingly evident that the blood or urine concentration of hormone is only one of several important guides. Normal endocrine function depends not only upon the secretory activity of a given gland but also upon the feedback effect of one hormone as opposed to another, the mechanism for transport in the circula-

tion, the response of the target organ, and the enzyme activities influencing the cellular response.

■ Diabetes mellitus

The steady increase in the number of patients with diabetes complicating pregnancy during the past three decades is the result of (1) insulin therapy, (2) recognition of obstetric problems peculiar to diabetic mothers, and (3) the hereditary tendency of the disease. In the preinsulin era the reproductive potentialities of women with diabetes were incredibly poor. Menstrual disturbances were common, and sterility was the rule. The maternal mortality rate in the few patients who did conceive was 25% to 30%, and the fetal loss was as high as 60% to 70%. At present the perinatal mortality rate ranges from 10% to 30% in clinics throughout the United States. The danger to the mother, although reduced, is still slightly increased over the normal.

Incidence. The investigation of Pincus and White indicates that diabetes is transmitted through mendelian recessive genes. With the outcome of pregnancy in diabetic women becoming more regularly successful, an increasing frequency of this complication must be expected in the future. The incidence of frank diabetes is now about 1 to 300 deliveries. Total screening of all prenatal patients reveals a much higher incidence of a latent disorder. O'Sullivan screened 20,070 pregnancies and found abnormalities in carbohydrate tolerance that met the criteria for diagnosis of gestational diabetes in 1 in 116 prenatal registrants. Progression to frank diabetes occurred in 28.5% of these patients within 5½ years.

Diagnosis. Pregnancy may precipitate rapid onset of diabetic symptoms, leading to acidosis in a previously unknown diabetic patient. Consequently the presence of reducing substances in the urine of gravid women should be regarded as abnormal unless proved otherwise. Lactosuria is rare until the last few weeks of pregnancy, but it is not uncommon after delivery. Lowering of the renal threshold for sugar does occur during pregnancy and may account for many cases of recurrent glycosuria, but this can be ascertained only by determination of blood sugar levels. Fasting values for true blood glucose exceeding 110 mg./100 ml. or values exceeding 170 mg./100 ml. 2 hours after ingestion of 100 Gm. of glucose are diagnostic of a diabetic state.

Influence of pregnancy upon diabetes. Metabolic control is more difficult during pregnancy. *Vomiting* disturbs chemical balance, and acidosis may develop with little warning. *Lowering of the renal threshold for glucose* is variable; a large amount of sugar may be excreted even though the blood sugar concentration is only slightly elevated; hence urine tests for sugar may fail to provide an accurate index upon which to base insulin dosage. *Carbohydrate tolerance is altered,* but the direction and the degree of change is unpredictable. As a rule, glucose tolerance is reduced in the latter half of pregnancy. In relatively few patients the status is unchanged or improved.

Insulin requirements are increased in approximately 70% of our patients, beginning about the twenty-fourth week of gestation. Speculations regarding the mechanism by which this diabetic challenge is evoked have been logically focused on the hormonal changes of pregnancy, although the emphasis on specific endocrine factors has shifted. Until recently, increased levels of adrenocorticosteroid hormone, thyroxin, and growth hormone were considered the factors chiefly responsible. New techniques that permit more discriminating studies of fetoplacental function indicate that the conceptus is specifically implicated. Anabolic and diabetogenic properties of a lactogenic growth hormone–like substance (HPL) are now well recognized. Contrainsulin effects of HPL and, in addition, active degradation of insulin by placental proteolysis may well account for the increased insulin demands of pregnancy.

Evidence for placental degradation of insulin is clear-cut. Freinkel and Goodner localized a proteolytic enzyme (insulinase) in the soluble cytoplasm of placental elements and demonstrated its ability to cleave insulin into constituent peptide and amino acid residues. Inactivation or increased destruction of insulin is only part of the picture. It now appears that human placental lactogen (HPL) plays a key role in the metabolic adjustments of pregnancy. The actions of HPL are similar but not identical to those of human growth hormone (HGH). In fact Grumbach and co-workers have designated HPL as the chorionic growth hormone-prolactin (CGP), or the "growth hormone" of the second half of pregnancy. Large amounts of HPL secreted by the syncytiotrophoblast pass unidirectionally into the maternal circulation. Minimal amounts are transferred to the fetus. In the maternal circulation, then, the concentration of HPL is high and that of HGH is relatively low, whereas in the fetal circulation the situation is reversed and fetal HGH is high and the concentration of HPL is low. The two hormones act synergistically to promote growth, and both HPL and HGH stimulate release of free fatty acids, but certain of their biologic properties are quite different. Whereas hypoglycemia induces a rise in serum HGH and hyperglycemia induces a fall, the secretion of HPL remains fairly constant, showing little if any fluctuation with oral intake.

Based on these facts the following sequence of events can be presumed to take place during pregnancy. The rise in plasma free fatty acids (FFA) is HPL-induced. In normal pregnancy, mobilization of fat stores provides an alternate pathway of metabolism so that the needs of the conceptus for glucose and gluconeogenic precursors can be met. Elevated FFA acts as a specific peripheral antagonist to insulin in normal gravid women, but in diabetic mothers insulin resistance is exaggerated. This hypothesis is particularly convincing in light of known biochemical changes in normal and diabetic pregnancies. In normal pregnant women, fasting glucose levels are approximately 20 mg./100 ml. lower than in nonpregnant subjects, a reflection of the increased glucose space and the mandate of the fetus, in addition to the maternal brain, for glucose. A decrease in peripheral utilization of glucose is demonstrable in diminution of the normal degree of hypophosphatemia after an intravenous glucose load. Plasma FFA levels are considerably elevated in the maternal circulation during late pregnancy, whereas fetal plasma FFA levels are low. Concurrently an increase in maternal insulin resistance is clearly evident in lower reactivity to both insulin and tolbutamide tests.

Reduction in insulin requirements after delivery is the usual pattern because the contrainsulin effects of hormones and placental destruction are halted abruptly. Hypoglycemic shock occurs more often in the immediate postpartum period than at any other time in pregnancy. This reaction can be prevented by appropriate reduction in insulin dosage and by frequent chemical and clinical observations.

Influence of diabetes upon pregnancy. The adverse effects of diabetes upon pregnancy can be greatly reduced but not entirely prevented by good chemical control. Maternal *acidosis* is frequently disastrous to the fetus. Although chemical derangement may occur at any stage, particularly if vomiting or infection develops, it is most common during the last half of pregnancy when insulin demands are increased. Jones regards acidosis as the major cause (40%) of fetal loss but at the same time the most preventable. *Water balance* is readily disturbed. Both fetal and maternal edema are common complications. *Hydramnios* occurs in 10% of diabetic mothers—an incidence twenty times that observed in nondiabetic mothers. The incidence of *toxemia* may be as high as 50% but can be kept much lower by improved care, including dietary sodium restriction and judicious timing of delivery. The risk to the mother with severe diabetes is greatly increased if vascular sclerosis or renal damage already exists. Fetal loss associated with toxemia per se is increased in diabetic pregnancies.

The harmful effects of diabetes may be demonstrable in the fetus of the patient exhibiting the earliest manifestations of the disease. *Excessive size of the infant* is so common a finding that unrecognized maternal diabetes should be suspected in patients who deliver babies weighing over 9 pounds. Infants of diabetic mothers present a typical appearance that Hoet aptly describes as "Cushing-like" because of the distribution of fat and the edema. In addition, there is an actual increase in both splanchnic and somatic growth. The cause for macrosomia in the infant of a diabetic mother is as yet unproved. Bergquist believes that it may well be related to an increased insulin production by the fetus acting independently or in synergism with fetal growth hormone. Insulin per se is capable of promoting growth in experimental animals, and *hyperplasia of the islets of Langerhans* is a consistent finding in postmortem examinations of affected infants. The combination of increased HGH common to all newborns and the fetal islet cell hyperplasia with significant hyperinsulin response to glucose, characteristic of the newborn infant of a diabetic mother, bears certain similarities to the situation found in studies of growth hormone and serum insulin levels demonstrated by Karam, Grodsky, and Forsham in obese subjects. Insulin antibodies have been found in the umbilical cord blood of diabetic offspring but not in the infants of normal controls. Spellacy and Goetz showed that an abnormal amount of I^{131} insulin is bound by the serum of newborn infants of insulin-dependent diabetic mothers and that the antibody disappears from the child's blood by approximately 3 months of age. The antibody appears to be passively transferred to the fetus. According to Vallance-Owen and Lilley an insulin antagonist, polypeptide in nature and linked with the albumin fraction of plasma protein, inhibits the uptake of glucose by muscle. According to Lowy and associates, this antagonist does not inhibit uptake of glucose by adipose tissue. Vallance-Owen postulated that because of its low molecular weight this substance may pass the maternal barrier and may account for the weak condition and fat habitus of the infant of the mother with either overt or latent diabetes. Goodner and Freinkel found that I^{131} insulin is transported across the rat placenta in small amounts. In the human, insulin does not freely pass the placental barrier, and therefore it is unlikely that the increased fetal insulinogenesis is of much significance to the diabetes of the mother. On the contrary, glucose is readily transferred, and thus hyperglycemia in the mother probably serves as an important stimulus for pancreatic islet cell hyperplasia in the fetus. Hyaline membrane disease occurs more commonly in the infant of a diabetic mother than in the infant of a comparable gestational age born of a nondiabetic mother.

Stillbirth and *neonatal death rates* are increased early in the course of maternal disease. The risk of intrauterine fetal death rises sharply after the thirty-sixth week. Prediction of impending fetal death is extremely difficult if not impossible on a clinical basis. Reduction of fetal activity may be noted by the mother, but this is not infallible evidence. Serial 24-hour urinary estriol excretion rates are now used as an objective means of assessing placental function and fetal well-being. High values in excess of 12 mg./24 hr. are reassuring in almost all cases of pregnancies of diabetic women except those in whom Rh isoimmunization exists as an added complication. Falling values require prompt reassessment of clinical and laboratory findings because, in general, the life of the fetus is threatened when values fall 50% or more below their previous levels. Other indices of fetoplacental function that show promise of serving as guides to the conduct of late pregnancy and delivery include serial plasma or amniotic fluid estriol, diamine oxidase level, or HPL level. These are discussed in Chapter 10.

The newborn infant who becomes ill in the neonatal period exhibits characteristic signs of diabetic embryopathy. At birth the baby frequently appears normal except for edema, but within an hour or two, hypotonia (a change in muscle tone or reflexes) develops, respirations become rapid (over 60 per minute), periorbital cyanosis appears, and a tendency toward bleeding may be noted by slight ooze from the cord or petechial hemorrhages in the skin. The infant may convulse. The cause of this disturbance is the subject of considerable controversy. Reardon and others have demonstrated two consistent alterations in blood chemical constituents in live-born infants who subsequently became ill: acidosis at birth, as evidenced by low pH and high P_{CO_2} in umbilical arterial blood, and hypoglycemia at 2 to 4 hours after birth that is more profound and more persistent than the hypoglycemia common to infants of normal mothers.

Stimmler and co-workers found significantly higher concentrations of plasma immunoreactive insulin in infants of diabetic mothers than in those of normal women. They also noted that increased insulinogenesis is associated with the early onset of hypoglycemia.

The occurrence of *congenital anomalies* is approximately six times the normal. Defects are not selective of any particular body system and are not necessarily incompatible with life. In Taylor's opinion the high rate of anomalies is related to inadequate diabetic control in the early weeks of pregnancy, since maternal acidosis of even mild degree provides an unfavorable environment for the developing fetus.

Management. The principles for successful management of diabetic mothers must include good control of the metabolic disturbance, early and adequate treatment of obstetric complications, removal of the fetus from an abnormal environment at a time optimal for survival, and special care of the newborn infant after delivery.

Study of each patient early in pregnancy, best conducted in the hospital, should include the laboratory tests essential to metabolic regulation and those necessary for detection of cardiovascular or renal disease. The blood pressure record, 24-hour urine protein determination, and funduscopic examination are requisite base-line studies of the vascular system. Electrocardiographic study is indicated when evidence of vascular disease is found or in any case of long-standing diabetes. Renal function tests are mandatory in women with kidney disease because the prognosis is determined in large measure by the ability of the kidney to respond to the demands of pregnancy. The outlook for the diabetic patient with severe renal damage is so unfavorable that termination of pregnancy is advisable. All prenatal patients with diabetes should be examined by the obstetrician and the internist at least every 2 weeks during the first half of pregnancy and weekly thereafter.

Diet. Total caloric allowance must be adjusted in accordance with the patient's nutritional status. For those of ideal weight, 1,800 to 2,000 calories per day usually permits a normal controlled gain throughout pregnancy. A daily intake of approximately 1,200 calories may be safely used in the obese diabetic patient without compromising the required protein intake of 1.5 grams per kilogram of standard body weight. An example of such a diet is 90 grams of protein, 50 grams of fat, and 100 grams of carbohydrate, but ketosis must be avoided. The necessary caloric energy is derived partially from maternal fat depots. For the patient of average weight the distribution is in the range of 100 grams of protein, 75 to 80 grams of fat, and 200 grams of carbohydrate. Supplementary vitamin and mineral preparations should be prescribed with these diets. Sodium intake should be restricted to 1 to 2 grams in all diabetic diets during pregnancy.

Insulin. It is of utmost importance to maintain a blood sugar concentration at as nearly normal levels as possible throughout pregnancy. Even the mildly diabetic patient whose fasting blood sugar is maintained within the normal range by strict adherence to diet but whose 2-hour postprandial value exceeds 150 mg./100 ml. should be given sufficient insulin to achieve a physiologic level. The patient should check urine samples daily for the presence of acetone as well as sugar and report for blood sugar determinations on the morning of each office visit.

Hormones. The value of hormone therapy remains the most controversial aspect of the management of diabetic pregnancies. Nelson, Gillespie, and White administer estrogen and progesterone in gradually increasing dosage throughout pregnancy to patients with all but the mildest form of diabetes. These authors consider substitutional therapy an important aid in improving fetal salvage. In their series, which included a high percentage of patients in whom the diabetes was at an advanced stage, the fetal loss was 10%. Results achieved by other investigators whose regimen did not include the use of hormones are as follows: Reis and associates reported a 13.6% fetal loss; Pedowitz and Shlevin, 8.2%. Whether good results obtained without hormone therapy could be further improved by the use of these preparations still remains to be proved.

Delivery. All patients with overt diabetes should be admitted to the hospital at the thirty-second to thirty-fourth week of pregnancy. Daily observations and adjustments in diet and insulin dosage can prevent many mishaps common to the late stages of diabetic pregnancy. Optimal timing of delivery is the critical issue. Since the risk of intrauterine death rises sharply as gestation approaches term, delivery is advisable by about the thirty-seventh week in the patient with otherwise uncomplicated symptoms. On the other hand many babies have been lost due to hyaline membrane disease when delivery has been carried out needlessly early. A number of objective guides are now available to determine fetal maturity (Chapter 17).

The threat to the fetus is greatly increased at any stage of pregnancy if the diabetes is complicated by maternal acidosis, toxemia, progressive hypertension, proteinuria, or hydramnios. If these disturbances cannot be controlled and if the gestation period is over 33 weeks, termination of pregnancy is likely to prove more rewarding than a further conservative course of treatment. Under such circumstances the harmful effects upon the fetus in utero are greater than the hazards of prematurity. This is a serious decision. It is in connection with these problems that serial estriol determinations have proved a valuable aid, particularly when estriol values remain within the normal range and unduly early termination of the pregnancy is thereby prevented. On the other hand, a precipitous fall in estriol levels reinforces the clinical decision to intervene.

Vaginal delivery may be both difficult and dangerous because of the size and fragility of the infant and the need for early intervention. Delivery by the normal route is feasible if the diabetes is uncomplicated, if the pelvis is normal, if the size of the infant is not excessive, and if the cervix is favorable for induction. *Cesarean section* is indicated if the disease is severe, if pregnancy complications exist, if induction is unsuccessful, or if the progress in labor is poor. Respiratory distress is the most frequent as well as the most serious problem in the newborn infant. For this reason *regional anesthesia* is preferable, and narcotics should be withheld until the baby is delivered.

Readjustment of insulin dosage is necessary during labor, delivery, and the puerperium, when wide fluctuations are inevitable. This can be accomplished by substituting regular insulin for long-acting preparations or by modifying the dosage of depot insulin. In our experience the following program is most satisfactory. Because of the reduced insulin requirement that follows delivery the patient receives only one half to two thirds of the usual dose of depot insulin on the day of delivery. Intravenous glucose in water is administered to replace the carbohydrate equivalent of the diet. At the time of delivery the concentration of glucose is raised from 5% to 10% to further preclude the possibility of hypoglycemia. Adjustments in insulin dosage after delivery are made principally on the basis of daily blood glucose determinations. In addition, urine samples are checked for sugar and acetone four times daily in order to detect unexpected fluctuations promptly.

Subsequent course. Despite the difficulties encountered during the course of pregnancy and the immediate puerperium, frank maternal diabetes is generally not worsened by the pregnancy. Furthermore, a previous intrauterine or neonatal loss should not discourage the mother from attempting another pregnancy unless her diabetes is complicated by cardiovascular renal disease. Although perinatal losses may be repeated, meticulous management of the prenatal course, early delivery, and skillful care of the newborn infant can provide the diabetic mother with a reasonably good prognosis.

Management of the newborn infant. Infants of diabetic mothers are often of necessity subjected to the cumulative effects of prematurity, delivery by cesarean section, and acidosis and hypoglycemia. Since the incidence of hyaline membrane disease is increased, every effort should be made to prevent or reduce respiratory distress. Treatment begins at delivery and consists of aspiration of mucus and other material from the respiratory passages, administration of oxygen, removal of the gastric contents by suction through a small rubber catheter, and transfer to an isolette with oxygen inflow of 40 to 50 vol.%, humidity of 55% saturation, and incubator temperature that does not exceed 85° F.

Pedersen in Denmark and Pedowitz and Shlevin in the United States fast all infants of diabetic mothers for 24 to 48 hours. Reis and associates offer a few drops of 50% glucose in water by dropper every 30 minutes if clinical evidence of hypoglycemia is observed. Carrington, Reardon, and Shuman demonstrated good results in critically ill infants after the administration of 5% glucose in 0.45 gram% saline solution, with a total fluid intake of 30 ml. per pound per 24 hours.

■ Subclinical diabetes

The concept of a prediabetic state stems from the fact that women who subsequently develop diabetes tend to produce oversized infants and to suffer a high fetal loss for many years before their disease becomes apparent. In 1944 Miller and associates analyzed 252 such pregnancies and found that the incidence of stillbirths and neonatal deaths was 19.8% during the 20 years preceding the onset of diabetes; the loss of viable infants rose to 35.4% in the immediate 5 years before the onset of clinical disease. Perinatal mortality can be reduced to 2% or 3% if the metabolic disorder is recognized and treated and if good pediatric care is given.

The factors contributing to excessive size of the infants and intrauterine fetal deaths during these years before maternal hyperglycemia, acidosis, or other evidence of diabetes appears are unknown. It is becoming increasingly clear that diabetes is a generalized process and that the time relationship between the appearance of hyperglycemia and the development of retinopathy or vascular changes, for instance, can vary widely. It is apparent that a characteristically affected offspring can be the earliest manifestation of the maternal disease process.

The following classification of progressive stages of diabetes mellitus is based on the extensive work of Conn and Fajans in this field and modified in accordance with our experience.

1. *The prediabetic stage.* The predisposition to diabetes is genetically determined and present from conception. There is no evidence of reduced carbohydrate tolerance during this period. Clues provided by the obstetric or family history should arouse suspicion and should require the testing of the patient for insulin reserve. Patients exhibiting such features as oversized stillborn infants, particularly if the family history is positive for diabetes, are advisedly considered *suspect,* even if the glucose tolerance test is normal at this time. Such patients should be retested during any subsequent stress period.

2. *Subclinical diabetes* is the term applied to temporary derangements in which hyperglycemia is found only during stress such as pregnancy, infection, emotional crises, or after cortisone administration.

3. *Chemical diabetes* is a more advanced stage in which the glucose tolerance test is abnormal in the absence of stress.

4. *Overt, or clinical, diabetes* is the stage in the dynamic disease process in which hyperglycemia is permanent and symptoms arise. The interval between the appearance of subclinical diabetes and the development of clinical diabetes may be very short or may take many years. Some apparently susceptible individuals may escape metabolic deterioration altogether during their lifetime.

Infants born during the latent diabetic years of their mothers may exhibit embryop-

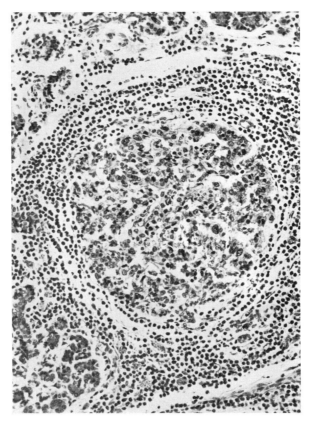

Fig. 19-1. Hyperplasia of pancreatic islets in infant of prediabetic mother. (×231.)

athy identical to that found in infants born of true diabetic mothers, indicating that the abnormal environment for the fetus is similar in both groups (Fig. 19-1). The newborn infant may be large, edematous, and plethoric. Respiratory disturbances are common. Infants who die show hyperplasia of the pancreatic islets, hematopoiesis of the immature type, and a tendency to hyaline membrane formation.

Diagnosis. Because diabetic symptoms in the mother are virtually absent in the early stages of the disease, a glucose tolerance test should be performed in patients whose records include one or more of the following: (1) a family history of diabetes, (2) previous stillbirth or unexplained neonatal loss, (3) oversized infants, (4) glycosuria during pregnancy, (5) hydramnios, and (6) repeated abortions. The presence of obesity in a patient with any of these disorders is often significant.

Criteria for an abnormal test are met if any two of the following values obtained by the Somogyi-Nelson method are equaled or exceeded: fasting blood sugar 110 mg.—at 1 hour 170 mg./100 ml., at 2 hours 120 mg./100 ml., at 3 hours 110 mg./100 ml. It should be remembered that the abnormality improves rapidly after the uterus is emptied, in the same way that insulin requirements are decreased after delivery in the patient with clinical diabetes. Hence, glucose tolerance tests obtained post partum are usually uninformative of conditions existing during pregnancy (Fig. 19-2). In general, an abnormality in carbohydrate metabolism found during one pregnancy tends to become increasingly abnormal in a subsequent pregnancy (Fig. 19-3).

The cortisone glucose tolerance test performed in the nonpregnant state may confirm the existence of subclinical diabetes. Plasma insulin levels in response to glucose loading are also significantly increased during the early stages of diabetes (Fig. 19-4). It is likely that immunoassay of circulating insulin will be used for diagnosis of early diabetes with increasing frequency in the future.

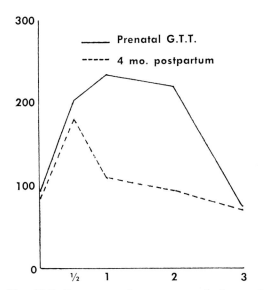

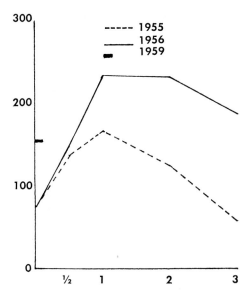

Fig. 19-2. Postpartum improvement of abnormal glucose tolerance curve (4 months). (From Carrington, E. R.: Clin. Obstet. Gynec. **3**:911, 1960.)

Fig. 19-3. Progressive abnormality in carbohydrate metabolism during 3 successive pregnancies. (From Carrington, E. R.: Clin. Obstet. Gynec. **3**:911, 1960.)

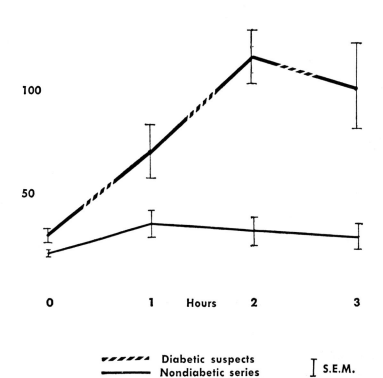

Fig. 19-4. Serum insulin levels in normal and in subclinical diabetic gravidae. (From Carrington, E. R., and McWilliams, N. B.: Amer. J. Obstet. Gynec. **96**:222, 1966.)

Management. Many patients can be controlled by dietary restrictions alone during the early stages of diabetes. Insulin should be added if the 2-hour blood sugar cannot be kept within normal range on the prescribed diabetic diet. The status of treatment of gravid women with oral hypoglycemic agents, which in contrast to insulin pass the placental barrier with ease, has been clarified neither with respect to consistency of metabolic control nor the effects on the fetus, and they are therefore better avoided. Many patients with subclinical diabetes can be carried to term uneventfully and delivered normally. Early delivery is justifiable in patients with a previous poor obstetric history, those in whom obstetric complications arise that cannot be readily reversed, and those in whom a significant fall in estriol levels gives evidence of failing fetoplacental function.

■ Diabetes insipidus

Diabetes insipidus is seldom associated with pregnancy because the disease is relatively rare. However, the reproductive capacity of patients with this condition is not necessarily reduced. Symptoms may be aggravated, improved, or unchanged during pregnancy. But for the most part these alterations can be met by adjusting the dosage of antidiuretic hormone. The disease may appear transiently during the course of pregnancy and must be differentiated from psychogenic polydipsia. In 3 of their own cases Blotner and Kunkel found labor and delivery normal, although other authors have reported an increased incidence of uterine inertia and stillbirths in association with this disturbance.

Pitressin should be used for treatment throughout pregnancy instead of pituitary extract, because Pitressin lacks the oxytocic principle. If the mechanism of labor proves faulty, Pitocin can be given as is indicated.

■ Diseases of the thyroid gland

The adverse effects of thyroid disorders upon the course of pregnancy are far more commonly associated with reduced function than with overactivity of the gland.

SIMPLE COLLOID GOITER

The basic disturbance in simple goiter is an iodine deficiency resulting in reduced transport of thyroxin to the tissues. In re-sponse, thyrotropic stimulation is increased, and the thyroid undergoes hypertrophy followed by involution and increased storage of colloid. As a rule, thyroid function remains within normal limits. Under these circumstances neither the pregnancy nor the condition of the infant at birth is affected, although the gland frequently undergoes further enlargement during the gestation period when iodine intake is borderline. If the basal metabolic rate or the protein-bound iodine level is low, patients with colloid goiter should receive thyroid substance as well as iodine supplement throughout pregnancy in order to prevent congenital goiter or frank cretinism in the infant.

HYPOTHYROIDISM

Menstrual disturbances, sterility, and repeated abortions are common in women with thyroid deficiency. In some cases conception and maintenance of the pregnancy proceed uneventfully, but untreated hypothyroidism in the mother is a potential cause for cretinism or congenital goiter in the infant. Preconceptional diagnosis and replacement therapy continued throughout the prenatal period are highly effective in preventing pregnancy complications because of thyroid deficiency. When pregnancy is established, accurate evaluation of thyroid activity may be difficult. The basal metabolic rate normally increases during the gestation period, but the range is variable and affected by extraneous factors. Blood cholesterol values are normally increased. The serum protein-bound iodine level is probably the most reliable index of thyroid function during pregnancy. Protein-bound iodine values should exceed 6 μg. /100 ml. within 3 to 6 weeks after conception. The research of Peters and associates has demonstrated that abortion is likely if an early rise in protein-bound iodine does not occur. These authors suggest that low protein-bound iodine levels may indicate an antecedent hypothyroidism or an improper reaction of the thyroid to the state of pregnancy—in effect, a temporary hypothyroidism. Substitution therapy with desiccated thyroid or thyroxin is indicated.

MYXEDEMA

Infertility rate is so high that only a few cases of pregnancy in women with proved myxedema have been reported. The outstanding features of 6 offspring of a myxedematous mother described by Hodges and co-workers were multiple congenital anomalies and mental retardation.

HYPERTHYROIDISM

The incidence of hyperthyroidism complicating pregnancy is about 0.2%. Views concerning the influence of pregnancy upon the development of this disorder differ. In Mussey's series the initiation of hyperthyroidism during the gestation period was rare. Dailey and Benson, on the other hand, reported the onset of symptoms concurrent with pregnancy in 12 of their 21 patients. In either event the course of hyperthyroidism is essentially the same in gravid and in nongravid patients, but the pregnancy may be affected. Fetal loss is higher, particularly in early pregnancy if the disease is untreated.

Diagnosis. The recognition of mild degrees of hyperthyroidism may be difficult. Nervousness, some increase in pulse rate, and thyroid enlargement are frequently found in normal pregnant women. The increase in basal metabolic rate may be as much as 25% to 30% above the prepregnancy level, and the serum protein-bound iodine value may occasionally reach 10 to 12 μg./100 ml. However, a similar or higher protein-bound iodine level in a patient with clinical symptoms indicates true hyperthyroidism. Herbst considers in vitro measurements of radioactive uptake of triiodothyronine by red cells or resin in excess of 10% or 25%, respectively, the most reliable diagnostic criteria. Since amenorrhea is not an uncommon symptom of hyperthyroidism, radioactive iodine should not be used for diagnosis of this condition until pregnancy has been ruled out. Fetal tissues have higher avidity for I^{131} than do maternal tissues. Ill effects in fetal life have resulted not only in hypothyroidism and mental retardation but also in increased incidence of congenital anomalies and in the occurrence of thyroid carcinoma during childhood.

Treatment. Thyrotoxicosis can be adequately controlled during pregnancy and therefore does not provide an indication for therapeutic abortion. Certain safeguards must be observed in the interest of the fetus. In general these are concerned with avoidance of overtreatment, causing myxedema in the mother and thus increasing the risk of abortion or of inducing goiter in the infant. On the contrary, hyperthyroidism in the mother does not produce permanent effects upon the fetus, although the newborn infant may exhibit symptoms of hyperthyroidism at birth and may require antithyroid treatment temporarily. Subtotal thyroidectomy after medical preparation with iodine or antithyroid drugs seldom affects the pregnancy, particularly if surgery is performed during the second trimester. Postoperative deficiency should be anticipated and corrected by the administration of desiccated thyroid. Effective control can be achieved with antithyroid therapy alone, but careful regulation of dosage is necessary to prevent depression of the fetal thyroid.

Antithyroid drugs such as propylthiouracil may be used during pregnancy without resorting to surgery, but they must always be used with caution. These drugs cross the placental barrier with ease. On the contrary, thyroxin and triiodothyronine are transferred to the fetus slowly. For this reason Astwood believes that antithyroid compound should be used without thyroid supplementation in dosages limited to the amount just necessary to control thyrotoxicosis. Such meticulous regulation is difficult; most authorities recommend a combination of antithyroid drugs and thyroid substance. This treatment consists of administering antithyroid drugs until normal pregnancy levels of protein-bound iodine are reached (8 to 9 μg./100 ml.), then adding thyroid in amounts sufficient to protect the fetus against hypothyroidism and associated abnormal development (120 to 180 mg. daily). Striking results were obtained by Herbst and Selenkow using combined therapy in 24 hypothyroid patients during 32 pregnancies. Breast-feeding is inadvisable in patients taking antithyroid compounds or iodines, since these drugs are secreted in maternal milk and may produce goiters in nursing infants.

The clinical diagnosis of mild or moderate degrees of hypothyroidism and mental retardation is admittedly difficult in the newborn infant. Cord blood or blood levels of protein-bound iodine (PBI) or butyl-extractable iodine (BEI) should be obtained in any newborn infant in whom potential depression exists. These levels should be only slightly lower than those obtained in the mother. Benson and co-workers found that the difference between maternal and cord BEI of 3.5 and 4.5 μg./100 ml. or more can mean the difference between serious sequelae in the infant and normal development.

■ Diseases of the parathyroid glands

TETANY

Changes in calcium metabolism during pregnancy and lactation may predispose to parathyroid tetany. Calcium requirements are doubled after the fourth month of gestation, and consequently the need for parathyroid hormone is increased. Relative deficiency of parathormone may interfere with phosphorus excretion and permit the serum level of ionized calcium to drop below 6 mg./100 ml. Latent tetany is aggravated by inadequate intake or low absorption of calcium and by hyperventilation, which causes a diminution in ionizable calcium through alkalosis. A history of renal calculi prior to or during pregnancy is a sufficiently recurrent complaint in this disorder to warrant investigation of maternal hyperparathyroid function.

An increase in fetal morbidity and mortality is associated with this disease. A number of cases of tetany in the infant have been reported that led to the diagnosis of previously unrecognized maternal hyperparathyroidism. This complication is fully reviewed by Ludwig.

Treatment consists of regulation of the intake, using a high-calcium, low-phosphorus diet supplemented by calcium lactate, 2 to 4 Gm. daily. Aluminum hydroxide can be used to reduce the absorption of phosphorus from the gastrointestinal tract. During an acute attack, 10 to 20 ml. of 10% calcium gluconate given intravenously will effect prompt temporary control.

■ Diseases of the adrenal glands

ADRENAL INSUFFICIENCY
(ADDISON'S DISEASE)

In 1953 Plotz collected data on maternal mortality in 72 persons with Addison's disease complicated by pregnancy. Maternal death occurred in 78% when no hormonal treatment was given, in 29% when early adrenal cortical extracts were used, and in 11% when potent adrenal cortical extracts

and desoxycorticosterone acetate were used. The outlook is very much improved with cortisone therapy.

Difficulties in control are encountered early in pregnancy if nausea and vomiting ensue and again during labor and delivery. Adrenal crisis, however, occurs most frequently in the immediate postpartum period. Acute vascular collapse at this time is caused by a combination of several factors, including poor tolerance to the stress of labor or cesarean section, depletion of carbohydrate reserves, blood loss superimposed upon low blood volume, and removal of placental hormones.

Treatment is by substitution therapy with special provision made for salt and carbohydrate replacement during labor and delivery. Because of the specific salt- and water-retaining properties of desoxycorticosterone acetate, cortisone plus additional salt in the diet is preferable for control during the prenatal period. A daily maintenance dose of 30 mg. of cortisone is usually sufficient. At the onset of labor 200 mg. of cortisone should be given orally, since administration by this route is more rapid than intramuscular injection, and 100 mg. of hydrocortisone should be given intravenously at delivery.

Patients with hypoadrenalism have an exceedingly low tolerance to analgesics and anesthetics. Oversedation occurs if more than one half the usual dosage of narcotics is administered. An intravenous drip of 5% or 10% glucose in physiologic saline solution offers protection against hypoglycemia and dehydration common to these patients under stress. Local anesthesia is advisable for delivery. Cortisone should be reduced gradually after delivery until the maintenance dose is reached on the sixth or seventh day. The infant is unaffected by the maternal disorder.

ACUTE ADRENOCORTICAL FAILURE

Sudden collapse, persistent shock, and finally death can occur as a result of acute adrenal failure during pregnancy or in the puerperium. This rare condition should be considered when severe obstetric shock occurs because death can be prevented by recognition and prompt treatment of adrenal failure. The pathologic lesions found in 53 women who died of adrenal insufficiency were hemorrhage, necrosis, or infarction of the adrenal glands. Preeclamptic toxemia, late vomiting, hemorrhage, and infection frequently were precipitating causes, but at autopsy each of these 53 deaths proved to be primarily of adrenal etiology. In addition to treatment with hydrocortisone and with other measures, as outlined in the discussion of Addison's disease, it may be necessary to administer norepinephrine 1:10,000 intravenously by slow drip as a temporary measure to maintain blood pressure.

ADRENAL ATROPHY

The administration of adrenal cortical hormones may suppress adrenal function and induce adrenal atrophy presumably through inhibition of pituitary production of ACTH. Impairment of adrenal function persists long after hormone therapy is discontinued. The increasing use of cortisone and similar drugs for many varied disorders is cause for concern. Suppression of the patient's own adrenal function may be sufficient to prevent a normal response to sudden stress. Death has followed relatively simple operations in patients with induced adrenal atrophy. Patients who have taken cortisone-like drugs for any protracted period, even if discontinued within 3 months, should be treated prophylactically with 200 mg. of cortisone at the onset of labor and treatment continued in gradually decreasing dosage after delivery.

ADRENAL HYPERFUNCTION

Adrenocortical hyperplasia (Cushing's syndrome). Although patients with adrenocortical hyperplasia are relatively infertile, Hunt and McConahey reported 7 pregnancies in 4 patients with this disturbance. The chief threat to pregnancy was chronic hypertension, and the resultant fetal loss was high (43%).

Medullary hyperfunction (pheochromocytoma). Maternal and fetal mortality rates associated with pheochromocytoma are appalling. Peelen and De Groat reviewed 30 pregnancies in 20 patients with this condition. Ten mothers died, 1 died undelivered, and the other 9 died within 72 hours post partum. There were 8 stillborn and 3 non-viable fetuses. Hypertension is extreme, may be paroxysmal or persistent, and is likely to progress during pregnancy. The usual symptoms are headache, anxiety, substernal pain, and nausea and vomiting followed by exhaustion and profuse sweating. Profound and irreversible vascular collapse is the great threat and occurs most commonly soon after delivery.

When symptoms are found in late pregnancy, they are usually confused with those of severe preeclampsia, and since pheochromocytoma is generally a benign tumor, it is important to make the diagnosis before its effects are disastrous. Pharmacologic tests are helpful but not definitive. Histamine vasopressor test and phentolamine tests are associated with severe side reactions, particularly in pregnancy. However, side reactions are not severe with tyramine test and false positives are rare, although false negative reactions do occur. Final diagnosis is dependent upon increased production of catecholamines or their major metabolites, the metanephrines (MN) or vanillylmandelic acid (VMA). Accuracy of diagnosis is so important that specific tests for these substances must be used, and no reliance should be placed upon some of the crude screening tests currently available. Values must be elevated distinctly above the normal pregnancy levels for these substances.

References

Anderson, G. W., and Musselman, L.: Treatment of tetany in pregnancy with brief review of literature, Amer. J. Obstet. Gynec. **43:**547, 1942.

Baird, J. D., and Farquhar, J. W.: Insulin-secreting capacity in newborn infants of normal and diabetic women, Lancet **1:**71, 1962.

Becker, W. F., and Sudduth, P. G.: Hyperthyroidism and pregnancy, Ann. Surg. **149:**867, 1959.

Benson, R. C., Pickering, D. E., Kontaxis, N. E., and Fisher, D. A.: Thyroid function in pregnancy, Obstet. Gynec. **14:**11, 1959.

Bergquist, N.: The influence of pregnancy on diabetes, Acta Endocr. **15:**166, 1954.

Bishop, E. H., and Corson, S.: Estimation of fetal maturity by cytologic examination of amniotic fluid, Amer. J. Obstet. Gynec. **102:**654, 1968.

Blotner, H., and Kunkel, P.: Diabetes insipidus and pregnancy, New Eng. J. Med. **227:**287, 1942.

Carrington, E. R., Shuman, C. R., and Reardon, H. S.: Evaluation of the prediabetic state during pregnancy, Obstet. Gynec. **9:**664, 1957.

Carrington, E. R., and Messick, R. R.: Diabetogenic effects of pregnancy; a 10-year survey, Amer. J. Obstet. Gynec. **85:**669, 1963.

Carrington, E. R., and McWilliams, N. B.: Investigation of serum insulin activity during pregnancy in normal and subclinically diabetic mothers, Amer. J. Obstet. Gynec. **96:**922, 1966.

Clinical Staff Conference National Institutes of Health: Pheochromocytoma; current concepts of diagnosis and treatment, Ann. Intern. Med. **65:**1302, 1966.

Conn, J. W., and Fajans, S. S.: The prediabetic state; a concept of dynamic resistance to a genetic diabetogenic influence, Amer. J. Med. **31:**839, 1961.

Dailey, M. E., and Benson, R. C.: Hyperthyroidism in pregnancy, Surg. Gynec. Obstet. **94:**103, 1952.

Davis, M. E., and Plotz, E. J.: Hormonal interrelationships between maternal adrenal, placental and fetal adrenal functions, Obstet. Gynec. Survey **11:**1, 1956.

Freiesleben, E., and Kjerulf-Jensen, K.: The effect of thiouracil derivatives on fetuses and infants, J. Clin. Endocr. **7:**47, 1947.

Freinkel, N., and Goodner, C. J.: Carbohydrate metabolism in pregnancy. I. Metabolism of insulin by human placental tissue, J. Clin. Invest. **39:**116, 1960.

Gellis, S. S., and Hsia, D. Y. Y.: The infant of the diabetic mother, J. Dis. Child. **97:**1, 1959.

Greene, J. W., Smith, K., Kyle, G. C., Touchstone, J. C., and Duhring, J. L.: The use of urinary estriol excretion in the management of pregnancies complicated by diabetes mellitus, Amer. J. Obstet. Gynec. **91:**684, 1965.

Grumbach, M. M., Kaplan, S. L., Sciarra, J. J., and Burr, I. M.: Chorionic growth hormone-prolactin (CGP); secretion, disposition, biologic activity in man, and postulated function as the "growth hormone" of the second half of pregnancy. In Sonenberg, M., editor: Conference on growth hormone, Ann. N. Y. Acad. Sci. **148:**501, 1968.

Haworth, S. G., Milic, A. B., and Adamsons, K.: Biochemical indices of fetal condition, Clin. Obstet. Gynec. **11:**1182, 1968.

Herbst, A. L., and Selenkow, H. A.: Hyperthyroidism during pregnancy, New Eng. J. Med. **273:**627, 1965.

Hodges, R. E., Hamilton, H. E., and Keettel, W. C.: Pregnancy in myxedema, Arch. Intern. Med. **90:**863, 1952.

Hoet, J. P. (translated by Lukens, F. D. W.): Carbohydrate metabolism during pregnancy, Diabetes **3:**1, 195⁴.

Hunt, A. B., and McConahey, W.: Pregnancy associated with diseases of the adrenal glands, Amer. J. Obstet. Gynec. **66:**970, 1953.

Jørgensen, K. R., Deckert, T., Pedersen, L. M., and Pedersen, J.: Insulin, insulin antibody and glucose in plasma of newborn infants of diabetic women, Acta Endocr. **52:**154, 1966.

Kinsell, L. W., Balch, H. E., and Michaels, G. D.: Accentuation of human diabetes by "pituitary growth hormone," Proc. Soc. Exp. Biol. Med. **83:**683, 1953.

Kvale, W. F., Roth, G. M., Manger, W. M., and Priestley, J. T.: Present-day diagnosis and treatment of pheochromocytoma, J.A.M.A. **164:**854, 1957.

Lowy, C., Blanshard, G., and Phear, D.: Antagonism of insulin by albumin, Lancet **1:**802, 1961.

Ludwig, G. D.: Hyperparathyroidism in relation to pregnancy, New Eng. J. Med. **267:**637, 1962.

Miller, H. C., Hurwitz, D., and Kuder, K.: Fetal and neonatal mortality in pregnancies complicated by diabetes mellitus, J.A.M.A. **124:**271, 1944.

Myant, N. B.: Passage of thyroxine and triiodothyronine from mother to fetus in pregnant women, Clin. Sci. **17:**75, 1958.

Nelson, H. B., Gillespie, L., and White, P.: Pregnancy complicated by diabetes, Obstet. Gynec. **1:**219, 1953.

O'Sullivan, J. B.: Gestational diabetes; unsuspected, asymptomatic diabetes in pregnancy, New Eng. J. Med. **264:**1082, 1961.

O'Sullivan, J. B., and Mahan, C. M.: Criteria for the oral GTT in pregnancy, Diabetes **13:**278, 1964.

Pedersen, J.: Blood sugar in newborn infants of diabetic mothers, Acta Endocr. **15:**33, 1954.

Pedowitz, P., and Shlevin, E. L.: The pregnant diabetic patient, Amer. J. Obstet. Gynec. **69:**395, 1955.

Peelen, J. W., and De Groat, A.: Pheochromocytoma complicated by pregnancy, Amer. J. Obstet. Gynec. **69:**1054, 1955.

Peters, J. P., Man, E. B., and Heinemann, M.: Pregnancy and the thyroid gland, Yale J. Biol. Med. **20:**449, 1948.

Plotz, J.: Nebennereninsuffizienz und Schwangerschaft, Klin. Wschr. **31:**831, 1953.

Rand, C. W.: Two cerebral complications of pregnancy; brain tumors and spontaneous subarachnoid hemorrhage, Clin. Neurosurg. **3:**104, 1957.

Reardon, H. S., Field, S., Vega, L., Carrington, E., Arey, J., and Baumann, M. L.: Treatment of acute respiratory distress in newborn infants of diabetic and "prediabetic" mothers, J. Dis. Child. **94:**558, 1957.

Reis, R. A., DeCosto, E. S., and Allweiss, M. D.: Management of the pregnant diabetic woman and her newborn infant, Amer. J. Obstet. Gynec. **60:**1023, 1950.

Russell, K. P., Rose, H., and Starr, P.: Effects of radioactive iodine on maternal and fetal thyroid function during pregnancy, Surg. Gynec. Obstet. **104:**560, 1957.

Sandberg, A. A., and Slaunwhite, W. R., Jr.: Transcortin; a corticosteroid-binding protein of plasma. II. Levels in various conditions and the effects of estrogens, J. Clin. Invest. **38:**1290, 1959.

Slaunwhite, W. R., Jr., and Sandberg, A. A.: Transcortin; a corticosteroid-binding protein of plasma, J. Clin. Invest. **38:**384, 1959.

Spellacy, W. N., Goetz, F. C., Greenberg, B. Z., and Ells, J.: The human placental gradient for plasma insulin and blood glucose, Amer. J. Obstet. Gynec. **90:**753, 1964.

Steinke, J., Soeldner, S., Davalos, R. A. C., and Renold, A. E.: Studies on serum insulin-like activity (ILA) in prediabetes and early overt diabetes, Diabetes **12:**502, 1963.

Stimmler, L., Brazie, J. V., and O'Brien, D.:

Plasma insulin levels in the newborn infants of normal and diabetic mothers, Lancet 1:137, 1964.

Vallance-Owen, J., and Lilley, M. D.: Insulin antagonism in plasma of obese diabetics and prediabetics. Preliminary communication, Lancet 1:806, 1961.

White, P., Gillespie, L., and Sexton, L.: The use of female sex hormone therapy in pregnant diabetic patients, Amer. J. Obstet. Gynec. 71:57, 1956.

Wilkerson, H. L. C.: Pregnancy and the prediabetic state, Ann. N. Y. Acad. Sci. 82:219, 1959.

20

Diseases of the circulatory system and blood during pregnancy

Diseases affecting the heart, the blood vessels, and the hematopoietic system are encountered in only a small percentage of pregnant women, but they are potentially more serious than are many other complications. Most disorders affecting the cardiovascular system are not difficult to recognize and can be detected by the usual prenatal studies.

■ Diseases of the circulatory system
HEART DISEASE

As the total number of maternal deaths has decreased, those due to heart disease have assumed a more prominent role. Heart disease is responsible for about 10% of all deaths of pregnant women and is exceeded only by hemorrhage, toxemia, and infection. About 2% to 3% of all pregnant women have an organic heart lesion, and except in the hot, dry areas of the United States, over

95% are of rheumatic origin. According to Mendelson about 75% of rheumatic lesions in pregnant women are confined to the mitral valve, and in 10% to 15% of pregnant women mitral and aortic lesions are combined. About 2% to 3% are congenital, and only an occasional instance of hypertensive cardiopathy is encountered.

Diagnosis. The diagnosis of heart disease is based upon clinical history and examination, electrocardiographic recordings, and cardiac x-ray examination. A more precise diagnosis can be made with cardiac catheterization. It may be difficult to make an accurate diagnosis of heart lesions during pregnancy by clinical examination alone. At least one half of all women develop systolic murmurs during pregnancy, and the heart sounds, particularly those of the apex, are altered. The changes, which are caused by the increase in plasma volume and cardiac output and altered viscosity, begin during the early second trimester and reverse rapidly after delivery.

Patients suspected of having a cardiac lesion should be treated as are those who actually do have one, even though a precise diagnosis cannot be made until after delivery. The lesions are classified according to the functional and therapeutic classifications of the New York Heart Association.

Functional classification:
Class I: Patients with cardiac disease that does not limit activity. Ordinary physical activity does not cause discomfort. The patients have no symptoms of cardiac insufficiency nor do they have anginal pain.
Class II: Patients with cardiac disease that produces slight limitation of activity. They are free from symptoms while at rest, but ordinary activity is accompanied by undue fatigue, palpitation, dyspnea, or anginal pain.
Class III: Patients with cardiac disease that produces marked limitation of activity. Less than ordinary activity is accompanied by undue fatigue, palpitation, dyspnea, or anginal pain.
Class IV: Patients with cardiac disease that prevents them from carrying out any activity without discomfort. Symptoms of cardiac insufficiency or anginal pain are present at rest, and any activity increases them.

Therapeutic classification:
Class A: Patients with cardiac disease whose physical activity need not be restricted.
Class B (functional class I): Patients with cardiac disease whose ordinary physical activity need not be restricted, but who should be ad-

vised against unusually severe or competitive efforts.

Class C (functional class II): Patients with cardiac disease whose ordinary physical activity should be moderately restricted and whose more strenuous habitual efforts should be discontinued.

Class D (functional class III): Patients with cardiac disease whose ordinary physical activity should be decidedly restricted.

Class E (functional class IV): Patients with cardiac disease who should have complete rest in bed or in a chair.

Prognosis. The prognosis for a patient with cardiac disease is determined by the functional capacity of the heart and its ability to meet the increased demands placed upon it by the normal physiologic changes of pregnancy, the most important of which are the expanded plasma volume and the great increase in the total vascular bed in the enlarging uterus. Other physiologic changes that add to the cardiac load include a gradual rise in heart rate, with a maximum increase of 8 to 10 beats per minute by about the thirty-fifth week, and the possibility that the choriodecidual space acts as arteriovenous fistula.

In order to maintain an adequate circulation the cardiac output begins to rise at about the tenth week of pregnancy and reaches a maximum, at least 35% above that of nongravid women, during the last weeks of the second trimester, after which it decreases. The changes in output occur mostly in response to alterations in stroke volume. The curve for cardiac output roughly parallels that for plasma volume until about the twenty-eighth week of gestation, at which time output begins to diminish. Plasma volume, however, remains elevated until at least the middle of the third trimester, when it begins to decrease. If an adequate output can be maintained, the patient will progress through pregnancy and delivery without difficulty, but if cardiac reserve is limited, the heart will be unable to respond to the increasing demands.

Most deaths are caused by cardiac failure, which can occur at any time but which is most frequent when the blood volume is at maximum. The majority of deaths occur in women with mitral lesions because these are the most common and because of the characteristic accompanying circulatory changes, which are exaggerated by the physiologic alterations of pregnancy. The normal heart has no difficulty in increasing its output as the plasma volume expands, but a stenotic mitral valve may present enough obstruction to prevent the necessary increase in blood flow from atrium to ventricle. With mitral stenosis the pressure in the left atrium must increase excessively to force enough blood through the constricted valve. If the opening is too small to permit an adequate flow, the pulmonary vascular pressure gradually increases, and congestion, pulmonary edema, and cardiac decompensation inevitably follow. During the last few weeks of pregnancy both cardiac output and plasma volume diminish, consequently the cardiac load is reduced and decompensation is less likely to occur.

Few women develop heart failure during labor. The heart has already proved its capacity to respond to the demands of maximum plasma volume and cardiac output. Hendricks observed a 30% increase in cardiac output during each first-stage uterine contraction. The systolic blood pressure increased 10 to 20 mm. Hg during each contraction, and there were consistent changes in heart rate and stroke volume. The heart rate rose at the onset, decreased below the resting level at the peak of the contraction, and then returned to normal as the uterus relaxed. Stroke volume first fell and then rose significantly at the peak of the contraction.

Ueland and Hensen described similar changes but also noted alterations due to position. Cardiac output during a contraction increased 24.8%, and stroke volume increased 33.1% with the patient in the supine position but only increased 7.6% and 7.7%, respectively, when the patient was on her side. They attribute the change to compression of the vena cava and aorta by the heavy uterus and the consequent alterations in venous return and in arterial pressure when the patient lies on her back. The changes that occur may be because 250 to 300 ml. of blood is forced from the uterine vessels into the general circulation during a contraction. Comparable changes in cardiac output, arterial pressure, and pulse rate can be produced by the rapid infusion of blood or plasma expanders into experimental animals.

According to Ueland and Hansen, cardiac output reaches a maximum during labor and delivery but declines somewhat, although it is still well above the prelabor level, during the first few postpartum hours. The changes in stroke volume are similar. This probably can be attributed to the expanded plasma volume due to the drastic reduction in uterine circulatory capacity at delivery and the consequent redistribution of blood in the general circulation.

Parity is far less important than age as a causative factor in decompensation; there is a sharp increase in deaths from heart disease in pregnancy after the age of 35 years. There is a high incidence of failure and death in women who have experienced previous episodes of decompensation or atrial fibrillation.

If the patient survives the pregnancy, the course of her heart disease and her life expectancy should not be altered. Chesley traced 259 of 263 women with heart disease who had been delivered at the Margaret Hague Maternity Hospital, Jersey City, N. J., during a 5-year period ending in August, 1942. He was unable to detect any effect of the original or subsequent pregnancies on the course of rheumatic heart disease or on death rates. Maternal heart disease alone does not increase *perinatal mortality,* but intrapartum death from hypoxia may occur from circulatory changes accompanying decompensation, paroxysmal tachycardia, and similar complications.

Treatment during pregnancy. The patient with heart disease should be examined before she becomes pregnant so that the lesion can be accurately diagnosed and cardiac function evaluated. A patient with a serious lesion, certainly one in functional class III or IV, should usually be advised against pregnancy. If she is first seen during pregnancy, it often is wise to admit her to a hospital for study; this is particularly important with severe lesions. In most instances consultation with a cardiologist is indicated, but the fact that the cardiologist offers a good prognosis should not alter the physician's care of the patient because she may decompensate during pregnancy even though the lesion seems relatively innocuous. With proper treatment the mortality should be minimal, even in those with advanced lesions, but if the patient is ignored or if she cannot or will not follow instructions, the death rate will be high.

Hospital care would be ideal for all pregnant women with heart disease, but actually it is not essential for those of functional classes I and II. All persons with class IV lesions should remain in the hospital if possible, and any patient who decompensates should be hospitalized for the remainder of the pregnancy. Acute infections, particularly those of respiratory origin, often precipitate failure; consequently most women with active infections should be treated in the hospital until they have recovered. It is usually recommended that patients with heart disease, except those with minimal asymptomatic lesions, be admitted 10 to 14 days before delivery is anticipated for controlled rest and diet in preparation for labor. Unless there is infection or evidence of decompensation, this is not strictly necessary because at this stage the demands on the heart are significantly less than they were during the preceding several weeks. It would seem much more logical to suggest hospital care between the twenty-sixth and thirty-fourth weeks, when the cardiac load is greatest.

Rest is of utmost importance, and a specific plan should be developed for each individual. Rest periods each morning and afternoon and at least 10 hours in bed each night are advisable. Although light tasks around the home are permissible if they do not produce symptoms, unusual activity such as stair climbing, shopping, and heavy cleaning should be avoided; this is particularly true after the middle of pregnancy. Patients who have decompensated or those in whom slight exertion causes symptoms should remain in bed or in a chair at the bedside almost all the time. If the cardiac reserve is limited, coitus should be avoided after the twentieth week.

The diet should be low in salt to prevent fluid accumulation, and diuretics such as chlorothiazide or hydrochlorothiazide or mercurial preparations can be prescribed if necessary. Calories should be limited for those who are overweight. An *iron supplement* is important because anemia increases the demands on the heart. Digitalis is used when indicated. Women with class III lesions must be considered to be partially decompensated; consequently they, as well as those with class IV lesions, should usually be taking digitalis throughout the entire pregnancy.

Therapeutic abortion. Termination of

pregnancy is unnecessary in women with milder lesions and even in those of classes III and IV if they can be provided proper care throughout the entire pregnancy. Unfortunately this is not always possible, and if a patient cannot or will not follow advice, the risk from continuing pregnancy may offer a serious threat to her life. If proper treatment cannot be administered, termination of pregnancy and tubal ligation are justifiable for the following patients:

1. Those who have decompensated previously, particularly those who have been in failure between pregnancies (about two thirds of these will decompensate during pregnancy)
2. Those with atrial fibrillation
3. Those in functional classes III and IV (the incidence of failure is high, particularly with the more advanced lesions)
4. Those over age 35 years with serious lesions

Interruption should be performed as early as possible because a major operative procedure may prove too much for the heart already burdened with gestational demands. In fact, the operation may actually contribute to the patient's death. Interruption should never be performed in a patient who is already in failure; the decompensation should be corrected first.

Valvulotomy. Operations to correct heart lesions are seldom necessary during pregnancy, as is indicated by the excellent results that can be obtained by medical treatment alone. Occasionally, however, mitral commissurotomy is warranted in a woman with stenosis if the constricted opening prevents the necessary increase in blood flow through or from the heart. The mortality is less than 3% and there should be no effect on the fetus if all phases of the operative procedure are managed properly. Whenever possible, the operation should be performed during the first trimester, but when necessary, it can be done later.

Valvulotomy, even those performed between pregnancies, does not always permit cardiac function that is adequate for normal gestation. Schenker and Polishuk, reporting on 182 patients who had mitral valvulotomies, found increased rates of spontaneous and therapeutic abortions and of intrauterine and neonatal deaths. In addi-

tion, 10 of 18 deaths (55%) occurred as a result of pregnancy and delivery. Decompensation occurred in 42% of patients who delivered for the first time after the operation. Atrial fibrillation developed in 35 patients (18%) during pregnancy; 5 patients (14.2%) died, 48.8% developed congestive failure, and 20% had thromboembolic phenomena. It seems evident that patients who have had valvulotomy are poor candidates for pregnancy.

Care during labor. Induction of labor for heart disease alone is contraindicated. If the patient is allowed to start labor spontaneously, the physician can be assured that the blood volume and cardiac output will both be reduced as much as possible and that labor will more likely be short and normal than if induction is attempted early. This is particularly true if there is any question of decompensation. Heart disease does not alter the length of labor.

Although failure does not often occur during labor, it may set in soon after delivery, and in most instances there is adequate warning that cardiac function is deteriorating. The best index of the condition of the heart during labor is offered by the pulse and respiratory rates. Failure is likely to occur if the pulse rate increases above 110 and the respiratory rate above 24 during the first stage. These, as well as the blood pressure, should be checked and recorded every 15 minutes. The patient remains in bed, preferably on her side. If there are any signs of beginning decompensation, oxygen should be administered by mask or tent and the patient should be digitalized rapidly unless she has been receiving an adequate dosage of digitalis.

Pain, anxiety, and muscular activity add to the burden on the heart, and the physician should try to eliminate them. This is best achieved with a caudal or epidural anesthetic if one or the other can be administered safely. These techniques usually have little effect on blood pressure; therefore oxygenation is maintained. The anesthetic is started when the patient becomes uncomfortable, if she is making satisfactory progress in labor, and can be continued for delivery. If caudal or epidural anesthesia is not available, the discomfort can be relieved with morphine sulfate, 0.01 to 0.016 Gm., or meperidine (Demerol), 75 to 100 mg. as needed. Scopolamine may increase both heart rate and muscular activity and is best avoided. Phenothiazine derivatives should be used with caution because they may cause hypotension, particularly when general anesthesia also is administered.

An occasional patient will develop subacute bacterial endocarditis as a result of pregnancy and labor; consequently 1.5 million units of penicillin and 0.5 Gm. of streptomycin should be given intramuscularly when labor begins. This can be repeated every 12 hours.

Delivery. Vaginal delivery is usually preferable to cesarean section unless there is an obstetric reason for the latter. Ueland, Gills, and Hansen found increases in cardiac output of 52% and in stroke volume of 67% and a decrease in heart rate of 11% after delivery by cesarean section under spinal anesthesia. Despite this, a test of labor is ordinarily contraindicated for patients with moderate or severe cardiac disease because it increases the risk of infection or decompensation if labor is prolonged or if cesarean section becomes necessary after several hours of ineffectual labor.

Bearing-down efforts raise intravascular pressure and increase the possibility of decompensation; consequently they should be prevented by eliminating the perineal phase of labor as completely as possible. This can be accomplished by low forceps extraction soon after the head begins to bulge the perineum and should be performed in most primigravidas. It is not necessary in multiparas who will deliver with a few second-stage contractions. Caudal, spinal, or pudendal block anesthesia will obliterate the perineal sensation, thereby eliminating bearing-down efforts, and they do not interfere with oxygenation when properly administered. Ether is most satisfactory for general anesthesia and can be administered with a high concentration of oxygen. Both cyclopropane and trichlorethylene may produce cardiac arrhythmias and are best avoided.

Ergotrate sometimes produces transient but severe hypertension and should not be used. If an oxytocic is necessary, oxytocin can be given safely.

Postpartum care. The heart is more likely to decompensate during the early puerperium than during labor, but the incidence can be kept low by meticulous care during pregnancy and labor. Those with cardiac symptoms should usually remain in bed a week or more, but ambulation for those in functional classes I and II usually need not be delayed. Penicillin and streptomycin are continued until it seems certain that the danger from infection is passed. Breast-feeding is tiring, so that patient with heart disease usually should not attempt to nurse her infant. The patient may be discharged whenever the physician is certain that the danger from decompensation is past. Most patients should remain in the hospital longer than normal women, particularly if they must assume complete responsibility for the care of the child and the home.

Reproduction in women with heart disease should usually be limited, the size of the family being determined by the functional capacity of the heart and the desires of the patient and her husband. The patient should be instructed about a reliable contraceptive method when she returns for her postpartum examination. Tubal ligation may be considered if the patient and her husband desire no more children and if the operation can be performed with only slight risk.

SUBACUTE BACTERIAL ENDOCARDITIS

Pedowitz and Hellman analyzed the pregnancies of 85 women who conceived after they had recovered from subacute bacterial endocarditis and 35 who were pregnant when this complication developed. The mortality was 3.5% and 14.2%, respectively. They conclude that if the endocarditis is well healed, the prognosis for pregnancy depends almost entirely upon the heart lesion and its effect upon cardiac function. The treatment of active endocarditis is not altered because of pregnancy.

CORONARY ARTERY DISEASE

Coronary occlusion or thrombosis does not occur often during pregnancy, but when it does, the mortality is high. Pregnancy usually is contraindicated in women who have had coronary occlusion, particularly if the blood pressure is elevated; therefore, therapeutic abortion can justifiably be advised. Acute coronary occlusion in a gravid woman should be treated as though she were not pregnant. If it is thought wise to terminate the pregnancy, the procedure should usually be delayed until the lesion is healed, but it may be preferable to permit the pregnancy to continue. In most instances vaginal delivery is permissible if precautions are taken to prevent pain, unusual muscular activity, and hypoxia during labor and delivery.

CONGENITAL HEART LESIONS

Most women with the milder forms of congenital heart disease have little difficulty during pregnancy, but the prognosis is less favorable for those with reduced cardiac function, particularly if they are cyanotic. The highest mortality is associated with coarctation of the aorta, with which the death rate is about 7%. The most frequent causes of death are heart failure and, in women with septal defects and patent ductus arteriosus, bacterial endocarditis; rupture of the aorta is common in women with coarctation.

The mortality with coarctation is so high that therapeutic termination of early pregnancy is often justifiable. Abortion need not usually be considered for other lesions unless cardiac reserve is so limited that failure can be anticipated as pregnancy advances. The basic principles of management are similar to those for women with other types of heart disease.

With the exception of coarctation, most women with congenital heart lesions can be delivered vaginally unless cesarean section is indicated for obstetric reasons. Abdominal delivery often is safer for those with advanced coarctation because the changes in circulatory dynamics accompanying uterine contractions and bearing down are likely to rupture the defective or recently repaired aorta.

Pregnancy should offer less hazard if disturbed cardiac function has been corrected by surgical repair of the defect. In most instances cardiac operations should be performed between pregnancies. Congenital heart lesions in the mothers may be duplicated in their offspring. There is evidence to suggest that this is caused by a recessive chromosomal abnormality.

KYPHOSCOLIOTIC HEART DISEASE

The collapsed rib cage in women with kyphoscoliosis reduces vital capacity by compressing the lungs and limiting their ability to expand. The enlarging uterus exaggerates the difficulty. The right ventricle hypertrophies to maintain an adequate pulmonary circulation, and cardiac failure may occur if the heart is unable to meet the increased demands as pregnancy advances.

Since the pelvis, as well as the spine, usually is deformed, cesarean section may be necessary. Therapeutic abortion is justifiable for those with limited cardiac reserve.

VARICOSE VEINS

Venous varicosities in the legs and vulva are common during pregnancy and are particularly likely to occur in women whose general supporting tissues are weak. In many women a history of similar defects in other members of the family can be elicited. The veins begin to distend during the first trimester and become progressively larger as pregnancy advances. The engorgement of the pelvic veins and delayed circulation through the lower part of the body exert increasing pressure on the vein walls; if the walls are not strong enough to resist the internal force, they stretch, producing the typical large tortuous veins of pregnancy.

Some women have no symptoms related to the enlarged veins, but many complain of heaviness and discomfort that become progressively worse the longer they remain in an upright position. Vulvar varicosities are particularly uncomfortable. The veins begin to improve within a few days after delivery and may disappear completely, only to recur and become worse with the next pregnancy. In many women the vulvar varicosities remain but become smaller between pregnancies.

The treatment during pregnancy is to compress the distended vessels with elastic stockings or bandages, which are best applied before the patient arises in the morning while the veins are collapsed and empty. It is more difficult to compress vulvar varicosities, but supporting pads and garments are available in surgical supply stores. It is seldom necessary to operate upon varicose veins during pregnancy.

NOSEBLEEDS

Mild nosebleeds occur frequently during pregnancy and can usually be controlled with pressure. Occasionally it may be necessary to cauterize the bleeding area.

OTHER VASCULAR CHANGES

Spider nevi and palmar erythema are common during pregnancy and disappear after delivery. Both are thought to result from the elevated estrogen level.

■ Diseases of the blood

Unlike the normal nonpregnant individual whose blood picture remains relatively stable, the blood of pregnant women undergoes great qualitative and quantitative alterations. The *plasma volume* begins to increase during the first trimester and reaches a maximum of at least 30% above the level during early pregnancy and about 6 weeks before term, after which it again decreases. The *red blood cell mass* and, as a consequence, the *total blood volume* also increase. If iron intake is adequate, the *total hemoglobin* content increases, and serum iron, erythrocyte protoporphyrin, and iron-binding capacity remain normal.

The body of a normal woman contains about 4 grams of iron; 60% to 70% of this is carried in hemoglobin, about 30% is stored in the liver, spleen, bone marrow, and other cells, and most of the rest is carried as transport iron in the iron-beta globulin complex. During pregnancy an additional gram or more of iron is required: at least 400 mg. for the expanded red cell mass, 500 mg. for fetal hemoglobin, and at least 100 mg. to replace that lost through bleeding during and after delivery. Even though iron is absorbed from the intestinal tract more readily during pregnancy (probably 1 to 2 mg. daily), the dietary intake provides less than that required; the estimated deficit averages about 400 mg.

The iron deficit may not be obvious in women whose iron stores are reasonably adequate. The hemoglobin concentration of a patient with normal total body iron will change little during pregnancy, even though she ingests no iron other than that in the diet. If iron stores are reduced, but there is still enough to supply the demand for extra hemoglobin, the hemoglobin concentration may decrease only slightly, but the storage iron will be even more depleted after delivery. If storage iron is considerably reduced, the hemoglobin concentration may fall as pregnancy advances and plasma volume expands because there is too little iron available to meet the demands for increased hemoglobin.

Every woman, even those with normal hemoglobin concentrations, should be given supplemental iron during pregnancy.

The *white blood cell* count is slightly increased during pregnancy, but it seldom exceeds 12,000 in normal women. The differential cell count is unaltered except for a slight decrease in eosinophils.

Iron-deficiency anemia. Iron-deficiency anemia is the most common form of anemia in pregnant women. It is caused by an iron deficit from rapidly recurring pregnancies, abnormal blood loss, or nutritional inadequacies.

There may be slight reductions in hemoglobin concentration and in hematocrit because plasma volume may increase more rapidly than red blood cell mass, but the change should be slight if the body iron content is normal. Holly believes that a decrease in hemoglobin below 12 grams, in hematocrit below 35%, and in red blood cell count below 3.75 million at any period of pregnancy indicates anemia. In such patients serum iron is diminished and iron-binding capacity and erythrocyte and protoporphyrin are increased. In most instances the red blood cells are normocytic aind hypochromic and the bone marrow is hyperplastic.

Whenever possible, iron-deficiency anemia should be corrected prior to conception. As a general rule, supplemental iron should be prescribed for all menstruating women because the cumulative iron loss from month to month is significant, and an effective iron preparation should be prescribed for all pregnant women even though the diet is considered to be adequate. Ferrous gluconate or ferrous sulfate, 1 Gm. daily, will usually provide an adequate amount of iron. Gastrointestinal disturbances can almost always be avoided if the preparation is ingested in small amounts three or four times each day.

Parenteral administration of iron is seldom necessary, but it may be considered for those who cannot take iron orally. Blood transfusions are seldom necessary, particularly if the patient is several weeks from term, because the anemia can be improved by the ingestion of iron. In those at term or in labor with hemoglobin readings below 7 or 8 grams, transfusion may be warranted; at least compatible blood should be available to compensate for excessive bleeding during delivery. Iron should also be prescribed.

Megaloblastic anemia. Megaloblastic anemia is far less common than is that due to iron deficiency, but it is usually much more severe. It is also called pernicious anemia of pregnancy or macrocytic anemia, but it has few of the characteristics of pernicious anemia and it is not always macrocytic.

The diagnosis usually is made during late pregnancy in women who are chronically undernourished. The hemoglobin, hematocrit, and red blood cell count fall rapidly, and the patient is pale, dyspneic, and may be edematous. Megaloblasts can often be found in the peripheral blood smear, but red cell size may be normal at the onset. The diagnosis is best made by demonstrating megaloblastic proliferation in the bone marrow.

The precipitating cause appears to be a deficiency in folic acid, but a deficiency in vitamin C, which is necessary for folic acid metabolism, is also an important factor. Iron alone will not correct the anemia, but folic acid, 0.5 to 1 mg. daily, will correct it, particularly when given with ascorbic acid and an iron preparation. Nutritional deficiencies also must be corrected.

Sickle cell disease. For many years sickle cell anemia was recognized as a serious complication of pregnancy, but the various types were not appreciated until electrophoresis became available. This test differentiates normal hemoglobin A from sickle hemoglobin S, fetal hemoglobin F, and hemoglobin C. *Sickle cell trait* occurs with an S-A pattern, *sickle cell anemia* with homozygous S-S pattern, and *sickle cell hemoglobin C disease* with the heterozygous S-C combination. *Sickle cell hemoglobin F disease* (S-F) and homologous *hemoglobin C disease* (C-C) occur less often. For practical purposes all these conditions are found only in women of Negroid ancestry.

Sickle cell anemia (S-S) has usually been diagnosed before the patient first conceives, and almost all patients have been chronically ill, with histories of typical symptoms and recurrent crises. Most of these women become progressively more anemic as pregnancy advances, and they may experience crises, but the crises do not increase in frequency or in severity. The complications are similar to those in nonpregnant women.

Sickle cell hemoglobin C disease (S-C) is more serious. Many patients are unaware of the disease until the symptoms begin during a pregnancy. Crises are common during the later weeks of the gestation period, and anemia becomes progressively more severe. The incidence of aseptic bone necrosis and embolism are far higher than with sickle cell anemia, and most of the deaths occur in this form of the condition. Of Curtis' 18 patients with S-C disease, unquestionable pulmonary embolism occurred in one third, and 3 died. None of the 15 patients with S-S disease died.

Sickle cell trait (S-A), the sickling of red blood cells with an S-A electrophoretic pattern, is present in about 8% of black women, but the outlook for pregnancy is much more favorable than with S-S or S-C disease. According to Whalley, Pritchard, and Richards, the incidence of pyelonephritis is significantly increased in women with sickle cell trait, but abortion, toxemia, prematurity, and perinatal mortality occur with a frequency similar to that in a comparable group of normal black women.

The sickling trait can be demonstrated by adding 1 drop of 2% sodium metabisulfite to a drop of blood on a coverslip preparation. The characteristic change occurs within a half hour. A sickling test should be run on every black patient. The genetic pattern of each patient whose red cells sickle should be determined by electrophoresis.

The course of the disease in those with S-S pattern is not usually altered, and activity of S-C disease is not likely to appear until the latter part of pregnancy. All patients should be maintained on a high-protein diet supplemented with iron and vitamins. Since infection may precipitate an acute crisis, each patient should be encouraged to report the development of an infectious process, and if it is severe, hospitalization often is indicated. Antibiotics, glucose, and packed red blood cell transfusions should be administered during the crisis.

Most women with the sickle cell diseases can be permitted to deliver normally unless cesarean section is warranted because of an obstetric complication. *Tubal ligation* for multiparas with sickle cell disease, particularly those with an S-C pattern, is justifiable.

Leukemia. The outlook for chronic leukemia does not appear to be altered by pregnancy; hence there is no reason to consider abortion. Treatment is the same as that in nonpregnant women, but the effects on the fetus of x-ray and antimetabolites, particularly antifolic acid compounds, must be considered.

Hodgkin's disease. Pregnancy does not alter the course of Hodgkin's disease, nor does the condition have any effect on pregnancy or the growth of the fetus. If x-ray therapy is administered, the uterus must be shielded. Abortion is not necessary.

Thrombocytopenic purpura. Thrombocytopenic purpura is rarely encountered in gravid women. The bleeding tendency and the reduced platelet count are not affected by pregnancy. The infant may have a transient thrombocytopenia, which can usually be corrected by the administration of adrenal corticosteroids. The mother is usually best treated with adrenal corticosteroids during pregnancy. If this medication does not correct the bleeding tendency, splenectomy is indicated.

References

Adams, J. Q.: Cardiovascular physiology in normal pregnancy, Amer. J. Obstet. Gynec. **67:** 741, 1954.

Adams, J. Q., and Alexander, A. M.: Alterations in cardiovascular physiology during labor, Obstet. Gynec. **12:**542, 1958.

Bunim, J. J., and Appel, S. B.: Principle for determining prognosis of pregnancy in rheumatic heart disease, J.A.M.A. **142:**90, 1950.

Chesley, L. C.: The remote prognosis for pregnant women with rheumatic cardiac disease, Amer. J. Obstet. Gynec. **100:**732, 1968.

Curtis, E. M.: Pregnancy in sickle cell anemia, sickle cell-hemoglobin C disease and variants thereof, Amer. J. Obstet. Gynec. **77:**1312, 1959.

Cutforth, R., and MacDonald, C. B.: Heart sounds and murmurs during pregnancy, Amer. Heart J. **71:**741, 1966.

Espino-Vela, J., and Castro-Abreu, D.: Congenital heart disease associated with pregnancy; a study of 53 cases, Amer. Heart J. **51:**542, 1956.

Hamilton, B. E., and Thomson, K. J.: The heart in pregnancy and the childbearing age, Boston, 1941, Little, Brown & Co.

Holly, R. G.: Dynamics of iron metabolism in pregnancy, Amer. J. Obstet. Gynec. **93:**370, 1965.

Long, J. H.: The usefulness of serial vital capacity determinations in the management of the pregnant patient with heart disease, Amer. J. Obstet. Gynec. **69:**715, 1955.

Lowenstein, L., Pick, C., and Philpott, N.: Megaloblastic anemia of pregnancy and puerperium, Amer. J. Obstet. Gynec. **70:**1309, 1955.

Mendelson, C. L.: The management of delivery in pregnancy complicated by serious rheumatic heart disease, Amer. J. Obstet. Gynec. **48:**329, 1944.

Mendelson, C. L.: Pregnancy and kyphoscoliotic heart disease, Amer. J. Obstet. Gynec. **56:**457, 1948.

Mendelson, C. L.: Cardiac disease in pregnancy, Philadelphia, 1960, F. A. Davis Co.

Mendelson, C. L., and Pardee, H. E. B.: The pulse and respiratory rates during labor as a guide to the onset of cardiac failure in women with rheumatic heart disease, Amer. J. Obstet. Gynec. **44:**370, 1942.

Pedowitz, P., and Hellman, L. M.: Pregnancy and healed subacute bacterial endocarditis, Amer. J. Obstet. Gynec. **66:**294, 1953.

Schenker, J. G., and Polishuk, W. Z.: Pregnancy following mitral valvulotomy, Obstet. Gynec. **32:**214, 1968.

Smith, R. B. W., Sheehy, T. W., and Rothberg, H.: Hodgkin's disease in pregnancy, Arch. Intern. Med. **102:**777, 1958.

Ueland, K., Gills, R. E., and Hansen, J. M.: Maternal cardiovascular dynamics. I. Cesarean section under subarachnoid block anesthesia, Amer. J. Obstet. Gynec. **100:**42, 1968.

Ueland, K., and Hansen, J. M.: Maternal cardiovascular dynamics. II. Posture and uterine contractions, Amer. J. Obstet. Gynec. **103:**1, 1969.

Ueland, K., and Hansen, J. M.: Maternal cardiovascular dynamics. III. Labor and delivery under local and caudal analgesia, Amer. J. Obstet. Gynec. **103:**8, 1969.

Whalley, P. J., Pritchard, J. A., and Richards, J. R., Jr.: Sickle cell trait and pregnancy, J.A.M.A. **186:**1132, 1963.

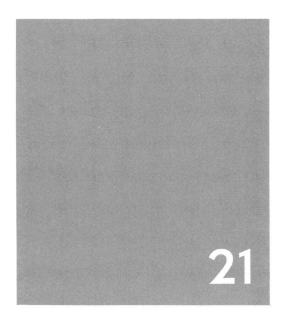

21

Digestive tract disorders during pregnancy

The structural and functional changes that occur in the digestive organs during pregnancy may account for many disturbing symptoms. In the majority of gravid women the secretion of free hydrochloric acid and pepsin decreases and gastric motility is reduced. The stomach is pushed upward and to the left by the enlarging uterus, and the tone of the entire intestinal tract is reduced.

■ Gingivitis

Occasionally the gums of pregnant women hypertrophy and become inflamed, spongy, and friable. This may be the result of vitamin C deficiency, in which event ascorbic acid, 1 Gm. daily, will produce improvement. In some women no change occurs as a result of the ingestion of vitamin C; in these persons the condition regresses spontaneously after delivery. Astringent mouthwashes may provide symptomatic relief.

■ Ptyalism

Excessive salivation is occasionally encountered. It usually corrects itself spontaneously by the middle of the second trimester, but during the peak of saliva production more than 1 L. may be secreted daily. Although tincture of belladonna, atropine, and other drugs may be prescribed, they alter the salivary secretion only slightly. Psychotherapy may prove beneficial when an emotional disturbance is the cause of salivation.

■ Nausea and vomiting

The nausea and vomiting experienced by at least one half of all women during the first trimester of pregnancy varies in degree from mild, transient morning nausea to severe constant vomiting that endangers the life of the patient. The symptoms usually appear about 2 weeks after the period has been missed, reach a maximum in about 2 more weeks, and then begin to regress by the tenth to twelfth week of gestation. They usually disappear completely by the fourteenth week, but in a few women nausea persists throughout the entire pregnancy. *Nausea and vomiting that begin after the tenth or twelfth week are more likely to be caused by a medical or surgical condition than by pregnancy alone.* Nausea and vomiting usually reappear and, in fact, may become worse with each pregnancy.

The nausea is most likely to occur when the stomach is empty, on arising in the morning or before meals, and it may be precipitated by certain odors or foods. In many women it is present upon awakening and may persist until they have eaten breakfast. In others the symptoms are somewhat more pronounced, with vomiting on arising or during the morning. A few will be nauseated all day long, whereas an occasional patient develops true *hyperemesis gravidarum,* with constant nausea and frequent vomiting that may seriously affect health.

The less severe degrees of nausea do not interfere with nutrition, and weight loss is slight, but hyperemesis may produce serious physiologic disturbances. The patient may lose 20 or more pounds and become severely dehydrated and depleted of essential electrolytes. The pulse increases to 110 to 120, and the temperature rises to 100.5° to 101° F. The serum electrolyte concentrations are reduced because of the unreplaced loss of sodi-

267

um, chloride, and potassium in the vomitus. Blood urea nitrogen increases, and a metabolic acidosis develops. The degree of change is determined by the duration and severity of the vomiting and the food and fluid ingestion.

The histopathologic changes in women who die of hyperemesis are like those that occur with starvation and include centrilobular fatty infiltration of the liver, sometimes with necrosis, degenerative changes in the renal tubules, punctate hemorrhages in the brain and retina, and degenerative neuritis in the peripheral nerves.

Etiology. The underlying etiologic factors are not completely clear, but it seems likely that the disturbance is caused by the addition of some substance new to the patient rather than the sudden development of a deficiency of vitamins, hormones, or other substances. The symptoms appear at a time during which the trophoblastic tissue is actively invading and destroying the decidua and when the function of the endocrine organs and hormone production are being drastically altered. Nausea is most pronounced when gonadotropin production reaches a maximum during the first trimester of normal pregnancy and is likely to be more troublesome with hydatidiform mole and multiple pregnancy, with which gonadotropin levels are even higher. Some substance produced during the period of tissue growth and destruction might well be responsible for the symptoms.

It is not likely that nausea is initiated by an emotional disturbance, but women with such disturbances are more likely to vomit, and the nausea can certainly be aggravated by psychic stimuli. In all probability most instances of severe nausea and vomiting (hyperemesis gravidarum) develop as a result of an emotionally stimulated increase of the "normal" pregnancy nausea. Psychiatric studies indicate that many women with hyperemesis unconsciously wish not to be pregnant, even though they may profess to want children. Some have even undergone extensive studies and treatment for infertility, which also may have had an emotional component. Others give evidence, such as frigidity, dyspareunia, and aversion to coitus, of rejecting a feminine role.

Treatment. Since the basic cause for nausea and vomiting during pregnancy has not yet been established, treatment must of necessity be directed toward reducing the severity of the symptoms. Each patient should understand that the symptoms are temporary and that they not only can be controlled but should disappear within a short time.

The nausea in the mild cases, which appears when the stomach is empty, can usually be eliminated by asking the patient to eat two or three soda crackers as soon as she awakens and before she gets out of bed. After 15 or 20 minutes she arises and eats a light breakfast, and if there is no recurrence of the nausea during the day, no other treatment is necessary.

Nausea that is constant throughout the day often can be controlled by frequent small feedings, keeping something in the stomach at all times. The patient is directed to eat in small amounts at least every 2 hours from the time she arises until bedtime. Dry foods such as crackers, toast, baked potato, white meat of chicken, and cereal are preferable because they are more likely to control the nausea. Hard candy frequently is effective. Highly spiced foods, tomato juice, orange juice, and any except bland vegetables are usually not tolerated. Liquids should be taken between feedings rather than with the solid food; tea, ginger ale or other carbonated beverages, or anything else the patient can retain are permitted. It usually is not possible for these patients to adhere to a full pregnancy diet.

Many types of medication have been used in patients with nausea and vomiting during pregnancy, but none is uniformly effective. The mild symptoms can usually be controlled with diet alone, so drugs are unnecessary. If, however, the symptoms are more severe and do not respond to diet therapy, some sort of medication may be prescribed. Mild sedation with phenobarbital, 0.032 Gm. four times daily, may be helpful, but the newer antiemetic drugs are more effective. There is no evidence to suggest that these drugs interfere with the early development of the human fetus. Prochlorperazine dimaleate (Compazine) 5 or 10 mg. three or four times daily, will often relieve the symptoms completely. It usually is unnecessary to continue the medication for more than 2 to 4 weeks.

The patient who has lost considerable

weight and is dehydrated because of hyperemesis must be admitted to the hospital for a period of active therapy to control the vomiting and correct the effects of the fluid and electrolyte loss. The important factors in the treatment of hyperemesis are (1) to control the vomiting, (2) to replace the fluid, (3) to replace water-soluble vitamins, and (4) to restore electrolyte balance. Interruption of pregnancy, which has been resorted to frequently in the past, is almost never necessary.

Upon admittance to the hospital, general physical and neurologic examinations are performed and blood is drawn for determinations of hematocrit and the concentrations of sodium, potassium, chloride, urea nitrogen and creatinine. Oral food and fluid are prohibited.

Fluid is administered intravenously, initially in the form of 10% dextrose in physiologic saline solution. The type and amount of fluid necessary to hydrate the patient and restore chemical balance will be determined by the urine volume and serum electrolyte concentrations, which should be repeated daily. It usually is necessary to supplement potassium as well as sodium and chloride. Ascorbic acid and vitamin B complex should be administered in the parenteral fluids, and a protein hydrolysate solution can also be given if the patient is seriously depleted. Parenteral administration of fluids is continued for 3 or 4 days until the patient begins to eat again. It usually is unnecessary to maintain intravenous therapy for more than 48 hours after vomiting has stopped.

Compazine can be administered intramuscularly in doses of 5 to 10 mg. every 6 or 8 hours. If Compazine alone does not control the vomiting, it may be necessary to reinforce its *sedative action* with intramuscular injections of Amytal sodium, 0.4 to 0.6 Gm. every 6 to 8 hours. It is seldom necessary to continue heavy sedation for longer than 48 to 72 hours.

The *diet* must be limited until the vomiting is controlled, after which small amounts of food can be ordered. At first small feedings of dry foods such as toast, crackers or zwieback every 2 hours are tolerated best. if there still is no recurrence of nausea, the diet is gradually increased by the addition of baked potato, chicken, roast beef, lamb, bland vegetables, cereals, Jello, and puddings. Fluids such as tea, water, or ginger ale are added 30 ml. at a time and are best given between feedings. One should proceed slowly with the addition of foods because the vomiting may recur if the progression toward a normal diet is too rapid.

Psychiatric treatment is seldom necessary for the immediate control of hyperemesis, even though it seems probable that an emotional disturbance plays an important part in the production of severe vomiting.

Once the vomiting has been stopped and chemical balance has been restored, the pregnancy usually progresses without a recurrence of the symptoms. Occasionally the vomiting does recur when the patient leaves the protective environment of the hospital, only to be easily controlled by readmittance. In such instances an emotional cause is likely, and an attempt should be made to identify the responsible factor in the patient's home situation.

■ Heartburn

Heartburn is a common complaint during pregnancy and varies in severity from occasional mild discomfort to constant incapacitating pain accompanied by nausea and vomiting. It is caused by regurgitation of stomach contents into the lower esophagus and, according to Lind and co-workers, is a result of changes in the pressure relationships in the stomach and in the esophagus at the level of the gastroesophageal sphincter. In normal nonpregnant subjects the mean resting intragastric pressure was 12.1 cm. H_2O, the spincter pressure was 34.8 cm. H_2O, and the stomach-to-sphincter gradient was 22.7 cm. H_2O. In pregnant women without heartburn the mean intragastric pressure was 17.2 cm. H_2O, the maximum sphincter pressure was 44.8 cm. H_2O, and the stomach-to-sphincter gradient was 27.6 cm. H_2O the latter being comparable to the controls. There was a striking difference in the pregnant women with heartburn: The intragastric pressure was unaltered, being 16.5 cm. H_2O, but the maximal sphincter pressure was only 23.8 cm. H_2O. The stomach-to-sphincter gradient of 7.3 cm. H_2O was obviously not high enough to prevent reflux of stomach contents. The management is similar to that described for hiatus hernia.

■ Hiatus hernia

Hiatus hernia can be demonstrated in about 12% of women during the last half of pregnancy. It is more often present in multiparas than in primigravidas and may produce annoying or even serious symptoms. Heartburn, which usually begins before the middle of pregnancy, is almost always present with hiatus hernia. It is usually made worse by lying down; therefore it often is noted at night and may interfere with sleep. Belching, hiccoughing, and regurgitation of sour material into the mouth also occur, but nausea and vomiting are somewhat less characteristic. The anatomic defect can be demonstrated by fluoroscopic and x-ray studies of the esophagogastric junction as the patient swallows barium.

Since the hernias almost always disappear after delivery, treatment should be directed toward controlling symptoms; surgical correction is almost never necessary. The regimen should include frequent small bland feedings, antacids such as aluminum hydroxide gel, 8 to 16 ml., or magnesium trisilicate tablets taken whenever necessary. Prostigmine bromide, 15 mg. taken orally three or four times daily, will increase gastric and intestinal motility and relieve heartburn. Elevation of the head on several pillows when the patient lies down will reduce regurgitation through the relaxed esophagogastric junction. It is seldom necessary to terminate pregnancy because of the symptoms produced by hiatus hernia.

■ Jaundice

It is commonly stated that liver function is unaffected by normal pregnancy, but there is considerable evidence to suggest that significant alterations do occur. Although no definite histopathologic changes can be observed in liver cells by light microscopy, certain liver functions are altered. The excretion of Bromsulphalein (BSP) is significantly impaired during pregnancy, and serum activity of nonspecific alkaline phosphatase, 5-nucleotidase, and leucine aminopeptidase is increased over that of nonpregnant women. These changes are most pronounced during the third trimester.

A small percentage of women become jaundiced during the last trimester of pregnancy without having definite evidence of viral hepatitis or other liver disease. Icterus usually is preceded by anorexia, nausea, with or without vomiting, and pruritus. The liver may be enlarged and tender, and liver function tests demonstrate the alterations just described. The histopathologic changes, which are characteristic of intrahepatic cholestasis, include centrilobular bile staining of the liver cells, canalicular bile plugs, and occasionally slight parenchymal cell necrosis. This condition, which is known as *idiopathic cholestasis* of *pregnancy,* clears promptly after delivery and there is no demonstrable residual.

Pruritus gravidarum, with which there is generalized itching that is difficult to relieve by any form of medication, is probably the same basic condition, but with less impairment of hepatic function since there is no accompanying jaundice.

Both cholestasis and pruritus gravidarum occur during late pregnancy and are thought to be caused by the response of the liver cells to estrogen and progesterone, which reach their maximum concentration during this period of the gestation. Kreek and co-workers treated a group of nonpregnant women who previously had pruritus or cholestasis during pregnancy with large doses of ethinyl estradiol and reproduced the symptoms they had experienced. Normal controls noted only mild morning nausea or had no symptoms during the treatment period.

■ Infectious hepatitis

The incidence of acute viral hepatitis in pregnant women has increased considerably in recent years. The virus responsible for acute infectious hepatitis may be introduced into the body by blood or plasma transfusion or by ingestion of contaminated food. The initial symptoms consist of anorexia, nausea, vomiting, headache, lassitude, and fever. Jaundice becomes evident in about 1 week and may last as long as 1 month or 6 weeks. The recovery period may extend over a 2- or 3-month period.

The mortality rate is low for those who were in good health at the time they contracted the disease. Five of 29 pregnant women treated by Zondek and Bromberg died, but all had been vomiting excessively and were undernourished. In a more recent series of 349 women with hepatitis during pregnancy, only 5 died. The nutritional state of the patient may be one of the most important prognostic factors. Roth reported 14 fetal and 17 neonatal deaths and 9 congenital anomalies in children born of 378 women with acute hepatitis.

Treatment is primarily of a supportive nature and includes a diet high in carbohydrate, protein, and vitamins. If the patient is vomiting or has severe anorexia, nutrition can be maintained temporarily by intravenous administration of these substances. Termination of pregnancy is not necessary.

■ Peptic ucler

The symptoms of peptic ulcer often subside during pregnancy, since both gastric acidity and motility are reduced. Clark reported that 44.8% of 118 women with peptic ulcer were free from symptoms during 313 pregnancies, whereas 43.4% were improved; pregnancy had no effect on 11.8%. Perforation and hemorrhage are rare, but either may occur. Medical treatment can be continued during pregnancy, but it may be necessary to alter the diet to meet the added nutritional requirements. Low-sodium antacid preparations should be prescribed.

■ Pancreatitis

Acute pancreatitis is rare in pregnant women, and when it does occur, it often is not diagnosed. The clinical course is similar to that in nonpregnant women, but the presence of an advanced pregnancy may prejudice the medical attendants. The basic confirmatory study, an elevated serum amylase, is as valid during pregnancy as in nonpregnant women.

Pancreatitis may occur in pregnant women being treated with thiazide preparations and with tetracycline and should be considered when a patient under treatment with these preparations develops abdominal pain.

The treatment is supportive, and operation is contraindicated if the diagnosis of pancreatitis is confirmed.

■ Ulcerative colitis

Ulcerative colitis has little effect on pregnancy, but the course of the condition in pregnant women is unpredictable. In some women the symptoms are exaggerated, but in others they remain the same or improve.

Colitis that first begins during pregnancy may run a fulminating course, ending in death. Bacon collected 208 cases from the literature and found that of these pregnancies only 18 terminated in spontaneous abortion and 5 in premature labor. Therapeutic abortion was performed in 11, 2 were delivered by cesarean section, and 172 were delivered normally.

It is particularly important that nutrition be maintained by the addition of a protein supplement when necessary and of vitamins and iron. Therapeutic abortion should be recommended if the life of the mother is endangered by the pregnancy. Most women can be delivered normally, even though the rectum and colon have been removed. Cesarean section is performed only for obstetric reasons.

References

Adams, R. H., and Combes, B.: Viral hepatitis during pregnancy, J.A.M.A. **192**:195, 1965.

Bacon, H. E.: Ulcerative colitis, Philadelphia, 1958, J. B. Lippincott Co.

Clark, D. H.: Peptic ulcer in women, Brit. Med. J. **1**:1254, 1953.

Fairweather, D. V. I.: Nausea and vomiting in pregnancy, Amer. J. Obstet. Gynec. **102**:135, 1968.

Felsen, J., and Wolarsky, W.: Chronic ulcerative colitis and pregnancy, Amer. J. Obstet. Gynec. **56**:751, 1948.

Johnston, J. L.: Peptic ulcer and pregnancy, Obstet. Gynec. **2**:290, 1953.

Kappas, A.: Biologic actions of some natural steroids on the liver, New Eng. J. Med. **278**:378, 1968.

Kreek, M. J., Weser, E., Sleisenger, M. H., and Jefferies, G. H.: Idiopathic cholestasis of pregnancy, New Eng. J. Med. **277**:1391, 1967.

Lind, J. F., Smith, A. M., McIver, D. K., Coopland, A. T., and Crispin, J. S.: Heartburn in pregnancy—a manometric study, Canad. Med. Ass. J. **98**:571, 1968.

Menzies, D., and Prystowsky, H.: Acute hemorrhagic pancreatitis during pregnancy and the puerperium associated with thiazide therapy, J. Florida Med. Ass. **54**:564, 1967.

Mixson, W. T., and Woloshin, H. J.: Hiatus hernia in pregnancy, Obstet. Gynec. **8**:249, 1956.

Rabkin, R. N.: Acute pancreatitis in pregnancy, Obstet. Gynec. **31**:508, 1968.

Roth, L. G.: Infectious hepatitis in pregnancy, Amer. J. Med. Sci. **225**:139, 1953.

Sheehan, H. L.: Jaundice in pregnancy, Amer. J. Obstet. Gynec. **81**:427, 1961.

Zondek, B., and Bromberg, J. M.: Infectious hepatitis in pregnancy, J. Mount Sinai Hosp. N. Y. **14**:222, 1947.

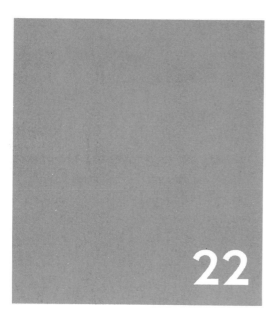

22

Urinary tract disorders during pregnancy

The structure and function of the urinary organs are altered considerably during pregnancy, but unless the tissues are seriously damaged by infection or direct injury, they return to normal during the puerperium.

The renal blood flow and the glomerular filtration rate begin to increase as early as the tenth week of pregnancy and reach a maximum during the first few weeks of the last trimester, after which they fall. At term they have returned to levels near those for normal nonpregnant women. These changes roughly parallel the rise and fall in plasma volume. The tubular reabsorption of electrolytes is increased during pregnancy. This change is at least in part due to the increased production of adrenal corticosteroid substances, which act at the tubular level to promote reabsorption. The specific gravity

of the urine often is as low as 1.010, and the kidney may be unable to excrete concentrated urine even when a concentration test is performed. This does not necessarily indicate disturbed function because the concentrating ability returns to normal after delivery. The normally functioning kidney does not permit the passage of more than 500 mg. of protein daily.

Renal function tests such as the phenolsulfonphthalein, the results of which are dependent upon measuring the amount of a foreign substance excreted during a specific period of time after a single injection, are not reliable during pregnancy. The kidney may excrete the material at a normal or even an increased rate, but the results of the test may fall into an abnormal range if urine transportation to the bladder is delayed because of stasis of urine resulting from dilatation and diminished peristalsis. This is less likely to occur when normal substances such as endogenous creatinine are measured or when a high blood level of a foreign substance such as inulin is maintained by constant infusion. The products of nitrogen metabolism are excreted more efficiently during pregnancy. The concentration of *urea nitrogen* in the serum is usually between 8 and 12 mg./100 ml. and that of *creatinine,* about 0.5 mg./100 ml. Urea nitrogen concentrations above 15 mg./ml. and of creatinine much above 1 mg./ml. must be considered as abnormal.

Cystoscopy can be performed throughout pregnancy, but during the last 4 to 6 weeks it may be relatively uninformative. At this period of gestation the bladder is pulled upward and the presenting part descends, making insertion of the instrument and inspection of the interior of the bladder difficult.

Pyelography should rarely be performed during pregnancy, particularly in the first trimester, because of possible radiation effects on the fetus. In most instances when a urinary tract disorder develops, x-ray examination can be deferred until postdelivery involution is complete.

It is important that physicians be completely familiar with the structural and functional changes that occur in the urinary tract during pregnancy; otherwise they will be unable to assess the risks of pregnancy for women with renal diseases, and they may interpret physiologic alterations as abnormalities.

■ Infection

Urinary tract infections do occur frequently during pregnancy and after delivery, but almost all of them can be prevented. From 7% to 10% of all pregnant women have a significant but asymptomatic bacteriuria (more than 100,000 colonies per milliliter of a catheterized or clean-voided urine specimen). About 40% of these will develop symptomatic urinary tract infections during late pregnancy or the puerperium. Whalley, Martin, and Pritchard found bacteriuria in 13.9% of 475 pregnant women with sickle cell trait as compared to 6.9% of a control group. One third of the bacteriuric women with sickle cell trait developed symptomatic infections during pregnancy and 13.6% after delivery. Comparable figures for control bacteriuric patients were 18.7% and 12.3%. Nineteen of 33 women with sickle cell trait had radiographic evidence of chronic pyelonephritis.

The bacteria appear early, most often during the first few weeks of the second trimester, and there usually is no accompanying pyuria. The reason for the bacteriuria is not always obvious, but chronic pyelonephritis or lower tract infections can be demonstrated in some women, particularly those who have had repeated symptomatic urinary tract infections. *Escherichia coli* is the organism most often found, but others, particularly streptococci, may be present in women with chronic or recurring infections.

It has been suggested that premature labor is more prevalent in women with bacteriuria, but most investigators have not found this to be true. It is possible, however, that infants born of mothers who have had urinary tract infections during pregnancy may have a decreased immunity toward the responsible bacteria. Wallach, Brody, and Oski found positive urine cultures in 27 (9.6%) of 279 pregnant women, *E. coli* being the responsible organism in 23. The infants of 12 women with *E. coli* bacilluria were studied for lymphocyte mitogenesis in response to *E. coli* antigen in vitro during the first 48 hours after delivery; the same test was run on 10 infants whose mothers had negative cultures. Ten of the infants of bacilluric mothers responded with the development of lymphocyte mitosis (the other two cultures were contaminated), whereas only 2 of 10 controls were positive. One infant of a bacilluric mother had *E. coli* omphalitis, and 8 others had other complications. This study suggests that *E. coli* organisms, or products of degeneration, cross the placenta and affect the baby. This initial contact with *E. coli* may be a factor in the development of neonatal infection by that organism.

Symptomatic infections and chronic pyelonephritis can be prevented if pregnant women with bacteriuria are identified and treated. Whalley, Martin, and Peters found that bacteriuria persisted after delivery in 90 (81%) of 111 women who had positive cultures during pregnancy but who were not treated; it persisted in only 45 (39%) of 115 women who were treated for bacteriuria. Bacteria can usually be detected by Gram stain of the sediment of a clean-voided specimen. The exact organism should be identified by culture of the urine containing bacteria so that appropriate treatment can be administered. An attempt should be made to eradicate the infection whenever possible. A urine culture should be obtained after delivery in every woman who has had bacteriuria or a symptomatic infection during pregnancy. Urologic study, including pyelograms, is indicated for women who have had repeated infections or those in whom bacteriuria persists.

PYELONEPHRITIS

Infection of the upper urinary tract may develop initially during pregnancy, or women with chronic pyelonephritis may conceive.

Acute pyelonephritis. Acute upper urinary tract infections may develop during pregnancy, usually late in the second trimester, early in the third, or after delivery. They occur in from 1% to 3% of all pregnant women, and even though they are treated intensively they may recur in subsequent pregnancies.

The infection may be a descending one, the organisms invading the kidney from the adjacent colon. At the onset the renal parenchyma alone is involved, but within a short time the process descends to the kidney pelvis, the ureter, and finally to the bladder. The organisms can also reach the upper uri-

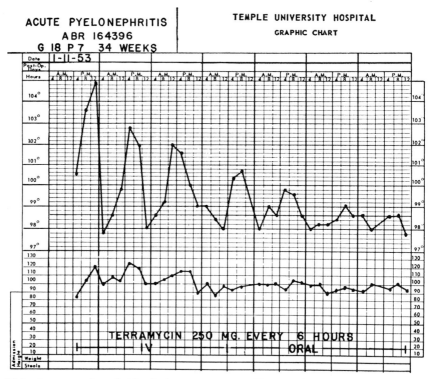

Fig. 22-1. Acute pyelonephritis during pregnancy. (From Willson, J. R.: Management of obstetric difficulties, ed. 6, St. Louis, 1961, The C. V. Mosby Co.)

nary tract by hematogenous spread, or they can ascend through the ureteral lymphatics.

During the early stages the patient may have none of the usual symptoms of urinary tract infection, but the involvement of the kidney and the resultant edema may cause flank pain and backache. At this period malaise and low-grade fever usually are present. Within 2 or 3 days the pain becomes more severe and may radiate downward toward the pelvis or the groin, the temperature rises, and the patient may have shaking chills. There may be nausea and vomiting, but it usually does not persist and the bowel habits are not much changed. Dysuria and frequency appear as the infection descends, and the urine may be dark and cloudy or even red if there is hematuria. At the peak of the infection the fever swings from high levels of 104° to 106° F. to 97° to 98° F.

Diagnosis. The patient looks ill and she may be dehydrated. Palpation of the kidney areas produces severe pain, and there may also be tenderness along the course of the ureter and over the bladder.

The diagnosis is confirmed by examina-

tion of a catheterized specimen of urine, which will contain many pus cells, singly or in clumps, red blood cells, and bacteria. Early in the course of the disease, if the infection is confined to the kidney parenchyma, the urine may be normal and remain so until the renal pelvis and ureter are involved. This stage of the disease is more often observed in the hospitalized postpartum patient than during pregnancy.

At the peak of the infection the white blood cell count may be as high as 20,000 to 30,000.

The *differential diagnosis* can be difficult, particularly in the delivered patient. The pain may begin in the right lower quadrant, and since nausea and vomiting are frequently encountered in association with urinary tract infections, appendicitis may be suspected. In urinary tract infections there is no muscle spasm, and the urine is infected. Puerperal infection must also be ruled out as a cause for the symptoms.

Treatment. Since most urinary infections are caused by *E. coli,* they can be treated more effectively with one of the sulfonamide preparations or a broad-spectrum antibiotic than with penicillin. A urine specimen should be obtained for culture before the drug is given, but the physician should not wait for the report before ordering the medication. The drug can be changed if the responsible organism is resistant to it and the clinical response is poor.

Gantrisin is effective, and because it is highly soluble it produces less crystalluria than do some of the other sulfonamide preparations. It is administered by mouth in an initial dose of 2 Gm. followed by 1 Gm. every 4 hours.

Ampicillin, a semisynthetic penicillin, is active against a number of gram-negative bacilli, other gram-negative organisms, and gram-positive cocci. It has been used successfully in the treatment of urinary tract infections in doses of 500 mg. every 6 hours.

Chloramphenicol is given orally in an initial dose of 500 mg. followed by 250 mg. every 6 hours. It can also be given intravenously in dosages of 250 to 500 mg. in 500 ml. of fluid every 12 hours. Tetracyclines should not be given because of their effect on fetal teeth and bones.

Nitrofurantoin (Furadantin) is an effective urinary antiseptic, but it is more likely to cause nausea and vomiting than are the other drugs. It is particularly effective in infections caused by the *Proteus* strains. The dosage is 50 to 100 mg. three or four times daily.

The patient should be encouraged to ingest at least 3,000 ml. of fluids daily unless she is vomiting, in which case an equivalent amount of 5% dextrose should be given intravenously. Aspirin, 0.65 Gm., and codeine, 0.065 Gm., or Demerol, 50 to 100 mg., can be given every 3 hours for pain.

The temperature usually falls to normal after 3 to 5 days of treatment, but the medication should usually be continued for at least 14 to 21 days. If there is no evidence of infection in the urine at this time, treatment can be stopped, but the patient ought to maintain a high fluid intake.

Recurrences usually mean that treatment has been discontinued before the infection is eradicated or that the fundamental cause of the infection is still present. If the infection does recur or if bacteriuria persists, an antibiotic or chemotherapeutic agent should be continued until after delivery. It is seldom

necessary to terminate pregnancy because of repeated episodes of pyelonephritis, but occasionally if the patient has several attacks in spite of adequate antibacterial treatment, the physician should consider the possibility of inducing labor as soon as it can be accomplished safely. This may prevent permanent damage to the kidney.

The urine should be examined for the presence of infection during the early puerperium and again after involution in all women who have had acute pyelonephritis during pregnancy. If the infection has been recurrent, pyelograms should be made 2 or 3 months after delivery in an attempt to demonstrate a lesion that could have caused the attacks or any damage that may have been produced by the infection.

Chronic pyelonephritis. If acute pyelonephritis is inadequately treated, the symptoms may subside but the infection may never be completely eradicated, and the patient may experience recurrent acute attacks. These can in time produce extensive tissue destruction and impaired kidney function. In some instances hypertension and renal insufficiency eventually occur. Chronic pyelonephritis can usually be prevented by treating acute infections with an effective antibacterial agent until the process has resolved completely.

Chronic infection does not necessarily preclude pregnancy if kidney function is normal, but it adds to the danger because acute attacks are likely to occur, thus increasing the possibility of permanent damage. Women with chronic urinary tract infections can be treated prophylactically with small daily doses of sulfonamides throughout pregnancy to prevent acute recurrences. If renal function is impaired and the blood pressure is elevated, pregnancy usually is contraindicated because the kidney often is functioning at almost maximum capacity and will be unable to meet the increasing demands as pregnancy advances.

URETHROCYSTITIS

Infection of the lower urinary tract occurs far more often than does pyelonephritis. It is diagnosed more frequently during the puerperium than before delivery and often develops in women who have had symptomatic bacteriuria during pregnancy.

The principal symptoms are frequency of

urination, dysuria, and bladder pain. The temperature may be elevated to 100° to 101° F., and many pus cells, red blood cells, and bacteria can be seen in a catheterized specimen of urine. *E. coli* is most often the offending organism.

Gantrisin, 1 Gm. every 4 hours, will usually eradicate the infection promptly, but before treatment is started a urine specimen should be sent for culture and drug sensitivity studies. If there is no response to the sulfonamide, an appropriate medication can then be selected.

TOXIC EFFECTS OF DRUGS

The physician must be aware that certain of the drugs used to treat urinary tract infections may cause undesirable reactions in both the mother and her baby.

Tetracyclines. Several instances of acute toxic reactions and even death after the administration of tetracycline to pregnant women with pyelonephritis have been reported. In most of them vomiting persisted or first appeared after treatment was started, and azotemia and jaundice developed. Whalley, Adams, and Combes found fine-droplet fatty metamorphosis of the liver and pancreatitis in 5 patients, one of whom died. The toxicity may be a result of reduced renal function, allowing accumulation of high concentrations of tetracycline in the tissues. This can be prevented by using smaller doses and by stopping the medication if urinary output is reduced, if the blood urea nitrogen concentration is elevated, or if there are other evidences of renal failure.

Tetracycline may also affect the infant because of its propensity to accumulate in embryonic bone. Tetracycline hydrochloride added to cultures of embryonic bone is deposited throughout the calcified area, preventing normal mineralization. Maldeveloped bones result.

Tetracycline can also be deposited in the enamel of fetal teeth, giving them a permanent yellow, mottled, fluorescent appearance. This only occurs if the drug is ingested after the fourth month of pregnancy.

Sulfonamides. Sulfonamide preparations should be used with caution in women who are about to deliver, particularly those in or likely to have premature labor. Sulfonamide dissociates bilirubin from its binding to albumin, permitting bilirubin to circulate freely and to diffuse into extravascular areas of the body. Under such circumstances the incidence of kernicterus in the newborn infant is definitely increased.

Chloramphenicol. Chloramphenicol may depress maternal bone marrow; total white blood cell and differential counts should be obtained twice weekly in an attempt to detect the first evidence of depression. This drug probably has no harmful effect on the fetus in utero, but in large doses it causes the "gray syndrome" in newborn infants.

Nitrofurantoin. Furadantin may cause hemolysis of red blood cells and megaloblastic erythropoiesis in pregnant black women with glucose-6-phosphate dehydrogenase deficiency.

RENAL TUBERCULOSIS

Tuberculosis of the kidney occurs rarely during pregnancy and may produce no symptoms unless the bladder is involved. It should be suspected if the urine contains white blood cells and red blood cells but no bacteria. The tubercle bacilli may be grown by a suitable culture technique. The characteristic lesions in the renal calyces can usually be demonstrated by pyelography.

Streptomycin, para-aminosalicylic acid, and other antituberculosis drugs can be administered safely during pregnancy. Nephrectomy, when indicated, can be performed. It is not necessary to terminate pregnancy because of renal tuberculosis.

■ Urinary calculi

Calculi seldom occur in pregnant women, even when urinary stasis and infection are present. These changes, which often influence the development of stones, are relatively transient, being present only until delivery. Thus, calculi do not have time to form.

Ureteral and renal calculi may produce fewer symptoms in pregnant than in nonpregnant women because of the decreased muscle tonus and dilatation in the urinary tract. Small stones in the ureter may be passed spontaneously as the pregnancy changes develop.

Treatment depends upon the size and position of the stones and the symptoms they cause. It may be necessary to remove obstructing calculi or those producing severe pain. Large, irregular vesical calculi should be removed because they may injure the bladder during labor and delivery. It is rarely necessary to terminate pregnancy in women with stones.

■ Hematuria

Blood in the urine can come from a lesion at any level of the urinary tract. Thus, a complete investigation is necessary. Cystoscopy can be performed at any stage of pregnancy, but the value of pyelography is limited when the infant is near term size. In such instances x-ray examination should usually be delayed until 3 or 4 weeks after delivery. The possible causes of hematuria are severe infection, rupture of small varicosities of the bladder, calculi, acute glomerulonephritis, tuberculosis, tumors, and other rare lesions.

■ Nephritis

ACUTE GLOMERULONEPHRITIS

An initial attack of glomerulonephritis is uncommon in gravid women, but when it does occur, the pregnancy adds an additional complicating factor. Urinary output is diminished or ceases completely, and the urine is smoky or bloody, of high specific gravity, and contains large amounts of protein and many cellular casts. The blood pressure usually is elevated, there is generalized edema, and the patient feels and looks sick.

Spontaneous abortion may occur during the acute phase. The place of therapeutic abortion is not clearly defined, but with moderately severe involvement, termination of pregnancy may be considered as the acute phase begins to subside. The elimination of the pregnancy may permit more complete healing of the renal lesions because kidney function must increase as pregnancy advances, and the abnormal kidney may not be able to respond.

CHRONIC GLOMERULONEPHRITIS

Fortunately the combination of chronic nephritis and pregnancy is seldom encountered. The abnormal renal function and the accompanying changes in the cardiovascular system increase the hazards for both mother and baby considerably.

Chronic nephritis should be suspected when protein is discovered in the urine, even in the event of a negative history, and the diagnosis can be confirmed if the physician can find red blood cells, white blood cells, and casts in a catheterized urine specimen. Hypertension and degenerative vascular changes may also be present.

The prognosis depends in a large measure upon whether or not the kidney is able to respond to the increasing demands as pregnancy advances; consequently, when chronic nephritis is discovered during pregnancy, the patient should be admitted to the hospital for evaluation. Minimal basic studies should include (1) history and physical examination, (2) examination of the retinal vessels, (3) daily blood pressure determinations, (4) determination of hemoglobin or hematocrit, white blood cell count, and red blood cell count, (5) measurement of blood urea nitrogen and creatinine concentrations, (6) complete examination of several catheterized urine specimens, (7) determination of daily urinary protein excretion, (8) urea and creatinine clearances, and (9) urine concentration tests.

If the renal impairment is minimal and the blood pressure is normal, pregnancy may be allowed to continue as long as the patient remains reasonably normal, but if the blood pressure rises progressively or if renal function diminishes as pregnancy advances, termination should be considered for the sake of the infant as well as of the mother.

The perinatal mortality is much higher than that for normal pregnancy, the principal causes of death being abruptio placentae, placental insufficiency caused either by an unusually small placenta or extensive infarction—which is characteristic of hypertensive cardiovascular disease—and premature labor. Babies born of mothers with chronic nephritis are usually smaller than the infants of normal women at a comparable stage of pregnancy. A relatively small uterus, therefore, should not influence the physician to delay delivery if the vascular renal status is deteriorating because under such circumstances the baby usually dies in utero.

Therapeutic termination of early pregnancy is advisable if the blood pressure is elevated or if renal function is impaired. Glomerular filtration and renal blood flow must increase progressively during pregnancy; if the kidney is unable to respond to the increasing demands as pregnancy advances, the mother will die. Since the kidney lesions are irreparable, pregnancy will be no less hazardous in the future; consequently tubal ligation should also be advised.

■ Congenital polycystic kidney disease

Congenital polycystic kidneys are only rarely encountered in pregnant women. Landesman and Scherr report that the diagnosis was made in 114 of 390,000 patients admitted to the New York Hospital. Only 28 were pregnant. The diagnosis is often overlooked in young women because clinical signs and symptoms usually do not appear until after the age period in which most women bear children. The occurrence of polycystic kidney disease in other members of the family should suggest the possibility.

Unless renal function is depressed, women with polycystic kidneys usually do well during pregnancy. Blood pressure elevation alone does not contraindicate pregnancy, but if proteinuria is present and renal function is depressed, prompt termination usually is warranted.

■ Single kidney

The lack of a kidney is no contraindication to pregnancy if the function in the remaining one is normal. Renal function should be evaluated before pregnancy is contemplated or as soon as possible after conception. Therapeutic abortion should be considered only if renal function is impaired, if there is a large calculus with infection, or if the patient has chronic pyelonephritis or has repeated urinary tract infections that cannot be controlled.

■ Renal transplants

Few women who have had renal transplants have become pregnant, but undoubtedly the number will increase in the future. Murray and associates reported on the results of 2 pregnancies in a woman who received a kidney from her twin sister because of preterminal glomerulonephritis.

Renal function was normal and her pregnancies were uneventful; she was delivered by cesarean section about 2 years and again about 4½ years after the transplant. Her sister, meanwhile, had 3 normal pregnancies.

The pelvic position of the transplanted kidney may place it in some jeopardy during pregnancy if it is located where pressure from the growing fetus can alter its blood supply. Cesarean section probably is preferable to vaginal delivery to protect the kidney from pressure during labor.

References

Baird, D.: Anatomy and physiology of the upper urinary tract in pregnancy: relation to pyelitis, J. Obstet. Gynaec. Brit. Comm. **38:**516, 1931.

Kass, E. H.: Bacteriuria and pyelonephritis of pregnancy, Arch. Intern. Med. **105:**194, 1960.

Kittredge, W. E., and Crawley, J. R.: Surgical renal lesions with pregnancy, J.A.M.A. **162:**1353, 1956.

Kline, A. H., Blattner, R. J., and Lunin, M.: Transplacental effect of tetracycline on teeth, J.A.M.A. **188:**178, 1964.

Landesman, R., and Scherr, L.: Congenital polycystic kidney disease in pregnancy, Obstet. Gynec. **8:**673, 1956.

Murray, J. E., Reid, D. E., Harrison, J. H., and Merrill, J. P.: Successful pregnancies after human renal transplantation, New Eng. J. Med. **269:**341, 1963.

Saxen, L.: Tetracycline; effect on osteogenesis in vitro, Science **149:**870, 1965.

Schaefer, G., and Markham, S.: Full-term delivery following nephrectomy, Amer. J. Obstet. Gynec. **100:**1078, 1968.

Wallach, E. E., Brody, J. I., and Oski, F. A.: Fetal immunization as a consequence of bacilluria during pregnancy, Obstet. Gynec. **33:**100, 1969.

Whalley, P. J., Adams, R. H., and Combes, B.: Tetracycline toxicity in pregnancy, J.A.M.A. **189:**357, 1964.

Whalley, P. J., Martin, F. G., and Pritchard, J. A.: Sickle cell trait and urinary tract infection during pregnancy, J.A.M.A. **189:**903, 1964.

Whalley, P. J., Martin, F. G., and Peters, P. C.: Significance of asymptomatic bacteriuria detected during pregnancy, J.A.M.A. **193:**879, 1965.

Whitelaw, M. J., Cobb, S. W., and Mengert, W. F.: Puerperal involution of urinary tract, Amer. J. Obstet. Gynec. **60:**192, 1950.

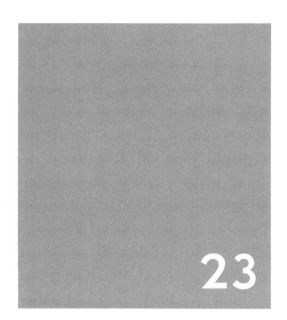

23

Genital tract disorders during pregnancy

Pathologic conditions originating in the genital tract may complicate the course of pregnancy, labor, or delivery. These disturbances include (1) local infections or infestations, (2) neoplasms, (3) uterine malpositions, and (4) congenital malformations. Some of these disorders become evident for the first time during pregnancy, particularly if gestation is threatened or if growth of the uterus and other local physiologic changes result in the development of symptoms. Careful prenatal pelvic examination, preferably during the first trimester, offers the best opportunity for diagnosis of genital tract disturbances and makes possible timely planning for the management of these conditions.

■ Vulvovaginal disorders

Mucoid secretion from the vagina is increased during pregnancy because of vascu-

larity and increased activity of the cervical glands. In the absence of symptoms or of evidence of inflammation, treatment of vaginal discharge is unnecessary. These changes and the increased glycogen content of the vaginal epithelium during pregnancy are conducive to the development of persistent local disturbances.

Vulvitis. Local irritation and itching are frequently secondary to some form of vaginitis. The vulva may become swollen, red, and edematous. Intertrigo extending over the inner aspect of the thighs is common in obese women. Treatment consists of local cleansing and the application of a bland ointment such as equal parts of Lassar's paste (plain) and boric acid ointment. If an allergic etiology is suspected, a hydrocortisone ointment is useful until the responsible factor is found and removed.

Condylomas. Condylomata acuminata may increase in size during pregnancy, occasionally attaining proportions sufficient to interfere with vaginal delivery. If the condylomas are not too large, they can be readily removed by the local application of 25% podophyllin ointment to each growth. The surrounding tissue should be protected against the irritating action of podophyllin by use of a bland ointment. Large lesions should be removed by electrosurgical or sharp excision as early as possible in pregnancy.

Condylomata lata are highly infectious secondary syphilitic lesions that appear in isolated areas over the vulva as flat warty plaques. The lesions disappear when antisyphilitic treatment is given.

Infection of Bartholin's glands. Acute lower genital tract infection caused by gonococcus or other pyogenic microorganisms may occur during pregnancy and involve the vulvovaginal glands. An abscess that develops despite antibiotic therapy should be drained, even during the last few weeks of pregnancy. Drainage prevents the inevitable rupture and genital tract contamination during delivery. Excision of an asymptomatic Bartholin cyst is usually better avoided during pregnancy because of the great increase in vulvar vascularity.

Gonorrhea. The presence of pregnancy offers no protection against acute gonorrhea, but the infection is usually limited to the lower genital tract. Extension of a newly

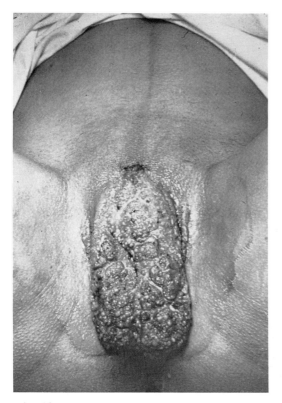

Fig. 23-1. Condylomata acuminata.

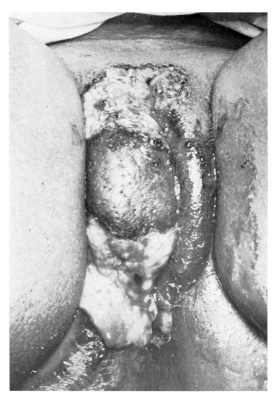

Fig. 23-2. Granuloma inguinale.

acquired infection upward to the tubes is uncommon during pregnancy, but upper genital tract infection may develop during the puerperium if the disease is not eradicated beforehand. During labor and delivery, infected material squeezed from cervical, Skene's, or Bartholin's glands may cause *ophthalmia neonatorum* in the infant. The diagnosis and treatment of gonorrhea are discussed in Chapter 40.

Lymphopathia venereum. Lymphopathia venereum, a veneral disease of viral origin, may give rise to obstetric complications in the advanced stages of the disease. The infection is found mostly in black women, although white women are not immune. It begins as a small papular or pustular lesion of the mucous membrane, generally in the region of the fourchet, and spreads via the perirectal and pelvic lymphatics, causing ulceration, edema, and extensive fibrosis of the soft tissues of the pelvis. Rectal and vaginal strictures are characteristic of chronic lymphopathia venereum.

The disease itself has no effect upon the

pregnancy or vice versa, but the dense pelvic fibrosis may make vaginal delivery hazardous. Trauma at delivery may produce hemorrhage, infection, or rupture into the rectum. Cesarean section is indicated if pelvic fibrosis is severe.

Granuloma inguinale. The lesions of granuloma inguinale tend to remain more superficial than those of lymphopathia venereum unless secondary infection is severe. In such cases the extent of the infectious process and the resultant soft tissue deformity may be sufficient to interfere with vaginal delivery. The primary lesion is a papular eruption usually in the region of the labia minora, the surface of which becomes ulcerated and spreads over the entire vulvoperineal area. The surface is weeping, foul, and granulomatous. Diagnosis is confirmed by the demonstration of Donovan bodies in scrapings obtained directly from the surface of the ulcers. The treatment of lymphopathia venereum and granuloma inguinale is discussed in Chapter 45.

Trichomonas vaginalis vaginitis. The

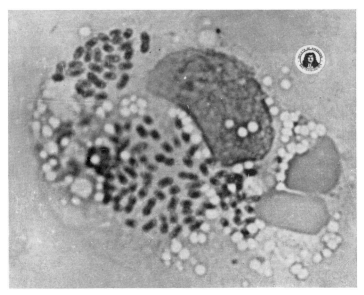

Fig. 23-3. Donovan bodies—direct ulcer scrapings. (S.A.B. No. 292.) (From Dougherty, J. M., and Lamberti, A. J.: Textbook of bacteriology, St. Louis, 1954, The C. V. Mosby Co.)

presence of vaginal trichomoniasis is a source of great annoyance throughout the entire prenatal period.

Metronidazole (Flagyl) is a singularly effective trichomonocidal agent, particularly since the drug can be administered orally to both male and female partners, but its use during the first trimester of pregnancy has been questioned. Peterson and associates administered the drug to 206 gravid women in full dosages of 250 mg. three times daily for 10 days. Side effects, occurring in 21%, were mild. Although direct cause-and-effect relationships could not be established, the slightly higher congenital anomaly rate noted in patients treated in the first trimester led the authors to recommend avoidance at this stage of gestation.

A vaginal douche can be employed, but special precautions must be taken during pregnancy. The nozzle should be inserted just inside the introitus and the solution permitted to flow gently by gravity. The use of any apparatus that requires manual pressure such as bulb syringe or a powder insufflator is contraindicated in the gravid patient because of the danger of air embolus.

Mycotic vulvovaginitis. The yeastlike fungus *Candida (Monilia) albicans* is a frequent cause of vaginitis in pregnant women. The increased glycogen content of the va-

ginal epithelium is conducive to the development of candidiasis because growth of the organisms is enhanced by carbohydrate. Intense itching is usually the first symptom. Vaginal discharge may be scant, but upon speculum examination, thick white plaques are often visible over a reddened mucous membrane. Secondary infection is common. *Monilia* organisms transferred to the infant during delivery are a usual cause of thrush in the newborn. The diagnosis and treatment are discussed in Chapter 44.

■ **Neoplastic growths**

Various benign neoplasms involving the generative organs and occasionally malignant tumors are found in gravid women. Their existence during pregnancy presents certain diagnostic and therapeutic problems. Opinions have been divided as to whether or not pregnancy has an accelerating effect upon the rate of neoplastic growth, but certainly early diagnosis serves the best interest of the mother, and usually her unborn child as well.

Cervical polyps. Cervical polyps tend to increase in size during pregnancy because of edema. The usual symptom is bleeding. The polyp, including the base, should be excised and sent to the laboratory for tissue examination. Polypectomy is unlikely to cause

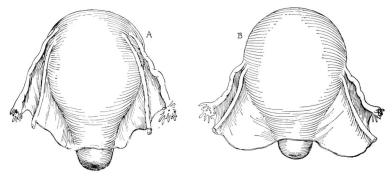

Fig. 23-4. Relationship of insertions of round ligaments and tubes to the fundus in, **A,** gravid uterus and, **B,** nongravid uterus, with symmetric enlargement due to fundal fibroid.

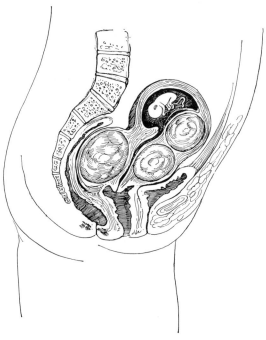

Fig. 23-5. Pregnancy in the myomatous uterus.

abortion. Bleeding almost always can be controlled by the application of a hemostatic agent such as Surgicel or the use of a tampon kept firmly in place for several hours.

Cervical carcinoma. Speculum examination and vaginal smears are innocuous regardless of the stage of gestation, and conization of the cervix, which should be done when suspicious smears are found, seldom disturbs the pregnancy. There has been considerable controversy regarding the interpretation of cytologic and histologic material in gravid women, especially with respect to the diagnosis of preinvasive carcinoma of the cervix. Greene and co-workers have presented ample evidence that when the histologic criteria are present for diagnosis of carcinoma in situ, the diagnosis can be made whether or not the patient is pregnant. Carcinoma of the cervix, including lesions complicating pregnancy, is discussed in detail in Chapter 43.

Uterine fibromyomas. The coexistence of uterine fibromyomas and pregnancy is relatively common. Small tumors are of little consequence unless their location is submucus, in which case the abortion rate is doubled. Although tumors of any size may produce symptoms of pain or pressure, surgical intervention is rarely necessary during the course of pregnancy. Complications are principally related to the size and location of the tumors, to degenerative changes in the fibroid, or to torsion of a pedunculated tumor.

Diagnosis. The main problem in diagnosis is the recognition of the existence of pregnancy in a fibroid uterus. This is particularly difficult when implantation bleeding or threatened abortion complicates the early course. Nevertheless, an accurate menstrual history is an important early guide. Delayed or abnormal bleeding, symptoms of early pregnancy, softening of the cervix, or recent increase in size of a fibroid uterus should suggest the possibility of pregnancy in every case. If any doubt remains, a biologic test for pregnancy, fetal electrocardiography, or x-ray examination of the abdomen for skeletal parts should be done before an ill-advised laparotomy is performed.

When a symmetrically enlarged uterus is discovered at operation, the differential diagnosis must be made between a soft myoma and an intrauterine pregnancy. If pregnancy is present, the resistance is less because of the fluid content. In addition, the tubes and round ligaments are elongated, since the relationship of their attachments to the fundal portion of the uterus is retained. The tubes and round ligaments are usually attached low on the uterus if the symmetric enlargement results from a soft, fundal leiomyoma. If these evidences are inconclusive, needle aspiration should be done in an attempt to detect amniotic fluid. Neither laparotomy nor needle aspiration is likely to disturb pregnancy if the uterus is not unduly manipulated.

Complications. Uterine fibroids tend to enlarge during pregnancy and diminish again as involution takes place. Their apparent growth results chiefly from edema and to a lesser extent from the hormonal stimulation of pregnancy. Degenerative changes are likely to occur during pregnancy, the hemorrhagic variety *(red degeneration)* being most common. Pain, local tenderness, and slight elevation of temperature are the usual symptoms. The pathologic process is ordinarily limited to the substance of the fibroid proper and tends to subside spontaneously in 2 or 3 days. Hence conservative treatment employing bed rest, local application of heat, and mild analgesics such as aspirin, 0.65 Gm., and codeine, 0.065 Gm., will control the symptoms in most instances. Myomectomy is rarely necessary and is frequently followed by abortion if the uterine wall is incised. An exception is found in *pedunculated tumors,* which may twist and become necrotic as the uterus enlarges and rises out of the pelvis. If torsion occurs, laparotomy is imperative before gangrenous changes and general peritonitis develop. Fortunately this type of tumor can usually be removed with impunity if wedge incision through the pedicle and imbrication of the cut edges can be accomplished without invading the myometrium.

The major complications resulting from fibroids arise during labor and delivery. These include (1) obstruction of the birth canal, (2) an increased incidence of dysfunctional labor, (3) fetal malpositions, (4) faulty placental separation, and (5) postpartum hemorrhage. Tumors blocking the inlet may make cesarean section necessary. Those situated low in the anterior wall are usually pulled up out of the pelvis as the lower uterine segment lengthens, but if the tumor is situated posteriorly, elevation may be prevented by the promontory of the sacrum. Vaginal examintion should be performed early in labor before deciding upon the route of delivery. If the birth canal is not obstructed and the fetal position does not preclude vaginal delivery, a trial of labor should be given. Occasionally the presence of fibroids alters uterine contractility and induces dysfunctional labor or postpartum hemorrhage. In rare instances the placenta is attached over a submucous or deep intramural fibroid, which may interfere with the normal process of separation and expulsion.

Despite the various potential hazards, vaginal delivery is frequently uneventful even in the presence of multiple uterine fibroids. If cesarean section is necessary because of pelvic obstruction or abnormal labor, hysterectomy may or may not be indicated, but myomectomy should be avoided. Except for the removal of a pedunculated tumor, cesarean section followed by myomectomy is attended by higher mortality and morbidity rates than cesarean section alone or cesarean section followed by hysterectomy.

During the puerperium the blood supply to uterine myomas may be suddenly reduced. Red degeneration is more common in the postpartum period than at any other time. Laparotomy is indicated if symptoms of degeneration develop and persist during the stage of uterine involution. Since complications including bleeding, infection, and postoperative bowel obstruction are more common if the uterus is allowed to remain, hysterectomy is preferable to myomectomy when surgical intervention is necessary during the puerperium.

Ovarian neoplasms. Ovarian neoplasms occur once in every 500 to 1,000 pregnancies. Their existence may be unsuspected prior to the prenatal examination, at which time the finding of an ovarian enlargement may present considerable diagnostic and therapeutic difficulties.

Diagnosis. The ovary containing the corpus luteum may be enlarged during the first trimester, but upon reexamination at 2- or 3-week intervals it becomes progres-

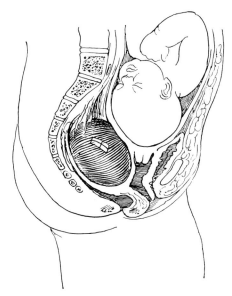

Fig. 23-6. Obstruction of birth canal by ovarian cyst.

sively smaller after the eighth to tenth week of pregnancy. *True ovarian neoplasms* are usually larger than 5 cm. in diameter and do not decrease in size upon repeated examinations. Discovery of an adnexal mass is much easier if the first prenatal pelvic examination is done in the first trimester. As pregnancy advances, an ovarian cyst is displaced by the enlarging uterus. If it is displaced laterally or is trapped in the cul-de-sac, it is still palpable upon bimanual examination, but often the cyst is carried upward above the uterus. In this case it is felt only upon abdominal examination. In most instances the diagnosis can be made clinically and the treatment is operative. Roentgenography is rarely necessary.

Complications and management. Ovarian tumors in puerperal women cannot be viewed with complacency because the incidence of malignancy is approximately 5%. Small cysts found early in pregnancy should be reevaluated at 2- or 3-week intervals. Those larger than 5 cm. that do not regress and all solid ovarian tumors require laparotomy. The time in pregnancy considered most favorable for their removal is during the fourth month for the following reasons: (1) nausea and vomiting of pregnancy are less likely to complicate the postoperative course; (2) the uterine size does not inter-

fere with whatever surgery is necessary; (3) a corpus luteum cyst will have shown regression; and (4) placental hormone production is adequate to support the pregnancy. How long the corpus luteum is essential for maintenance of the pregnancy is debatable. There have been numerous instances of its removal in early pregnancy without abortion ensuing. Pratt reported two cases of persons in whom the corpus luteum was removed at 21 and 30 days after the last normal menstrual period without disturbing the pregnancies. Delivery occurred at 272 and 279 days, respectively, verifying the history and clinical findings of very early gestations at the time of surgery. Grimes and co-workers reported 28 cysts removed in the first trimester, 16 containing the corpus luteum, and one abortion occurred. Tulsky and Koff performed total excision of the corpus luteum early in pregnancy in 14 women in whom therapeutic abortion was ultimately done. There were only two spontaneous abortions, and 10 of the 14 continued to excrete normal quantities of pregnanediol after complete lutectomy.

Immediate removal of the cyst is necessary regardless of the stage of pregnancy if symptoms of torsion or hemorrhage arise or if rapid growth of the mass is detected. If the neoplasm is diagnosed late in pregnancy and the birth canal is not obstructed, vaginal delivery is preferable, but cystoophorectomy should be carried out in the immediate postpartum period. Torsion of the elongated pedicle is common as the uterine size decreases. If the cyst obstructs the pelvis, it or the uterus may rupture during labor. No attempt should be made to evacuate the cyst by cul-de-sac aspiration or drainage, since leakage into the peritoneal cavity may result in widespread peritonitis, shock, or dissemination of malignant cells. Cesarean section and cystectomy are preferable. Since ovarian lesions are frequently bilateral, examination with biopsy of the opposite ovary is indicated in every case.

■ Malpositions of the uterus

Anterior displacement. Early in pregnancy the uterus is anteflexed, but it straightens as the uterus rises from the pelvis and meets the resistance of the anterior abdominal wall. Significant anterior displacement occurs if the rectus abdominis muscles are widely separated or extremely lax. The uterus falls directly forward, producing sharp angulation at the cervicouterine junction.

Apart from the patient's discomfort, effects upon the pregnancy are minimal until labor begins. Dystocia is common if the position is uncorrected, since the force of uterine contractions is misdirected, driving the presenting part toward the sacrum rather than into the pelvis. In addition, the anterior portion of the cervix is compressed; hence retraction and dilatation may be impaired. The difficulties can be overcome by the application of a good support during pregnancy and a firm abdominal binder during labor.

Ventrofixation of the gravid uterus. Ventrofixation of the gravid uterus is relatively rare, since fixation operations for the correction of uterine retroversion during the childbearing years have fortunately become obsolete. Occasionally, firm adhesions develop between the uterus and anterior abdominal wall after myomectomy or cesarean section. Abortion is the usual result because the growing uterus is incapable of uniform distention. If the pregnancy continues, the uterus enlarges almost entirely by stretching of the posterior uterine wall. This becomes remarkably thin, forming a *posterior sacculation* of the uterus. Cesarean section is usually necessary for delivery.

Retrodisplacement. Some degree of uterine retroversion or retroflexion is observed in at least 20% of normal women. Ordinarily, the fertility rate is not affected if the retroversion is uncomplicated. Spontaneous correction is the rule as the uterus gradually enlarges and rises out of the pelvis. This is true even in those instances in which posterior adhesions resulting from previous inflammatory disease or endometriosis are present. Adhesions of this type usually stretch or undergo dissolution, permitting spontaneous restitution by the twelfth week of pregnancy. Once the fundus rises above the sacral promontory, there is no danger of recurrence.

Occasionally the retrodisplaced uterus is held in the pelvis by dense adhesions or by a fibroid situated posteriorly and becomes impinged beneath the sacral promontory. Abortion occurs if the uterine circulation is significantly reduced by compression. Pressure

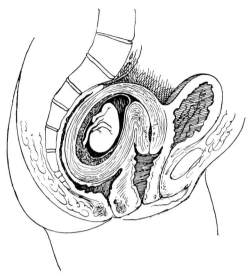

Fig. 23-7. Incarceration of the gravid uterus.

symptoms may develop acutely if the condition is uncorrected by the thirteenth or fourteenth week, and the pregnant uterus becomes incarcerated in the pelvis. The rectum is compressed posteriorly, whereas the cervix is pulled sharply forward, exerting pressure against the urethra and vesicle neck. The patient may have difficulty urinating and may even develop urinary retention with overflow.

Manual replacement is indicated early in pregnancy when symptoms arise or in those persons approaching the twelfth week in whom spontaneous correction has not taken place. This is more readily accomplished with the patient in the knee-chest position. Should gradual bimanual manipulation alone fail to elevate the fundus, simultaneous traction against a tenaculum applied to the cervix is usually effective. A pessary should then be inserted in order to maintain the correction. This can be removed by the sixteenth week. Manual reposition is more difficult in the rare instances of incarceration, but there is no need for hasty or traumatic procedures. The bladder should be kept empty by means of an indwelling catheter and bimanual manipulation repeated after knee-chest exercises have been done. Anesthesia may be necessary to dislodge and elevate the uterus, but laparotomy is seldom indicated.

Prolapse of the gravid uterus. Prolapse

of the uterus occurs occasionally in association with pregnancy. Descensus may be present before conception or may develop after pregnancy is established. Spontaneous correction will sometimes occur at about the sixteenth week when the uterus becomes too large to enter the pelvis, but mechanical replacement will provide earlier relief and prevent progressive elongation, edema, and congestion of the cervix. If the prolapsed uterus becomes incarcerated in the pelvis, abortion is likely to occur. Obviously ulceration and infection increase the hazard of delivery, but if treatment has been instituted beforehand, labor and delivery should be relatively uncomplicated.

Management. Replacement of the uterus is indicated at whatever stage of pregnancy prolapse appears. Bed rest in slight Trendelenburg position is advisable for a few days if cervical edema is severe. If prolapse occurs during the first trimester, a properly fitting pessary can then be introduced and left as long as is necessary. Klawans and Kantor believe that replacement of the pessary immediately after delivery reduces puerperal complications associated with recurrence of the prolapse, in particular subinvolution, bleeding, and infection.

■ Congenital anomalies

The müllerian ducts make their first appearance by the sixth week of embryonic life. Growth of the paired ducts and fusion of their lower portions forming the uterus and vagina should be complete by the sixteenth week. Failure of development on the one hand or failure of fusion on the other will result in absence or reduplication of related structures. Because of the close embryonic association, anomalies of the genital tract are frequently accompanied by malformations of the urinary apparatus. For example, when double uterus is observed, absence of one kidney is common. Minor deviations may have no effect whatever upon

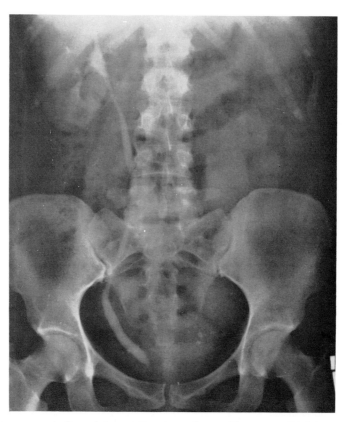

Fig. 23-8. Pregnancy at 6 weeks' gestation in patient with uterus didelphys and congenital absence of one kidney.

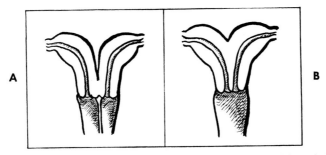

Fig. 23-9. A, Uterus didelphys bicollis (septate vagina). B, Uterus bicornis bicollis (vagina simplex).

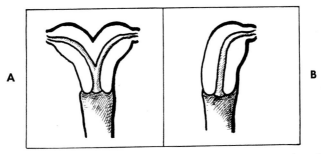

Fig. 23-10. A, Uterus bicornis unicollis (vagina simplex). B, Uterus unicornis.

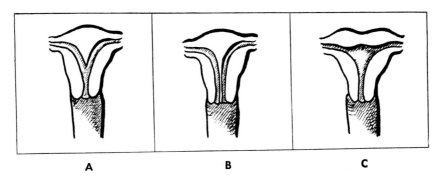

Fig. 23-11. A, Uterus subseptus. B, Uterus septus. C, Uterus arcuatus.

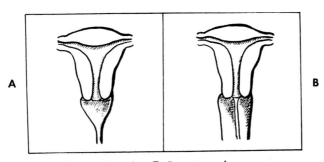

Fig. 23-12. A, Congenital stricture of vagina. B, Septate vagina.

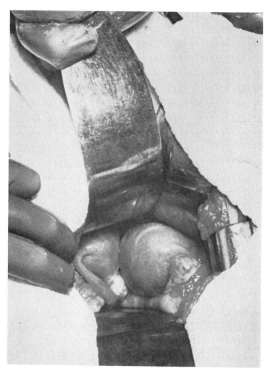

Fig. 23-13. Double uterus showing pregnancy in right uterus.

sexual function, and as a consequence many remain undetected. On the contrary, the patient with pronounced uterine malformation is subject to many complications of pregnancy, labor, and delivery and consequently suffers a higher fetal loss. Early recognition, regardless of the gradation of the abnormality, is the best preventive measure.

Types. Various types of uterine malformations are graphically demonstrated according to a modification of Jarcho's classification.

1. Uterus didelphys bicollis (septate vagina)
2. Uterus duplex bicornis bicollis (vagina simplex)
3. Uterus bicornis unicollis (vagina simplex)
4. Uterus septus (complete)
5. Uterus subseptus (partial)
6. Uterus arcuatus (concave fundus)
7. Uterus unicornis

Early complications. Genital malformations do not ordinarily reduce fertility, and although many pregnancies continue un-

eventfully, spontaneous abortions and premature labors are significantly increased. These accidents occur because the deformed uterus is less likely to provide a normal implantation site or to supply adequate nutrition for the early conceptus. In addition, the influence of underdeveloped uterine musculature may become apparent by lack of distensibility or accommodation, with premature contractions and early rupture of the membranes, or by ineffectual contractions after labor begins in those who are approaching term.

Pregnancy in one side of a double uterus is frequently associated with vaginal bleeding during the first trimester. Philpott and Ross encountered this symptom in over 50% of their 56 reported cases. Since the ovarian cycle is suspended by a viable pregnancy regardless of its location, this bleeding does not represent continued menstruation but rather the casting off of decidua from the nonpregnant side. Recognition is important in order to avoid unnecessary medical treatment or surgical interference.

Late complications. Vaginal delivery can often be accomplished with little or no difficulty, and the opportunity should be afforded as long as conditions during labor remain satisfactory. Nevertheless, close observation is necessary because *malpositions* and *uterine inertia* are not uncommon complications. Occasionally the birth canal becomes obstructed by the nonpregnant portion of a double uterus, and abdominal delivery is necessary. *Obstructed delivery* caused by vaginal septa requires nothing more than local excision. The third stage of labor is often complicated by *retained placenta* requiring manual removal.

Diagnosis and management. Early diagnosis is difficult at best and becomes more so if the first prenatal examination is done after the fourteenth week of gestation. Discovery of a vaginal septum should arouse suspicion of other genital and urinary tract anomalies. Intravenous pyelography is indicated, except during pregnancy, whenever a malformation of the reproductive tract is discovered. Patients in whom preconception examination is suggestive and those with histories of repeated unexplained abortions, premature labors, or fetal deaths deserve further study by hysterosalpingography before another pregnancy is attempted.

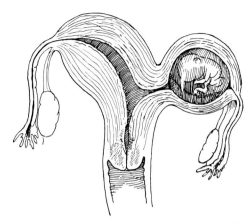

Fig. 23-14. Pregnancy in the rudimentary horn.

A sterile vaginal examination should be carried out early in labor. If the fetal position is normal, if there is no obstruction from an accessory organ, and if the mechanism of labor is not faulty, vaginal delivery can be expected. Incision of a vaginal septum is necessary only if descent of the presenting part is delayed. Bleeding from this procedure is usually minimal. Manual removal of the placenta is frequently necessary, and as a result of defective musculature, poor uterine contractions after the third stage increase the likelihood of postpartum hemorrhage.

Delivery by cesarean section for congenital malformations will be required when conditions for vaginal delivery cannot be met, but it should rarely be practiced as an early elective procedure. Corrective measures may be advisable several months post partum in selected cases, but malformations of the uterus do not provide an indication for therapeutic abortions or sterilization. The unification operation of Strassmann is highly effective in the treatment of double uterus. The occurrence of two or more consecutive abortions or pregnancy failures is ample indication for operation. A transverse incision in the fundus has the advantage of avoiding loss of valuable myometrial tissue, but in some cases elliptic wedge-shaped incisions directed anteroposteriorly are more feasible.

Pregnancy in the rudimentary horn of uterus didelphys presents a rare but urgent problem in which early diagnosis is of utmost importance. This condition differs from other uterine malformations in that the rudi-

mentary horn may have an inadequate opening into the more developed uterine cavity. The clinical course resembles that of ectopic pregnancy except that the musculature, although defective, may permit a more advanced gestation than implantation in the fallopian tube. As a consequence, rupture may occur somewhat later and incite more profuse intra-abdominal hemorrhage and shock.

Differential diagnosis usually rests between uterine myoma, ovarian cyst, and ectopic pregnancy. Treatment is surgical with complete removal of the rudimentary horn.

References

Barter, R. H., and Parks, J.: Myoma uteri associated with pregnancy, Clin. Obstet. Gynec. 1: 519, 1958.

Boutselis, J. G., and Ullery, J. C.: Intraepithelial carcinoma of the cervix in pregnancy, Amer. J. Obstet. Gynec. 90:593, 1964.

Capraro, V. J., Chuang, J. T., and Randall, C. L.: Improved fetal salvage after metroplasty, Obstet. Gynec. 31:97, 1968.

Carter, B., Cuyler, K., Thomas, W. L., Creadick, R., and Alter, R.: Methods of management of carcinoma in situ of the cervix, Amer. J. Obstet. Gynec. 64:833, 1952.

Dougherty, C. M., and Lund, C. J.: Solid ovarian tumors complicating pregnancy, Amer. J. Obstet. Gynec. 60:261, 1950.

Fenton, A. N., and Singh, B. P.: Pregnancy associated with congenital abnormalities of the female reproductive tract, Amer. J. Obstet. Gynec. 63: 744, 1952.

Greene, R. R., Peckham, B. M., Chung, J. T., Bayly, M. A., Benaron, H. B. W., Carrow, L. A., and Gardner, G. H.: Preinvasive carcinoma of the cervix during pregnancy, Surg. Gynec. Obstet. 96:71, 1953.

Grimes, W. H., Jr., Bartholomew, R. A., Colvin, E. D., Fish, J. S., and Lester, W. M.: Ovarian cyst complicating pregnancy, Amer. J. Obstet. Gynec. 68:594, 1954.

Gustafson, G. W., Gardiner, S. H., and Stout, F. E.: Ovarian tumors complicating pregnancy, Amer. J. Obstet. Gynec. 67:1210, 1954.

Hertig, A. T., and Younge, P. A.: Debate: what is cancer in situ of the cervix? Is it the preinvasive form of true carcinoma? Amer. J. Obstet. Gynec. 64:807, 1952.

Jarcho, J.: Malformations of the uterus, Amer. J. Surg. 71:106, 1946.

Jones, H. W., Jones, G. E. S.: Double uterus as an etiological factor in repeated abortion; indications for surgical repair, Amer. J. Obstet. Gynec. 65:325, 1953.

Kaiser, I. H., and King, E. L.: Lymphopathia venereum complicating labor, Amer. J. Obstet. Gynec. 54:219, 1947.

Klawans, A. H., and Kantor, A. E.: Prolapse of the uterus and pregnancy, Amer. J. Obstet. Gynec. 57:939, 1949.

Lamb, E. J., and Greene, R. R.: Microscopic study of growth of leiomyomas of the uterus during pregnancy, Surg. Gynec. Obstet. **108:**575, 1959.

Mann, E. C., McLarn, W. D., and Hayt, D. B.: The physiology and clinical significance of the uterine isthmus, Amer. J. Obstet. Gynec. **81:**209, 1961.

Parks, J., and Barter, R. H.: The myomatous uterus complicated by pregnancy, Amer. J. Obstet. Gynec. **63:**260, 1952.

Peterson, W. F., Stauch, J. E., and Ryder, C. D.: Metronidazole in pregnancy, Amer. J. Obstet. Gynec. **94:**343, 1966.

Philpott, N. W., and Ross, J. E.: Congenital uterine anomalies and associated complications of pregnancy, Amer. J. Obstet. Gynec. **68:**285, 1954.

Pratt, J. P.: Corpus luteum in its relation to menstruation and pregnancy, Endocrinology **11:**195, 1927.

Schulman, H., and Ferguson, J. H.: Comparison of the behavior of intraepithelial carcinoma of the cervix in the pregnant and the nonpregnant patient, Amer. J. Obstet. Gynec. **84:**1497, 1962.

Tawa, K.: Ovarian tumors in pregnancy, Amer. J. Obstet. Gynec. **90:**511, 1964.

Tulsky, A. S., and Koff, A. K.: Some observations on the role of corpus luteum in early human pregnancy, Fertil. Steril. **8:**118, 1957.

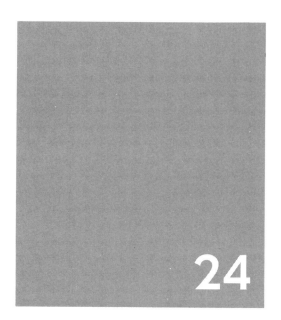

Disorders of the nervous system, the skin, and the bones and joints during pregnancy

With the exception of puerperal psychosis and possibly poliomyelitis, disorders of the nervous system do not differ appreciably in pregnant and nonpregnant women either from the standpoint of their incidence or their prognosis. Symptoms may be temporarily exaggerated, however, when the mechanical and physiologic burdens of pregnancy are added to chronic disease of the nervous system. In general, skin diseases also affect gravid and nongravid women similarly. On the contrary, disturbances of the bones and joints are most frequently related to the physiologic changes of pregnancy that are responsible for separation and increased mobility especially affecting the pelvic joints.

■ Disorders of the nervous system
PSYCHOSIS

Mental illnesses associated with pregnancy occur in predisposed women or in those whose pregnancies have been complicated by severe toxemia or infection. Thus the term *postpartum psychosis* does not imply a specific psychiatric entity but, rather, the occurrence of any type of psychiatric disorder in women who have recently borne infants. Boyd estimated the incidence of mental disturbances as 1 in 400 deliveries, of which 14% become obvious during the prenatal period, 54% in the first 14 days post partum, and 32% in the late puerperium.

Depressive psychosis appearing 1 or 2 weeks after delivery is the most frequent form, with rejection of the infant as the usual response. During this phase there is a danger of suicide or infanticide. *Schizophrenic reactions* are less common but most refractory to treatment. *Manic reactions* are almost exclusively related to toxic states.

Treatment. In many instances, prodromal signs can be observed early in pregnancy. Psychotherapy at this time may avert a more serious mental disorder later. Thorazine or one of the tranquilizing agents may be useful aids during the period of psychotherapy. Electroconvulsive shock therapy has been employed effectively during pregnancy as well as in the postpartum period. The risk of abortion or damage to the fetus is not appreciably increased, particularly when measures are taken to reduce anoxia. Oxygen may be administered during the postconvulsive stages of coma, and muscle relaxants may be used to modify the shock when necessary.

Prognosis. Early and complete recovery is the rule if mental disturbances are precipitated by infection or toxemia. Dieckmann observed 182 patients with eclampsia, 5 of whom developed psychosis post partum. In each instance, recovery was complete within approximately 4 weeks. Nearly all cases of depression psychosis can be cured, but only about 25% of schizophrenic reactions can be permanently reversed. Nevertheless the puerperal psychotic patient may respond so remarkably to treatment that a poor prognosis should be withheld unless deterioration is evident.

Foundeur and co-workers at the Westchester Division of the New York Hospital followed up 100 women in whom mental illnesses of various types were precipitated by childbirth. Three out of 4 women remained well in the average 4-year follow-up period. Twenty-two of these women were observed through 27 subsequent pregnancies; 1 in 7 had recurrence of psychosis.

EPILEPSY

Epilepsy has no remarkable influence upon the course or outcome of pregnancy, and, conversely, childbearing does not, as a rule, alter the epileptic status permanently.

Symptoms. Temporary effects of pregnancy are wholly unpredictable. In the majority of epileptic mothers, symptoms remain unchanged or become aggravated, but in some, seizures are reduced throughout the prenatal period and return with their usual frequency after delivery. Rarely, grand mal attacks make their first appearance during pregnancy or in the puerperium and must be distinguished from eclampsia. Positive water balance associated with pregnancy can increase epileptic attacks, presumably as a result of cerebral edema.

Treatment. Dilantin, phenobarbital, or other anticonvulsant drugs can be continued throughout pregnancy. In addition, sodium intake should be restricted in order that fluid retention be kept at a minimum. Attacks during labor are uncommon. Lactation does not increase convulsions, but nursing should be restricted or supervised to prevent injury to the baby if an attack occurs while it is at breast.

Direct genetic transmission of epilepsy is unusual. Because epilepsy does not significantly disturb the pregnancy, interruption is not indicated, but if mental deterioration is progressive or if status epilepticus has ever occurred, sterilization is advisable.

POLIOMYELITIS

Incidence. The incidence of poliomyelitis is significantly higher in pregnant than in nonpregnant women. There is some indication that the risk of infection is further increased in pregnant women directly in relation to the number of children in their immediate households. Attack rates during pregnancy were increased 59% above the expected incidence in a survey conducted by Siegel and Greenberg in New York City from 1949 through 1953.

Mortality rate, on the other hand, is not increased when the disease is complicated by pregnancy. In Horn's series of 447 patients, the maternal mortality was 4.7% and the total fetal loss was 18%. The abortion rate in this group was 11%.

Management. The treatment of poliomyelitis should not be altered because of the pregnancy. Since the uterine muscle is not involved, normal labor can be anticipated. Local anesthesia or pudendal block is preferable for delivery. Management of the pregnancy must be individualized in patients who develop bulbar poliomyelitis after the thirty-second week. Serial determinations of vital capacity and tidal air provide means of evaluating respiratory reserve. When increasing respiratory embarrassment is evident late in gestation, termination of pregnancy by induction of labor, if this can be readily accomplished, or cesarean section, if necessary, is in the best interest of both mother and baby.

Fetal effects. The greatest hazard to the fetus is the associated maternal anoxia. Positive pressure devices, administration of oxygen, and early tracheotomy will reduce this danger. Only a few cases of neonatal poliomyelitis have been reported, generally as a result of contamination with the mother's virus at the time of delivery. Shelokov and Weinstein isolated the same polio virus from a mother, from her infant born in a respirator, and from the substance of the placental villi—a finding that suggested the possibility of intrauterine infection.

Immunization. The susceptibility of pregnant women is of sufficient magnitude to warrant prenatal immunization with poliomyelitis vaccine. The safety of immunization during pregnancy has been shown in the large number of gravid women given Salk vaccine and, more recently, the Sabin oral live attenuated virus vaccine. The immunologic response is comparable to that of nonpregnant individuals. There is no increase in abortion rate in women vaccinated during the first trimester, and no teratogenic effects attributable to the administration of vaccine have been encountered.

POLYNEURITIS AND POLYRADICULOPATHY (GUILLAIN-BARRÉ)

Polyneuritis as a result of dietary deficiencies has all but disappeared in the United States. It is occasionally seen in connection with severe hyperemesis gravidarum, in which symptoms may be related to vitamin B deficiency. Multiple nerves are involved with resulting paresthesias, burning, dysesthesia, and muscle weakness. Central nervous system effects are seen in some cases, showing disorientation, ataxia, and cranial nerve involvement. Deaths have occurred with polyneuritis due to cardiac or phrenic nerve involvement and respiratory failure.

Polyneuritis due to other causes such as diabetes, alcohol, drugs, and heavy metals must be differentiated from the foregoing, the cause removed, and substitution therapy instituted promptly.

Guillain-Barré syndrome, or polyradiculopathy, simulates poliomyelitis or polyneuritis with multiple peripheral and cranial nerve involvement. High protein content of the cerebrospinal fluid with few or no cells present is characteristic. This is a temporary disorder, although remissions and exacerbations are known to occur. Supportive therapy of the paralyzed limbs and the temporarily embarrassed respiratory function is of great importance, and steroid therapy is often beneficial in this condition. Recovery rate is high.

CHOREA GRAVIDARUM

Chorea is a rare complication of pregnancy, occurring in approximately 1 in 3,500 deliveries.

Etiology. The cause is unknown, but it is likely that chorea gravidarum is a form of Sydenham's chorea associated with pregnancy. In over one half of the cases studied by Beresford and Graham a history of previous attacks of chorea or rheumatism could be obtained. It is not unusual, however, for the disturbance to make its first appearance during pregnancy. The primary attack may occur in women of any parity but is most common in young primigravidas. *Recurrences* with subsequent pregnancies are likely but not inevitable.

Course. The severity and duration of the disease vary. Mild cases may disappear in as little as 8 days, whereas severe cases many continue for 8 months. Evidence of cardiac lesions can be noted in approximately one third of the cases, but rheumatic manifestations are rare during pregnancy.

Treatment. Every effort should be made at conservative management. The major difficulty lies in the fact that generalized hypermotility and incoordination of movements interfere with the patient's nutrition and rest. External stimuli and anxieties accentuate the symptoms. Most attacks will respond favorably to sedation with barbiturates or tranquilizing agents, quiet surroundings, adequate carbohydrate intake as protection against liver damage, and supplementary vitamin therapy.

Complications. The most serious complication is acute carditis, which should be suspected if the course becomes febrile. Acute manic psychosis is occasionally encountered. If symptoms progress despite treatment and the patient develops fever, jaundice, incontinence, or mania, termination of the pregnancy should be considered.

Prognosis. The prognosis for both mother and baby has improved in recent years. Willson's series of 951 cases reported in 1932 showed a fetal mortality of 50% and a maternal mortality of 13% when the patient delivered spontaneously. The maternal mortality was increased to 33% in the grave cases terminated therapeutically. In contrast, of 144 cases reported by Beresford and Graham in 1950 there were 2 maternal deaths and a fetal loss of 3.3%.

MYASTHENIA GRAVIS

Myasthenia gravis reflects a disturbance in acetylcholine metabolism at the myoneural junction that results in weakness of the ocular, facial, pharyngeal, and laryngeal muscles and the muscles of respiration. Although the disease progresses through remissions and recurrences, many patients can be maintained for years by the use of Prostigmin. The dosage of anticholinesterase medication frequently must be adjusted during pregnancy and the puerperium.

Although the effect of childbearing upon the course of myasthenia gravis is not entirely predictable, in most instances the pregnancy is well tolerated and normal vaginal delivery can be anticipated. The disease rarely provides an indication for therapeutic abortion. In each of the 14 cases reported by Fraser and Turner uterine contractions were efficient and contrasted strikingly with the patient's voluntary muscle weakness. Sedatives should be used judiciously during labor because narcotic drugs are poorly tolerated and tranquilizing drugs may aggravate the weakness. Pudendal block is the preferred anesthesia for delivery. Relapse is most likely to occur during the first 3 weeks post partum. During a myasthenic crisis, symptoms are intensified, respirations may need the mechanical assistance of a positive pressure apparatus, and tracheotomy may be necessary. A myasthenic crisis must be differentiated from effects of overdose of anticholinesterase therapy in which weakness is also intensified, but salivation, abdominal cramps, and nausea are prominent symptoms. Atropine is usually effective in controlling the abdominal pain.

Occasionally the infant of a mother suffering with this disease will show evidence of neonatal myasthenia. The effects are usually transitory and tend to disappear within 2 to 4 weeks. Prompt treatment with Prostigmin is essential for survival and should be continued for as long as muscle weakness persists.

MULTIPLE SCLEROSIS

Multiple sclerosis is a disease of progressive demyelinization, characterized by exacerbations and remissions. At first only one or two nerve areas are involved in patchy distributions. Characteristic symptoms of the early stage are intention tremor, nystagmus, and scanned speech. The interval between these symptoms and the development of optic neuritis, paraplegia, and impairment of bowel and bladder control vary widely with the individual—pregnant or not. There is no evidence that exacerbations are increased or that the progress of the disease is accelerated during pregnancy. The fetus is not affected.

Normal labor and delivery can usually be expected. Because the disease is progressive and ultimately incapacitating, childbearing should be limited.

SUBARACHNOID HEMORRHAGE, CEREBRAL ANEURYSM, AND OCCLUSIVE CEREBRAL DISORDERS

Spontaneous subarachnoid hemorrhage and cerebral aneurysm may occur during pregnancy, but the incidence is not increased in gravid women as compared with others of the same age group.

Etiology. The usual cause is a bleeding aneurysm or angioma, and only rarely are cardiovascular or other disturbances such as blood dyscrasias, tuberculosis, or tumors responsible. Occasionally there is no discoverable disease.

Diagnosis. The onset is generally sudden with severe headache, vomiting, paralysis, and eventually coma. The blood pressure may be elevated, but the characteristic findings of nuchal rigidity, increased intraspinal pressure, and grossly bloody spinal fluid differentiate this lesion from coma of intracerebral or metabolic origin. The clinical course is determined by the size of the vessel involved and the extent of the hemorrhage.

Treatment. The mortality rate associated with spontaneous subarachnoid hemorrhage is high, amounting to almost 50% whether the victim is pregnant or not. About one half of the fatalities occur within the first 24 hours. Initial medical treatment is aimed at gaining control of bleeding, convulsions, and associated symptoms. Cerebral arteriography can be done when symptoms have subsided. Pregnancy is not a contraindication to the procedure. If an aneurysm is found and its location is accessible, surgical correction is advisable in order to prevent recurrence.

The method of delivery should be individualized, but if the vaginal route is chosen, the second stage of labor should be eliminated and forceps delivery carried out as soon as the cervix is fully dilated. Cerebrospinal fluid pressures are not much changed with uterine contractions alone, but as recordings obtained by McCausland and Holmes indicate, cerebrospinal fluid pressures may rise above 700 mm. H_2O when the patient bears down with contractions. If any delay or difficulty is anticipated, delivery by cesarean section is preferable.

Nonhemorrhagic stroke is also seen in gravid women. Cross, Castro, and Jennett at the Institute of Neurological Sciences at Glasgow found that strokes occurring in association with pregnancy were more frequently due to occlusive cerebral arterial disease than to cerebral venous thrombosis. They reported 31 cases of carotid territory ischemia all with hemoplegia and 16 with dysphasia. The onset was abrupt in 23 women. Prodromal headache, visual disturbances, epilepsy, and paresthesias were often noted. Since 5 of these patients had occlusion of the internal carotid artery in which surgery might have been corrective and since the clinical features per se do not distinguish between these two types of cerebral vascular disease, Cross believes that definitive diagnosis by angiography should not be deferred.

NEURITIS

Neuritic disturbances of varying severity are observed during pregnancy. Manifestations range from sensory effects such as paresthesias and pain, which are common, to sensory and motor changes, which are rare.

Etiology. Neuritis may be caused by the following factors:

1. Inadequate intake or utilization of vitamin B complex is responsible for most symptoms of numbness and tingling of the hands and feet and for the most severe form of polyneuritis.

2. Toxic factors are observed in trigeminal neuritis associated with carious teeth.

3. Mechanical factors are largely responsible for sciatic and traumatic neuritis.

Paresthesias. Paresthesias often persist throughout pregnancy despite therapy and disappear slowly thereafter. If foci of infection are found, these should be treated while supplementary vitamin therapy is continued.

ACRODYSESTHESIA. Acrodysesthesia (brachialgia statica dysesthetica) or numbness, tingling, and stiffness of the upper extremities may appear and persist during pregnancy. Symptoms are caused by stretching or pressure on the brachial plexus when relaxation of the ligaments allows greater motion of the shoulder girdle in both forward and backward direction. Discomfort is greatest when steady traction is exerted, and for this reason the patient usually complains of numbness, sometimes almost complete anesthesia of the hands, particularly in the distribution of the ulnar nerve upon awakening from sleep. Since this is purely a mechanical problem, relief is obtained only by supporting the shoulder in a favorable midposition by use of pillows at night and by assuming proper posture in the daytime. There is no permanent motor or sensory damage.

Polyneuritis. Polyneuritis is fortunately a rare complication. Actual degenerative nerve changes that occur result in diminished sensation, paralysis, and muscular atrophy. The process may be limited to a single nerve but can become generalized and rapidly fatal with bulbar involvement. Manifestations are similar to those of Landry's ascending paralysis. Treatment is preventive. Deficiency states developing in the course of severe hyperemesis or other depleting disorders should be avoided by early replacement of fluid, electrolytes, water-soluble vitamins, and carbohydrate. When nerve damage characteristic of polyneuritis develops, changes may be irreversible.

Sciatic neuritis. Pain and tenderness over the sciatic and occasionally the femoral distribution result from relaxation of the sacroiliac joints and subsequent tension or trauma to the nerves involved. Immobilization of the sacroiliac joints by use of a firm support and bed boards offers relief, but some discomfort may persist for several weeks after delivery.

Traumatic or maternal obstetric paralysis. Symptoms of pain, paresthesia, or muscle weakness developing in the lower extremities during labor or soon afterward suggest the syndrome of traumatic neuritis or maternal obstetric paralysis. Dorsiflexors of the foot are most frequently affected. Compression of the lumbosacral trunk by the fetal skull is the usual etiologic factor. This may occur spontaneously with arrest of the fetal head at the pelvic brim, particularly in the platypelloid pelvis with reduced anteroposterior diameter, or as a result of a difficult forceps delivery. In some persons protrusion of a lumbar intervertebral disk is the etiologic factor.

The peroneal nerve can be injured by undue pressure against the stirrups during delivery. Foot drop is the result. Since the nerve is superficial as it passes laterally around the fibular neck, this area should be protected by padding when the patient is positioned and by avoiding pressure against the knee when the patient is anesthetized.

Treatment of traumatic neuritis consists of splinting, active and passive exercises, and galvanic stimulation of the affected muscles. Prognosis for recovery is good.

■ Skin disorders

With one or two possible exceptions there are no cutaneous diseases that occur only during pregnancy. Any of the *acute skin eruptions* can occur coincidentally, but their course and treatment are not appreciably altered in gravid women. *Chronic skin dis-*

eases, however, are frequently influenced by pregnancy. Eczema, psoriasis, and various allergic skin manifestations may be improved in some patients and aggravated in others. Acne and hypertrichosis may be more apparent during pregnancy than otherwise.

HERPES GESTATIONIS

Herpes gestationis is a variant of dermatitis herpetiformis that usually occurs in gravid women and may recur with subsequent pregnancies. The disease is characterized by superficial vesicobullous or pustular lesions with an erythematous base. These occur in patches distributed over the extremities and trunk. An intense pruritus, which accompanies the eruption, persists throughout pregnancy and gradually disappears after delivery. Constitutional symptoms are not pronounced.

In the infant, infection with the virus of herpes is extremely serious and often fatal. Viremia occurs readily after skin lesions appear and spreads rapidly to internal organs, with liver and brain showing greatest susceptibility. Treatment with antihistaminics has provided minimal if any relief, but the daily administrations of corticosteroids or ACTH has resulted in significant improvement or cure. Fosnaugh believes that the disorder is related to an abnormality in tryptophan metabolism, and he obtained good results in 5 patients using pyridoxine in doses ranging from 50 to 300 mg. daily.

IMPETIGO HERPETIFORMIS

Impetigo herpetiformis is a rare inflammatory disease of the skin that occurs almost exclusively in association with pregnancy. The etiology is unknown. Characteristic lesions are miliary pustules arranged in irregular or circinate clusters. The pustules spread peripherally as the centers undergo desiccation. The usual sites are the inner aspects of the thighs and the genitocrural areas. The mucous membranes of the oral cavity may be involved with lesions that appear as grayish white plaques.

Symptoms include severe burning and itching of the skin, chills, fever, vomiting, diarrhea, and prostration. Mortality in reported cases has been high and often associated with septicemia. Antibiotic therapy and correction of dehydration should greatly improve the outlook.

LUPUS ERYTHEMATOSUS

Lupus erythematosus is of interest because it occurs most frequently in women during the reproductive years, and although the spontaneous abortion rate may be increased, it does not otherwise affect fertility. The disease is serious and unpredictable at best. The outcome in puerperal women depends more upon the severity of the disease than the existence of pregnancy. With the discoid type neither mother nor baby is much affected. With systemic lupus erythematosus, exacerbations or remissions may occur, remissions fortunately being more common. The incidence of preeclamptic toxemia is greater probably because of the renal lesions of disseminated lupus erythematosus.

Proteinuria is a serious manifestation of renal involvement in systemic lupus erythematosus. Since systemic lupus erythematosus can no longer be considered a rare disease, Mund and co-workers urge that it be considered in the diagnosis of otherwise unexplained proteinuria during pregnancy, especially in patients with fever, arthralgia, alopecia, or rashes.

Cortisone or adrenocorticotropic hormone provides the most effective form of treatment, and these can be administered during pregnancy without endangering the fetus. Bridge and Foley showed that the lupus erythematosus factor crosses the placental barrier. These and other investigators have found lupus erythematosus cells in cord and peripheral blood of infants whose mothers had systemic disease, although the babies appeared normal and healthy in each case. The lupus erythematosus cells are not demonstrable in the offspring after 7 weeks of life.

PRURITUS

Generalized pruritus is not an uncommon occurrence during pregnancy. Skin manifestations other than scratch marks are frequently absent, but occasionally urticarial reactions are visible. When there is no associated jaundice and no increase in blood bilirubin levels, a neurogenic etiology is most likely. In some patients the itching is related to idiopathic cholestasis. Symptoms range from mild discomfort to intolerable itching, restlessness, and fatigue. Treatment consists of antihistaminics, mild sedation, and local analgesic applications. In resistant cases specific psychotherapy may be necessary.

■ Bone and joint disorders

The bones forming the pelvic girdle are solidly united in the adult woman except during pregnancy, when hormonal effect upon the sacroiliac joints and the symphysis pubis permits varying degrees of motion. Roentgen evidence of relaxation can be observed as early as the first trimester, becoming maximal by the beginning of the third trimester.

SACROILIAC RELAXATION

Sacroiliac relaxation is the most common cause of low back pain in pregnant women. Backache may be limited to the lower lumbar region or radiate down the back of the legs in the distribution of the sciatic nerve. Occasionally pain follows the course of the femoral nerve over the anterior aspects of the lower abdomen and thighs. Although symptoms may be transitory, they frequently persist throughout pregnancy and for several weeks after delivery. Tenderness can be elicited by palpation over the posterior surface of the sacroiliac joint or by pelvic palpation below and lateral to the sacral promontory. X-ray examination is not particularly informative, since the degree of pelvic tilt at the sacroiliac joints is poorly correlated with symptomatology. Complete immobilization is impractical, if not impossible, during pregnancy, and accordingly few persons are cured, but relief can be obtained by the use of a firm sacroiliac support, bed boards, and increased periods of rest.

SYMPHYSIAL SEPARATION

Widening of the symphysis occurs regularly during pregnancy, and although the increase is sometimes remarkable, symptoms arise less frequently than might be expected. It is likely that acute or chronic trauma to the periosteum is necessary before characteristic signs appear. These may occur during the course of pregnancy but are far more common after a difficult forceps delivery or the birth of a large baby.

The patient experiences severe pain over the pubic and lumbar regions upon walking or in attempting to turn in bed. Efforts to reduce motion of the pelvic girdle result in a typical waddling gait. Motion of the pelvic bones can be demonstrated upon direct palpation of the symphysis while the patient transfers her weight from one extremity to the other or by x-ray examinations made under the same conditions of alternate weight bearing. The degree of disability, however, is not necessarily related to the amount of separation.

Treatment. Immobilization of the pelvic girdle by an encircling adhesive tape binder or tight support using protective pads over the symphysis and sacrum will permit gradual ambulation. In most cases symptoms disappear within 2 or 3 weeks, although some persist for months. Since recurrence in a subsequent pregnancy is possible, prophylactic use of a firm support is advisable.

SPINAL FUSION (SPONDYLOLISTHESIS)

Patients who have had orthopedic problems involving the spinal column, particularly those requiring spinal fusion, need special management during pregnancy and delivery. A detailed survey of these problems conducted by Trelford showed that a high proportion of patients who had fusion prior to pregnancy experienced exacerbation of symptoms and in 9 of 17 instances required repeat fusion subsequent to delivery. This complication can usually be avoided by use of a support or brace that provides 3-point fixation (symphysis pubis, lower sacrum, and upper lumbar–lower rib cage) and often hospitalization during the prenatal period.

The stress directed at the fifth lumbar and first sacral segments during late pregnancy may be a factor in the initiation or aggravation of spondylolisthesis in women. The lithotomy position can be detrimental. Human leg holders are preferable in the conduct of vaginal delivery. Trial of labor should not be protracted. If progress is not satisfactory after 6 to 8 hours, operative delivery is advisable.

ANKYLOSIS OF THE SACROCOCCYGEAL JOINT

Fusion or injury resulting in ankylosis of the sacrococcygeal joint may be suspected upon prenatal pelvic examination if the configuration is unusual or the joint rigid. No difficulties arise until the patient is in labor. Descent of the presenting part is delayed, but fracture of the coccyx during forceps extraction usually permits vaginal delivery. In this event, pain upon sitting or straining can be expected for several weeks. Rarely, symptoms are so persistent that surgical removal of the coccyx is advisable.

DISLOCATION OF THE COCCYX

Dislocation of the coccyx may cause excruciating pain that makes its appearance immediately after the parturient recovers from anesthesia. Replacement by rectal manipulation under morphine analgesia or light anesthesia affords startling and prompt relief.

OSTEOGENESIS IMPERFECTA

Osteogenesis imperfecta has a strong hereditary tendency, since it is transmitted by an autosomal dominant gene. The underlying process is a diffuse mesenchymal hypoplasia manifested by severe osteoporosis with fracture on minimal trauma, blue sclerae, and middle ear deafness. The disorder may be early in onset or latent. Neonatal osteogenesis imperfecta is often considered incompatible with life, but the outlook is not always so hopeless. We have delivered 3 infants of a family with paternal osteogenesis imperfecta. Fractures were demonstrable on x-ray examination before delivery. All infants survived. The risk of fracture and hematoma formation is greater with vaginal delivery. Cesarean section is indicated if predelivery x-ray examination shows involvement of the fetus in utero.

References

Baskin, J. L., Soule, E. H., and Mills, S. D.: Poliomyelitis of the newborn; pathologic changes in 2 cases, Amer. J. Dis. Child. 80:10, 1950.

Benson, R. C., and Inman, V. T.: Brachialgia statica dysesthetica in pregnancy, Western J. Surg. 64:115, 1956.

Beresford, O. D., and Graham, A. M.: Chorea gravidarum, J. Obstet. Gynaec. Brit. Comm. 57: 616, 1950.

Boyd, D. A., Jr.: Mental disorders associated with childbearing, Amer. J. Obstet. Gynec. 43:148, 335, 1942.

Brew, M. F., and Seidenberg, R.: Psychotic reactions associated with pregnancy and childbirth, J. Nerv. Ment. Dis. 111: 08, 1950.

Bridge, R. G., and Foley, F. E.: Placental transmission of the lupus erythematosus factor, Amer. J. Med. Sci. 227:1, 1954.

Bryan, W. M., Jr.: Myasthenia gravis in pregnancy and in the newborn infant; review of literature and case report, Obstet. Gynec. 4: 339, 1954.

Chalmers, J. A.: Traumatic neuritis in the puerperium, J. Obstet. Gynaec. Brit. Comm. 56: 205, 1949.

Charatan, F. B., and Oldham, A. J.: Electroconvulsive treatment in pregnancy, J. Obstet. Gynaec. Brit. Comm. 61:665, 1954.

Cohn, S. L., Schreier, R., and Feld, D.: Osteogenesis imperfecta and pregnancy, Obstet. Gynec. 20:107, 1962.

Crawford, G. M., and Leefer, R. W.: Diseases of the skin in pregnancy, Arch. Dermat. Syph. 61: 753, 1950.

Cross, J. N., Castro, P. O., and Jennett, W. B.: Cerebral strokes associated with pregnancy and the puerperium, Brit. Med. J. 3:214, 1968.

Douglas, L. H., and Jorgenson, C. L.: Pregnancy and multiple sclerosis, Amer. J. Obstet. Gynec. 55:332, 1948.

Foldes, F. F., and McNall, P. G.: Myasthenia gravis; a guide for anesthesiologists, Anesthesiology 23:837, 1962.

Fosnaugh, R. P., Bryan, H. G., and Orders, R. L.: Pyridoxine in the treatment of herpes gestationis, Arch. Derm. 84:90, 1961.

Foundeur, M. A., Fixsen, C., Triebel, W. A., and White, M. A.: Postpartum mental illness, Arch. Neurol. Psychiat. 77:503, 1957.

Fraser, D., and Turner, J. W. A.: Myasthenia gravis and pregnancy, Lancet 2:417, 1953.

Hamby, W. B.: Intracranial aneurysm, Springfield, Ill., 1952, Charles C Thomas, Publisher.

Horn, P.: Poliomyelitis in pregnancy; a twenty-year report from Los Angeles County, California, Obstet. Gynec. 6:121, 1955.

Horn, P.: Obstetric management of poliomyelitis complicating pregnancy, Clin. Obstet. Gynec. 1: 127, 1958.

Katzenstein, L., and Morris, A. J.: Cortisone and ACTH in pregnancy, New Eng. J. Med. 250: 366, 1954.

Keynes, G.: Obstetrics and gynecology in relation to thyrotoxicosis and myasthenia gravis, J. Obstet. Gynaec. Brit. Comm. 59:173, 1952.

Lindeman, C., Engstrom, W. W., and Flynn, R. T.: Herpes gestationis, results of treatment with ACTH and cortisone, Amer. J. Obstet. Gynec. 63:167, 1952.

Martins da Silva, M., Prem, K. A., Johnson, E. A., McKelvey, L., and Syverton, J. T.: Response of pregnant women and their infants to poliomyelitis vaccine; distribution of poliovirus antibody in pregnant women before and after vaccination; transfer, persistence and induction of antibodies in infants, J.A.M.A. 168:1, 1958.

McCausland, A. M., and Holmes, F.: Spinal fluid pressures during labor. Preliminary report, Western J. Surg. 65:220, 1957.

McElin, T. W., Lovelady, S. B., and Woltman, H. W.: Chorea gravidarum; a review of recent literature and report of 5 cases, Amer. J. Obstet. Gynec. 55:992, 1948.

Mund, A., Simson, J., and Rothfield, N.: Effect of pregnancy on course of systemic lupus erythematosus, J.A.M.A. 183:917, 1963.

Pedowitz, P., and Perell, A.: Aneurysms complicated by pregnancy, Amer. J. Obstet. Gynec. 73:736, 1957.

Plass, E. D., and Mengert, W. F.: Gestational polyneuritis, J.A.M.A. 101:2020, 1933.

Robb, J. P.: Neurologic complications of pregnancy, Neurology 5:679, 1955.

Sabin, M., and Oxorn, H.: Epilepsy and pregnancy, Obstet. Gynec. 7:175, 1956.

Shelokov, A., and Weinstein, L.: Poliomyelitis in

the early neonatal period; report of a case of possible intrauterine infection, J. Pediat. **38:**80, 1951.

Siegel, M., and Greenberg, M.: Incidence of poliomyelitis in pregnancy, its relation to maternal age, parity, and gestational period, New Eng. J. Med. **253:**841, 1955.

Strean, G. J., Gelfand, M. M., Pavilanis, V., and Sternberg, J.: Maternal-fetal relationships; placental transmission of poliomyelitis antibodies in newborn, Canad. Med. Ass. J. **77:**315, 1957.

Sweeney, W. J.: Pregnancy and multiple sclerosis, Amer. J. Obstet. Gynec. **66:**124, 1953.

Trelford, J. D.: Spondylolisthesis in pregnancy, Amer. J. Obstet. Gynec. **91:**320, 1965.

Walton, J. N.: Subarachnoid hemorrhage in pregnancy, Brit. Med. J. **1:**869, 1953.

Willson, P., and Preece, A. A.: Chorea gravidarum—a statistical study of 951 collected cases, Arch. Intern. Med. **49:**471, 1932.

Zakon, S. J., Leader, L. O., and Siegel, I.: Herpes gestationis, treatment with ACTH and cortisone, Obstet. Gynec. **2:**78, 1953.

Zuelser, W. W., and Stulberg, C. S.: Herpes simplex virus as the cause of fulminating visceral disease and hepatitis in infancy, Amer. J. Dis. Child. **83:**421, 1952.

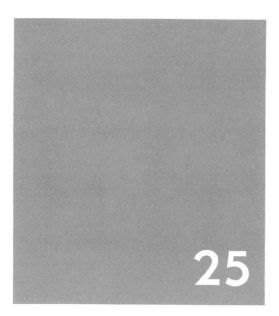

25

Surgical complications of pregnancy

Acute surgical emergencies occur no less frequently in gravid than in nongravid women of a like age and must be treated in the same manner. With prompt diagnosis and surgical intervention, the operative risk is not increased because of the pregnancy, but complications develop rapidly and the prognosis is more serious in the pregnant woman if a necessary operation is deferred. Physiologic changes associated with pregnancy can increase the difficulty of early diagnosis. Simple nausea and vomiting may be present during the early weeks, but they never begin after the first trimester and are not associated with abdominal pain. A leukocytosis of 12,000 or 14,000 is not uncommon, but granulocytosis with an increasing percentage of nonsegmental forms is abnormal. The sedimentation rate is normally increased in pregnancy

and is of no value in differential diagnosis. Pain must be distinguished from discomfort related to the enlarging uterus, the pelvic ligaments, the corpus luteum, or urinary tract disturbances.

Regional anesthesia is preferable during pregnancy because anoxia may damage the fetus. If inhalation anesthesia is used, a high percentage of oxygen must be administered. A gas mixture that contains less than 20% oxygen should not be permitted.

Endocrine therapy for prevention of abortion after operative procedures is rarely necessary. The incidence of abortion is low if the uterus is not manipulated and the serosa is not involved in an inflammatory process. If progesterone is used at all, particularly after surgical procedures that disturb the corpus luteum, the dosage should be adequate. At least 250 mg. should be given daily for the first few days and the amount reduced gradually thereafter.

Antibiotic therapy is neither necessary nor desirable as a prophylactic measure simply because of the pregnancy. However, these drugs may be lifesaving when an operation must be performed in a contaminated field or when the problem is already complicated by infection. They should then be used in full amounts for a sufficient time and in accordance with the culture and sensitivity patterns.

■ Appendicitis

Acute appendicitis occurs with the same frequency in pregnant as in nonpregnant women, but the diagnosis is more difficult and delay in treatment is hazardous. In 373 cases of acute appendicitis during pregnancy Black found no maternal deaths in the first trimester, 3.9% in the second trimester, 10.9% in the third trimester, and 16.7% intrapartum. The enlarged uterus may obscure the appendix, which tends to be displaced upward and laterally in the direction of the right iliac crest. Its ultimate position, however, is variable. Suppuration of the acutely inflamed appendix is rapid, and rupture occurs early. Diffuse spreading peritonitis results because the increased vascularity, lack of omental protection, and motion of the uterus hinder localization. Abortion or premature labor may occur if the inflammatory process involves the uterine serosa. Uterine contractions stimulated by peritoneal infec-

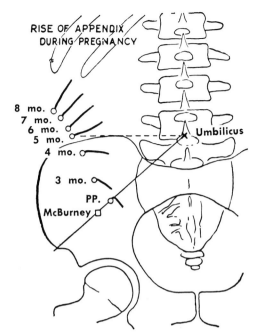

RISE OF APPENDIX
DURING PREGNANCY

8 mo.
7 mo.
6 mo.
5 mo.
4 mo.
3 mo.
PP.
McBurney

Umbilicus

Fig. 25-1. Rise of appendix at various stages of pregnancy. (From Baer, J. L., Reis, R. A., and Arens, R. A.: J.A.M.A. 98:1359, 1932.)

tion are frequently tetanic and predispose to fetal anoxia and intrauterine fetal death.

Diagnosis. Nausea and vomiting, epigastric pain localizing in the right side of the abdomen, and tenderness anywhere from McBurney's point to the right flank are suggestive. Evidences of infection including elevated temperature and more particularly an increased pulse rate are usually present. A single white blood count is of doubtful value in the questionable case because leukocytosis is physiologic during pregnancy. Serial studies at hourly intervals that reveal an increase in both total count and in young polymorphonuclear cells indicate the presence of an acute infectious process.

Differential diagnosis. Urinary tract infection or ureteral stone presents the greatest difficulty in the differential diagnosis. Examination of a catheterized urine sample is indicated in every case and should be repeated in an hour or two when the diagnosis is questionable. In the last trimester appendicitis must be differentiated from abruptio placentae or uncomplicated premature labor.

Treatment. Appendicitis complicating pregnancy requires operation as soon as the diagnosis can be established. Technical difficulties are increased late in pregnancy because of the large uterus and the position of the appendix. Tilting of the patient to the left side is helpful. If leakage or perforation has occurred, the peritoneal cavity should be lavaged with large quantities of warm saline solution, and large dosages of broad-spectrum antibiotics should be administered parenterally. *Abortion* is not likely to occur if infection is confined to the appendix, but labor can be initiated by peritonitis. Since abortion or premature labor after appendectomy is not related to changes in hormone levels, the administration of progesterone postoperatively is of little value. Sedation can be used as necessary and ambulation permitted at the usual time unless evidence of uterine irritability persists.

If labor ensues soon after operation, it should be conducted according to usual obstetric principles, but elimination of the second stage by low forceps delivery is advisable. Caudal or epidural anesthesia during labor and delivery can be a valuable aid in such circumstances.

Maternal mortality is no higher in gravid than in nongravid patients if there is no delay. After perforation the threat to the pregnant woman increases disproportionately. Fetal loss associated with peritonitis is high.

■ Intestinal obstruction

Because of the inordinately high morbidity and mortality, intestinal obstruction should be suspected in any pregnant woman with a history of previous abdominal operation or inflammatory disease in whom abdominal pain is accompanied by nausea, vomiting, and constipation. Changes in size and shape of the uterus, which then exerts tension on intraperitoneal adhesive bands, or kinking and constriction of adherent bowel is the usual etiology. Volvulus accounts for 15% to 25% of all cases of intestinal obstruction.

Early in pregnancy valuable time may be lost if the symptoms are regarded as simple nausea and vomiting, but examination of the patient should clarify this problem since pain, tenderness, and distention are not characteristic of any physiologic process. Vomiting that makes its first appearance after the twelfth week must be considered as caused by some condition other than pregnancy it-self. During late pregnancy recurrent colicky pains must be differentiated from labor.

Metabolic imbalances can occur in as little as 4 hours after obstruction and are very pronounced within 1 or 2 days. Procrastination may be disastrous. Decompression, correction of blood volume deficits with fluid, electrolytes, and plasma as indicated are essential first steps in management, but the necessary surgery should be performed as soon as possible thereafter. Operation should be aimed at removing the cause of obstruction without disturbing the pregnancy, even though labor ensues within a few hours, but if exposure cannot be otherwise obtained, the uterus must be emptied irrespective of the gestation period.

■ Rectal operations

Hemorrhoids. Because of pressure from the enlarging uterus and the tendency to constipation during pregnancy, the hemorrhoidal veins are frequently dilated. Medical treatment is preferable during the prenatal and puerperal periods except for the acutely painful thrombotic hemorrhoid, which can be incised under local anesthesia and the clot evacuated. Hemorrhoidectomy is indicated only in the rare instance in which bleeding is persistent and depleting despite conservative therapy.

Rectal carcinoma. Cancer of the rectum is an unusual but serious complication of pregnancy. In Bacon and Rowe's experience therapeutic abortion is not essential during the first trimester; they advise radical surgical removal of the cancerous rectum with regional lymph node dissection but without hysterectomy. During the second trimester the enlarged uterus interferes with visibility and should be removed intact. After the twenty-eighth week hysterectomy is preceded by cesarean section. Of 21 cases operated upon during pregnancy the fetal salvage was 85% and the maternal mortality 10%.

■ Gallbladder disease

Physiologic changes accompanying pregnancy exert some influence upon gallbladder function. Cholecystographic studies carried out by Gerdes and Boyden in normal pregnant women indicate that gallbladder empty-ing time is retarded in the second and third trimesters when serum cholesterol and cholesterol esters are also increased. It is possible that gallstone formation can be accelerated under these conditions.

Symptoms usually appear in the latter half of pregnancy during the period corresponding to physiologic or gestational biliary stasis, but they may be encountered at any stage. In early pregnancy, pain and jaundice, if present, serve to differentiate cholecystitis and cholelithiasis from simple nausea and vomiting. In late pregnancy, gallbladder disease must be differentiated from severe preeclampsia, in which vomiting, upper abdominal pain, tenderness over the liver, and occasionally jaundice may be present. Cholecystography is less reliable in establishing diagnosis during the third trimester because the enlarged uterus and fetal skeleton may distort or obscure the gallbladder shadow.

Medical management is preferable during pregnancy, and in most cases regulation of the diet and antispasmodic drugs provide adequate control. Operation should be performed if medical treatment fails or in patients with impacted common-duct stone or empyema. Reevaluation at 4-hour intervals is indicated during an acute attack. Operative difficulties are greatly increased by the gravid uterus after the twenty-sixth or twenty-eighth week.

■ Hernia

Hernias may appear or increase in size during pregnancy. Inherently weak fascial structures are further weakened by the pressure of the enlarging uterus and from the hormonal effects of relaxin.

Inguinal or *femoral hernias* rarely give rise to serious complications. The enlarging uterus pushes the bowel upward and tends to occlude the defect.

Umbilical hernias are most common. If the ring is small, adherent omentum may fill the sac. Tension often produces pain, but obstruction is unusual. Large umbilical defects and ventral hernias are more likely to contain bowel, but these can be readily reduced. During labor the use of an abdominal support adds to the patient's comfort and prevents the uterus from protruding through a large ventral defect. Except in the rare instance in which strangulation occurs, herniorrhaphy should be delayed until after delivery.

■ Carcinoma of the breast

Carcinoma of the breast during pregnancy or lactation is fortunately rare. Pregnancy does not predispose to mammary cancer, but growth, extension, and metastasis may be accelerated by the physiologic expansion of vascular and lymphatic channels and possibly by the elevated levels of estrogen.

Diagnosis. Diagnosis during pregnancy or lactation is frequently delayed because a small mass in the hypertrophied breast may be difficult to detect or may be misinterpreted. Regular prenatal examinations of the breasts and prompt biopsy of palpable nodules are mandatory if early lesions are to be discovered.

Prognosis. The outlook for the patient with coincidental mammary cancer and pregnancy is not hopeless. The pessimistic view of inoperability of these lesions in gravid women has been revised in recent years, and early adequate treatment has resulted in a significant number of cures. In Adair's report of 102 pregnancy cases, 44.1% were alive at the end of 5 years.

Management. Radical mastectomy and axillary dissection at the earliest possible moment offers the only chance for cure. The criteria of operability should be the same for pregnant as for nonpregnant patients, but the need for immediate intervention without as much as a week's delay is more imperative during pregnancy.

Subsequent pregnancies usually cause no complications if the patient is well and without evidence of recurrence after 3 or 4 years. Axillary metastasis does not preclude cure, although the 5-year survival rate in such cases has been less than 10%. Whether this poor prognosis is influenced by the increased vascularity and the hormonal stimulation of pregnancy or by the frequent delay in detection and treatment in gravid women is not yet clear. As a consequence, the value of terminating pregnancy as soon as possible after radical mastectomy is still a moot question. In Cheek's survey most of the 55 physicians dealing with this problem believed that immediate interruption would improve the prognosis. On the other hand, White found little to recommend the procedure in 78 persons in whom therapeutic abortion was carried out. When a malignant lesion of the breast is discovered early in pregnancy and when the mother must therefore be exposed to high levels of circulating ovarian and placental steroids over a long period of time, interruption of the pregnancy seems justifiable. Obviously the management of this problem must be individualized. No benefit is derived from interference with the pregnancy in late-stage inoperable carcinoma of the breast. Irradiation therapy can be applied to the breast and to axillary or chest metastases if the fetus is shielded, but castration and other palliative procedures should be deferred until a viable infant is delivered.

■ Melanoma

Pigmented moles frequently become more obvious during pregnancy, just as increased pigmentation of other areas of the skin may be noted at that time. The question of which of these innumerable lesions, most of which are benign, should be removed often arises. On the basis of their wide experience with 1,050 patients with malignant melanoma, including 32 cases complicated by pregnancy, Pack and Scharnagel recommend removal of pigmented moles in the following circumstances: (1) those on the trunk that are subject to irritation and all those on the genitals and feet where true melanomas are disproportionately more common, (2) moles that are smooth and blue-black in color, and (3) those exhibiting growth, ulceration, or pain. These should be excised wide of the lesion and never removed by desiccation since each specimen requires microscopic examination.

If malignant melanoma is found, prompt and radical surgical treatment is just as essential and just as rewarding in gravid as in nongravid women, the prognosis for a 5-year survival being 42% and 45%, respectively. Therapeutic interruption of pregnancy does not improve the outlook. Placental metastases have been reported, but even in these, transmission to the fetus is rare. In Freedman and McMahon's patient numerous tumor cells were found in the intervillous space but none within the villi, indicating that the placenta acts as a barrier to these cells unless a melanotic lesion erodes and invades the villous circulation.

■ Dental operations

Dental operations do not cause abortion or other pregnancy complications. On the contrary, it is to the patient's advantage to have cavities corrected and infected teeth extracted regardless of the gestation period. When extraction is necessary, it is our policy to administer an antibacterial drug, usually sulfadiazine, for several days starting the day before operation. Okell and Elliott took blood cultures before and after extraction and demonstrated transient bacteremia, usually alpha hemolytic streptococci, in 76% of persons when extractions were done under nitrous oxide anesthesia. Burket found bacteremia in only 17% when local anesthesia with epinephrine was used. He attributed this difference to vasoconstriction of the surrounding vessels. Most normal patients can combat this bacterial shower without difficulty, but treatment is particularly important in patients with rheumatic or congenital heart disease because of the ever-present danger of subacute bacterial endocarditis. The high concentrations of nitrous oxide ordinarily used in dentistry are contraindicated because of the danger of fetal anoxia. Local anesthesia should be used whenever possible.

■ Special surgical procedures

A number of operations previously avoided in pregnant women are now quite feasible when necessary. The indications for surgical intervention during pregnancy in the treatment of cerebral aneurysms, valvular and congenital heart lesions, renal calculi, and lesions of the endocrine and reproductive organs are described in other chapters.

References

Adair, F. E.: Carcinoma of the breast, Surg. Clin. N. Amer. 33:313, 1953.

Bacon, H. E., and Rowe, R. J.: Abdominoperineal proctosigmoidectomy for rectal cancer complicating pregnancy; report of four cases, Southern Med. J. 40:471, 1947.

Baer, J. L., Reis, R. A., and Arens, R. A.: Appendicitis in pregnancy, J.A.M.A. 98:1359, 1932.

Barter, R. H., and Rovner, I. W.: Surgical complications of pregnancy, J.A.M.A. 165:317, 1957.

Black, W. P.: Acute appendicitis in pregnancy, Brit. Med. J. 1:1938, 1960.

Burket, L. W.: Oral medicine, diagnosis and treatment, Philadelphia, 1957, J. B. Lippincott Co.

Cheek, H. J.: Survey of current opinions concerning carcinoma of the breast during pregnancy, Arch. Surg. 66:664, 1953.

DeVor, R. W., and Ferris, D. O.: Pregnancy at term complicated by ruptured appendix, Mayo Clin. Proc. 22:135, 1947.

Freedman, W. L., and McMahon, F. J.: Placental metastasis; review of the literature and a report of a case of metastatic melanoma, Obstet. Gynec. 16:550, 1960.

George, P. A., Fortner, J. G., and Pack, G. T.: Melanoma with pregnancy; a report of 115 cases, Cancer 13:854, 1960.

Gerdes, M. M., and Boyden, E. A.: The rate of emptying of the human gallbladder in pregnancy, Surg. Gynec. Obstet. 66:145, 1938.

Gerwig, W. H., Jr., and Thistlewaite, J. R.: Cholecystitis and cholelithiasis in young women following pregnancy, Surgery 28:983, 1950.

Harer, W. B., Jr., and Harer, W. B., Sr.: Volvulus complicating pregnancy and the puerperium, Obstet. Gynec. 12:399, 1958.

Hoffman, S., and Suzuki, M.: Acute appendicitis in pregnancy; a ten year survey, Amer. J. Obstet. Gynec. 67:1338, 1954.

Journey, R. W., and Payne, F. L.: Nonobstetric surgical complications during obstetric care; a review of the recent literature, Amer. J. Med. Sci. 232:695, 1956.

Montgomery, T. L.: Detection and disposal of breast cancer in pregnancy, Amer. J. Obstet. Gynec. 81:926, 1961.

Nabatoff, R. A.: The management of varicose veins, New York J. Med. 58:1691, 1958.

Okell, C. C., and Elliott, S. D.: Bacteriaemia and oral sepsis, with special reference to aetiology of subacute endocarditis, Lancet 2:869, 1935.

Pack, G. T., and Scharnagel, I. M.: The prognosis for malignant melanoma in the pregnant woman, Cancer 4:324, 1951.

Pulaski, E. J.: Discriminate antibiotic prophylaxis in elective surgery, Surg. Gynec. Obstet. 108: 385, 1959.

Snyder, W. H., and Chaffin, L.: Emergency conditions in obstetrics and general surgery, Obstet. Gynec. 13:683, 1959.

Steffen, E., and Grace, H.: Pregnancy subsequent to radical mastectomy of the breast for cancer, Amer. J. Obstet. Gynec. 58:180, 1949.

Turell, R.: Obstetrical and gynecological aspects of proctology; review of literature with comments, Obstet. Gynec. Survey 5:159, 1950.

Walter, R. I.: Intestinal obstruction complicated by pregnancy, J. Mount Sinai Hosp. N. Y. 17: 625, 1951.

White, T. T.: Carcinoma of the breast in the pregnant and the nursing patient; review of 1375 cases, Amer. J. Obstet. Gynec. 69:1277, 1955.

White, T. T.: Prognosis of breast cancer for pregnant women; analysis of 1413 cases, Surg. Gynec. Obstet. 100:661, 1955.

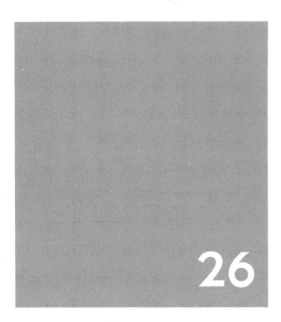

26

Toxemias of pregnancy

The term *toxemia of pregnancy* is non-specific, indicating an entire group of conditions that have similar signs and symptoms but that actually are quite different.

■ Classification and diagnosis

I. Acute toxemia
   A. Preeclampsia
      1. Mild
      2. Severe
   B. Eclampsia
II. Chronic vascular disease and pregnancy
   A. Chronic hypertensive vascular disease without superimposed toxemia
      1. Known hypertension before pregnancy
      2. Hypertension before the twenty-fourth week of pregnancy
   B. Chronic hypertensive vascular disease with superimposed toxemia
III. Unclassified toxemias

Preeclampsia. In preeclampsia the patient appears normal during early pregnancy, but hypertension, edema, and pro-teinuria appear after the twenty-fourth week. The following standards have been established by the Committee on Maternal Welfare, with the suggestion that pre-eclampsia can be diagnosed whenever one of the signs can be detected, but in general at least two of the three should be present before a diagnosis of preeclampsia is made.

Hypertension. A systolic blood pressure of at least 140 and/or a diastolic pressure of at least 90 mm. Hg or an increase in systolic pressure of at least 30 points and/or in diastolic pressure of at least 15 points is abnormal. The levels must occur on 2 occasions at least 6 hours apart.

Edema. Weight gain of at least 5 pounds in 1 week when accompanied by edema of the face and hands can be considered caused by toxemia.

Proteinuria. Plus 1 qualitative protein in a catheterized or clean-voided urine specimen or the excretion of more than 500 mg. daily on at least 2 successive days is abnormal.

Severe preeclampsia. If any one of the following is present, the preeclampsia is severe:

   1. Systolic blood pressure at least 160 mm. Hg or diastolic pressure at least 110 mm. Hg on 2 or more occasions at least 6 hours apart with the patient in bed
   2. At least 5 grams of protein in 24 hours (qualitative plus 3)
   3. Less than 400 ml. urinary output in 24 hours
   4. Cerebral or visual symptoms
   5. Edema of lungs or cyanosis

Mild preeclampsia. The absence of the criteria just listed indicates mild preeclampsia.

Eclampsia. Covulsions and/or coma in a pregnant or puerperal woman with characteristic signs of preeclampsia is indicative of eclampsia.

Chronic hypertensive vascular disease. An abnormal elevation in blood pressure must be present before the twenty-fourth week of pregnancy or between pregnancies and persist indefinitely after delivery.

Chronic hypertension with superimposed toxemia. The diagnosis of chronic hypertension with superimposed toxemia can be made in a patient with chronic hypertension who develops edema, proteinuria, or an increase in blood pressure of at least 30 mm. Hg systolic pressure and/or 15 mm. Hg diastolic pressure during pregnancy.

Recurrent toxemia. Recurrent toxemia is the "toxemia" that recurs in pregnancies subsequent to that in which an acute toxemia was diagnosed if (1) no signs are present between pregnancies or (2) if the signs are not evident 6 weeks after termination of the pregnancy in which the diagnosis of recurrent toxemia is considered.

Unclassified toxemias. Those not falling into the groups just discussed are termed unclassified toxemias.

■ Incidence

From 7% to 10% of all pregnancies are complicated by one of the toxemias of pregnancy, and of these, approximately one half are hypertensive disease and one half preeclampsia. The incidence of primary renal disease as a complication of pregnancy has been considered to be low, but renal biopsy studies suggest that it occurs relatively frequently. Spargo, McCartney, and Winemiller found histologic changes characteristic of chronic renal disease in 15 of 62 primigravidas in whom a diagnosis of preeclampsia had been made and in 32 of 152 multiparas diagnosed as having chronic vascular disease with a superimposed acute toxemia.

■ Preeclampsia-eclampsia

Preeclampsia-eclampsia is the true toxemia of pregnancy. It occurs only in pregnant human beings and has not been reproduced in experimental animals or in nonpregnant female or male human beings; it has no exact counterpart in the hypertensive states in nonpregnant persons. The signs appear after the twenty-fourth week of pregnancy except in the rare instances in which it is associated with hydatidiform mole. It is more common in young primigravidas than in older multiparas and is characterized by *edema, proteinuria,* and *hypertension.*

Clinical course. The first evidence of an abnormality is usually an excessive gain in weight, more than 1 pound a week. After a period of abnormal weight gain the other signs appear together or one slightly in advance of the other. If the condition is untreated, it may progress until the patient develops eclampsia, which is simply the most advanced stage of acute toxemia of pregnancy.

Edema. From 8 to 10 pounds of the weight gained during normal pregnancy can

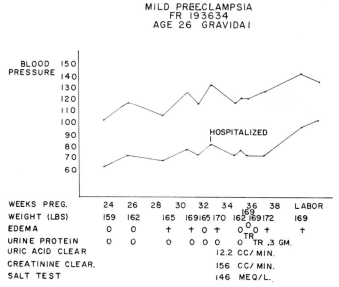

Fig. 26-1. Course of mild preeclampsia. Abnormal weight gain is evident early, whereas blood pressure, although gradually rising, is still within normal range. (From Willson, J. R.: Med. Clin. N. Amer. **39:**1781, 1955.)

be accounted for by the increased plasma volume and by fluid in the extravascular compartments. Most observers agree that the basic reason for fluid retention is delayed excretion of sodium and the other electrolytes, which are held in the tissues with enough water to maintain a normal concentration. The physiologic high levels of both total body water and exchangeable sodium are increased whenever a pregnant woman develops preeclampsia-eclampsia. Whether this represents an exaggeration of the normal mechanism or is a new process has not yet been determined. Nonetheless a rapid increase in body weight usually precedes the other clinical signs of toxemia by days or weeks. Even edema cannot be detected until a considerable amount of tissue fluid has accumulated.

Although the exact mechanism by which salt and water retention is exaggerated in women with acute toxemia is unknown, it seems likely that it is a result of imbalance between tubular reabsorption and glomerular filtration. During normal pregnancy tubular reabsorption increases to balance the rise in glomerular filtration, thereby preventing excessive electrolyte loss in the urine. One of the important changes in renal function with acute toxemia is a progressive diminution in glomerular filtration; as a consequence less sodium is presented to the tubules. If this and other electrolytes are reabsorbed at the usual high pregnancy rate, excessive amounts of sodium and water will be returned to the blood. This will reduce urine output and favor the development of edema. The action of adrenal cortical substances in the regulation of renal function is not yet clear, but it seems likely that they play an important role. Adrenal cortical activity is increased during normal pregnancy, and in patients with preeclampsia-eclampsia the corticoid levels are even higher.

The results of this alteration in salt metabolism can be demonstrated by injecting hypertonic saline solution intravenously and measuring the urinary output of sodium and chloride (Dieckmann salt test). The excess electrolytes and water are eliminated less rapidly in normal pregnant women than in nonpregnant women, but there is a further delay in those with preeclampsia. In normal pregnant women the sodium excretion during the first 2 hours after the administration of 1,000 ml. of 2.5% salt solution averaged 267 mEq./L., and in those with preeclampsia, 158 mEq./L. Eighty-eight percent of the normal women eliminated the excess fluid rapidly, returning to the pretest weight within 48 hours; 70% of those with preeclampsia had not returned to the pretest weight within 96 hours.

Hypertension. The blood pressure rise as-

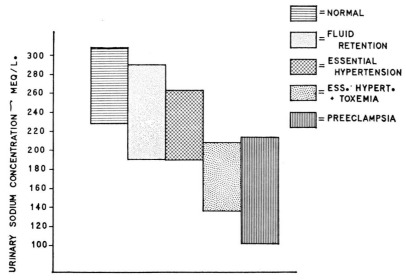

Fig. 26-2. Results of Dieckmann salt test. Urinary excretion of sodium is reduced with preeclampsia and essential hypertension with acute toxemia superimposed.

sociated with preeclampsia is not necessarily severe, and hypertension is seldom the initial sign of toxemia. The height of the blood pressure does not indicate the overall severity, the average systolic blood pressure in preeclampsia being only about 160 mm. Hg. Although any blood pressure over 140/90 mm. Hg is considered to be abnormal, the physician should not wait for the blood pressure to reach this level before suspecting that something is wrong. Since the blood pressure during normal pregnancy should remain at the prepregnancy level or even fall slightly, a gradual but persistent rise should arouse his suspicions. An increase of over 30 mm. Hg in systolic pressure and/or over 15 mm. Hg diastolic pressure, even though it remains within the limits of normal, is suggestive that preeclampsia is developing.

The rise in blood pressure is undoubtedly a response to widespread precapillary arteriolar spasm and the consequent increase in peripheral resistance. The vascular changes can be seen in the retinal and conjunctival vessels and can be measured in the kidney and in the brain. Renal blood flow becomes progressively more reduced as preeclampsia progresses. The alteration is a result of increased resistance in the afferent glomerular arterioles and narrowing of the lumina of the glomerular capillaries. McCall observed increased vascular resistance in cerebral vessels, although blood flow and cerebral oxygen consumption remained normal. Uterine blood flow also is reduced, although precise methods for measuring it in human beings are not yet available. The mechanism by which vasospasm is initiated is unknown, but it seems likely that the stimulus is some substance produced by the trophoblastic cells or in the decidua.

Proteinuria. The third important sign of preeclampsia is the excretion of protein in the urine. This makes its appearance at about the same time as the hypertension and increases in severity as the disease progresses. This also may be a result of hypoxia, since proteinuria can be produced experimentally by reducing renal blood flow.

The examination of the urine in patients with early preeclampsia reveals no abnormality except for the presence of protein. The amount increases with the severity of the condition, and eventually 10 grams or more may be excreted daily. One of the important prognostic signs is the amount of urinary protein. A qualitative measurement of protein is likely to be misleading because a given amount of protein diluted in a large amount of urine may be read 1 plus, whereas the same amount in a small quantity of urine may give a 3 or 4 plus reaction. By measuring the total excretion in successive 24-hour periods, the physician has an accurate means of evaluating changes in renal function. This simple test should be part of the study of every patient with toxemia.

Urine microscopy. As the toxemia progresses, the urinary findings increase: In the severe case large amounts of protein, red blood cells, white blood cells, and all kinds of casts may be found. At this stage the urine examination is of little value in the differential diagnosis of the condition.

Renal function. The renal function in early preeclampsia is slightly reduced as evidenced by inulin, creatinine, and uric acid clearances that are below those for normal pregnancy. As the disease becomes severe, there is progressive diminution both in renal function, as evidenced by a further depression in the excretion of the various testing substances, and in urine volume. Women with severe preeclampsia and eclampsia may excrete only 100 to 200 ml. of urine in a 24-hour period or may even be completely anuric. That the decreased function is not directly related to the height of the blood pressure is evidenced by the fact that after delivery the renal function is reestablished, with the blood pressure at a level that usually is at least as high as in the predelivery period.

Plasma volume. A progressive *hemoconcentration* that is the result of the abnormal flow of fluid from the bloodstream into the tissue spaces and cells accompanies severe toxemia. As the blood volume decreases, so does the amount of urine excreted; the patient with severe preeclampsia or eclampsia may be anuric. There can be no diuresis without a reversal of the flow of fluid back into the bloodstream from the tissue spaces and reestablishment of blood flow through the glomerular capillaries.

Uric acid. Uric acid metabolism also is disturbed. As preeclampsia becomes more severe, the renal clearance of uric acid becomes progressively more reduced and the serum level rises. The maximum normal serum uric acid concentration is 6 mg./100 ml., and the minimum normal uric acid clearance is 10 mg./min. The increase in serum uric acid is probably a result of decreased renal excretion, but liver metabolism may also be altered. The serum uric acid concentration may be elevated in women who have been taking a chlorothiazide preparation.

Eclampsia. Eclampsia is the most severe stage of toxemia of pregnancy and represents a progression of preeclampsia with the addition of convulsions and/or coma.

The physiologic changes are simply a continuation of those found in severe preeclampsia. There is a further increase in blood pressure, but this need not be to exceedingly high levels; the systolic blood pressure is often below 200 mm. Hg except during the actual convulsions. The oliguria increases to anuria, and there is a further increase in the hemoconcentration, the hemoglobin at times reaching 125%. A retention of nitrogenous waste material accompanies the depression of kidney function, and for the first time a rise in blood urea nitrogen may be noted.

Eclampsia may develop prior to the onset of labor, during labor, or within the first 24 hours following delivery.

Etiology. The etiology of preeclampsia-eclampsia has not been clearly established, but it is evident that the condition can develop only in women with active trophoblastic tissue. Toxemia occurs more often during multiple pregnancy (increased amount of placenta) and with hydatidiform mole (abnormally functioning placenta) than in single pregnancy with a normal infant. The incidence is increased in patients with chronic cardiovascular renal disease, diabetes mellitus, and severe anemia.

The role of dietary deficiency in the development of preeclampsia-eclampsia is not clearly defined, but it seems likely that malnutrition is an important factor. Toxemia develops more often in women of lower socioeconomic classes who are chronically undernourished than in middle and upper class women. Their diets are likely to be low in protein and high in salt. Although diet is important, it probably is not the sole cause of toxemia. Bryans and Torpin studied 243 women who previously had eclampsia; 188 had 565 pregnancies subsequent to the one complicated by convulsive toxemia. Although 56.4% of the women developed toxemia during at least one subsequent pregnancy, only 36% of the 565 pregnancies were toxemic. Eclampsia recurred in only 4.8%. If diet alone were the most important causative factor, the recurrence rate should have been considerably higher because few if any changes could have been made in dietary, economic, or environmental factors. Many attempts have been made to correlate geographic and climatic conditions with its development. So far no convincing evidence has been advanced.

The most tenable current theory is that of uterine ischemia. A reduction in blood flow to the choriodecidual space could alter placental function, permitting the trophoblast or the decidua to produce thromboplastin or thromboplastin-like material, pressor polypeptides, or other substances that might initiate the characteristic vascular changes. The basic theory has much in its favor. Preeclampsia-eclampsia occurs most often in young primigravidas, particularly those with twins, and in women with hydatidiform moles. In each of these the uterus tends to be either tense or more distended than usual. This could cause a reduction in blood flow through the smaller vessels. The incidence in women with preexisting hypertensive disorders and with diabetes, particularly those with vascular degeneration, also is high. In these women, too, uterine blood flow is reduced.

Page has set up an interesting table of "rates" for hypothetical "antitoxemia insurance," which vary according to the incidence of preeclampsia-eclampsia in individuals with various vascular or metabolic conditions (Table 9).

Prophylaxis. It probably will not be possible to prevent the development of acute toxemia until more is known about its basic cause. The serious advanced stages with their high perinatal and maternal mortality can be avoided if the alert physician detects the earliest evidence of fluid retention or of minor blood pressure changes at their onset. It has been suggested that toxemia will not develop if the protein intake throughout pregnancy is adequate. Although this seems to be an unduly optimistic attitude, every attempt should be made to correct nutritional deficits. Equally enthusiastic claims

Table 9. "Antitoxemia Insurance Premiums" per each $100 policy*

	Primipara	*Multipara*
Average body build	8.00	2.50
Short and obese	20.00	10.00
Tall and thin	2.00	.75
Twins	27.00	10.00
Triplets	50.00	25.00
Hydramnios, acute	35.00	17.50
Essential hypertension	33.00	33.00
Chronic nephritis	25.00	25.00
Diabetes mellitus	50.00	25.00
Severe anemia (untreated)	40.00	20.00
Beriberi	65.00	65.00
Hydatid mole (after fourth month)	70.00	50.00
Obese, diabetic, chronic hypertensive woman with twins	95.00	95.00

*From Page, E. W.: Hypertensive disorders of pregnancy, Springfield, Ill., 1953, Charles C Thomas, Publisher.

have been made for the use of diuretics throughout pregnancy, but the study of Kraus, Marchese, and Yen failed to confirm this.

Treatment. Dieckmann divided the signs and symptoms of preeclampsia into groups that indicate progressive severity of the condition and that may be utilized as an aid in guiding treatment:

Group A
Edema (weight), hypertension, proteinuria

Group B

Cerebral	*Visual*
Headache	Diplopia
Dizziness	Scotomas
Tinnitus	Blurred vision
Drowsiness	Amaurosis
Change in respiratory rate	
Tachycardia	
Fever	
Gastrointestinal	*Renal*
Nausea	Oliguria
Vomiting	Anuria
Epigastric pain	Hematuria
Hematemesis	Hemoglobinuria

Group C
Convulsions, coma

Office treatment of preeclampsia. Although preeclampsia cannot be cured until the pregnancy is terminated, the careful treatment of the condition early in its course may prevent its progression, at least until labor can be induced. The early recognition and treatment of fluid retention before the other signs appear is important. Every patient with edema will not develop preeclampsia, but it is impossible to determine in advance who will, and so all patients with edema must be managed as potential preeclamptic patients. The treatment of the earliest stage of toxemia can usually be initiated in the office if the patient can follow a carefully outlined regimen and if she can be examined frequently.

Since fluid accumulation in the tissue spaces is a direct result of abnormal retention of electrolytes, a reversal may be anticipated if the sodium chloride content can be reduced, thus freeing the water. This can be accomplished by a diet that contains 2 to 4 grams of sodium chloride daily. If the patient adheres strictly to this diet, the tissue electrolytes will be utilized by the body, and the excess water that was holding them in solution will be excreted by the kidney. Blood pressure determinations, weight checks, and measurement of the 24-hour protein excretion should be made at least twice weekly.

The effectiveness of the office treatment of the patient with fluid retention can be gauged by (1) control of weight (edema), (2) stabilization of blood pressure, (3) maintenance of urine output, (4) stabilization of the 24-hour protein excretion, and (5) absence of symptoms. Failure of office treatment is indicated by (1) progressive increase in blood pressure, (2) progressive gain in weight or an increase in the amount of edema, (3) increase of proteinuria, and (4) development of symptoms (group B). Such a failure makes hospitalization and the institution of more active therapy imperative.

Hospital treatment of preeclampsia. The initial hospital treatment of preeclampsia concerns itself primarily with the classification of severity of the condition and the initiation of a regimen designed to control the signs and symptoms. With the exception of an evaluation of the duration of pregnancy, the size and position of the fetus, and the adequacy of the pelvis, the pregnancy is, at the onset, ignored. The excessive fluid retention can usually be reversed by a carefully prepared low-sodium diet (less than 2 grams).

The *blood pressure* should be checked at least twice daily and the patient *weighed* each morning at the same time. The *fluid intake* and *urine output* are carefully measured and recorded daily, and the amount of edema is evaluated. Daily quantitative determination of the *total urinary protein excretion* likewise is of prognostic significance. A steady increase or a constant excretion of more than 3 to 5 grams daily is a grave sign, indicating a failure of medical treatment to control the disease. Daily protein excretion greater than 5 grams is associated with a definite increase in intrauterine fetal death. The *serum uric acid* and the *uric acid and creatinine clearances* should be checked twice a week. The *retinal vessels* should be examined at regular intervals for evidence of increasing spasm and alterations in the vessel walls.

Success in therapy is determined by control or reversal of the abnormal signs (weight, blood pressure, and proteinuria) and by the absence of symptoms. If the response to this regimen is favorable, that is, if an adequate urine output (at least 1,500 ml.) is maintained, the proteinuria does not increase, the blood pressure is controlled, and the weight is stabilized, the patient may be carried until the cervix is "ripe," at which time labor can be induced.

Advance in severity of the toxemia is characterized by increasing weight and edema, a progressive diminution in urinary output with an increase in total protein, an increase in serum uric acid, a decrease in uric acid and creatinine clearances, further elevation of blood pressure, hemoconcentration as indicated by an increase in hemoglobin and hematocrit, progressive change in the retinal arterioles, and in many cases the appearance of symptoms that become progressively more pronounced. It is important to recognize that weight loss and regression of edema can occur while the other signs indicate an increasingly severe process; hence evaluation on the basis of a change in one sign alone is impossible.

STIMULATION OF RENAL FUNCTION. The maintenance or promotion of urinary output is one of the most important steps in treating severe preeclampsia, but it cannot always be achieved. If the toxemia is advancing rapidly and the urinary output is diminishing or if the patient has symptoms, haste is important. Reversal of fluid flow by diet may not be possible at this stage, and even though it is, no significant effect can be expected for 36 to 48 hours. Diuretics may be tried, but since glomerular blood flow and filtration are remarkably reduced at this stage, those acting at a tubular level probably will not help.

SEDATION. Sedatives are important in the management of severe or progressing preeclampsia but are unnecessary during the mild phases of the condition. Oversedation should be avoided because if too much is given, hypoxia may be increased and it may be difficult to differentiate the lethargy or coma produced by the drug from that due to the disease.

The cerebral depressant action of *magnesium sulfate* produces general sedation; this, its ability to decrease vascular tone, and its depression of the myoneural junction tend to lower blood pressure and help to prevent convulsions. McCall, studying cerebral hemodynamics in pregnancy toxemia, found that magnesium sulfate not only lowers blood pressure but relieves cerebral vasospasm, increases cerebral blood flow, and increases oxygen utilization by brain tissue. All these tend to reverse the changes of preeclampsia-eclampsia.

Magnesium sulfate can be given intramuscularly as a 50% solution, or it can be given intravenously. Intramuscular injection has the disadvantages of being painful and of the unpredictable absorption rate due to vascular spasm. When given intravenously, the dosage is about 1 Gm./hr.

as a 10% solution. Magnesium intoxication is possible but is unlikely to occur if the patient is being observed properly. Magnesium is excreted in the urine, consequently an adequate urinary output is essential; if the urine volume decreases below 30 ml./hr., the dosage of magnesium sulfate must be reduced. Magnesium sulfate also decreases hyperactive reflexes, thereby decreasing the possibility of convulsions. The reflexes can be used to monitor dosage; as long as the patellar reflexes are present, there is no immediate danger of magnesium toxicity. They should be checked about every 30 minutes.

Morphine sulfate, 10 to 16 mg., *Luminal sodium,* 0.3 Gm. intramuscularly every 6 to 8 hours, or *Amytal sodium,* 0.3 Gm. intravenously, have been used extensively but are much less effective than magnesium sulfate and need not be used.

CONTROL OF BLOOD PRESSURE. Unless the blood pressure is greatly elevated, hypotensive drugs ordinarily are unnecessary in the treatment of severe preeclampsia because the magnesium sulfate will usually depress the blood pressure to a reasonably safe level. If the pressure falls to an unusually low level or sometimes even to the normal range, the output of urine may be greatly reduced.

If the systolic blood pressure is rising rapidly or is over 160 to 180 mm. Hg, a definite effort should be made to control it. Hydralazine hydrochloride (Apresoline), 20 to 30 mg. diluted to 20 ml. and given slowly intravenously, will often lower the blood pressure and maintain it at a safe level for several hours. This is particularly effective during labor. The effect of Apresoline on cerebral blood vessels and blood flow is similar to that of magnesium sulfate but more pronounced. When given by mouth, the drug has much less effect. Reserpine in 5 mg. doses is also effective.

It is possible to control blood pressure over relatively long periods of time with the hypotensive drugs, but there is little point in allowing a pregnancy of 36 or more weeks' duration to continue; the only reason for delaying delivery in a patient with toxemia is in the interest of the baby. If the condition can be controlled and the delivery of a small premature infant can be avoided, infant mortality will be decreased.

TERMINATION OF PREGNANCY. The decisive cure for preeclampsia-eclampsia is termina-tion of pregnancy at a carefully chosen time. No method of treatment is uniformly effective in controlling advancing preeclampsia; consequently unless the symptoms are all stabilized or reversed, eclampsia with its high maternal and infant mortality can only be prevented by delivery. Patients with mild toxemia that progresses despite treatment or with severe preeclampsia that does not respond to medical treatment should be delivered regardless of the duration of pregnancy.

Controlled preeclampsia in a patient 30 to 32 weeks pregnant presents a more serious problem. It is desirable to delay delivery in the interests of the infant if possible. One can wait as long as the blood pressure is controlled, renal function—as evidenced by urinary output and protein excretion and clearance studies—is improving or has stabilized at a reasonably normal level, and the patient is free from symptoms. The patient should be delivered promptly if medical control of the disease is lost or soon after the thirty-sixth week, even though the process still appears to be stabilized.

Labor can often be induced in these women, even though the cervix may feel unfavorable; hence in most instances the membranes should be ruptured and oxytocin given as an initial procedure. If labor has not begun within 6 to 12 hours, cesarean section can be performed.

Hospital treatment of eclampsia. If the patient develops convulsions, either through failure on her part to report to her physician or through failure on the part of the physician to interpret the signs of advancing preeclampsia correctly, the prognosis at once becomes grave.

Unless the natural tendency to overtreat the patient with eclampsia is curbed, the mortality may be increased. Before any medication is ordered for a convulsing patient, she must be examined to be certain that she actually has eclampsia and to evaluate her general condition. If she is comatose, as most women with eclampsia are, large doses of sedative drugs may be harmful.

The aims in the treatment of eclampsia are (1) to promote adequate renal function, (2) to control convulsions, and (3) to lower blood pressure.

GENERAL TREATMENT. The patient is placed in a dark, quiet room with an attendant constantly present. A *mouth gag* prepared by wrapping gauze around a tongue blade should be available to insert between the teeth during convulsions to prevent injury to the tongue. Facilities for *aspiration of mucus* from the pharynx and trachea should be available. Recordings of *blood pressure, urine volume, temperature, pulse, respirations,* and *response to treatment* should be made hourly. Nothing is given by mouth until after delivery, and the stomach should be aspirated if the patient is vomiting. Since there is always hypoxia associated with hemoconcentration, the administration of *oxygen* by tent, mask, or catheter is a valuable aid in therapy. Copious pulmonary secretions may fill the bronchi and lower trachea, thereby obstructing the airway. Oxygenation can be improved by performing *tracheotomy* whenever pulmonary edema is diagnosed, when respirations are labored, or when there is a suggestion of cyanosis. Most women with eclampsia should be *digitalized.*

PROMOTION OF RENAL FUNCTION. An indwelling catheter is inserted into the bladder, and hourly urine outputs are recorded. The urinary diuretic preparations are completely valueless because the anuria is a result of decreased glomerular filtration, and most diuretics act at a tubular level. Since the decrease in glomerular filtration is at least in part a result of glomerular arteriolar spasm, the most important part of the treatment is to decrease peripheral vascular spasm, which can best be accomplished with magnesium sulfate and other antihypertensive agents. The injection of large amounts of hypotonic glucose should be avoided, since it tends to increase edema because of delayed excretion. Sodium-containing fluids are contraindicated.

CONTROL OF CONVULSIONS. Sedation and control of convulsions are important steps in treatment. Magnesium sulfate, administered as described for severe preeclampsia, will usually provide adequate sedation and control the convulsions.

Morphine has been extensively utilized in eclampsia, but it has certain pharmacologic effects that may be disadvantageous: the production of acidosis, concentration of the blood, and an increase in intracranial pressure.

CONTROL OF BLOOD PRESSURE. Depression of blood pressure is not necessarily an important factor in the treatment of eclampsia. In fact in some patients even a moderate fall in pressure may result in a reduction of urine output. Magnesium sulfate or other sedatives will often reduce blood pressure to a reasonable level. However, another hypotensive agent should be administered if there is no response to magnesium sulfate and if the pressure is high enough to cause concern over the possibility of cerebral hemorrhage.

Apresoline, 20 to 30 mg. diluted to 20 ml. and given slowly intravenously or 50 to 100 mg. in 1,000 ml. of 5% dextrose as an intravenous drip, may be given if the blood pressure remains too high. *Reserpine,* 5 to 10 mg., or *Unitensen,* 0.25 to 1 mg. intramuscularly, may also be used. It is advisable to start with a small dose until the response can be evaluated. The medications can be repeated as often as necessary to maintain the hypotensive effect.

TERMINATION OF PREGNANCY. Although termination of the pregnancy is the decisive step in the treatment of both preeclampsia and eclampsia, ill-advised attempts at delivery at an inopportune time may result in the death of a patient who otherwise might have survived. Initial treatment by delivery by any method without a preliminary period of medical control of the disease is accompanied by an alarming maternal mortality; hence control of convulsions and reestablishment of renal function must precede delivery. In certain instances it may become necessary to terminate pregnancy in patients with severe eclampsia who are responding poorly to treatment, but ordinarily they should be delivered soon after convulsions are controlled, hemoconcentration has been corrected, and a satisfactory urinary output has been established. Delivery from below is preferable if there are no contraindications. Cesarean section is to be considered only in those in whom there is contraindication to vaginal delivery or in those in whom labor cannot be induced by rupturing membranes and administering oxytocin.

POSTDELIVERY CARE. Any patient with severe preeclampsia may develop eclampsia during the first 48 hours after delivery. During this time diuresis should begin, and if this occurs it is unlikely that the toxemia will progress. Should the anuria continue, however, the patient is in danger of convulsing. The same careful observations and the same treatment given the undelivered, severely preeclamptic patient is continued after delivery until the disease process has reversed itself. The urine output is carefully measured at hourly intervals. Sedation should be continued for about 48 hours after delivery but in diminishing amounts. These patients should not be allowed out of bed until the process has definitely reversed itself.

Pathologic changes in preeclampsia-eclampsia. The morphologic changes accompanying toxemia are mostly the result of the characteristic circulatory changes. Fibrin emboli and the acute degenerative changes that can be observed in the small vessels and the hemoconcentration of eclampsia certainly disturb the blood flow through the tissues and may lead to local anoxia and functional or anatomic disruption.

Kidney. Acute degenerative changes and fibrin deposition may be observed in the smaller vessels. The size of the glomerular capillary lumina is reduced by swelling of the endothelial cells, by the deposition of amorphous material beneath the normal basement membrane of the capillaries, and by proliferation of the intercapillary cells that lie between the vascular loops. These changes, called glomerular endotheliosis, which formerly were thought to be from thickening of the capillary basement membrane, have been clarified by electron microscopy. The tubular cells appear to be degenerated, but the changes probably are caused by excessive absorption of protein. Cortical necrosis may occur in women with severe abruptio placentae.

Adrenal glands. Adrenal hemorrhage and necrosis occur frequently, particularly in the patients who die in a state of vascular collapse.

Liver. Fibrin thrombi in the vessels and exudates and hemorrhage or actual tissue necrosis in the periportal areas may be found with severe preeclampsia-eclampsia. Liver involvement is minimal or absent with mild preeclampsia.

Brain. The same vascular changes may be observed in the brain as elsewhere. Hemorrhage from the rupture of large cerebral vessels is the cause of death in about 15% of women with eclampsia. Cerebral edema may be a postmortem change.

Retinal vessels. Narrowing of the vessels and retinal edema may be observed relatively early. As the toxemia advances, hemorrhages and complete retinal detachment may occur. Recovery usually is complete.

Mortality in preeclampsia-eclampsia. The maternal mortality for preeclampsia is low in general, and in the early stages there should be no mortality from the disease itself. As it progresses in severity, there may be mortality from toxemia and also from the treatment. The mortality rate for eclampsia in the United States is probably about 10%, but it can be kept much lower than this by proper care. The mortality rate with proper treatment may be less than 5%. The principal causes of death are congestive heart failure, cerebral hemorrhage, and liver necrosis. Others are infection and adrenal cortical necrosis with vascular collapse. Hemorrhage is even more lethal than with normal delivery because of hemoconcentration, which is so characteristic of eclampsia; much more hemoglobin is lost in concentrated than in normal blood.

The perinatal mortality also is high, and although in some instances the fetus can be saved, a high death rate goes along with the condition and its treatment. The main causes of death are intrauterine anoxia, the complications of prematurity, toxemia, and infection.

Relationship of eclampsia to chronic hypertension. There has been much discussion concerning the relationship between eclampsia and the subsequent development of chronic vascular disease. Most studies have suggested that there is no direct relationship, but the numbers of women who could be included in such studies are small because so frequently the immediate prepregnancy blood pressure is unknown. Chesley, Annitto, and Cosgrove traced 268 of 270 women who had been treated for eclampsia in the Margaret Hague Maternity Hospital, Jersey City, New Jersey, between 1931 and 1951. They found that women who had eclampsia in the first pregnancy carried to viability had the same prevalence of hypertension 15 or more years later as did an unselected control group of the same ages. The remote mortality for white women who had eclampsia in the first pregnancy carried to viability was like that of the control group, but death rates were increased 2.6 to 3.8 times in all black women who had eclampsia and in white women whose eclampsia occurred after the first pregnancy. They suggest that this represents an increased basic tendency to the development of vascular disease rather than an effect of eclampsia and conclude that there is no relationship between eclampsia and the subsequent development of chronic vascular disease.

An unexpected finding in this study was that diabetes was increased five times in women who had eclampsia during the first pregnancy and ten times if eclampsia developed in multiparous women.

■ Hypertensive cardiovascular disease in pregnancy

Essential hypertension may be present in a woman who becomes pregnant or may first manifest itself during pregnancy. It may become a serious complication jeopardizing the lives of both mother and infant.

Diagnosis. If the patient has a history of hypertension either between pregancies or repeatedly during pregnancy, it is likely that the present episode is a chronic vascular disease. The blood pressure elevation usually is present before the twenty-fourth week of pregnancy, and there may be other evidences of chronicity of the condition such as organic changes in the retinal vessels. Cardiac enlargement and serious renal pathology are seldom encountered in hypertensive pregnant patients because they are usually young women who have not had severe hypertension long enough to produce these changes. Ordinarily if the elevation in blood pressure is not accompanied by edema (abnormal weight gain) and proteinuria, a diagnosis of essential hypertension is likely.

Effect of pregnancy on hypertension. Pregnancy often has no effect on the hypertension, but this cannot be relied upon. In about one third of all pregnant women with essential hypertension, acute toxemia is superimposed upon the chronic condition. This presents a much more serious problem than preeclampsia in the normal patient, and the incidence of both fetal and maternal death is increased. In another one third of patients with chronic hypertension the blood pressure falls, occasionally, but not usually, to normal levels during the pregnancy.

Effect of hypertension on pregnancy. In most women with essential hypertension the pregnancy progresses uneventfully, but the complications that can develop are severe.

Effect on the fetus. There is a great increase in perinatal mortality associated with hypertension. The fetus is almost always smaller than in normal pregnancies of the same duration. This may be because the placenta is small and infarcted, probably because the vascular disease in the placental site interferes with its growth and development. The small placenta limits the amounts of oxygen and food that can be supplied the baby, and if it is compromised enough, it may die in utero. Early abortion is increased and adds to the fetal loss. The patient who begins pregnancy with a systolic blood pressure near 200 mm. Hg has only about a 50% chance of having a living healthy infant.

Abruptio placentae. About one half of all cases of severe premature separation of the placenta occur in women with vascular disease. This is associated with a high fetal and an increased maternal mortality.

Acute toxemia. Thirty to forty percent of all women with vascular disease will develop signs characteristic of preeclampsia during pregnancy. The complication usually appears late in the second trimester at about the period of viability and is associated with a high fetal and maternal mortality. This may progress rapidly to the convulsive state, further increasing the mortality.

Cerebral hemorrhage. Intracranial hemorrhage is a more common cause of maternal death than in eclampsia because the vessels may have undergone an organic degenerative change and because the arterial blood pressure usually is much higher.

Renal cortical necrosis. Renal cortical necrosis is sometimes encountered in women with hypertension and premature placental separation.

Treatment. Patients with severe hypertension should be admitted to the hospital for a period of observation when first seen. The examination should include (1) general physical examination, (2) frequent blood pressure recordings, (3) eye examination for evidence of retinitis, (4) renal function studies such as fluid intake and urine output, urea, creatinine, and uric acid clearances, daily quantitative protein determinations, and microscopic urine examination and concentration test, (5) blood urea nitrogen determination, and (6) cardiac evaluation. A base line is thus established for repeat examinations during pregnancy, and a decision can be made as to whether or not pregnancy should continue.

Interruption of pregnancy. If the systolic blood pressure is above 180 to 200 mm. Hg and remains elevated after a period of bed rest, if there are degenerative changes in the retinal arterioles, if the patient has had a previous cerebral hemorrhage, or if renal function is reduced, pregnancy is dangerous and interruption should be recommended.

Test of pregnancy. If the pregnancy is allowed to continue, the patient is informed of her condition and advised of the possibilities. She is told to be prepared to enter the hospital at any time and to remain in the hospital for a long period. As long as the pregnancy remains uneventful, it is to be allowed to continue, but should the patient develop an acute toxemia that does not respond to treatment, interruption must be considered.

Prenatal care. Patients with chronic hypertension should be seen at least every 2 weeks and often more frequently. They should rest every morning and afternoon and spend at least 10 hours in bed each night. A low-salt diet is prescribed, and for the patient who is obese caloric intake should also be reduced.

The hypotensive drugs such as reserpine (Serpasil) may serve a useful purpose, particularly if the patient is taking them when she conceives. If they are started after she is already pregnant, the infant mortality rate may still be high because of abnormal placentation.

Any prenatal patient with hypertension should be admitted to the hospital at once if (1) the blood pressure rises, (2) protein appears in the urine, (3) she gains weight abnormally or develops edema, or (4) symptoms appear.

Termination of pregnancy. If the patient with hypertension develops an acute toxemia that cannot be controlled with medical treatment, the pregnancy must be terminated even though the infant is not yet viable. The indications for termination of

pregnancy are (1) rising blood pressure that fails to respond to treatment, (2) increasing evidence of retinal vascular damage, or (3) decreasing renal function. Since these women frequently are multiparas, labor often can be induced by amniotomy if the cervix is effaced; otherwise cesarean section may be necessary.

If the blood pressure remains stable throughout the pregnancy or falls slightly and if an acute toxemia does not develop, the prognosis is reasonably good. Such patients can continue to term, and spontaneous delivery can be anticipated.

Care during labor. Magnesium sulfate is less effective in lowering blood pressure in essential hypertension than in preeclampsia-eclampsia. Apresoline may be given if the blood pressure is unusually high or rises during labor. *Local anesthesia* is preferable for delivery.

Postpartum care. During the immediate postdelivery period the blood pressure must be taken at regular intervals because it may either rise rapidly or fall precipitously, and the output of urine must be recorded every hour until diuresis has been established. Mild sedation with Amytal sodium, 0.2 to 0.4 Gm. during the first day or two, may help to control the hypertension.

Special problems. Special problems involve fetal death, abruptio placentae, and future pregnancies.

Previous fetal death. Some of the women may have had previous intrauterine fetal deaths at about the same time in each pregnancy. If the infant can be delivered either vaginally or by cesarean section while it is still alive, it may survive even though it is premature. Serial urinary estriol determinations during the last trimester may be helpful in evaluating placental function.

Abruptio placentae. Placental separation usually is severe and may be associated with a high mortality. The prompt transfusion and treatment of such patients will reduce the maternal mortality.

Future pregnancies. Tubal ligation should be considered for any patient with essential hypertension who has evidence of degenerative vascular changes in the retinal vessels, decreased renal function, or cardiac enlargement. Those whose blood pressure is higher after each pregnancy and those who have had repeated intrauterine fetal deaths and premature placental separation also are poor risks for further pregnancy. If more pregnancies are not contraindicated, the deliveries should be spaced about 18 months apart in order to complete childbearing while the patient is young and before the degenerative vascular changes appear.

Mortality. The maternal mortality is increased ten to twenty times over that of the normal patient, and the fetal loss is as high as 30% to 40%. The principal causes of death are abruptio placentae, eclampsia, cerebral hemorrhage, postpartum collapse, renal cortical necrosis, and infection. The mortality can be reduced by recognition of the fact that hypertension is a serious complication of pregnancy requiring special attention. Careful prenatal care and interruption of pregnancy at any time the vascular signs progress and fail to respond to treatment will contribute most to this reduction in deaths. Tweedie and Mengert, whose program is similar to this, reported a maternal death rate of 0.3% and a perinatal mortality of 6% in 368 women with uncomplicated chronic hypertension. In 71 women with chronic hypertension and superimposed acute toxemia the maternal death rate was 1.4% and the perinatal mortality 21.1%.

References

Acosta-Sison, H.: The relationship of hydatidiform mole to pre-eclampsia and eclampsia, Amer. J. Obstet. Gynec. 71:1279, 1956.

Altchek, A.: Electron microscopy of renal biopsies in toxemia of pregnancy, J.A.M.A. 175:791, 1961.

Bryans, C. I., and Torpin, R.: A follow-up study of two hundred and forty-three cases of eclampsia for an average of 12 years, Amer. J. Obstet. Gynec. 58:1054, 1949.

Carrington, E. R., and Willson, J. R.: Eclampsia as a cause of maternal death in Philadelphia, Amer. J. Obstet. Gynec. 65:12, 1953.

Chesley, L. C., Annitto, J. E., and Cosgrove, R. A.: Long-term follow-up study of eclamptic women, Amer. J. Obstet. Gynec. 101:886, 1968.

Chesley, L. C., and Cosgrove, R. A.: Remote deaths following eclampsia, Obstet. Gynec. 4:165, 1954.

Dawson, B.: The prevention of eclampsia; an Australian experiment, J. Obstet. Gynaec. Brit. Comm. 60:80, 1953.

Dieckmann, W. J.: Toxemias of pregnancy, St. Louis, ed. 2, 1952, The C. V. Mosby Co.

Hayashi, T. T.: Uric acid and endogenous creatinine clearance studies in normal pregnancy and toxemias of pregnancy, Amer. J. Obstet. Gynec. 71:859, 1956.

Hayashi, T. T.: Uric acid and endogenous creatinine clearances after normal and toxemic pregnancy, Amer. J. Obstet. Gynec. 73:23, 1957.

Kraus, G. W., Marchese, J. R., and Yen, S. C.: Prophylactic use of hydrochlorothiazide in pregnancy, J.A.M.A. 198:1150, 1966.

McCall, M. L.: Cerebral blood flow and metabolism in toxemias of pregnancy, Surg. Gynec. Obstet. 89:715, 1949.

Mengert, W. F., and Tweedie, J. A.: Acute vasospastic toxemia; therapeutic nihilism, Obstet. Gynec. 25:662, 1964.

Page, E. W.: The relation between the hydatid moles, relative ischemia of the gravid uterus, and the placental origin of eclampsia, Amer. J. Obstet. Gynec. 37:291, 1939.

Page, E. W.: The hypertensive disorders of pregnancy, Springfield, Ill., 1953, Charles C Thomas, Publisher.

Spargo, B., McCartney, C. P., and Winemiller, R.: Glomerular capillary endotheliosis in pregnancy, Arch. Path. 68:593, 1959.

Tillman, A. J. B.: Effect of normal and toxemic pregnancy on blood pressure, Amer. J. Obstet. Gynec. 70:589, 1955.

Tweedie, J. A., and Mengert, W. F.: Hypertensive disease and pregnancy, Obstet. Gynec. 25:188, 1965.

Willson, J. R.: The recognition of the early toxemias of pregnancy, Med. Clin. N. Amer. 39:1781, 1955.

Willson, J. R., Carrington, E. R., Hadd, H. E., and Boutwell, J.: Pregnancy edema; chemical and hormonal constituents of blood, urine, and edema fluid in patients with fluid retention and pre-eclampsia, Obstet. Gynec. 3:651, 1954.

Willson, J. R., and Hayashi, T. T.: Laboratory aids in diagnosis and treatment of pregnancy toxemia, Clin. Obstet. Gynec. 1:723, 1958.

Willson, J. R., Williams, J. M., and Hayashi, T. T.: Hypertonic saline infusions for the differential diagnosis of the toxemias of pregnancy, Amer. J. Obstet. Gynec. 73:30, 1957.

Zuspan, F. P., and Ward, M. C.: Improved fetal salvage in eclampsia, Obstet. Gynec. 26:893, 1965.

27

Bleeding during late pregnancy

Although the majority of women who bleed from the vagina during late pregnancy do not have a serious lesion, others may have. Since bleeding of any type is abnormal, the physician should attempt to determine its source whenever it occurs.

■ Placenta previa

About once in every 100 to 150 deliveries the entire placenta or part of it is implanted in the lower portion of the uterus rather than in the upper active segment. This is called *placenta previa*. Whenever a portion of the lower edge of the placenta separates from its attachment, bleeding may occur. Synonymous terms are *premature separation of the abnormally implanted placenta* and *unavoidable hemorrhage.*

Types. The types of placenta previa are determined by the relationship of the placenta to the internal cervical os. In *complete* or *total placenta previa* the entire cervical os is covered by placental tissue,

whereas in *incomplete placenta previa* the os is only partially covered. The incomplete types can be subdivided into *marginalis,* in which the edge of the placenta extends to the edge of the cervical canal, and *lateralis,* in which the edge of the placenta covers a part of the cervical opening. With a *low-lying placenta* a portion of the placenta is implanted in the lower uterine segment, but the placental border may be several centimeters above the internal os.

The classification is made on the basis of the findings at the initial examination and may change as labor advances. For instance, the edge of the placenta may extend across the entire cervical opening during early labor when the cervix is only dilated 2 or 3 cm. (complete placenta previa). However, as labor progresses and the cervix reaches 6 to 8 cm. dilatation, the placenta will have been drawn upward with the retracting lower uterine segment so that it covers only part of the opening. If the patient were first examined at this time, the diagnosis would be incomplete placenta previa.

Etiology. The reasons why the ovum implants in the lower segment are not always obvious. Placenta previa occurs more often in multiparas than in primigravidas. The suggestion that atrophic or inflammatory changes in the decidua because of defective blood supply or repeated pregnancies cause abnormal placentation is probably not valid because placenta previa rarely recurs. If decidual changes of this type were responsible, repeated episodes should be encountered more frequently. It seems more likely that the fertilized ovum reaches and implants in the lower segment by chance. The relatively large uterine cavity of the multipara might favor this.

Signs and symptoms. Bleeding is the most reliable single sign of placenta previa. Characteristically it is painless and bright red in color and occurs first at about the thirty-second week of pregnancy without a precipitating cause such as trauma or unusual activity. The initial episode of bleeding usually is slight and consists of spotting or a brief gush of bright red blood. Overwhelming hemorrhage rarely occurs at the onset unless the placental edge is separated from the uterine wall by digital examination or during coitus. Each bleeding episode usually subsides, only to recur in a few days or at

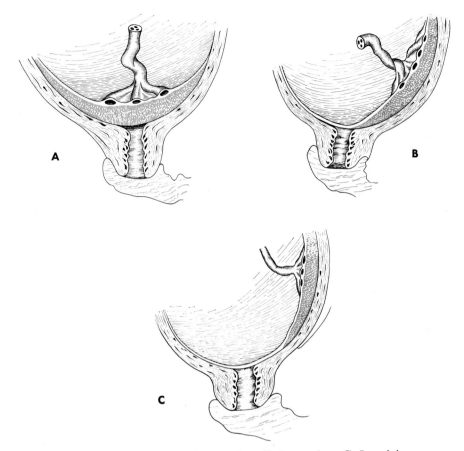

Fig. 27-1. Types of placenta previa. **A,** Complete. **B,** Incomplete. **C,** Low lying.

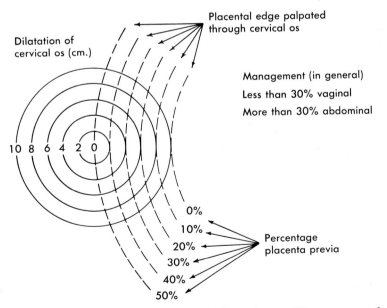

Fig. 27-2. Relationship of placental edge to cervical opening at different stages of dilatation. (From Tatum, H.: Amer. J. Obstet. Gynec. **93:**767, 1965.)

the most after a week or two. Subsequent bleedings are likely to become progressively heavier until finally profuse hemorrhage may occur. Occasionally placenta previa produces no symptoms until late in pregnancy or even until labor begins. A few patients with placenta previa may have had bleeding suggesting threatened abortion during the first half of pregnancy.

The source of bleeding is the maternal uterine sinuses, and the cause is the mechanical separation of a portion of the placenta from its uterine attachment as the lower segment lengthens during late pregnancy. It could also come from the marginal sinus that is injured as the lower edge of the placenta is retracted upward with the developing lower uterine segment. Bartholomew and co-workers have suggested an additional cause for the bleeding with complete placenta previa. They believe that the circulation of maternal blood through the intervillous spaces to the chorionic plate and then back to the general circulation is dis-

turbed because the placenta is implanted over the cervix. The pressure within the intervillous spaces overlying the cervical opening is less than in those that are implanted in the intact uterine wall, and the blood tends to flow toward the area of reduced pressure. If the cervical canal is open, the blood is forced out of the intervillous circulation and is lost in the vagina.

Diagnosis. Placenta previa can be suspected from a history of painless bleeding that begins during the last part of pregnancy. The physician should consider such bleeding to be caused by placenta previa until another reason is found.

Examination. The reason for bleeding can be determined only by examining the patient. Systematic application of the available methods for locating the placental implantation site will usually demonstrate the placentas that are situated low in the uterus.

ABDOMINAL EXAMINATION. An exact diagnosis cannot be made by abdominal examination alone, but it may provide suggestive

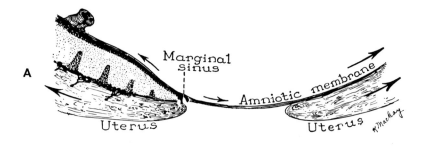

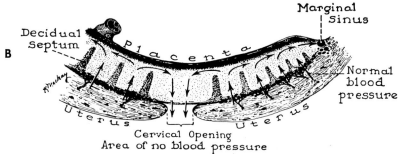

Fig. 27-3. Possible causes of bleeding with placenta previa. **A,** Rupture of marginal sinus with incomplete placenta previa. **B,** Bleeding caused by differences in pressure relationships with complete placenta previa. (From Bartholomew, R. A., Colvin, E. D., Grimes, W. H., Jr., Fish, J. S., and Lester, W. M.: Obstet. Gynec. **1:**41, 1953.)

information. Transverse lie and breech positions occur frequently with placenta previa. If the vertex is high above the inlet and deviated anteriorly or laterally and cannot be pushed into the pelvic inlet, the placenta may be preventing its descent. The location of the placental souffle is of little value in determining placental site.

VAGINAL EXAMINATION. A digital examination must be made at some time on every patient suspected of having placenta previa to confirm the diagnosis and to determine the degree of involvement and the condition of the cervix so that an appropriate method for delivery can be selected. If the patient is bleeding profusely, vaginal examination should be performed as soon as arrangements can be made in the operating room because it undoubtedly will be necessary to deliver her regardless of the stage of the pregnancy.

Immediate vaginal examination for those who are several weeks from term and are bleeding only slightly is usually contraindicated because the manipulations necessary to make an accurate diagnosis may separate

enough placenta to cause an alarming hemorrhage and force immediate delivery. Under such circumstances it is preferable to obtain an x-ray or isotope study and to withhold vaginal examination until the baby has grown large enough to survive outside the uterus.

Vaginal examination should only be performed after the following preparations have been made:

1. The patient and doctor must be prepared as carefully as for delivery.

2. The examination must be performed in an operating room that is ready for any type of treatment necessary to control the bleeding and deliver the patient.

3. Carefully cross-matched blood, 1,000 ml., should be available for use before the examination is made, or if there is no blood bank, donors of proved compatibility must be in the hospital.

4. Enough doctors and nurses must be available to meet any situation.

If the cervix is soft and patulous, the index finger is carefully introduced in an attempt to feel the cotyledons of a complete

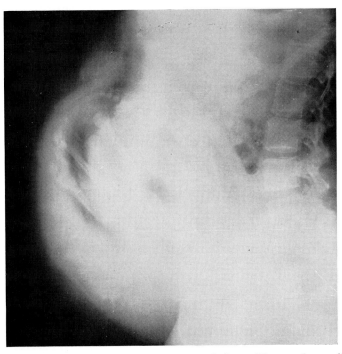

Fig. 27-4. Localization of placenta by soft tissue technique. The uterine wall can be seen posteriorly, and the placenta is implanted low on the anterior wall.

placenta previa covering the opening or the edge of an incomplete variety. If the amnion and the presenting part are felt directly above the cervical os, the examining finger is swept around the lower segment in an attempt to reach the edge of the placenta. As soon as the placenta is felt, the finger is withdrawn because vigorous manipulation will certainly separate more of it and initiate bleeding. If the cervix is closed, no attempt should be made to force the finger through it. The physician can sometimes clarify the situation by attempting to palpate the presenting part through the lower segment. If the uterine wall is thin, he can often feel the suture lines of the fetal head, unless a bulky placental mass lies between the uterus and the presenting part. This method is relatively inaccurate.

RECTAL EXAMINATION. Rectal examination should never be performed in a patient who is bleeding until placenta previa has been eliminated as a cause. Digital examination may separate the placenta and produce extensive bleeding.

X-RAY EXAMINATION. Placenta previa can be demonstrated by x-ray examination, but the amount of placenta over the cervical os and the condition of the cervix itself cannot be determined by this method. X-ray study

in patients suspected of having placenta previa need not be performed routinely, but it is particularly helpful in those who bleed during the early weeks of the third trimester. It is difficult to make the diagnosis by digital examination at this stage of pregnancy, and if bleeding is precipitated by the examination, the physician may be forced to deliver a small infant who has minimal chance to survive. If the placental site can be visualized by an x-ray study, the physician will have a better idea as to how to proceed. If the placental shadow can be seen in the upper segment, if there is no cervical lesion visible by speculum examination, and if the bleeding is slight and does not recur, no further investigation is necessary. If the placenta is implanted in the lower segment, the cervix should be inspected, but digital examination should not be performed until delivery becomes necessary.

1. Soft tissue technique: The placental shadow can be demonstrated unless it is obliterated by the bony pelvis. The absence of placental shadow in the upper segment is evidence for placenta previa.

2. Relation of the fetal head to the pubis and sacral promontory: If the shadow of the skull is close to the pubis or the promontory, there probably is no placental tis-

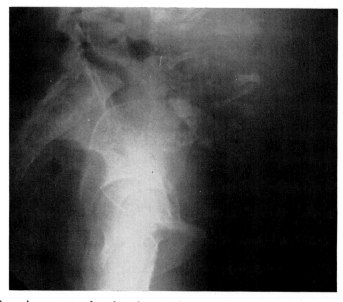

Fig. 27-5. There is no room for the placenta between the head and the sacral promontory or pubis.

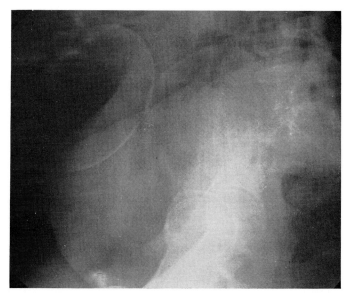

Fig. 27-6. Head is displaced upward and anteriorly by placenta in lower uterine segment.

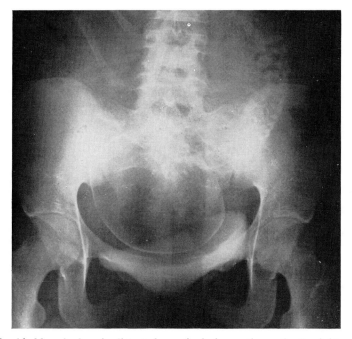

Fig. 27-7. The bladder shadow is distorted, particularly on the patient's right, and the head is separated from the bladder by placental tissue.

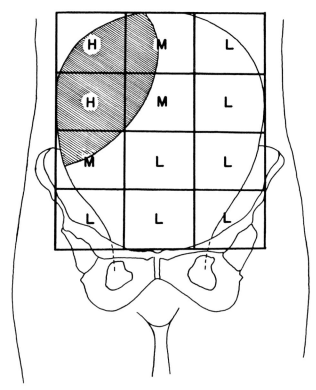

Fig. 27-8. Radioisotopic placental localization. The count is highest (**H**) in the area of placental implantation, moderately elevated (**M**) near the implantation site, and low (**L**) in the rest of the uterus.

sue in that area. If there is a considerable space either anteriorly or posteriorly, placenta previa may be present.

3. Radiopaque material in the bladder may help to demonstrate placentas implanted on the anterior wall. If the vertex is presenting, it will be centered in the inlet and in contact with the bladder shadow unless the placenta extends into the anterior portion of the lower segment. The placenta in this position prevents the presenting part from approximating the uterine wall; consequently the head will be separated from the bladder by several centimeters.

RADIOISOTOPE METHOD. The placental site can be determined with considerable accuracy by the use of radioactive iodinated human serum albumin (RISA). When this material is injected intravenously, it is disseminated throughout the maternal blood, but the amount in the slowly moving pool of blood in the choriodecidual space will be greater than that in the rest of the uterine circulation. The position of the placenta can

be mapped with reasonable accuracy by checking each of 12 areas over the anterior surface of the uterus with a scintillation counter. The counts will be higher over the placental site, where the activated albumin is concentrated, than over the rest of the uterus.

This method has several advantages over x-ray placental localization: it is more accurate, particularly during the last weeks of the second trimester and with abnormal presentations, it costs less, and it subjects the mother and the baby to much less radiation than do the conventional methods. At the moment the main disadvantage is that it requires an isotope laboratory and an individual experienced in the use of isotopes to prepare the material and to supervise the examinations.

Differential diagnosis. Bleeding such as that in placenta previa can also be produced by benign or malignant lesions of the cervix, rupture of the marginal sinus, rupture of placental vessels, premature labor, premature separation of the normally implanted placenta, bladder or bowel lesions, and other causes. These can be excluded during the course of the examination.

Treatment. To maintain a low maternal and infant mortality in patients with placenta previa the treatment must be planned individually for each patient. The fundamentals of the management of any patient with bleeding during pregnancy include determining the source of bleeding and controlling it, replacing the lost blood, and terminating the pregnancy at the proper time.

Delayed treatment. Under certain circumstances termination of the pregnancy may be delayed in the interests of the fetus. Since placenta previa manifests itself as early as 30 to 32 weeks of gestation, immediate delivery is associated with a high fetal loss. This may be reduced if the pregnancy can be allowed to continue until a later date. It is seldom necessary to delay termination if the pregnancy is of at least 36 weeks' duration.

X-ray or isotope placentography is obtained and the cervix is inspected with a sterile speculum, but no digital examinations are performed. If the placental shadow is in the lower segment and the bleeding ceases, active treatment of placenta previa can be delayed until it is made necessary by recurrence and a progressive increase in bleeding or by the onset of labor, or until the pregnancy reaches the thirty-seventh week, when the patient should usually be delivered.

Delayed treatment is feasible only if the bleeding is slight and if compatible blood and facilities for rapid treatment of hemorrhage are constantly available. Delay is contraindicated if the bleeding is profuse, if the fetus is abnormal, if the pregnancy is of at least 36 weeks' duration, if the supply of blood is uncertain, or if treatment facilities are inadequate.

Active treatment. If the pregnancy is near term, if the bleeding is profuse, or when it becomes necessary to terminate pregnancy after a period of delay, the physician must decide how to proceed. At this time vaginal examination, performed with the precautions outlined previously, is necessary to determine the condition of the cervix and type of placenta previa so that

the proper method for delivery can be selected.

Incomplete placenta previa. Cesarean section is the best method for terminating pregnancy in most women with incomplete placenta previa. This is particularly true when delivery becomes necessary while the cervix is closed and unsuitable for induction. If the fetus is dead, the bleeding has been controlled, and vaginal delivery is possible, there is no reason to perform cesarean section, but abdominal delivery is justifiable, even though the baby has died, if bleeding cannot be stopped.

Vaginal delivery may be possible in an occasional multipara with a soft, effaced, and partially dilated cervix and a minor degree of placenta previa. If the membranes are ruptured, the head will descend, exert pressure against the placenta, and compress the bleeding uterine sinuses beneath it. Vaginal delivery usually increases the hazard for the infant because compression of the placenta by the presenting part obstructs fetal vessels. If a large enough area of fetal circulation is eliminated, the infant will die of anoxia. Vaginal delivery, therefore, is most appropriate before the thirty-fourth week, when the baby has little chance of surviving. Under these circumstances if labor can be induced and bleeding controlled until the infant is delivered, the potential problems of a uterine scar during subsequent pregnancies will be avoided.

When vaginal delivery is selected, there are several possible methods for reducing maternal blood loss, but all increase the risk for the infant; they are only appropriate when the baby has little chance of surviving. *Scalp traction* may be used if simple rupture of the membranes does not suffice. The force necessary to compress the maternal sinuses is supplied by manual traction or a weight. When the breech presents and the cervix is partially dilated, one or both legs can be pulled down, permitting the *buttocks to tamponade the placenta.*

Whenever the placenta is implanted in the lower segment, the tissues in that part of the uterus and in the cervix are far more vascular and friable than in normal pregnancy. They are easily torn by the manipulations designed to control bleeding from the placental site, and many deaths have occurred as a result of ill-advised attempts to

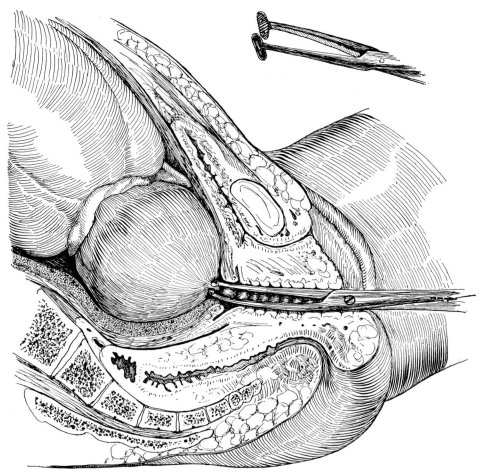

Fig. 27-9. Compression of vessels at the placental site by scalp traction to control bleeding with placenta previa. (From Titus, P.: Atlas of obstetric technic, St. Louis, 1949, The C. V. Mosby Co.)

effect delivery through the vagina simply to avoid cesarean section.

Complete placenta previa. In almost every instance the patient with complete placenta previa should be delivered by cesarean section.

Supportive treatment. Blood lost must be replaced with blood. No other fluid will do. If blood is not promptly and adequately replaced, the mortality will be high. No examination is to be made or treatment started on a bleeding patient unless blood is available. In an emergency, Rh-negative type O blood may be administered without cross matching. Plasma, glucose, or saline solution may be used only as a temporary measure while blood is being obtained.

Effect of placenta previa on mother and

infant. Low implantation of the placenta can be responsible for *early abortion,* but it usually does not disturb the course of pregnancy in any other respect. *Postpartum hemorrhage* occurs more often because the lower segment does not contract and control bleeding as well as the upper part of the uterus. *Puerperal infection* may occur because of the proximity of the placental site to the vagina, from which organisms may be introduced directly into the uterus during the manipulations for delivery and the control of bleeding. Unreplaced blood loss predisposes to the development of infection.

Maternal mortality should be less than 1%. The principal causes of death are hemorrhage and infection.

Perinatal mortality may be as high as

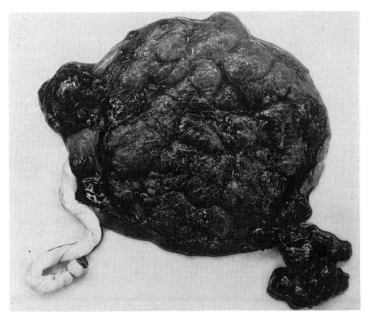

Fig. 27-10. Abruptio placentae. Note organized clots and dark, depressed areas of separation involving more than one half of the total placental surface.

30%. The principal causes of death are *prematurity; intrauterine anoxia* secondary to maternal blood loss, placental separation, and prolapsed cord; *respiratory distress syndrome; injury;* and occasionally *bleeding from placental injury. Development anomalies* are thought to be more common with placenta previa. Some reduction in premature deaths can be achieved by delayed treatment, but in many instances delay is precluded by profuse or continued bleeding. The lowest infant mortality rates that have been reported are about 12%.

■ Abruptio placentae

The term *abruptio placentae* indicates a complication of late pregnancy in which the placenta separates from its normal implantation site in the upper segment of the uterus before the birth of the baby. The mild types that ordinarily occur during labor are almost as common as placenta previa. The more severe ones, however, usually occur before the onset of labor and are encountered approximately once in 500 deliveries. This complication is also called *premature separation of the normally implanted placenta, ablatio placentae,* or *accidental hemorrhage.* If the placenta is completely de-tached from the uterine wall, *complete separation* can be diagnosed, but if a portion of it retains its connection, it is termed *partial separation.*

Etiology. The etiology of placental separation is not always obvious, but trauma plays a minor role in its production. *Chronic vascular renal disease,* such as long-standing hypertension or glomerulonephritis, is present in one third to one half of the women who develop complete placental separation, and the most serious instances are encountered in these patients. In all probability the hemorrhage and subsequent separation of the placenta occur as the result of abnormalities in the vessels of the placental site.

Howard and associates described the *supine hypotensive syndrome,* which occurs in about 10% of women during the last weeks of pregnancy and sometimes may be a factor in the production of premature placental separation. This circulatory change occurs as the vena cava is compressed by the weight of the pregnant uterus when the patient lies on her back. The flow of blood to the heart is impeded, and the venous pressure below the block, including that in the intervillous spaces, is increased. The pulse rate rises, the arterial blood pressure falls, and the resultant cerebral hypoxia causes unpleasant symptoms like those of a syncopal attack. The increasing pressure in the intervillous spaces may result in local hemorrhage and placental separation. Mengert and co-workers produced placental separation by compressing the vena cava before opening the uterus at the time of cesarean section. A protective mechanism must exist to prevent excessive pressures within the choriodecidual spaces in all pregnant women. These probably consist of extensive collateral circulation through the ovarian, renal, and vertebral veins.

Folic acid deficiency has been suggested as a cause for abruptio placentae. Hibbard and Hibbard's study, in which they found a folic acid deficiency in almost all women with premature placental separation, has been questioned because the diagnosis was made by the FIGLU test, which is not entirely specific. Streiff and Little studied serum and red blood cell folate activities in nonpregnant and normally pregnant women and in 16 women with abruptio placentae. In 15 of the latter the serum folate activity was deficient, as was red blood cell folate activity in the 9 who were tested. Although these figures suggest that a relationship exists between folic acid deficiency and abruptio placentae, further study is necessary to clarify it.

Accidents of labor. Any sudden decrease in size of a uterus overdistended by hydramnios or multiple pregnancy may produce partial placental separation. Traction on a short umbilical cord as the fetus descends through the birth canal may have the same effect, but this is unusual.

Mechanism of separation and clinical course. The vascular lesion in the decidual vessels that appears to be responsible for the disintegration and the resulting hemorrhage in women with chronic hypertensive disease is an acute degenerative arteriolitis. The extent of placental separation is determined by the amount of decidual bleeding. If the area is small and the bleeding is readily controlled by the pressure from the surrounding tissues, a small infarct may develop. If the bleeding is more extensive, part or all of the placenta may be dissected off the uterine wall. As the bleeding continues, the blood may remain in the retroplacental area, gradually dissecting the placenta off the

uterine wall without any visible hemorrhage at the onset. This is known as *concealed bleeding*. The blood may also remain concealed if it dissects upward between the membranes and the uterus rather than downward toward the cervix. In most instances the blood escapes from beneath the placenta, dissects the membranes off the uterine wall, and flows through the cervix, producing *external hemorrhage*. In rare instances the amniotic membrane may rupture within the uterine cavity, permitting the blood to collect inside the fetal sac.

With severe bleeding the patient may demonstrate signs of blood loss that often are much more pronounced than would be expected from the amount of visible bleeding. With complete placental separation, particularly in those patients with vascular renal disease, a *clotting defect* may develop, and bleeding may occur from the uterus, beneath the serosal surfaces, from the mucous membranes, from needle punctures, and directly into the uterine wall *(Couvelaire uterus or uteroplacental apoplexy)*. The clotting defect is usually caused by a disturbance in the fibrinogen-fibrin conversion mechanism. Thromboplastin from the abnormal subplacental decidua enters the bloodstream through the damaged vessels at the placental site and initiates the normal intravascular clotting process. Fibrinogen is converted to fibrin, which may occlude the small vessels throughout the body and cause local tissue anoxia. As more and more thromboplastin is introduced into the circulation and more and more fibrinogen is converted, the plasma fibrinogen concentration is progressively reduced until it is seriously depleted; the blood then becomes incoagulable, and abnormal bleeding is evident. The normal plasma fibrinogen concentrations during pregnancy range between 300 and 700 mg./100 ml.; when the concentration falls below 100 mg./100 ml., abnormal bleeding is likely to occur.

Although hypofibrinogenemia is the most frequent cause of coagulation defects with abruptio placentae, the AC globulin and prothrombin concentrations and blood platelets also may be reduced. A fibrinolytic process may also occur with severe abruptio placentae but plays a minor role in blood incoagulability. The clotting defects are almost never encountered with mild degrees of separation.

If the patient with severe abruptio placentae survives the initial bleeding and does not develop a clotting defect, she may develop anuria caused by disruption of the kidney tubules or by bilateral renal cortical necrosis, the effect of which is almost uniformly fatal.

The less severe types of placental separation usually occur during the latter part of the first stage or in the second stage of labor and may be the result of mechanical separation of a portion of placenta. This can be suspected if the patient develops more pain than she has been experiencing, particularly if the fetal heart tones become a bit irregular, the vaginal bleeding increases, and the labor becomes tumultuous. This type of separation ordinarily does not affect either maternal or infant mortality.

Page and co-workers have divided abruptio placentae into three grades: mildly severe, moderately severe, and severe. With the *mild* forms bleeding is minimal and none may be obvious; the uterus is slightly tender and irritable but not tetanically contracted. The conditions of the mother and infant are good, and the clotting mechanism is undisturbed. With *moderately severe* types bleeding usually is heavier and may be concealed. The uterus is hypersensitive and may be tetanically contracted. The maternal pulse rate is elevated and the infant may be dead. A soft clot forms, but it may disintegrate within an hour. With the *severe* types bleeding often is excessive but may be concealed. The uterus is tender to light pressure and firmly contracted. The mother is in shock and the infant is dead. A clotting defect has developed.

Signs and symptoms. Bleeding associated with pain that varies in severity is characteristic of premature separation of a normally implanted placenta. The pain may come on suddenly and be severe when there is a major separation or be milder and intermittent with a less severe lesion. The blood is usually dark or even clotted because it is retained within the uterus for a period of time before it is discharged into the vagina. This is in contrast to the bright red bleeding in placenta previa, which comes from the placental site just within the cervical opening. If there is a considerable amount of concealed bleeding, the pain will increase in severity as the uterus becomes distended with blood.

Diagnosis. Ordinarily it is not difficult to recognize the severe forms of abruptio placentae, but the milder degrees may be less obvious.

Clinical examination. In most instances the diagnosis can be made by history and clinical examination of the patient.

ABDOMINAL EXAMINATION. The abdominal findings change as the condition progresses in severity, but in general the uterus feels firm and is tender to the touch. At the onset the tenderness often is confined to a small area of the uterine wall, but eventually the gentlest palpation at any point produces pain. If there is a considerable amount of concealed bleeding, the uterus will gradually enlarge as the blood collects within its cavity and infiltrates the muscular wall. At the onset intermittent uterine contractions can usually be palpated, but eventually they may no longer be discernible.

FETAL HEART RATE. The fetal heart tones may be normal if only a small amount of placenta is separated, or they may be completely absent in the more severe forms. Slow and irregular fetal heart tones suggest severe intrauterine anoxia.

VAGINAL EXAMINATION. Vaginal examination should usually be performed as an aid in diagnosis and to determine how delivery will be effected. In contrast to placenta previa, placental tissue will not be felt within the cervical canal, and the presenting part may be deep in the pelvis rather than high, as it is with an abnormally implanted placenta. Vaginal examination should be performed under aseptic conditions.

LABORATORY EXAMINATIONS. The hemoglobin may be reduced, the level depending upon the amount of bleeding. The white blood cell count often is elevated to 20,000 or 30,000, whereas in placenta previa it is more likely to be within the normal range.

A *clotting defect* can be demonstrated by the Lee-White clotting time and by observing the type of clot and its stability. Hodgkinson and Neufeld state that the clot observation test can be used as a rough indication of the fibrinogen concentration. If the blood fails to clot, the fibrinogen concentration is below 60 mg.; a flimsy clot in which lysis completely takes place within 1 hour indicates a concentration between 60 and 120 mg. If the clot is firmer and lysis only partially occurs in 2 hours, the concentration is between 120 and 150 mg. If the concentration is above 150 mg., a firm clot forms and remains intact.

Laboratory methods for measuring fibrinogen levels are more accurate than the clot observation test, particularly because the latter does not become positive until after fibrinogenopenia develops; it does not detect falling concentrations. The chemical method for measuring fibrinogen concentration is the most accurate but takes too long to be of practical value in patient management. The fibrin index test, with which the plasma to be tested is added to thrombin, is rapid, simple, and more informative than the clot observation test and is commercially available. It can be used to guide clinical management.

Differential diagnosis. Abruptio placentae can be confused with placenta previa, but in most instances it is possible to differentiate between them (see below).

PLACENTA PREVIA

1. The bleeding is painless.
2. The blood is bright red.
3. Observed bleeding and signs of shock are comparable.
4. Bleeding is usually slight at the onset.
5. The uterus is soft, not tender, and may be contracting.
6. The fetus can be felt easily, and fetal heart tones usually are present.
7. The placenta may be felt.
8. There is no evidence of toxemia.
9. The urine usually is normal.
10. The blood usually clots normally.

ABRUPTIO PLACENTAE

1. The bleeding is accompanied by pain.
2. The blood usually is dark.
3. Signs of shock may be out of proportion to visible bleeding.
4. The first bleeding usually is profuse.
5. The uterus is firm, tender, and tetanically contracted.
6. The fetus may be difficult to feel, and fetal heart tones may be absent or irregular.
7. The placenta cannot be felt.
8. The patient may have toxemia, but the blood pressure may be low because of excessive bleeding.
9. The urine may contain protein, or the patient may be anuric.
10. A clotting defect may be present.

Treatment. The principles of treatment of abruptio placentae are simple: control the bleeding, replace the lost blood, and empty the uterus. Each patient must be carefully evaluated before a plan for treatment is evolved.

Complete placental separation. Complete placental separation usually occurs before the onset of labor in women with chronic vascular renal disease. The infant often is dead, and the patient is in poor condition from blood loss. The first step in treatment is to improve the general condition by treating shock with oxygen and intravenous fluid, followed as rapidly as possible by large amounts of compatible blood.

As soon as a diagnosis of abruptio placentae is suspected, blood is drawn for *clot observation* and *fibrin index tests*. If the blood fails to clot or if an unstable clot forms and soon disintegrates, hypofibrinogenemia can be diagnosed. From 2 to 6 Gm. of fibrinogen given intravenously will usually correct the defect. Blood must also be administered. It often is necessary to give 3 L. or more of blood to replace that lost from premature placental separation. The clotting tests should be rechecked at least every 2 hours until delivery because hypofibrinogenemia may develop during labor, even though it was not present initially. It may also recur in patients who have received fibrinogen because thromboplastin may continue to enter the circulation from its retroplacental source until the uterus is empty.

Delivery. Even though the cervix is uneffaced, vaginal delivery may be possible. Therefore, after blood transfusions have been administered and the clotting defect corrected, a sterile vaginal examination should be performed *to rupture the membranes.* The reduction in intrauterine pressure and the retraction of the uterine muscle fibers that follow amniotomy may reduce the rate of thromboplastin infusion into the maternal circulation. Dilute oxytocin solution can also be administered intravenously to stimulate uterine contractions. Oxytocin solution must be given with even more than the usual care because the uterus is likely to rupture. This is especially true if it is infiltrated with blood. If labor does not begin within a few hours in spite of amniotomy and stimulation, cesarean section can be performed. Vaginal delivery is more often possible in multiparas than in primigravidas, but one may be surprised by the rapidity with which many primigravidas deliver. If labor has already begun, the membranes should be ruptured to hasten its progress.

Uteroplacental apoplexy is caused by the coagulation defect, and the bleeding into the uterine wall and from serous surfaces should respond to the administration of fibrinogen. Hysterectomy should seldom be necessary to control bleeding.

Incomplete placental separation. Incomplete placental separation usually occurs during labor and is much less severe than the complete one. The only treatment usually necessary is to hasten labor by rupturing the membranes, to administer oxygen to the mother, and to complete the delivery as soon as it can be done safely. If the fetal heart tones remain normal, no particular haste is necessary, but if the infant does show signs of hypoxia, low forceps extraction as soon as it can be accomplished safely usually is advisable. The uterus almost always contracts well, and bleeding is not excessive because clotting defects rarely, if ever, occur with milder types of premature separation.

Infant mortality. The perinatal mortality is at least 50% with abruptio placentae, the main cause of death being anoxia, injury, maternal toxemia, and the complications of prematurity. With the most severe forms the infant loss is 100%.

Maternal mortality. The maternal death rate should be about 1%. It has been suggested that the results with vaginal delivery are better than those with cesarean section, but this is not borne out by the experience in most clinics. Most of the patients with more serious abruptio placentae are delivered by section, whereas those with the less severe forms are delivered vaginally, thus weighting the statistics in favor of vaginal delivery. Those patients who are given liberal blood transfusions and in whom coagulation defects are recognized and corrected are most likely to survive. In many instances more blood must be given than the patient lost. It should be administered early and in large amounts, and for the patient in shock it ordinarily is given under pressure.

Anuria may follow abruptio placentae. This occurs most often in association with the severe lesions occurring in hypertensive patients. The cause of the failure to produce urine may be renal cortical necrosis, in which event treatment appears to be valueless, or may be from lower nephron syndrome, the course of which may be influenced by adequate care. It may be possible to prevent renal complications by prompt recognition and treatment of coagulation defects and by early and adequate blood replacement.

■ Bleeding from marginal sinus

The marginal sinus is a discontinuous duct at the periphery of the placenta through which some of the blood circulating through the intervillous spaces is returned to the maternal circulation. It is continuous with the intervillous spaces, and maternal uterine veins open into it. It is not a blood vessel per se but is formed from the chorionic membrane and the trophoblastic plate. According to Ramsey, blood enters the intervillous spaces in intermittent spurts from 20 to 30 spiral arterioles, which are perpendicular to the uterine wall. The blood, which is forcibly injected, circulates between the branching villi in all directions. Most of it is returned to the maternal circulation through the basal veins, but some is forced laterally into the marginal sinus or marginal lakes and then into the veins.

It is possible that these spaces at the margin of the placenta represent a mechanism by means of which unusual fluctuations in pressure within the intervillous spaces can be controlled. Whenever the pressure increases too much—for instance, when the basal veins are occluded by uterine contractions—the blood is forced laterally into the marginal lakes. If the pressure rise is temporary, as with normal uterine activity, the filling of these areas may suffice to control the situation until the uterus relaxes. If, however, the pressure continues to rise because blood flows into the spaces and cannot leave, the marginal lakes may rupture at one or more points. The escaping blood will lower the pressure within the intervillous spaces, thereby reducing the risk of placental separation. No further bleeding will occur if the pressure relationships return to normal, but if the abnormality persists, bleeding from the defect in the sinus will continue, or if the pressure continues to rise, the entire placenta will separate.

The bleeding associated with rupture of a marginal sinus may be concealed or visible, depending upon the amount of blood escaping, the area from which it comes, and whether the implantation site is in the lower segment or in the upper segment of the uterus. It occurs most often during the last weeks of pregnancy and during labor. At these times the stress on the placental attachment is greatest and the pressure in the intervillous spaces reaches a maximum. The bleeding usually is painless and is similar to that of placenta previa. Profuse hemorrhage is not likely to occur if the placenta is implanted normally.

It is impossible to make a diagnosis of marginal sinus bleeding without inspecting the placenta; therefore a clinical diagnosis can be only a tentative one. The diagnosis is made by finding an opening into the marginal sinus through which an adherent clot protrudes. There may also be a small area of placental separation adjacent to the sinus defect.

In most cases no treatment is necessary because the bleeding is slight, but the site of placental implantation should be determined. With more severe bleeding, treatment is like that for placenta previa.

■ Other causes of bleeding

Cervical lesions. Benign or malignant lesions of the cervix may bleed during late pregnancy, particularly if the cervix is manipulated. The cervix should be inspected as part of the examination of any pregnant woman with bleeding. Tissue should be taken for biopsy from any cervical lesion that bleeds. Lesions other than carcinoma ordinarily need not be treated.

Rupture of a placental vessel. In the rare abnormality of rupture of a placental vessel the blood comes from the fetus; the membranes must be ruptured to permit blood to appear externally. If immature red blood cells are present in the stained smear of blood taken from the vagina, the diagnosis is to be suspected. If the bleeding is profuse, the infant must be delivered promptly. It may be necessary to give the baby a blood transfusion.

Bladder and bowel lesions. The source of the bleeding may not always be obvious to the patient and may come from bladder or bowel lesions. Hemorrhoids often bleed during pregnancy, and occasionally a pregnant woman will bleed from benign or malignant rectal lesions. Bladder hemorrhage can be detected by examining a catheterized specimen of urine.

References

Adams, J. Q., Henry, L. C., and Schreier, P. C.: Management of premature separation of the placenta, Obstet. Gynec. **14:**724, 1959.

Ball, R. P., and Golden, R.: A roentgenologic sign for the detection of placenta previa, Amer. J. Obstet. Gynec. **42:**530, 1941.

Bartholomew, R. A., Colvin, E. D., Grimes, W. H., Jr., Fish, J. S., and Lester, W. M.: Hemorrhage in placenta previa; a new concept of its mechanism, Obstet. Gynec. **1:**41, 1953.

Bishop, P. A.: Radiologic studies of the gravid uterus, New York, 1965, Paul B. Hoeber, Inc., Medical Book Department, Harper & Row, Publishers.

DeValera, E.: Abruptio placentae, Amer. J. Obstet. Gynec. **100:**599, 1968.

Fish, J. S.: Marginal placental rupture, Clin. Obstet. Gynec. **3:**599, 1960.

Green, G. H.: Placenta previa; a review of 242 cases and the principles of management, J. Obstet. Gynaec. Brit. Comm. **66:**640, 1959.

Hibbard, B. M., and Hibbard, E. D.: Aetiological factors in abruptio placentae, Brit. Med. J. **2:**1430, 1963.

Hodgkinson, C. P., and Neufeld, J.: Premature separation of the normally implanted placenta, Clin. Obstet. Gynec. **3:**585, 1960.

Howard, B. K., Goodson, J. H., and Mengert, W. F.: Supine hypotensive syndrome in late pregnancy, Obstet. Gynec. **1:**371, 1953.

Laros, R. K., Thaidigsman, J., and Schulman, H.: Clinical application of placental scanning using RISA, Obstet. Gynec. **26:**388, 1965.

Mengert, W. F., Goodson, J. H., Campbell, R. G., and Haynes, D. M.: Observations on the pathogenesis of premature separation of the normally implanted placenta, Amer. J. Obstet. Gynec. **66:**1104, 1953.

Page, E. W., Fulton, L. D., and Glendenning, M. B.: The cause of the blood coagulation defect following abruptio placentae, Amer. J. Obstet. Gynec. **61:**1116, 1951.

Page, E. W., King, E. B., and Merrill, J. A.: Abruptio placentae; dangers of delay in delivery, Obstet. Gynec. **3:**385, 1954.

Pritchard, J. A., and Brekken, A. L.: Clinical and laboratory studies on severe abruptio placentae, Amer. J. Obstet. Gynec. **97:**681, 1967.

Ramsey, E. M.: Vascular adaptations of the uterus to pregnancy, Ann. N. Y. Acad. Sci. **75:**726, 1959.

Rigby, E.: An essay on the uterine hemorrhage which precedes the delivery of the full-grown fetus, London, 1776.

Streiff, R. R., and Little, A. B.: Folic acid deficiency in pregnancy, New Eng. J. Med. **276:**776, 1967.

Weiner, A. E., Reid, D. E., and Roby, C.: Incoagulable blood in severe premature separation of the placenta; a method of management, Amer. J. Obstet. Gynec. **66:**475, 1953.

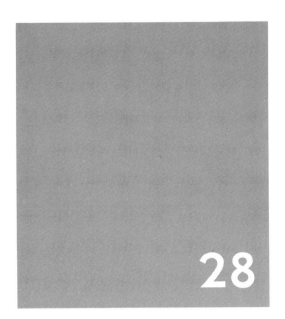

Determination of position and lie

The position of the fetus within the uterine cavity is of no importance during pregnancy, but it must be favorably situated if labor and delivery are to progress normally.

The term *lie* refers to the relationship between the long axis of the mother and the long axis of the infant. In a *transverse lie* the infant's spine crosses that of the mother at a right angle, whereas in a *longitudinal lie* the fetal and maternal spines are parallel. In an *oblique lie* the baby's spine crosses the mother's at an acute angle.

The *presenting part* is the part of the fetus that descends first through the birth canal. It is, therefore, the part that can be palpated through the cervix with the examining finger. *Presentation,* which has been used as a synonym of lie, is now generally used to indicate the intrauterine situation of the fetus somewhat more accurately and simply. For example, the term *face* or *breech presentation* is used to indicate a longitudinal lie in which the face or the breech is the presenting part.

The exact fetal *position* is determined by the relationship of some definite part of the baby (the guiding point) to a fixed area of the maternal pelvis. The guiding point may be directed anteriorly toward the symphysis, posteriorly toward the sacrum, laterally toward the acetabula, obliquely anteriorly toward the area between the symphysis and the acetabula, or obliquely posteriorly toward the area between the sacrum and the acetabula. The possible positions clockwise around the pelvis are therefore direct anterior, left anterior, left transverse, left posterior, direct posterior, right posterior, right transverse, and right anterior.

Attitude refers to the relationship of the parts of the fetus to each other. This ordinarily is one of complete flexion with the chin resting on the chest, the spine flexed in a smooth curve, the arms folded across the chest, and the hips and knees flexed. With the *deflexed attitude* the head is extended and the curve of the spine is reduced.

The position and presentation vary considerably during pregnancy because the fetus can move freely within the amniotic cavity, particularly when there is a relatively large amount of fluid. During the last 8 weeks of pregnancy the fetal mass expands rapidly and the volume of amniotic fluid is relatively decreased. As a consequence the fetus fills the uterine cavity more completely, it can no longer move freely, and its position becomes more stable. Some portion of the head is the presenting part in about 96% of women at term, but this is not true during the earlier

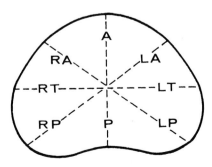

Fig. 28-1. Directions of fetal position in maternal pelvis from below.

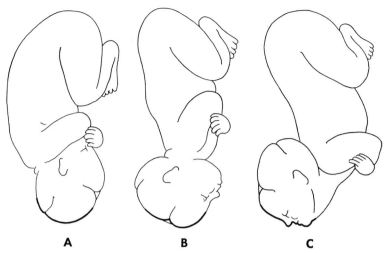

Fig. 28-2. Degrees of deflexion of the head. **A,** Flexed (occiput position). **B,** Partially deflexed (brow position). **C,** Completely deflexed (face position).

weeks. Breech presentation can be diagnosed in over one third of all women at the middle of pregnancy, but the incidence gradually decreases to 3% or 4% at delivery. Transverse lies are encountered in only 0.25% to 0.5% of deliveries at term, but the total incidence at some time during pregnancy is far greater.

Of all the reasons that have been advanced to account for the preponderance of vertex positions, the most logical is that the infant can accommodate itself most comfortably to the shape of the uterine cavity with its head down. The buttocks, thighs, and feet are more bulky than the head and fit better in the comparatively wide uterine fundus than in the lower segment. Further evidence that this is a factor is that in most breech positions the placenta is implanted in the region of one of the uterine horns, thus reducing the amount of room in this portion of the cavity.

■ Methods for determining position and lie

The physician can usually determine position by clinical examination alone, particularly if the pregnancy is well advanced. Until about the thirtieth week, however, diagnosis is less accurate because the fetus is small and there may be a relatively large amount of amniotic fluid. Fortunately, precise diagnosis of position is of little importance before the last 8 weeks because it

changes frequently and because abnormalities in presentation are far less formidable complications of labor at this period than they are later, when the infant is much larger.

Abdominal palpation. A reasonably accurate diagnosis of the position of the infant can be made by abdominal palpation unless the abdominal wall is unusually resistant, the uterus is tender or irritable, or there is an excessive amount of amniotic fluid. Any of these may prevent the physician from outlining the fetal structures.

Abdominal examination should be performed systematically and gently with the physician standing on the right side of the patient as she lies in the dorsal position on the examining table. The examiner first determines which fetal pole occupies the fundus of the uterus. The head is round, firm, smooth, and can be ballotted between the fingers if there is enough fluid, whereas the breech is softer, less regular, more pointed, and not ballottable. The back is located by palpating through the sides of the uterus with the palmar surfaces of the fingers of each hand. The fetal spine presents a smooth convex curve in contrast to the ventral surface, which is concave, soft, and irregular; the motion of the extremities can usually be felt on the side opposite the back.

The fetal pole that lies over the inlet should be felt next to identify the presenting part; it is easier to identify if it has not yet

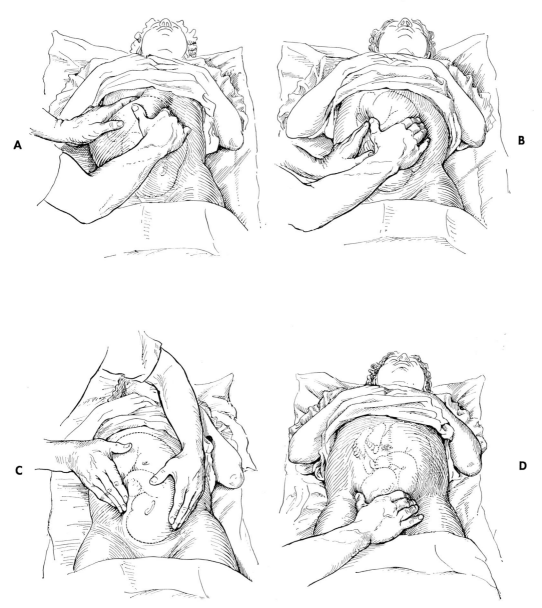

Fig. 28-3. Diagnosis of fetal position. **A,** Palpation of superior pole. **B,** Palpation of fetal back and small parts. **C,** Palpation of cephalic prominence. **D,** Ballottement of presenting part.

entered the pelvic inlet than if it is deeply engaged. If the vertex is presenting, it usually is possible to palpate the *cephalic prominence* which is, as the name implies, the part of the fetal head that is most readily felt. This area, which is opposite the back if the head is flexed and on the same side as the back in deflexed attitudes, can usually be felt without difficulty unless the face is pointed almost directly posteriorly. The position of the cephalic prominence is de-

termined as shown in Fig. 28-3, *C*. The examiner can tell how deeply the head has descended through the inlet by grasping it between the fingers of one or both hands and attempting to move it back and forth or by palpating the anterior shoulder to determine how far it has descended toward the pubis.

Auscultation of the fetal heart is not an accurate method for determining position, although it is usually heard best above the level of the umbilicus with breech positions and in the lower quadrants when the head presents. The heart sounds are transmitted through the area of the fetal chest wall, which lies in contact with the uterine wall,

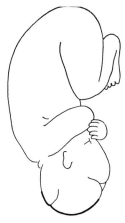

Fig. 28-4. Occiput position. Note smooth curve of flexed spine and head. Cephalic prominence (forehead) is on same side as fetal small parts.

and are usually loudest about one third of the distance from the mother's umbilicus to the anterior superior iliac spine in occiput anterior positions and more laterally in the occiput posterior positions. The heart may be inaudible in obese women or those with hydramnios, or if the infant's position is unfavorable.

Orificial examination. Identification of the presenting part by direct digital palpation will aid in establishing position. For greatest accuracy the cervix must be open enough to permit the insertion of the finger; consequently this method is more often used during labor than earlier in pregnancy. Vaginal examination provides far more accurate information than does rectal examination. The landmarks on the presenting part may be obscured by edema or intact membranes, and if there has been little descent, the physician may be unable to insert the finger deeply enough to reach it.

X-ray examination. Fetal position can be determined accurately by x-ray examination, but this procedure ordinarily is not necessary.

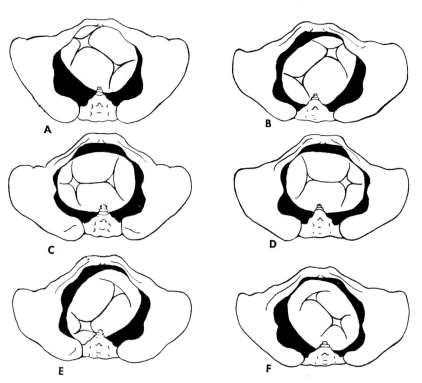

Fig. 28-5. Landmarks on fetal skull in various occiput positions: A, L.O.P.; B, R.O.P.; C, L.O.T.; D, R.O.T.; E, L.O.A.; F, R.O.A. (From Titus, P., and Willson, J. R.: The management of obstetric difficuties, St. Louis, 1955, The C. V. Mosby Co.)

■ Longitudinal lie

In longitudinal lies some portion of the head is almost always the presenting part.

Occiput positions. In the occiput positions, which comprise 95% of all vertex presentations, the fetal head is flexed and its occipital portion becomes the presenting part or guiding point. Upon abdominal examination the breech is felt in the fundus, the back on either the right or left side of the uterus, and the head in the inlet in a flexed attitude, with the cephalic prominence on the side opposite the back. The landmarks on the fetal skull and their relationships to the bony pelvis as they would feel on vaginal examination are illustrated in Fig. 28-5.

The possible occiput positions and their abbreviations are as follows:

Occiput anterior	O.A.
Left occiput anterior	L.O.A.
Left occiput transverse	L.O.T.

Left occiput posterior	L.O.P.
Occiput posterior	O.P.
Right occiput posterior	R.O.P.
Right occiput transverse	R.O.T.
Right occiput anterior	R.O.A.

Of these, approximately 60% are occiput transverse, 15% to 20% are oblique posterior, and the rest direct anterior or posterior positions when labor begins. The position is determined by the shape of the bony pelvic canal. The long anteroposterior axis of the oval fetal skull tends to accommodate itself to the long axis of the pelvic inlet, which is most often the transverse, thus accounting for the predominance of occiput transverse positions. In the direct occiput anterior or posterior positions the anteroposterior axis of the bony pelvis is usually longer than the transverse.

Brow positions. If the head is partially extended, some part of the vertex anterior to the occiput becomes the presenting part.

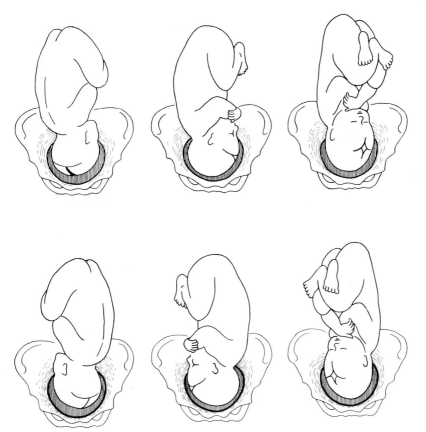

Fig 28-6. Varieties of occiput positions. From left to right, above, right occiput anterior, right occiput transverse, and right occiput posterior. Below, left occiput anterior, left occiput transverse, and left occiput posterior.

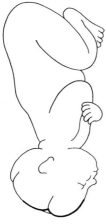

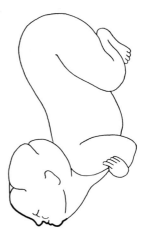

Fig. 28-7   **Fig. 28-8**

Fig. 28-7. Brow position. Note deflexion of head, extension of spine, and cephalic prominence on each side.

Fig. 28-8. Face position. Note extension of spine and complete deflexion of head with cephalic prominence on the same side as the fetal back.

The position is designated as a brow or frontum when the area of the head between the anterior fontanel and the supraorbital ridges descends first through the cervix. The possible brow positions and their abbreviations are as follows:

Frontum anterior	F.A.
Left frontum anterior	L.F.A.
Left frontum transverse	L.F.T.
Left frontum posterior	L.F.P.
Frontum posterior	F.P.
Right frontum posterior	R.F.P.
Right frontum transverse	R.F.T.
Right frontum anterior	R.F.A.

Face positions. If the head is completely deflexed to a point at which its occipital region lies in contact with the infant's back, the face descends through the birth canal first, and the chin (mentum) becomes the presenting part. The possible face positions and their abbreviations are as follows:

Mentum anterior	M.A.
Left mentum anterior	L.M.A.
Left mentum transverse	L.M.T.
Left mentum posterior	L.M.P.
Mentum posterior	M.P.
Right mentum posterior	R.M.P.
Right mentum transverse	R.M.T.
Right mentum anterior	R.M.A.

Breech positions. If the breech or buttocks present at the pelvic inlet, the sacrum becomes the guiding point, and the possible positions and their abbreviations are as follows:

Sacrum anterior	S.A.
Left sacrum anterior	L.S.A.
Left sacrum transverse	L.S.T.
Left sacrum posterior	L.S.P.
Sacrum posterior	S.P.
Right sacrum posterior	R.S.P.
Right sacrum transverse	R.S.T.
Right sacrum anterior	R.S.A.

■ Transverse lie

A transverse lie or shoulder presentation is one in which the long axis of the fetus lies at a right angle to that of the mother. The position is designated according to the quadrant of the pelvis toward which the scapula is directed. The possible positions and their designated abbreviations are as follows:

Left scapula anterior	L.Sc.A.
Left scapula posterior	L.Sc.P.
Right scapula posterior	R.Sc.A.
Right scapula anterior	R.Sc.P.

29

Normal labor and delivery

Labor is the mechanism by which the products of conception are expelled from the uterus and vagina and the beginning regression of the pelvic organs is initiated. This is accomplished almost entirely by the activity of the uterine muscle.

■ Changes preceding the onset of labor

According to Reynolds the growth of the uterus during pregnancy is divided into three phases:

1. A short period of preparation during which the progestational changes necessary for nidation develop.

2. A period of uterine enlargement characterized by hypertrophy of muscular and connective tissue elements, producing a rapid increase in the weight of the uterus. In human beings this phase ends at about the twentieth week.

3. A period of uterine stretching during which the rate of growth, as evidenced by a slower increase in weight, is much less rapid. The progressive enlargement of the cavity to accommodate the rapidly growing fetus is accomplished primarily by longitudinal stretching and thinning of the muscular walls so that the uterus becomes elongated rather than spherical. The uterus also becomes wider as the infant grows, but the lateral expansion is less than the longitudinal.

Gillespie states that until about the twentieth week of pregnancy the human uterus is spherical in shape and its walls are thick. During the last half of pregnancy the wall becomes progressively thinner and the increase in size of the uterus is predominantly due to elongation.

Certain other changes take place in the uterus during pregnancy. These consist of the demarcation of the uterus into two separate divisions: the *upper uterine segment,* which is composed of the active contracting muscle tissue that supplies the force necessary to complete delivery, and the thin, passive *lower uterine segment,* through which the presenting part passes into the pelvic cavity.

According to Danforth and Ivy the lower uterine segment is derived from the isthmus of the uterus—that area of the muscular corpus which is situated just superior to the histologic internal os of the cervix. The muscle tissue of the isthmus is indistinguishable from that of the rest of the body of the uterus in contrast to the fibrous cervix below it. Until about the sixteenth week of pregnancy it is almost impossible to identify the isthmus as a distinct entity, but at about that time the area of the isthmus begins to lengthen or *unfold* as an aid in providing room to accommodate the rapidly growing fetus. The entire fibrous portion of the cervix below the isthmus remains closed.

Uterine muscle fibers have certain characteristics that are essential for normal pregnancy and successful delivery. They must be able gradually to *elongate* to permit the progressive increase in uterine size necessary to accommodate the growing fetus. They must be *elastic* so they can return to their normal length after periods of uterine distention. Since labor and delivery are accomplished by the force generated by uterine muscle activity, they must be able to *contract* and force the products of conception from the uterus. It is evident that unless the uterus remains closely approximated to the fetus as

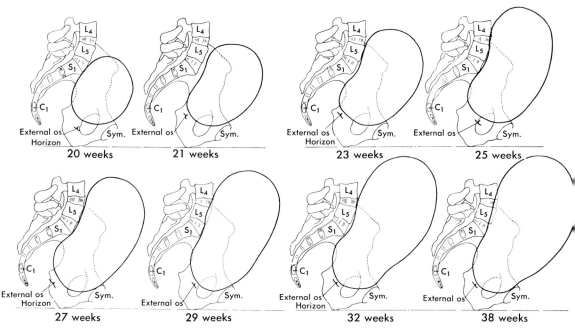

Fig. 29-1. Change in shape of uterus during pregnancy. (From Gillespie, E. C.: Amer. J. Obstet. Gynec. **59:**949, 1950.)

it is gradually expelled from the cavity, the effect of each successive contraction will be diminished. As labor advances and the fetus descends through the birth canal, the uterine cavity does gradually become smaller so that effective force is maintained. This is accomplished by *retraction,* or *brachystasis,* the unique ability of uterine muscle fibers to become progressively shorter and thicker while they retain their power to contract forcibly.

Muscular activity, which is present throughout pregnancy, has been studied extensively by recording the effects of the contractions on amniotic fluid pressure. The *uterine tonus,* the amniotic fluid pressure between contractions, is from 3 to 8 mm. Hg during normal pregnancy. Two types of spontaneous contractions can be identified: small contractions that occur in localized areas of the uterine wall and that increase the pressure by 2 to 4 mm. Hg, and Braxton Hicks contractions, which involve more uterine muscle and which increase pressure by 10 to 15 mm. Hg. Both are painless and only the latter can be felt by the pregnant woman. Braxton Hicks contractions occur irregularly during early pregnancy but become stronger and closer together as pregnancy advances.

Uterine activity increases during the last 8 or 10 weeks of pregnancy. The Braxton Hicks contractions gradually become stronger, and the small contractions can no longer be identified. By the time labor begins the intrauterine pressure during a contraction averages 28 mm. Hg. The increased muscle activity is responsible for the characteristic prelabor changes in the uterine corpus and cervix.

Since the fibers in the active upper segment shorten during each contraction, it is obvious that this portion of the uterine wall must become shorter and thicker during periods of muscle activity. Such a change would reduce the capacity of the uterine cavity unless a compensatory expansion of some other portion occurred during a contraction. This is in fact what happens. As the muscle fibers of the upper active segment shorten during a contraction, the inferior border of this portion of the uterus, which blends into the superior border of the lower segment, is drawn upward, exerting tension on the lower uterine segment. In response the relatively passive fibers in the wall of the lower segment elongate as they are pulled upward because the relatively firm cervix remains closed. The wall of the

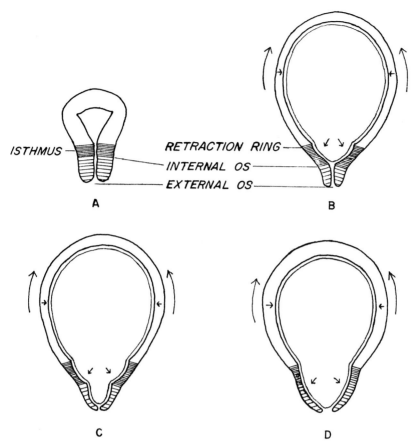

ISTHMUS —
RETRACTION RING —
INTERNAL OS —
EXTERNAL OS —

A

B

C

D

Fig. 29-2. **A,** The isthmus of the uterus occupies the area just superior to the histologic internal os. **B,** The isthmus begins to lengthen and retract, but there is little change in the rest of the cervix. **C,** The histologic internal os is retracted upward, and the cervical canal is shortened. **D,** Effacement is complete.

lower part of the uterus, therefore, becomes thinner during each contraction.

As the muscle of the upper segment relaxes at the end of the contraction, the individual fibers lengthen, the lower border of the upper segment returns almost to its original position, and the lower segment shortens and its wall thickens. Each individual contraction produces no perceptible permanent change, but the upper segment gradually becomes shorter and shorter and its wall thicker and thicker from progressive retraction of individual muscle fibers. As a consequence the lower segment gradually becomes longer and thinner.

The increased length of the lower segment is almost entirely a result of the expansion of the isthmus; the cervix remains closed until the last 2 or 3 weeks, or even the last few days, before labor begins. Eventually, however, the cervix is *effaced,* or *taken up,* by a process similar to that by which the isthmus is lengthened. As the isthmus is stretched by the contraction and retraction of the muscle fibers in the active segment, the internal cervical os begins to open, being gradually pulled upward around the presenting part and incorporated with the isthmus in the lower segment. As a result of the upward traction on the internal os against the resistance of the presenting part of the fetus, the cervix lengthens, becomes thinner, and assumes a funnel shape; as effacement continues and the internal os is pulled higher and higher, the cervical canal becomes shorter and shorter, until finally it is completely obliterated. The completely developed lower uterine segment is about 10 cm. long;

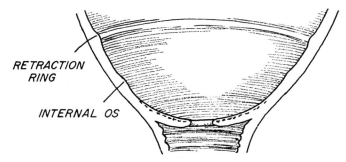

Fig. 29-3. Ripe cervix in primigravida. The retraction ring is at the junction of the isthmus and the active upper segment.

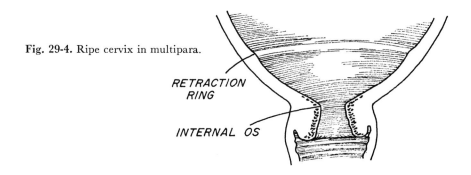

Fig. 29-4. Ripe cervix in multipara.

the thinned-out, elongated isthmus and the effaced cervix each make up approximately one half its length, although the cervical portion may be longer.

In primigravidas the cervix is usually well effaced before the contractions of true labor begin, but preparation of the cervix in multiparas differs slightly. In multiparas the cervix may be incompletely effaced when labor starts. The isthmus of the uterus elongates and the internal os is retracted and opened but less so than before the first labor. The cervical canal is wide and patulous and considerably shortened; it usually is possible to insert two fingers through it without difficulty. In many multiparas, however, the cervical canal is completely obliterated when labor begins. The changes in the cervix can be felt most accurately by vaginal palpation, and the physician should become thoroughly familiar with them because he must be able to recognize the *prepared,* or *ripe, cervix* before he can induce labor safely.

■ Forces in labor

Labor occurs as a result of the force of muscular contractions. The *primary force,* that produced by the involuntary contractions of uterine muscle, is more important than the *secondary force,* that produced by voluntary increase in intra-abdominal pressure. Labor can often be completed by the primary forces alone, but the secondary powers are effective only during the expulsive phase of late labor.

Primary force. Uterine muscle contractions during labor have certain distinctive characteristics. They are involuntary and recur intermittently and rhythmically, and they produce pain. At the onset of labor they may come irregularly and last only a few seconds, but they soon recur at shorter and shorter intervals, last longer, and produce more discomfort. Each uterine contraction is slight at its onset and can be palpated several seconds before the patient is aware of it; it gradually increases in intensity until the uterus becomes hard and cannot be indented with finger pressure. At this time the patient feels pain, which probably is caused by pressure of the presenting part against the cervix and the other structures in the pelvis. After reaching its acme the force of the contraction gradually subsides.

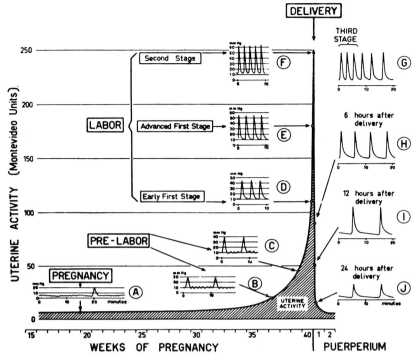

Fig. 29-5. The evolution of spontaneous uterine activity throughout the pregnancy cycle is illustrated by the striped area. Typical (schematic) tracings of uterine contractility at different stages of the cycle are shown. (From Caldeyro-Barcia, R., and Poseiro, J. J.: Ann. N. Y. Acad. Sci. **75:**813, 1959.)

Between contractions the uterus is soft and relaxed.

Caldeyro-Barcia, Alvarez, Reynolds, Hendricks and others have studied the effects of uterine muscle contraction during pregnancy and labor by measuring changes in amniotic fluid pressure or by recording the force of muscle contractions directly by means of recording devices placed at various places on the abdominal wall or within the myometrium. There is, therefore, considerable information concerning uterine muscle activity at various periods of pregnancy.

During the prelabor period Braxton Hicks contractions recur more often and become progressively stronger. They involve more and more uterine muscle as term approaches. Uterine contractions during labor are initiated by one of two *pacemakers* situated in the cornual areas of the fundus. One, usually the right, predominates, and during normal labor each contraction is initiated by a single pacemaker. The contraction is propagated downward from its site of origin

at a speed of about 2 cm./sec.; in about 15 seconds the entire uterus is contracting. The contraction mechanism is so well coordinated that the peak of contraction is reached in all parts of the uterus simultaneously. This means that the systolic phase of the contraction is longest in the region of the pacemaker and that it becomes progressively shorter in areas more distant from the fundus of the uterus. There is more muscle in the fundus than in the lower part of the uterus, hence the intensity of the contraction in this area is approximately twice that in the isthmus.

During early normal labor the contractions recur irregularly, but as labor advances they come at intervals of 2 to 4 minutes. According to Caldeyro-Barcia the intrauterine pressure ranges between 35 and 55 mm. Hg at the peak of a normal contraction. Between contractions the tonus is from 8 to 12 mm. Hg.

The exact duration of each contraction is difficult to determine without using precise recording devices. The uterine wall can be

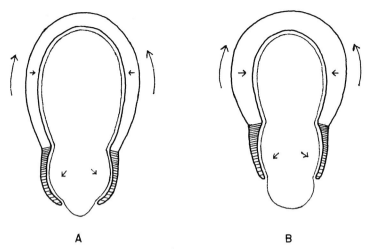

A   B

Fig. 29-6. **A,** The cervix is partially dilated and has not yet retracted around the presenting part. **B,** Cervical dilatation is complete, and the cervix is being pulled upward as the presenting part descends.

felt to contract after an increase in amniotic fluid pressure of about 10 mm. Hg, but the patient will feel no discomfort until the pressure rises at least 15 mm. Hg. The uterine wall can usually be indented until the pressure has increased by 40 mm. Hg, after which it is too firm to depress. After reaching its acme the force of the contraction gradually diminishes and the uterus softens. By clinical observation a normal contraction may last 90 seconds, but the pressure changes may extend over a period as long as 200 seconds.

The ultimate effect of the three principal characteristics of a normal labor contraction—propagation of the wave downward from a fundal source, a prolonged fundal systolic phase, a maximal fundal intensity—is a gradient of force directed from the fundus to the least active and weakest area of the uterus, the cervix. The force generated by each contraction is applied to the amniotic fluid and directly against the pole of the infant that occupies the upper segment. Each time the muscle contracts, therefore, the uterine cavity becomes smaller, and the presenting part of the infant or the forebag of waters lying ahead of it is pushed downward into the cervix. This tends to force it open, or *dilate* it. A more potent factor in cervical dilatation, however, is the retraction of the upper segment. As this area of the uterus becomes shorter and thicker, it pulls

the lower segment and the dilating cervix upward around the presenting part at the same time the uterus contracting directly against the infant tends to push it through the cervical opening. The cervix opens or is dilated by a combination of these two factors, but retraction is probably more important than the pressure of the presenting part, since dilatation will occur even though the presenting part does not descend into it. This can be observed with a transverse lie, with which the cervix may dilate completely even though the presenting part, the shoulder, cannot enter the pelvis. A *completely dilated cervix* that will permit a term infant to pass through it has a diameter of about 10 cm.

The total "uterine work" required to achieve complete cervical dilatation has been measured by Cibils and Hendricks, using an intrauterine recording apparatus during prelabor and throughout the first stage. Uterine work is calculated as the sum of intensities of all uterine contractions until complete dilatation has occurred. "Efficiency" of uterine work can be estimated by comparing the work in mm. Hg to the slope of cervical dilatation. Cibils and Hendricks' important work provides objective measurements demonstrating that in normal labor the driving force of contractions, or efficiency of uterine work, is greater in multiparas than in primigravidas and is significantly improved by rupture of the membranes and by occiput anterior rotation of the fetal head, which provides better mechanical adaptation to the birth canal.

Secondary force. Voluntary forceful contractions of the abdominal muscles with the diaphragm fixed after forced inspiration increases intra-abdominal and thereby intrauterine pressure. The secondary forces have no effect upon cervical dilatation, but they are of considerable importance in aiding the expulsion of the infant from the uterus and vagina after the cervix is open. Contractions of the abdominal muscles become almost involuntary when the patient feels the presenting part pressing on the rectum and distending the perineum. When the pressure sensation is eliminated by analgesic drugs or by anesthesia, the *bearing-down* efforts cease, and the second stage may be prolonged indefinitely if the primary forces are not strong enough to expel the infant.

■ Cause of labor

Why labor begins is not definitely known, but changes in the amniotic fluid, placenta, myometrium, cervix, and pituitary gland all seem to be important. For example, labor usually begins within 72 hours after the membranes rupture and amniotic fluid is released.

The uterus is active throughout pregnancy, but during the last 8 or 10 weeks the contractions increase in frequency and duration and in the immediate prelabor period are quite similar to those of the normal first stage. The effects of estrogen and progesterone on uterine muscle activity have not been clearly defined, but it seems likely that altered concentrations of these hormones are important factors in muscle contraction. The concentration of actomyosin, the contractile protein of muscle, in the uterus at term is about one fourth that of striated muscle, but that of the nonpregnant uterus is only one eighth. That the actomyosin content is in some way related to estrogen stimulation is suggested by these figures and by the fact that the concentration of this protein in uterine muscle of castrates is only one sixteenth that in striated muscle. Furthermore the concentration is increased by estrogen administration. Changes in the estrogen-progesterone ratio alter contractility of the uterus by altering the ratio of potassium to

sodium, thereby increasing or decreasing membrane potential; a contraction occurs as membrane potential decreases.

The progesterone concentration is not equal throughout the uterus. Progesterone is elaborated by the fetoplacental unit and is transmitted to the mother from the fetal circulation through the placenta; as a consequence the concentration in maternal blood in the intervillous spaces is greater than in the peripheral circulation. The concentration of progesterone in subplacental myometrium is greater than in the rest of the uterine muscle, and the sodium-potassium ratio in muscle cells reflect this difference. These findings suggest that progesterone, as well as estrogen, plays an important role in uterine muscle activity. It suggests a reason why the placenta remains attached as the uterus becomes more active. The placenta is rather loosely attached to the decidua and is easily separated at the completion of normal labor by firm contraction of the underlying myometrium. The placenta presumably remains attached during pregnancy because the high concentration of progesterone in this area prevents muscle activity. The muscle in the rest of the uterus, where progesterone concentration is lower, contracts.

According to the progesterone theory, labor begins because of the difference between the amount of area of the subplacental myometrium and that of the rest of the uterus and because of differences in progesterone concentration. The area of uterine wall beneath the placenta remains relatively unchanged, whereas that of the rest of the uterus increases as the fetus grows; thus the ratio between subplacental and extraplacental area changes. If progesterone production decreases, an excess will still accumulate in the subplacental muscle, but the concentration in the periphery will be reduced, permitting uterine activity to increase. At some critical point labor begins.

Although this theory is an intriguing one, much more information must be obtained before it can be accepted. There is no decrease in progesterone production before labor begins, and Taubert and Haskins could not alter the pattern of labor by the infusion of large amounts of progesterone. On the other hand Bengtsson has stopped uterine contractions in women who were aborting and in those with contractions following rupture of the membranes by injecting medroxy-progesterone (Provera) at several points in the uterine wall. Furthermore, patients with missed abortion or intrauterine fetal death may fail to go into labor because placental function continues.

Oxytocin, when properly administered, stimulates physiologic uterine contractions. Labor can usually be initiated at almost any period of pregnancy if oxytocin is given long enough and in the proper dosage. An attractive theory can be constructed to explain the onset of labor based upon the relationship of oxytocin production to that of placental oxytocinase, which destroys it, but unfortunately the roles of these substances in normal labor are so confusing that such a theory can properly be questioned.

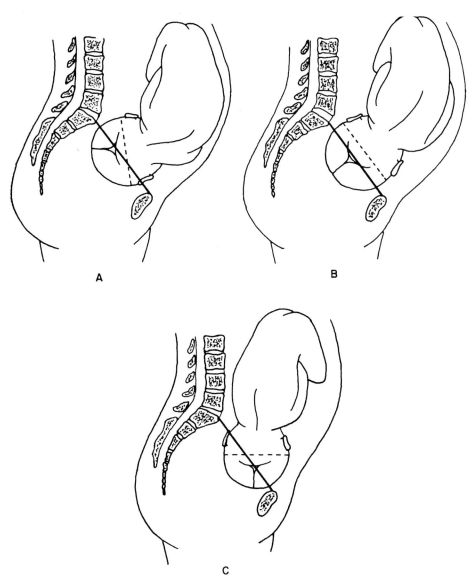

Fig. 29-7. Descent through the inlet. **A,** Anterior parietal bone presentation. The sagittal suture is in the posterior segment of the inlet. **B,** Synclitism. The sagittal suture is equidistant from sacrum and pubis. **C,** Posterior parietal bone presentation. The sagittal suture is in the anterior segment of the inlet.

Manipulation of the cervix may stimulate the onset of labor. Labor will often begin several hours after the membranes have been digitally stripped away from the lower uterine segment or when an operative procedure such as cone biopsy is performed on the cervix. This suggests that neurogenic factors play a part in normal labor. Stretching of the cervix stimulates uterine activity, but it probably is not related to the release of oxytocin from the posterior pituitary.

■ Mechanism of normal labor

The *mechanism of labor* is a term applied to a series of changes in the attitude and position of the fetus that permits it to progress through the irregularly shaped pelvic cavity. A complete understanding of how this is accomplished is fundamental if the physician is to practice intelligent obstetrics and is an absolute necessity for safe operative delivery, since the normal mechanism must be followed as closely as possible. If the physician has a clear understanding of the basic concepts of the mechanism of normal labor for the occiput positions, he can determine what to expect during any labor and what the probable mechanism will be for any position the fetus can assume.

The steps in the mechanism of labor for the occiput positions are *descent, flexion, internal rotation, restitution,* and *external rotation.* These do not occur as separate processes but are combined. For instance, descent through the pelvis, flexion, and internal rotation may all occur more or less simultaneously. The progress of labor is the result of the tendency for each uterine contraction to push the fetus downward through the pelvis and of the resistance of the soft tissue and the bony pelvis to its descent. The infant itself is entirely passive. With each uterine contraction the infant is pushed lower into the pelvic cavity, and its position gradually is altered to accommodate it to the varying shapes of the different parts of the pelvis.

Descent. The presenting part is propelled through the pelvis by the force of the uterine contractions. In occiput positions the longest diameter of the infant's head, the anteroposterior, enters the pelvis in the longest diameter of the inlet, the transverse, in almost every instance. If the sagittal suture is equidistant from the symphysis and the sacral promontory, the head is said to be entering the inlet in a *synclitic* manner. Some degree of *asynclitism* usually is present. If the sagittal suture lies closer to the sacrum than to the pubis and the anterior parietal bone lies over the inlet, an *anterior parietal bone presentation* can be diagnosed. If the sagittal suture lies closer to the pubis and the posterior parietal bone lies over the inlet, it is a *posterior parietal bone presentation.* The latter is usually present at the onset of normal labor.

When labor begins, the area of the infant's head just below the parietal eminence rests upon the sacral promontory, the opposite parietal eminence lies above the superior border of the pubis anteriorly, and the sagit-

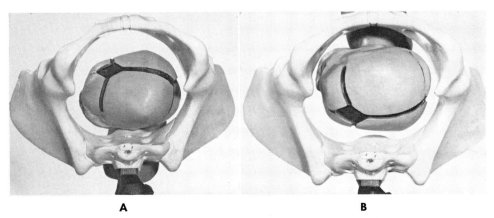

A   **B**

Fig. 29-8. Asynclitism. **A,** Posterior parietal bone presentation. **B,** Anterior parietal bone presentation.

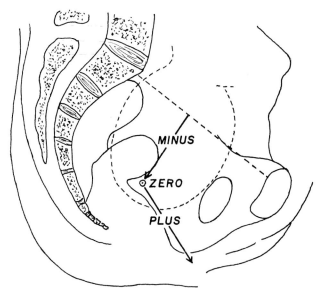

Fig. 29-9. Stations of the birth canal. The presenting part (dotted lines) is just below station zero. The biparietal diameter has passed the plane of the inlet.

tal suture is in the transverse diameter of the inlet, closer to the pubis than to the sacrum. As uterine contractions become more effective, the anterior parietal bone is slowly forced downward behind the pubis. During this process the sagittal suture gradually moves posteriorly as the head assumes a synclitic position in the inlet. The head *descends* through the inlet with its biparietal diameter approximately parallel to the plane of the inlet.

The head is said to be *engaged* after the widest transverse diameter, the biparietal, has passed the plane of the inlet. If the occiput is the presenting part and there is little molding and elongation of the head, engagement occurs when the occiput passes the level of the ischial spines. The fact that the lowest portion of the head is at the level of the spines does not always mean that engagement has occurred. If there has been considerable molding and elongation of the head to permit it to pass an inlet with reduced measurements, the biparietal diameter may still not have entered the true pelvis when the lowest portion reaches the level of the spines. When the head is completely deflexed, as in face positions, the biparietal diameter does not pass the pelvic inlet until the presenting part reaches the pelvic floor.

Descent can be delayed by an incompletely dilated cervix, resistant soft tissues, disproportion between the size of the infant and the pelvic cavity, and weak, ineffective uterine contractions. Descent usually occurs more gradually in primigravidas than in multiparas because the cervix dilates more slowly and the soft-tissue resistance is greater.

The degree of descent is gauged by the *station* of the presenting part, which is its relationship to the plane of the ischial spines. If the presenting part is at the level of the spines, it is at station 0; if 1 cm. above the spines, at station minus 1; if 2 cm. above the spines, at station minus 2, etc. If the lowest level of the presenting part is above station minus 3, it is said to be *floating*. If the presenting part is 1 cm. below the plane of the spines, it is at station plus 1, etc. When the presenting part reaches station plus 3, it usually is resting on the pelvic floor.

Flexion. The head usually lies in the pelvic inlet during late pregnancy in a flexed attitude, but the degree of flexion may increase during descent, particularly if the pelvis is small. The purpose of flexion is to substitute the suboccipitobregmatic diameter of 9.5 cm. for the occipitofrontal diameter, which measures 10.5 to 11 cm. Flexion

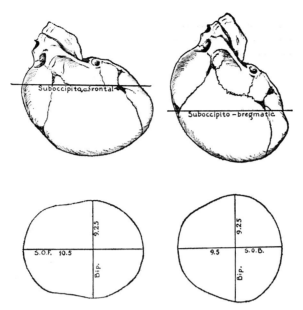

Fig. 29-10. As flexion increases, the anteroposterior diameter of the head, which must pass through the pelvis, becomes shorter. (From Beck, A. C.: Obstetrical practice, Baltimore, 1955, The Williams & Wilkins Co.)

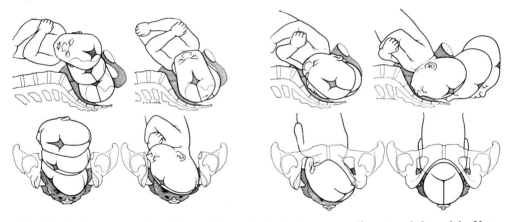

Fig. 29-11. Head enters the inlet and descends in the transverse diameter of the pelvis. Note that the occipital portion of the flexed head descends to the ischial spine before the anterior portion. The occiput then rotates anteriorly to a position beneath the pubic arch, and the head is born as it descends and extends. (From Steele, K. B., and Javert, C. T.: Surg. Gynec. Obstet. **75:**477, 1942.)

occurs because the force applied by the resistance of the bone and soft tissues to the anterior portion of the head is greater than that applied to the posterior portion. If the anteroposterior diameter of the infant's head is considered to be a lever with its fulcrum at the foramen magnum, where the spinal column joins the skull, one can see how this might occur. The anterior arm of the lever is longer than the posterior arm; consequently when equal force is applied to each, the resultant force anteriorly is greater and the head flexes. The smaller the pelvis the greater is the resistance and the more complete is the flexion. The head may flex only slightly if the pelvis is large and the baby is small.

Internal rotation. Rotation of the long

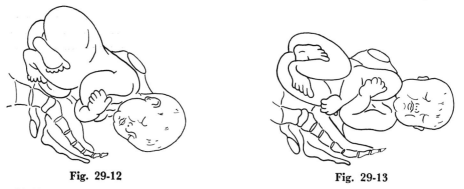

Fig. 29-12   **Fig. 29-13**

Fig. 29-12. Head has restituted to normal relationship with shoulders, which lie in the left oblique diameter.

Fig. 29-13. Anterior shoulder has rotated to position beneath the pubic arch (external rotation of head).

axis of the fetal head from the transverse diameter, in which it descended through the upper pelvis, to the anteroposterior diameter at the outlet is essential. The transverse diameters of the midpelvis and lower pelvis are too short to permit the passage of the unrotated head of a normal-size infant. Rotation begins at the level of the ischial spines but is not completed until the presenting part reaches the lower pelvis.

The bispinous diameter is too short to permit a normal-sized head to pass in the transverse diameter; consequently it is rotated slightly by simple pressure from one of the protruding spines. In an occiput left transverse position, for instance, the occiput descends through the upper pelvis on the left. As flexion increases, the occiput is lower than the frontal portion of the head and will reach the spine first. The spine lies slightly posterior and therefore will contact the posterior portion of the occipital area. Each time the uterus contracts and the head descends slightly, the occiput will be pushed anteriorly a bit more by the pressure of the ischial spine; eventually it will be able to pass the midpelvis.

Rotation is completed because the bony side walls of the lower pelvis slope anteriorly and slightly inward and because the levator ani muscles form a double-inclined plane, the resultant slope of which is anterior. As the flexed head descends, its presenting part, the occipital portion that already has been rotated slightly anteriorly by the spine, strikes the bony pelvis and the levator sling anteriorly and with each uterine contraction

slides further up the muscle plane until it lies in the midline beneath the pubic arch. The head is almost always rotated by the time it begins to distend the pelvic floor. The importance of the levators in anterior rotation is evidenced by the fact that in multiparas in whom the muscular support has been destroyed by previous childbirth injury, the head frequently fails to turn anteriorly.

Extension. The upper half of the pelvic canal is directed posteriorly toward the sacrum and the lower half anteriorly, making the canal a curved rather than a straight tube. The course of descent of the presenting part must therefore change to conform to the pelvic architecture. After the occiput has rotated to an anterior position, the suboccipital area impinges beneath the pubis, and the parietal bossae impinge on the levators and the descending pubic rami, where they remain while the forehead slides up the inclined plane formed by the perineum as the head extends. The forehead, face, and chin progressively emerge from the introitus, and the face then falls posteriorly, freeing the occiput. At this stage of labor the fetal spine is no longer flexed but is extended to conform to the contour of the birth canal.

Restitution. After the head is free from the introitus it rotates 45 degrees to the right or left of the midline to assume its normal relationship to the back and shoulders. If the fetal back is on the left, the occiput rotates in that direction, and if on the right, it rotates to that side.

External rotation. As the shoulders de-

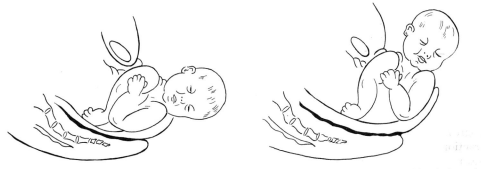

Fig. 29-14. Anterior shoulder remains beneath pubic arch, whereas posterior shoulder is forced anteriorly over the distended perineum.

scend and rotate within the pelvis, the occiput rotates further externally; this external rotation of the head actually indicates a change in position of the body of the fetus. With an occiput left transverse position the shoulders pass the inlet after the head is delivered and descend with the long bisacromial diameter in the left oblique diameter of the pelvis. The anterior shoulder, the right one, meets the levator sling first as descent continues and, like the occiput, is rotated 45 degrees anteriorly to a position beneath the pubic arch. The left shoulder then lies directly over the sacrum in the muscular gutter formed by the two levator muscles. The anterior shoulder remains impinged beneath the pubic arch, and the fetal spine bends laterally as the posterior shoulder is forced up over the perineum. When the posterior shoulder is free, it falls backward, and the opposite one is pushed out from beneath the pubic arch. The body of the infant is delivered without any particular mechanism.

The mechanisms for occiput right and occiput left positions are identical except that in the former the occiput and back descend down the right side of the pelvis and rotate from right to left.

■ Clinical course of labor

Prodromes. Certain symptoms and objective signs precede the onset of labor.

Lightening. In primigravidas the fetal head begins to settle into the upper pelvis from 2 to 3 weeks before labor begins. This coincides with the period of elongation of the lower segment and the progressive effacement of the cervix, which permits the head to descend. In multiparas, develop-

ment of the lower segment and effacement is less complete, and the head usually remains high until early in labor. If lightening fails to occur with the first pregnancy, the physician should consider the possibility of a contraction of the bony pelvis, placenta previa, a pelvic tumor, abnormal fetal position, or anything else that might prevent the head from descending.

As the infant "drops," the pressure on the diaphragm is reduced; consequently the patient breathes more easily, but she experiences more pelvic pressure, frequency of urination, and discomfort as the presenting part presses on the pelvic organs.

False contractions. There may be periods during which the uterine contractions are painful. They usually are irregular and of short duration, but the entire episode sometimes continues for several hours. It can usually be relieved by prescribing a sedative such as Nembutal, 0.2 Gm., or Amytal sodium, 0.4 Gm.

Vaginal discharge. As the cervix effaces and the pressure on it increases, the patient may note more vaginal discharge. Labor often begins a few days after this is observed.

Passage of mucous plug. As the cervix is obliterated, the thick mucus in the canal, the *mucous plug,* and portions of the hypertrophied glands are expelled. This often is blood streaked and is termed the *show.*

Onset and diagnosis of labor. As was noted previously, the contractions of true labor produce discomfort and thus are differentiated from the Braxton Hicks contractions during pregnancy. They occur irregularly at the onset but usually increase until they recur every 2 to 3 minutes and last from 60 to 90 seconds. *The contractions of* *true labor produce progress such as thinning of the cervix, dilatation of the cervical opening, or descent of the presenting part.* Labor begins when the patient first experiences recurring painful uterine contractions, which terminate in delivery.

The principal criterion necessary for the diagnosis and evaluation of labor, therefore, is progress rather than the character of the contractions. In some patients labor progresses rapidly, even though the contractions recur irregularly and feel weak. In others no progress can be detected despite the fact that the contractions are regular, feel forceful, and are painful. This is called *false labor.* The contractions of false labor usually stop after a few hours and can almost always be controlled by the administration of Amytal sodium, 0.4 Gm. False labor can be diagnosed, therefore, if no progress is made and if the contractions cease spontaneously or with medication.

Stages of labor. There are three stages of labor.

First stage. The first stage of labor lasts from its onset until the cervix is completely dilated. The membranes usually rupture during the latter part of the first stage, but they may rupture earlier or remain intact until delivery.

Second stage. The second stage begins when the cervix is completely dilated and ends with the delivery of the baby. Neither the first nor the second stage can be timed accurately unless the patient is examined frequently; during normal labor the exact duration of each of the two stages is not particularly important.

Third stage. The third stage begins when the baby leaves the uterus and ends with the delivery of the placenta.

■ Course and duration of labor

Busby, in a review of almost 15,000 deliveries, calculated the mean duration of labor in white primigravidas to be 13 hours, the median 11 hours, and the mode (the figure that occurs most often) 7 hours. The corresponding figures for white multiparas were 8, 6, and 4 hours. Friedman calculated the mean duration in primigravidas to be 14.4 hours and in multiparas, about 7.8 hours.

Calkins states that the second stage is concluded with no more than 20 uterine contractions in primigravidas and 10 or less in multiparas. This corresponds well with a median duration of 50 minutes for primigravidas and 20 minutes for multiparas reported by Hellman and Prystowsky.

Friedman made a major contribution to our understanding of labor by dividing the

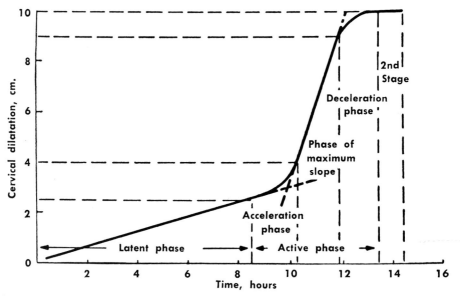

Fig. 29-15. Phases of labor in a primigravida. (From Friedman, E. A.: Obstet. Gynec. 6:567, 1955.)

first stage into a *latent* and an *active phase*. According to him the latent phase in primigravidas, during which the cervix is effaced and dilated to 2 cm., lasts about 8 hours. He subdivided the active phase into an *acceleration phase* of about 2 hours, a phase of *maximum slope* during which the cervix reaches 9 cm. dilatation, and a *deceleration phase* of slightly more than 1 hour during which dilatation is completed. We have used this method extensively in the management of both normal and abnormal labors; the duration of the two major phases in our patients correlates remarkably closely to those calculated by Friedman.

Schulman and Ledger, reporting on 1,500 patients, found effacement to be the principal change in the cervix during the latent phase; there was little increase in dilatation. They calculated the mean duration of the latent phase to be 7.26 hours in primigravidas and 4.14 hours in multiparas. Labors extending beyond the limits of two standard deviations of these means were considered as abnormal. By these criteria the maximum length of the normal latent phase is 17 hours in primigravidas and 11.5 hours in multiparas. They were unable to identify either acceleration or deceleration periods during the active phase, which began at 4 cm. dilatation, and calculated the mean maximum duration of the active phase to be 8.7 hours for primigravidas and 5.4 hours for multiparas. They suggest that active-phase progress can be accurately described in terms of *slope* of the curve (centimeters of dilatation per hour). They consider progress to be abnormal if cervical dilatation progresses at a rate less than 0.7 cm./hr. in primigravidas and less than 1.1 cm./hr. in multiparas.

The duration of labor in any given individual is determined by her parity, the size and position of the baby, the capacity of the pelvis, the consistency of the cervix, the efficiency of the uterine mechanism, and the patient's attitude toward pregnancy and womanhood.

■ Preparation for labor

During the prenatal period the physician should make every effort to eliminate misapprehensions and fears and to instill confidence into his patients. The primigravida, who has not yet experienced labor, is certain to be apprehensive, particularly if she has acquired a considerable amount of misinformation from her friends and relatives. As the weeks go by, much can be learned about the patient's attitudes by simple questions, and many of her fears can be allayed. Most women are concerned about the length of labor, pain, type of anesthetic, etc., and so usually it is helpful to discuss the procedures that will be carried out when she enters the hospital, who will examine her, and the like. It also is helpful to have her taken on a tour of the maternity division some time during the pregnancy. Many hospitals and community organizations conduct classes in which pregnancy, labor, delivery, and care of the infant are discussed with groups of husbands and wives.

Instructions to the patient. Some time during the last month the patient must be instructed as to how to recognize the onset of labor and what to do when the contractions begin.

When to enter the hospital. The normal primigravida should usually enter the hospital when the contractions are recurring regularly at about 5-minute intervals, but multiparas must come in earlier because so many have rapid labors.

Rupture of membranes. If the membranes rupture, the patient should be examined because the cord may have prolapsed or some other abnormality may be present.

Bleeding. Any vaginal bleeding, no matter how slight, should be reported.

Food. The gastric emptying time is prolonged during labor, and food may be vomited and aspirated during delivery. Patients should be warned against ingesting either solid food or liquids after the contractions begin or the membranes rupture.

■ Admittance to hospital

Most women should be delivered in a hospital rather than at home because in hospitals, particularly those with well-organized obstetric departments, there are trained personnel to care for the patients and facilities to cope with emergencies. The maternity division should be separated from the rest of the hospital, and its nursing staff should have no assignments other than those related to obstetric patients and their newly born infants. The delivery rooms should not be used for surgical procedures other than cesarean section or the treatment of uninfected abortion. Laboratory facilities for the rapid determination of hemoglobin or hematocrit levels and for urine examination are necessary. There should be a reliable source of anesthesia, and at least two bottles of Rh-negative type O blood should be available in the delivery room at all times.

Each patient should be seen by a physician as soon as she arrives at the hospital. Her prenatal record should be available for review. A brief interval history is recorded and a physical examination is made. The fetal position and presentation, the location, rate, and regularity of the fetal heart tones, the height of the fundus, and the frequency and duration of the uterine contractions are determined by *abdominal palpation and auscultation*. Unless there is bleeding, a *vaginal examination* is next made to confirm fetal position and to determine the amount of cervical dilatation and the station. The *blood pressure* is recorded, a *urine specimen* is examined, and a *hemoglobin* or *hematocrit* determination is made.

If the patient actually is in labor, orders are written to *shave the perineum*; it is not necessary to remove pubic hair. In the past an *enema* was administered routinely to women entering the hospital in labor, but one need not be given if the rectum is empty. If it is filled with fecal material, an enema will empty it and the colon, thereby helping to prevent contamination from the expulsion of feces as the presenting part descends and exerts pressure on the rectum. The enema is avoided in multiparas who enter late in the first stage of labor, in primigravidas in the second stage, or whenever the presenting part is deep in the pelvis. Under these conditions an enema is difficult to administer, and it may not be expelled until the patient is delivering. *An enema should never be administered to a patient who is bleeding until serious lesions such as placenta previa or abruptio placentae are eliminated as causes.* Patients who are in early labor may be given a *shower*.

■ Care during labor

Patients in labor, even though they are multiparas, are usually apprehensive and uncomfortable, and every effort must be made to allay fear and to make the entire experience as rewarding as possible. The attendants must refrain from laughing, joking, and loud conversation near the labor rooms because these are all annoying to the patients. The discussion of other patients and particularly of obstetric problems must be strictly avoided if there is any chance that the conversation can be overheard.

Private labor rooms are preferable, and they should be pleasant, comfortable, and dimly but adequately lighted. Minimum equipment should include a blood pressure manometer, a stethoscope, and sterilized gloves and lubricant for examinations. The bed should have crib sides that can be elevated after sedatives have been administered. A physician or an experienced labor nurse should remain with the patient at all times. The husband may also remain in the room if he and the patient so desire, but he cannot substitute for a professional attendant.

Observations during labor. The following observations will indicate the condition of the mother and her infant and the progress of labor.

Fetal heart. The fetal heart sounds are an index of the condition of the fetus and should be counted and recorded at least every 30 minutes during the first stage and at 5-minute intervals during the second stage of normal labor. They are checked during or immediately after a contraction as well as in the interval between contractions because changes caused by interference with fetal oxygenation are usually heard first during the period of uterine activity. It is not until hypoxia is well advanced that changes can be heard while the uterus is relaxed. The normal rate is from 120 to 160 beats per minute, and the rate slows at least 10 beats during a uterine contraction. A fall of more than 20 beats or a rate of less than 100 beats per minute suggests the possibility of hypoxia, the investigation and treatment of which are discussed in Chapter 32.

The fetal heart tones should be counted during several contractions after the membranes rupture because the cord may be washed through the cervix with the gush of fluid.

Blood pressure. The blood pressure is recorded at 30-minute intervals because it may rise to alarming levels during labor.

Contractions. The length, duration, and

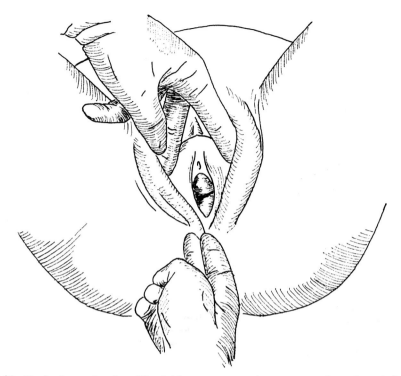

Fig. 29-16. Vaginal examination. The labia are separated to prevent them from being rolled into the vagina as the fingers are inserted.

intensity of uterine contractions, and the interval between them are recorded at 30-minute intervals. The length is determined by palpation rather than by the patient's statements because she cannot feel the contraction until several seconds after it has begun and the discomfort disappears before the uterus is relaxed. Intensity is estimated by the firmness with which the muscle contracts.

Examinations. The progress of labor is determined by various examinations.

Abdominal examination. Abdominal examinations are performed to evaluate the uterine contractions and to follow the descent of the presenting part into the pelvis. As descent occurs, the cephalic prominence and the shoulder, which can be palpated above the pubis, move downward. When the head is deep in the pelvis, the cephalic prominence can no longer be felt and the shoulder lies just above the pubis.

Perineal palpation. The presenting part can be palpated through the perineum after it has reached the pelvic floor. A bit later perineal bulging and crowning can be observed.

Vaginal examination. The progress of cervical dilatation and of descent can be determined by vaginal palpation. Since it is inevitable that bacteria are carried on the fingertips from the introitus and the vagina to the interior of the uterus, it is essential that vaginal examinations be performed properly and that they be limited in number. As a general rule no more than three or four are necessary during a normal primigravid labor; one is given when the patient is admitted, one when it appears that she may need sedation, and one or two more as labor advances.

Examinations made simply to determine position, station, and cervical dilatation can be performed in the labor bed with the patient in dorsal position. The examiner wears sterile gloves, and a hexachlorophene solution is used to cleanse the vulva and act as a lubricant. The labia are separated with the fingers of one hand, and the hexachlorophene-covered index and second fingers of the other are inserted into the vagina, palpating the fetal head and the cervical rim. If more information must be obtained, for example, if there is a question of cephalopelvic disproportion or of placenta previa, or if an abnormal presentation is suspected, the examination must be performed with the patient in lithotomy position because it is impossible to assess such situations accurately with the patient in bed.

It is essential that the physicians' examinations and the nurses' observations and treatment be recorded accurately in the labor record. The progress of labor is best appreciated if cervical dilatation, descent, and position are plotted on a labor graph. Labor is assumed to have begun when the patient first became aware of painful uterine contractions, even though they occurred irregularly for several hours. The results of the first and subsequent examinations are recorded on the labor graph at an appropriate hour of labor as determined by the time it began. On such a graph, deviations from the normal are obvious and can be appreciated much earlier than they are by other recording methods.

General care. General nursing care during labor is directed toward making the patient as comfortable as possible and protecting her from infection and injury.

Position. Patients in early labor may be out of bed if they wish, but they usually are more comfortable lying down when labor is advanced. Most are more comfortable on their sides than on their backs, and in fact the latter position may be potentially dangerous in that it is a possible cause for the supine hypotensive syndrome and placental separation. Those who have been sedated should be confined to bed.

Food. The gastric emptying time is delayed during normal labor, and the administration of analgesic and sedative drugs decreases it even more. The oral ingestion of fluids and food should be avoided during labor. Glucose solution can be administered intravenously if labor is prolonged.

Bladder. As the lower segment lengthens and the cervix is retracted, the bladder is pulled upward. This and the pressure from the descending presenting part may make spontaneous voiding impossible. The distended bladder can be seen and felt as a fluctuant mass in the lower abdomen. If the patient cannot void during labor, she should be catheterized at intervals.

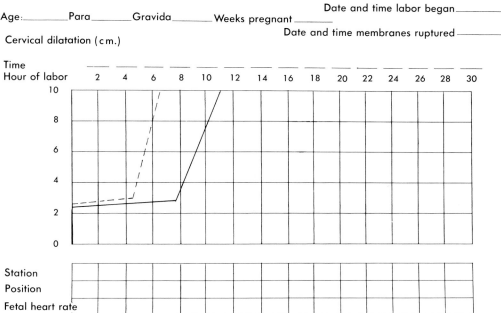

Labor record

Age:_____ Para_____ Gravida_____ Weeks pregnant_____

Date and time labor began_____

Cervical dilatation (cm.)

Date and time membranes ruptured_____

Fig. 29-17. Graphic labor record. The dotted line represents the average curve for multiparas; the solid line represents the average curve for primigravidas.

Transfer to delivery room. Patients should be taken to the delivery room in their beds in time to prepare them properly for delivery and to administer anesthesia. Primigravidas are moved when the presenting part begins to distend the perineum, and multiparas when they are 8 to 9 cm. dilated. As the presenting part descends deep into the pelvis and begins to exert pressure on the pelvic floor, the patient will feel as though she needs to evacuate her rectum and will ask for a bedpan. Soon after this she will begin to hold her breath, tense her abdominal muscles, and strain or *bear down* in an attempt to expel the baby each time the uterus contracts. As this occurs, the relatively high-pitched cry at the time of the contraction changes to a sustained grunt, which can be recognized as indicating the second stage whenever it is heard. Bearing down during the first stage serves no useful purpose and should not be permitted because it will only tire the patient. The bloody vaginal discharge usually increases as cervical dilatation is completed, and the pressure of the presenting part may force small amounts of fecal material from the rectum.

■ Normal delivery

Everyone in the delivery room should wear a cap and a face mask that covers both the nose and the mouth, and those participating directly in the delivery should wear sterile surgical gowns and gloves. Others wear clean surgical dresses or suits and no one is admitted in his street clothes.

When the patient is ready to deliver, she is placed in lithotomy position with her legs in suitable stirrups and her buttocks hanging slightly over the foot of the table. The stirrups should be padded to prevent pressure on the peroneal nerve. Certain multiparas, particularly those in whom there is no need for episiotomy, can be delivered in the dorsal position without stirrups. In this position there is less stretch on the perineum and it is less likely to tear. Episiotomy and forceps delivery cannot easily be performed in this position, and in general, lithotomy is to be preferred. The vulva and anus, the upper portions of the thighs, and the skin over the pubis and lower abdomen are cleaned with soap and water or a hexachlorophene solution, wiping from anterior to posterior and discarding the cotton sponge after each stroke. No attempt is made to cleanse the

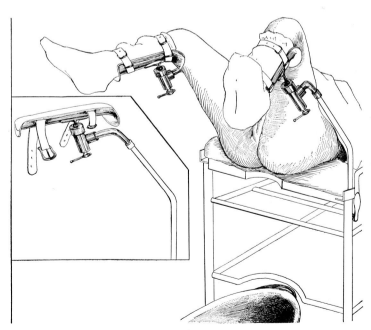

Fig. 29-18. Position on delivery table. (From Titus, P.: Atlas of obstetric technic, St. Louis, 1949, The C. V. Mosby Co.)

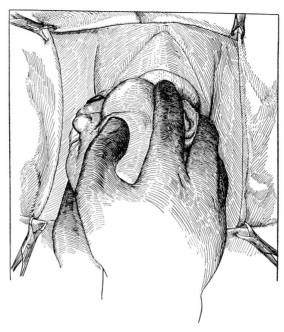

Fig. 29-19. Downward traction on the head to bring the anterior shoulder beneath the pubic arch. The brachial plexus can be injured by too much traction. (From Titus, P.: Atlas of obstetric technic, St. Louis, 1949, The C. V. Mosby Co.)

vagina; the constant discharge of amniotic fluid serves to keep it as clean as possible. Sterile leggings are placed over the feet and legs, and the abdomen is covered with a sterile sheet. In many hospitals a sterile sheet is also placed posteriorly covering the anus, but this is usually promptly saturated with blood and amniotic fluid and contaminated by fecal material expressed from the rectum. It is seldom necessary to catheterize the patient because the bladder has been pulled up entirely out of the pelvis.

Episiotomy, when necessary, is performed after the perineum has been well flattened out by the crowning head, and it should be deep enough to sever the fascia covering the lower surface of the levator muscles. With each contraction the head will extend and more of the scalp will be visible through the dilated introitus. Delivery of the head can be controlled by *Ritgen's maneuver,* with which upward pressure is applied through a sterile towel with the thumb and forefinger of the pronated right hand, or the first and second fingers with the hand supinated, first to the supraorbital ridges and later to the chin through the distended perineal body. The upward pressure, which increases ex-

tension and prevents the head from slipping back between contractions, is counteracted by downward pressure on the occiput with the fingertips of the other hand; this tends to prevent extension. With this maneuver the delivery of the head can be readily controlled, and its rapid expulsion, which causes perineal tearing, can be prevented. As soon as the head is delivered, the physician feels for a loop of cord around the neck. If a long, loose loop is present, it can be slipped over the head; a shorter, tighter one can be slipped over the advancing shoulder. If there are several tight loops, it may be impossible to slip them either way, in which event the cord is doubly clamped, cut, and unwound.

After the head is delivered the anterior shoulder descends and rotates to a position beneath the pubic arch. At this point the shoulder is said to be *impinged* beneath the pubis, but actually it can be considered to be delivered since it and the upper humerus are visible. Impingement of the anterior shoulder can be aided by downward traction on the head; little force should be applied to accomplish this because the brachial plexus may be stretched and injured by the maneuvers. After the shoulder is visible the physi-

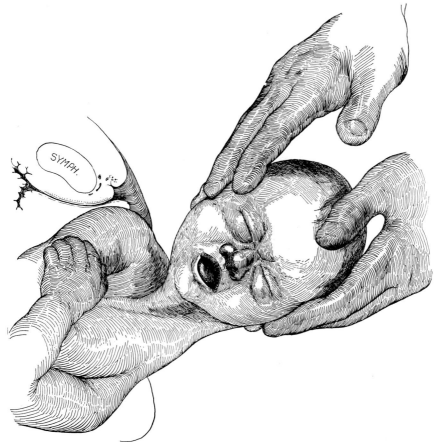

Fig. 29-20. Upward traction on head to deliver posterior shoulder over the perineum. (From Titus, P.: Atlas of obstetric technic, St. Louis, 1949, The C. V. Mosby Co.)

cian waits for about 30 seconds to permit the muscle fibers in the fundus to retract and reduce the size of the uterine cavity, from which part of the baby has been delivered. The head is then elevated toward the ceiling, and downward traction is applied simultaneously to deliver the posterior shoulder over the perineum. After another 30 seconds' wait the remainder of the body is slowly extracted by traction on the shoulders.

The baby is held with its head downward for a few seconds while the cord is stripped from the introitus toward the infant several times. This adds 75 ml. or more of blood, which would otherwise be discarded with the placenta, to the infant's vascular system. Two clamps are then placed on the cord, and it is cut between them. The infant is placed in a heated crib with its head slightly

lower than its body. The head-down position should not be too deep, nor should the infant be held upside down for any period of time because the pressure of the abdominal viscera against the diaphragm interfers with normal respiratory efforts.

■ **Premature labor and delivery**

The term *premature delivery* indicates the termination of pregnancy before the end of the thirty-sixth week. In the past a premature or a term delivery was based upon the birth weight of the infant. If the baby weighed less than 2,500 grams (the average for Caucasian infants at the end of the thirty-sixth completed week), a diagnosis of prematurity was made automatically. The term *low birth weight infant* (LOWBI) is preferable because many infants weighing less than 2,500 grams actually are not pre-

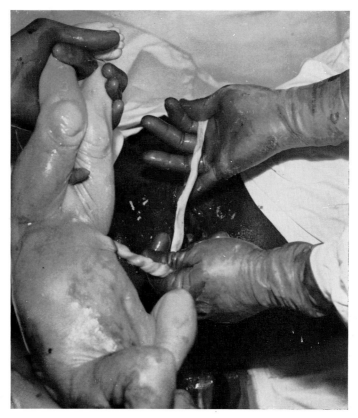

Fig. 29-21. Stripping the umbilical cord.

mature by date; their low weight is due to some other factor. By the same token the fact that an infant weighs more than 2,500 grams at birth is no guarantee of maturity. The babies of mothers with diabetes are excellent examples; some may weigh 3,500 to 4,000 grams at 35 or 36 weeks, but their development is comparable to that of babies of similar gestational age.

About 7% of all pregnancies terminate in the delivery of low birth weight infants; this occurs in from 3% to 5% of private and in about 15% of clinic patients. Low weight infants are born more often to black than to white women.

The significance of the delivery of low birth weight infants is discussed in Chapter 1.

Etiology. The causes of premature labor are not completely understood, but it may occur in women with placenta previa, abruptio placentae, multiple pregnancy, and hypertensive cardiovascular disease. It may be necessary to induce labor prematurely in the treatment of these as well as other conditions, notably preeclampsia. The membranes often rupture prematurely, after which labor begins; in some this may be caused by an old cervical laceration that permits early effacement, but in others the cervix is long, closed, and relatively firm. In such instances an abnormality in the membranes or infection from the cervix, which may weaken them, may be a responsible factor. The infants of women who smoke excessively weigh less at birth than the babies of nonsmokers, but they are normally developed. Low birth weight infants are born more often to women at extremes of the reproductive years, the young teenager, and those over 35 years than to those between the ages of 18 to 30 years. The part played by anemia, malnutrition, infection, general poor health, and inadequate medical supervision, all so characteristic of women of the lowest socioeconomic levels who have the highest rates of low birth weight delivery, has not been completely assessed.

Management. It is not always possible to prevent premature labor, but with complications such as mild hypertension, minor degrees of placenta previa, and similar problems, delivery often can be delayed until the infant has a good chance of surviving independently.

Sedative and analgesic drugs should be administered in small amounts because they enter the fetal circulation and depress cerebral function; if the infant is born during the period of depression, it may be unable to establish its vital functions. Morphine and meperidine often are given in an attempt to stop premature labor, but they have little effect on uterine contractions. Isoxsuprine, an epinephrine-like compound, will diminish uterine contractions temporarily or abolish them completely and has been used in an attempt to halt premature labor. When given during the early latent phase, it may prevent labor from progressing, but it rarely stops active labor. Isoxsuprine may depress maternal blood pressure and increase the pulse rate. It may also be possible to stop uterine contractions with alcohol. Fuchs and co-workers administered 9.5% alcohol in 5% dextrose in water intravenously to women 21 to 36 weeks pregnant who were having regular contractions. Uterine activity was inhibited in all; delivery was postponed in two thirds of those with intact membranes but in none whose membranes had ruptured. Further investigation of these and other substances known to alter uterine muscle contraction is necessary.

Caudal or epidural anesthesia, if available, is excellent for the control of pain during premature labor because they have no effect on the fetus; they can be continued during delivery. Paracervical and pudendal block anesthesia also can be used during labor and delivery, or saddle block can be given during the terminal part of the first stage. If inhalation anesthesia must be used, it should be administered with the highest possible oxygen concentration. Postpartum fetal apnea occurs much more frequently with a combination of a narcotic or barbiturate during labor and inhalation anesthesia for delivery than if pain is controlled with regional block.

The brain structures of premature infants are easily injured and should be protected during labor and delivery. The membranes should not be ruptured artificially if labor is progressing normally. Deep episiotomy should be performed when the presenting part begins to distend the perineum. It may be difficult to deliver the head in breech position because it is relatively larger than the body and may not be able to pass through a cervical opening that permitted passage of the body and shoulders without difficulty.

■ **Prolonged pregnancy**

Sometimes pregnancy is prolonged for several weeks past the due date, during which time the fetus may die. This is most often observed in primigravidas, and according to some authorities it is a more frequent cause of perinatal mortality with the first pregnancy than is prematurity. Browne reported that 12.4% of 15,116 pregnancies terminated after 41 weeks, and 3.5% after 42 weeks. After excluding those women with toxemia and antepartum hemorrhage the perinatal mortality at 40 to 41 weeks was 11 per 1,000; at 43 weeks it had doubled, and at 44 weeks it had trebled. The incidence of fetal distress doubled at 42 weeks in those without toxemia and at 41 weeks in those with toxemia. In some other studies no such increase in mortality was observed. The number of children with serious congenital anomalies, particularly those involving the central nervous system, is greater with prolonged than with normal-length pregnancies.

After the forty-second week of pregnancy the amount of amniotic fluid decreases and vernix disappears; in the affected infants the skin appears dry and cracked. Meconium, passed because of hypoxia, stains the placental surface, the umbilical cord, and the remaining vernix yellow green. In more advanced cases the fingernails and toenails of the infant are also stained. The babies weigh less than the usual term infant and appear to have lost weight. Studies on fetal blood oxygen levels in presumably postmature infants are contradictory and confusing.

The cause of the abnormality in the infant is chronic hypoxia from placental dysfunction. The placenta can maintain the requirements of the infant only until it reaches a certain size, which is determined by the amount of functioning chorionic tissue. If the placenta is small or a portion of it has been destroyed, as occurs with chronic hypertensive disease, the baby will be smaller than usual; it often dies in utero before term and shows the same changes as the so-called "postmature" infant. *Placental deficiency syndrome* is therefore a better term than postmaturity. Greene and Touchstone and others have studied estriol excretion during normal and abnormal pregnancy. Since estriol is produced by the fetus and the placenta and since there is a progressive increase in estriol production during the second and third trimesters of normal pregnancy, a consistently low level or a fall may indicate placental insufficiency. Repeated determinations are necessary to assess function.

Because of the danger to the infants in pregnancies that have gone beyond the calculated due date, induction of labor or even cesarean section has been advised at the forty-second week. These recommendations should not be accepted without reservation; in most instances of presumed post-term pregnancy the baby is normal, and the due date probably was miscalculated. This is particularly true in multiparas. If the cervix is ripe and labor has not begun by the forty-second week, the physician may consider inducing labor if there is no question as to the accuracy of the menstrual history and if there are no contraindications to induction. Cesarean section should be considered only under unusual circumstances—for instance, in a primigravida whose pregnancy is unquestionably prolonged and for whom there is x-ray evidence of fetal maturity, and then only if labor cannot easily be induced.

■ Pregnancy and labor in young primigravidas

Labor usually is normal in girls less than 16 years of age, and vaginal delivery can almost always be anticipated. The incidences of certain complications such as preeclampsia and prematurity are increased, partly because of inadequate supervision. Venereal disease is common.

Semmens, studying 12,847 pregnancies in teenagers, reported preeclampsia in 5.9% (17.7% in those under 15 years) and premature labor in 9.5%. In 30% labor terminated in less than 3 hours, but it was prolonged in about 8%. Only 1.4% were

delivered by cesarean section. Israel and Deutschberger found the highest incidence of prematurity to be in black women under age 16 years (23.7%), but the rates in girls of all races under age 20 years were increased.

■ Pregnancy and labor in elderly primigravidas

A woman more than 35 years of age and pregnant for the first time is called an "elderly primigravida." Almost all will deliver without difficulty, but cesarean section is necessary more often than in younger patients. A greater percentage of women of this age will have dysfunctional labor on an emotional basis either because psychologic problems prevented their marrying earlier or because a long period of infertility had a psychogenic basis. The indications for cesarean section may be liberalized slightly because these women are approaching the end of their childbearing careers, but abdominal delivery should not be performed unless there is a logical reason. The incidence of essential hypertension, preeclampsia-eclampsia, heart disease, uterine fibroids, and other conditions that appear during the fourth decade is higher than in younger women. Perinatal mortality is increased two or three times. The incidence of congenital anomalies is higher than in other age groups except the very youngest.

■ Labor in multiparas

Physicians tend to direct less attention toward multiparous women, particularly those who have had several children. This attitude cannot be justified because both maternal and perinatal mortality are increased. Disproportion, prolonged and obstructed labor, ruptured uterus, and fetal death may occur because babies tend to become progressively larger with each succeeding pregnancy and the uterine mechanism becomes less effective. The impaired uterine mechanism also is responsible for a high incidence of postpartum hemorrhage. Hypertension and degenerative vascular disease are more common in multiparas because they are often in the older age groups.

■ Precipitate labor and delivery

Precipitate labors, those lasting less than 3 hours, occur in only about 10% of all deliveries and are encountered more often in multiparas than in primigravidas. The baby may be injured during rapid, uncontrolled labor.

Patients who have delivered rapidly in previous pregnancies should enter the hospital at once if the membranes rupture or when contractions begin. Elective induction is indicated for those who live some distance from the hospital.

The physician should remain with the patient during her labor so that he will be available to conduct the delivery. It usually is wise to move her to the delivery room when she is about half dilated. If labor progresses so rapidly that it seems unlikely that she can be moved, it is safer to deliver her in bed than to risk the trip to the delivery room. Under no circumstances should the head be restrained forcibly or an anesthetic administered in an attempt to prevent delivery.

■ Induction of labor

Labor may be induced artificially by mechanical stimulation or by the administration of oxytocic drugs. In some patients, particularly those with conditions that might be aggravated by continuing pregnancy, induction serves an important purpose, but it is seldom necessary if pregnancy is normal.

Selection of patients. It is difficult to induce labor safely unless it is about to begin spontaneously. Many of the complications associated with induction occur because it is attempted in women who actually are not yet ready to start. In most instances the condition of the cervix is the best indication of whether attempted induction is likely to be successful. If the cervix is firm, uneffaced, and occupies a position in the posterior part of the vagina, attempts to induce labor are hazardous, and if immediate delivery is necessary, cesarean section should be considered. On the other hand, it usually is possible to initiate labor when the cervix is soft, effaced, partially dilated, and situated in the middle of the vagina.

Indications for induction. Most indicated inductions are performed for preeclampsia-eclampsia or chronic hypertension, bleeding complications, and premature rupture of membranes.

Preeclampsia-eclampsia or chronic hypertension. If advance in the severity of pre-eclampsia-eclampsia or chronic hypertension cannot be controlled by medical treatment, delivery is necessary. Most patients can be delivered vaginally after labor has been induced.

Bleeding complications. It may become necessary to deliver women with placenta previa or abruptio placentae to control bleeding. If this can be accomplished safely from below, it often is preferable to cesarean section.

Premature rupture of the membranes. Labor usually begins promptly after the membranes rupture if the patient is near term. If pregnancy is less advanced, there may be a long latent period between rupture of the membranes and the onset of contractions. During this time pathogenic bacteria may invade the uterus and placenta and infect the baby. An attempt should be made to induce labor within a few hours after the membranes rupture if contractions do not begin spontaneously. Cesarean section may be justified if the estimated weight of the baby is at least 2,000 grams and if effective labor cannot be induced and delivery cannot be anticipated within 24 hours after the membranes rupture. Cesarean section is seldom necessary if the baby weighs more than 2,500 grams. The difference in management is determined by the fact that the death rate from infection in small babies after prolonged rupture of the membrane is very high; this is not true at term.

Elective induction. The elective induction of labor is becoming more and more popular, but there is little information to indicate that it decreases either perinatal or maternal mortality. In fact, when it is carelessly performed, both may be increased. Elective induction may be justifiable in multiparas whose previous labors have been rapid and who live some distance from the hospital. It is rarely to be considered during the first pregnancy. If there is any question as to the duration of pregnancy, every effort should be made to make sure the baby is mature, even though the cervix is favorable, before induction is attempted.

Erythroblastosis fetalis. Under certain circumstances Rh sensitivity may constitute an indication for inducing labor. Early induction is quite justifiable in women whose infants have been severely affected at birth or who have died in utero during the last few weeks of pregnancy. Spectrophotometric examination of amniotic fluid will be helpful in assessing the severity of the disease and in indicating the need for early delivery.

Other indications. In patients with *recurrent pyelonephritis, diabetes mellitus, prediabetes,* or *repeated intrauterine fetal death,* early induction may be warranted.

Technique for induction. Labor can be induced by *artificial rupture of the membranes,* by the infusion of 1:1,000 *oxytocin solution* intravenously, or by a combination of both. If the head is well engaged and the cervix soft, effaced, and partially dilated, the membranes may be ruptured and labor will usually begin promptly. If the presenting part is high, the cord can prolapse when the membranes are ruptured; therefore, under such circumstances or if the breech presents, it usually is preferable to administer oxytocin, leaving the membranes intact. Oxytocin can also be used if labor has not begun within 6 hours after amniotomy has been performed.

Oxytocin must be administered with great caution, since the physician cannot determine in advance how responsive the uterus will be. An excessive dose may produce tumultuous contractions, which may injure the baby or even rupture the uterus. An intravenous infusion of 5% dextrose is started, and the needle is secured in the vein. The needle from a second 1 L. bottle of 5% dextrose to which 1 ml. (10 units) of oxytocin has been added is connected through an infusion pump to the tubing of the first intravenous infusion set. The flow from the bottle of plain 5% dextrose solution is adjusted to about 10 drops per minute, just enough to maintain a constant flow.

The dosage of oxytocin is calculated in milliunits (mU.). If 1 ml. of oxytocin (10 I.U. or 10,000 mU.) is added to 1,000 ml. of 5% dextrose, each milliliter of the resultant solution contains 10 mU. of oxytocin. The dosage necessary to stimulate contractions varies, but it may be as low as 0.5 mU./min.; consequently the constant infusion pump is set to deliver this dosage. If the uterus fails to respond within 20 or 30 minutes, the dosage can be increased to 1 mU./min. The dosage is gradually increased at regular intervals until the contractions are similar to those of normal labor, recurring at intervals

of 2 to 3 minutes and lasting 60 to 90 seconds.

It is important that someone remain with the patient during an induction, recording the duration of each contraction and checking the fetal heart rate and the patient's pulse and blood pressure frequently. If the contractions become tetanic, recur too frequently, or last too long, the infusion rate must be reduced.

As a general rule the uterus responds promptly and labor terminates rapidly. It often is wise to stop the infusion after an hour or two to see if labor will continue spontaneously. If effective contractions continue, there is no further need for the oxytocin.

The total dosage of oxytocin in any uninterrupted period should be limited. Large dosages of oxytocin administered in electrolyte-free fluids over long periods of time should be avoided because oxytocin may have an antidiuretic effect. This combination may produce edema or even water intoxication and convulsions.

References

Abramowicz, M., and Kass, E. H.: Pathogenesis and prognosis of prematurity, New Eng. J. Med. **275:**878, 1966.

Bengtsson, L. G.: Some aspects of the endocrine control of labor, Proceedings of Symposium, Advances in Oxytocin, New York, 1965, Pergamon Press.

Browne, J. C. McC.: Postmaturity, J.A.M.A. **186:**1047, 1963.

Busby, T.: The duration of labor: mean, median, and mode, Amer. J. Obstet. Gynec. **55:**846, 1948.

Caldeyro-Barcia, R., and Poseiro, J. J.: Greenhill's Obstetrics, Philadelphia, 1965, W. B. Saunders Co.

Caldwell, W. E., Moloy, H. C., and D'Esopo, D. A.: A roentgenologic study of the mechanism of engagement of the fetal head, Amer. J. Obstet. Gynec. **28:**824, 1934.

Caldwell, W. E., Moloy, H. C., and Swenson, P. C.: The use of the roentgen ray in obstetrics. III. The mechanism of labor, Amer. J. Roentgen. **47:**719, 1939.

Calkins, L. A.: The second stage of labor; the descent phase, Amer. J. Obstet. Gynec. **48:**798, 1944.

Cibils, L. A., and Hendricks, C. H.: Normal labor in vertex presentation, Amer. J. Obstet. Gynec. **91:**385, 1965.

Danforth, D. N., Graham, R. J., and Ivy, A. C.: Functional anatomy of labor as revealed by frozen sagittal sections in Macacus rhesus monkeys, Surg. Gynec. Obstet. **74:**188, 1942.

Danforth, D. N., and Ivy, A. C.: The lower uterine segment; its derivation and physiologic behavior, Amer. J. Obstet. Gynec. **57**:188, 1942.

Friedman, E. A.: Primigravid labor; a graphico-statistical analysis, Obstet. Gynec. **6**:567, 1955.

Friedman, E. A.: Labor in multiparas, Obstet. Gynec. **8**:691, 1956.

Fuchs, F., Fuchs, A. R., Poblete, V. F., and Risk, A.: Effect of alcohol on threatened premature labor, Amer. J. Obstet. Gynec. **99**:627, 1967.

Gillespie, E. C.: Principles of uterine growth in pregnancy, Amer. J. Obstet. Gynec. **59**:949, 1950.

Greene, J. W., Jr., and Touchstone, J. C.: Urinary estriol as an index of placental function; a study of 279 cases, Amer. J. Obstet. Gynec. **85**: 1, 1963.

Hellman, L. M., and Prystowsky, H.: The duration of the second stage of labor, Amer. J. Obstet. Gynec. **63**:1223, 1952.

Israel, S. L., and Deutschberger, J.: Relation of mother's age to obstetric performance, Obstet. Gynec. **24**:411, 1964.

Llauro, J.: Runnebaum, B., and Zander, J.: Pro-gesterone in human peripheral blood before, during and after labor, Amer. J. Obstet. Gynec. **101**:867, 1968.

Rydberg, E.: The mechanism of labor, Springfield, Ill., 1954, Charles C Thomas, Publisher.

Schneider, J.: Low birth weight infants, Amer. J. Obstet. Gynec. **31**:283, 1968.

Schulman, H., and Ledger, W. J.: Practical applications of the graphic portrayal of labor, Obstet. Gynec. **23**:442, 1964.

Semmens, J. P.: Implications of teen-age pregnancy, Obstet. Gynec. **26**:77, 1965.

Steele, K. B., and Javert, C. T.: Mechanism of labor for transverse positions of the vertex, Surg. Gynec. Obstet. **75**:477, 1942.

Taubert, H. D., and Haskins, A. L.: Intravenous infusion of progesterone in human females; blood levels obtained and effect on labor, Obstet. Gynec. **22**:405, 1963.

Woodbury, R. A., Hamilton, W. F., and Torpin, R.: The relationship between abdominal, uterine, and arterial pressure during labor, Amer. J. Physiol. **121**:640, 1938.

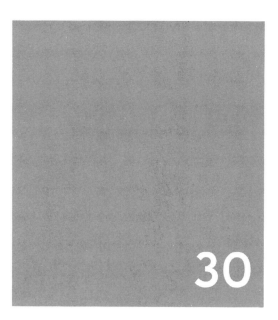

30

Obstetric analgesia and anesthesia

In 1847 the Scottish obstetrician James Y. Simpson reported to the Edinburgh Medical-Chirurgical Society that he had been able to abolish pain of delivery with chloroform and thereby initiated a new era in obstetrics. Strangely enough, among those most bitterly opposed to the use of anesthesia were some of the members of the clergy. They argued that according to the Bible women were meant to bring forth their children in "sorrow" as they had for thousands of years. Simpson countered with the point that anesthesia must be acceptable to God because He himself had put Adam to sleep to remove the rib from which Eve was created. Despite the controversy, chloroform was readily accepted by women in labor who were not particularly impressed by the theoretical arguments of the clergymen. The opposition was substantially reduced by Queen Victoria's acceptance of

chloroform for the delivery of her eighth child in 1853.

Since that time many other drugs have been given to make labor and delivery less painful, but unfortunately all have disadvantages that limit their usefulness. The "perfect" agent must provide relief from pain while it neither interferes with the progress of labor nor adds to the maternal or fetal risk. Such an agent has not yet been discovered.

The subject of pain relief as it is related to natural or normal childbirth is not always clearly understood. A few rabid proponents of so-called "natural" childbirth believe that because labor is a physiologic process it should be painless and that discomfort is an abnormal result of civilization. They believe that the need for sedation during labor and anesthesia for delivery can be eliminated by proper prenatal conditioning. They also state that the use of sedation increases infant morbidity and may even contribute to the development of subsequent emotional disturbance in both the mother and her child. Our concept of normal childbirth is not that it necessarily be painless but rather that labor proceed normally and that it terminate within a reasonable period of time in the birth of a healthy infant. This does not preclude the use of analgesics during labor, anesthesia for delivery, episiotomy, or even forceps extraction. All of these, when used intelligently, make labor and delivery safer for both mother and child.

■ Control of pain during labor

Most of the drugs given to control pain during labor pass through the placenta and affect the infant. This is not particularly important while the infant is within the uterus as long as the exchange of respiratory gases across the placenta continues at the usual rate. At birth, however, the situation changes. The infant must now breathe for itself, and if enough of the drugs given to the mother have crossed to the infant, its respiratory center may be considerably depressed.

It is seldom possible to eliminate pain during labor without compromising the fetus unless some form of conduction anesthesia is used. Systemic analgesics should usually be used in an attempt to reduce the discomfort to a tolerable level and to relax the patient enough to permit her to rest or even sleep during the pain-free interval between contractions. This can be accomplished without increasing the risk for the infant.

The need for pain relief during labor is in a large measure determined by the attitude toward pregnancy, delivery, and motherhood in general. Those who are most emotionally secure in their feminine roles and who approach delivery with a maximum of understanding and a minimum of apprehension usually require the least medication. A normal woman can achieve this state with the help of an understanding obstetrician who is willing to devote time and thought to individual prenatal supervision and instruction. The results of a similar program in women who are emotionally less well oriented toward pregnancy and motherhood often are unsatisfactory.

Women who have attended predelivery educational courses, such as those in which the Lamaze and similar methods are taught, can often go through labor and even delivery with a minimum of discomfort. In many instances the labor progresses more rapidly than is anticipated. It is essential that the physician understand that his principal role is supportive and that there is no need to interfere as long as labor is progressing normally and the mother is reasonably comfortable. It is equally essential, however, that the patient and the physician reach an understanding of the goals before labor begins. The physician must never force the patient to take an analgesic drug or anesthesia, nor must she feel that she cannot have one simply because she has chosen to try one of the psychoprophylactic methods. On the other hand, they must agree that should the labor not progress normally, the physician automatically has the prerogative of ordering whatever medication is necessary for the procedure required to correct the abnormality. The understanding, participation, and support of the physician, the nursing staff, and the husband are essential factors in a successful outcome.

There are many methods for providing analgesia during labor, no one of which is suitable for every individual. There can be no "routine" method because some women neither want nor need medication, and in others it may be contraindicated. Each dose should be ordered individually after the physician has satisfied himself that it will benefit the patient.

Since no single method can be applied to all women, it is necessary that the physician be familiar with more than one type. The techniques, however, must be ones that are safe in his particular environment. Certain methods that are permissible in large, well-staffed maternity hospitals may be too dangerous to use in smaller institutions or at home.

PRECAUTIONS

Never give an analgesic before labor is well established. Most women do not need as analgesic preparation during early labor when the contractions are relatively far apart and of short duration. At this stage an ataractic drug will usually relax her enough to permit her to rest or even sleep until labor is better established.

An analgesic should usually first be given to a *primigravida* when the contractions are recurring regularly at 3- to 4-minute intervals and the cervix is 3 to 5 cm. dilated. In *multiparas* it may be given somewhat earlier because labor progresses so rapidly.

Never give an analgesic too late. If medication is given too late in labor, the infant may be born during the period of its maximum effect and as a consequence may be depressed. In general, sedation should not be administered within 2 hours of delivery; this is much easier to gauge in primigravidas than in multiparas.

Give an analgesic only if the patient can be observed constantly. Medicated patients may be hyperactive and irrational and may injure themselves if left alone.

Be familiar with the physiologic effects of the preparations used. The physician must be reasonably certain that a drug will provide pain relief without being harmful.

SYSTEMIC ANALGESIA

If enough morphine, Demerol, or some similar substance is given to relieve pain completely, the infant's respiratory center may be so depressed that it will be unable to initiate respiration after delivery. Pain can be controlled with relatively small and safe dosages of narcotics, however, if they are combined with other drugs. In the past a combination of *morphine and scopolamine* was used extensviely. Scopolamine is a cerebral depressant that produces amnesia, thereby abolishing the memory of pain and even of the entire labor. It also causes excitement and hyperactivity, particularly when painful stimuli must be applied after its administration. It is now used infrequently during labor but may be given preoperatively to inhibit bronchial secretions.

Barbituric acid derivatives have no analgesic properties and therefore are not particularly important in programs for pain relief during labor. They exert a more profound depressant effect on the fetal respiratory center than do the narcotics, and they may produce considerable excitement in certain individuals. They are most helpful during preliminary or early labor because they will relax the patient and often permit her to sleep until the contractions become stronger. The pains of false labor often will stop after a barbiturate is given. For these purposes Amytal sodium, 0.2 to 0.4 Gm., or sodium pentobarbital, 0.2 to 0.4 Gm., can be given by mouth, by intramuscular injection, or by rectum.

Phenothiazine compounds relax the patient and are at least as effective as the barbiturates in inducing sleep, both during early labor and between contractions when they become more severe. The main danger is from hypotension, which is likely to occur if some of the drug is inadvertently injected intravenously or if too large a dose is given. Fifty milligrams of Sparine or Phenergan injected intramuscularly during early labor may suffice; it can be repeated, however, at 6-hour intervals if the patient becomes restless. Phenothiazine preparations have little analgesic effect themselves; consequently they are usually given with a narcotic. It is important to reduce the dosage of the narcotic to one half or less of the usual amount.

Drugs used to provide systemic analgesia should usually be injected intramuscularly or subcutaneously because gastric motility and emptying time are considerably reduced during labor, thus making absorption of oral medications uncertain. It is seldom necessary to inject these drugs intravenously.

Demerol (meperidine). Demerol relieves pain almost as well as morphine and in addition has an antispasmodic action, thought to be caused by depression of the parasympathetic nerve endings and of smooth muscle directly. It does not alter the course of labor significantly. It does cross the placenta, and if too much is given or if it is administered too late in labor, the infant may be depressed.

A combination of Sparine or Phenergan, 50 mg., and Demerol, 50 mg., provides excellent analgesia and relaxation without untoward effect on the infant. The patient often sleeps between contractions but can easily be aroused. Subsequent doses of Demerol when necessary vary between 25 and 50 mg. A second injection of the phenothiazine can be given in 4 to 6 hours if the patient is restless or uncomfortable.

Morphine sulfate. Morphine is an excellent analgesic for use during labor and exerts no peculiar untoward effect on the infant when it is administered in reasonable doses. It can be combined with a phenothiazine derivative quite effectively and is no more dangerous than meperidine. The initial intramuscular dosage of morphine sulfate is 6 to 10 mg., given with 50 mg. of Sparine or Phenergan. This can be repeated once or twice if necessary.

Complications from systemic analgesics. The most important complication accompanying the use of systemic analgesics is depression of the infant's respiratory center and subsequent apnea neonatorum, which is particularly likely to occur if general anesthesia is also administered. This can be prevented by using small doses of the drugs and by attempting to time the last injection to precede delivery by at least 2 hours. If the infant is narcotized by Demerol, morphine, or similar substances, the effect of the drugs can be neutralized by injecting Nalline (*N*-allyl-normorphine), 0.1 to 0.2 mg., into the umbilical vein. This drug must be used with caution since it is antagonistic only to morphinelike drugs. It increases the depression produced by barbiturates and inhalation anesthetics.

Oversedation may reduce the efficiency of the uterine contractions, particularly when sedation is given too early, and may prolong labor somewhat. The heavily medicated patient cannot cooperate during the second stage, thus the number of required operative deliveries is increased by excessive sedation.

INHALATION ANALGESIA

Almost all the volatile anesthetic agents have been used to relieve pain during labor, but none is entirely satisfactory. The most effective ones are nitrous oxide–oxygen mixtures or trichloroethylene (Trilene). These are usually administered intermittently during each contraction; between contractions the patient is allowed to breathe air or oxygen. It takes several seconds for the agent to pass through the lungs to the bloodstream and then to the brain. To achieve adequate pain relief the patient must start inhaling the anesthetic before she is aware that a contraction has begun. The anesthetist keeps his hand on the abdomen, and when he feels the first evidence of uterine activity, which is before the patient is aware of it, he asks her to start inhaling the gas. As the force of the contraction begins to wane, the mask can be removed. This method is most valuable at the end of the first stage in multiparas and during the second stage in both multiparas and primigravidas. The gas can be inhaled intermittently for some time without interfering with uterine contractions or compromising the infant, unless too high a concentration is used. The low concentration and intermittent use limits the accumulation of the agent in the maternal blood. When delivery becomes imminent, the agent can be administered continuously to provide anesthesia during the birth of the baby.

Nitrous oxide–oxygen. Nitrous oxide (75% to 80%) and oxygen (25% to 20%) when given intermittently will usually control pain well. If the concentration of oxygen is reduced below 20%, the infant may become hypoxic. A mixture of 50% of each gas provides an abundance of oxygen and does reduce pain.

Trichloroethylene (Trilene). Trichloroethylene, a volatile blue liquid with an odor similar to that of chloroform, may stimulate respiratory activity, but in the usual concentrations it does not alter the pulse rate or blood pressure. Its primary effect is to relieve pain rather than to produce unconsciousness, as a true anesthetic does.

It can be given intermittently during labor with an anesthetic machine or by means of a small hand inhaler attached to the patient's wrist, permitting her to regulate the amount she takes. Trichloroethylene

is of particular value when labor is progressing so rapidly that systemic analgesics cannot be used safely, but it is most effective when it is started relatively early, before delivery is imminent.

Trilene must not be used with soda lime because it breaks down to form phosgene in the presence of alkali. Pituitrin and vasopressors should not be given to patients receiving Trilene.

REGIONAL ANALGESIA

The transmission of pain impulses can be controlled by nerve block. With this type of analgesia the mother is awake and comfortable and the baby cannot be depressed. Most nerve block techniques require an experienced individual to administer the anesthetic

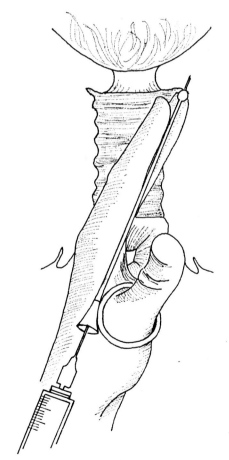

Fig. 30-1. Paracervical block. The needle is introduced through the guide until it penetrates the vaginal mucosa. The anesthetic agent is injected at 4 and at 8 o'clock.

and supervise the patient during the rest of her labor and delivery, and as a consequence some of these forms of analgesia are usually available only in large institutions. These techniques are accompanied by a high mortality if they are used carelessly.

Paracervical (uterosacral) block. The pain during the first stage of labor, which arises from the dilating cervix, can usually be controlled by blocking the sensory and autonomic nerves that supply the cervix. To accomplish this an anesthetic agent is injected at about the junction of the uterosacral ligaments, through which the nerve fibers pass, and the cervix. The block usually is administered when painful contractions are recurring regularly and the cervix is dilated 5 to 6 cm. in primigravidas and slightly earlier in multiparas.

A hollow metal guide, such as an Iowa trumpet, is inserted along the fingers into the vagina until its tip rests against the lateral fornix at about 4 o'clock. A 6-inch, 20-guage needle is passed through the guide until its point punctures the vaginal mucosa. The tip of the needle is inserted to a depth of about 0.5 cm. and, after aspiration to make certain that it has not punctured a blood vessel, 10 ml. of 1% Xylocaine is injected into the tissue. The procedure is repeated on the opposite side at 8 o'clock. It is important that the anesthetic agent be injected relatively superficially.

This technique provides prompt and effective pain relief in at least 75% of patients. The duration of action varies, but it often lasts an hour or two; the injection can be repeated if pain recurs and the patient is not yet ready for delivery.

In some patients uterine contractions stop for a short period of time after the injection, but when the contractions begin again, labor progresses normally. Fetal bradycardia, which has been observed frequently, is probably caused by absorption of the anesthetic agent into the fetal circulation. If the concentration of the drug in fetal tissues is high enough, the infant may be depressed at birth or even die. Paracervical block probably should not be used if there is any suggestion of placental insufficiency.

This technique is particularly effective for pain control in multiparas, but it also is suitable for many primigravidas. It does not anesthetize the lower vagina or the perineal structures; consequently pudendal block or local infiltration is necessary for delivery.

Caudal analgesia. The injection of an anesthetic drug through the caudal canal into the extradural space will control pain by blocking the transmission of painful stimuli along the sacral and coccygeal nerves without interfering with the muscular activity of the uterus. Control of the voluntary muscles in the legs is maintained, but the pelvic muscles are relaxed, making delivery easier for both the mother and her infant. Because caudal analgesia does not alter oxygenation it is particularly valuable during premature labor and in women with heart disease, diabetes, and pulmonary lesions.

A special needle is inserted through the sacral hiatus, and the anesthetic agent is injected when labor is well established and progressing normally and when the patient is uncomfortable. If the needle is secured in place or is replaced by a polyethylene catheter, subsequent injections can be made as needed to keep the patient comfortable until the baby is delivered. The technique is not difficult to master, and when it is used properly, the results are excellent.

Caudal analgesia should never be attempted unless an experienced individual can supervise the insertion of the needle and the injection of the anesthetic agent throughout the entire labor.

In about 25% of all women anomalies of the sacrum interfere with the insertion of the needle. Caudal analgesia is contraindicated if there is any skin infection near the proposed puncture site, if the patient has any sort of nervous or spinal disease, or if she is bleeding severely or is in shock. It is far more suitable for the delivery of primigravidas than of multiparas, particularly those who have had rapid easy labors in the past.

The complications, many of which are potentially lethal, can be kept at a minimum by strict observance of the necessary precautions. The most serious complications include *massive spinal anesthesia* from inadvertently injecting the agent into the subarachnoid space, *meningitis, epidural abscess, intravenous injection,* and *break of the needle or catheter.* In 1947 Hingson and colleagues found 43 maternal deaths in 200,-000 patients in whom caudal anesthetics were used, as reported in the literature.

They have personally supervised the administration of caudal anesthetics in 12,015 patients for delivery with 2 deaths: 1 from a peridural infection and 1 in a patient with acute leukemia. Evans, Morley, and Helder reported on the use of caudal anesthesia for control of pain during labor and delivery in 9,822 patients and for predelivery analgesia in an additional 920 patients. High levels of anesthesia were observed in 6 women, in 1 of whom respiration was arrested. The systolic blood pressure fell more than 35 mm. Hg in 1,238. One patient with diabetes mellitus, hypertension, intracapsular glomerulosclerosis, and bacteremia died.

Epidural analgesia. Epidural analgesia is similar to caudal analgesia except that the needle is inserted into the extradural space between two lumbar vertebrae rather than through the caudal canal. The same precautions are necessary.

■ Anesthesia for delivery

Relief of pain during the actual delivery of the infant plays an important part in modern obstetrics. It permits us to utilize methods for delivery that decrease maternal soft-tissue damage and, if properly used, it does not increase fetal mortality or morbidity. Pain relief is not worth an increase in maternal or fetal mortality, but such an increase is not necessary if the physician will select the anesthetic most suitable for each individual patient and will provide for its safe administration.

INHALATION ANESTHESIA

Many apprehensive women demand inhalation anesthesia to obliterate all consciousness of what is happening during delivery. Although this can be accomplished with relative safety by the proper selection and administration of the agent, there are certain hazards that accompany the use of inhalation anesthesia. *Vomiting* and *aspiration* are serious complications. Merrill and Hingson estimate that at least 100 maternal deaths from aspiration of vomitus occur each year. Patients should be cautioned against eating after the contractions begin, and nothing is allowed by mouth during labor. Regional anesthesia should be used for women who have eaten recently, or if this is not available, the stomach should be emptied. White has described the use of apomorphine to induce vomiting before an inhalation anesthetic is administered. A solution containing 6.5 mg. of apomorphine hydrochloride in 10 ml. of saline solution is slowly injected intravenously until the patient becomes nauseated and vomits; the nausea disappears promptly. The average emetic dose is 3.9 mg. Unfortunately, this does not always empty the stomach completely. Prolonged deep anesthesia may *interfere with uterine contractions,* thereby increasing the incidence of operative delivery and of bleeding during the third stage. Since the inhalation anesthetic agents cross the placenta, the infant may be anesthetized and *apneic at birth* if deep anesthesia has been induced. This need not occur during normal delivery, but prolonged anesthesia is a distinct hazard when the uterus must be relaxed with inhalation anesthesia to permit version and extraction or breech extraction.

Inhalation anesthesia should usually be avoided in women with acute and chronic respiratory disorders, those with severe heart disease, diabetes, many with toxemia of pregnancy, those in premature labor, and those who have eaten recently. This method usually is preferable to spinal or caudal anesthesia for women with hypotension from bleeding or other causes and those with disorders of the spine or nervous system. Inhalation anesthesia is essential whenever it is necessary to abolish uterine contractions and relax the uterine muscle to complete delivery as for version and extraction or breech extraction.

Nitrous oxide–oxygen. Nitrous oxide–oxygen mixtures are easy to administer, but they are not particularly potent anesthetic agents. They are most useful for the control of pain during the terminal phases of labor and for spontaneous delivery of multiparas. More profound anesthesia with nitrous oxide–oxygen alone can only be obtained by decreasing the oxygen content below 20% to 25%. This not only will increase intrauterine hypoxia and neonatal apnea but may be injurious to the mother. It usually is necessary to supplement nitrous oxide–oxygen with trichloroethylene or ether for forceps delivery or episiotomy.

Trichloroethylene. Trichloroethylene (Trilene) is an analgesic rather than an anesthetic, but when it is given with nitrous oxide and oxygen, it provides excellent pain relief and will permit the performance of forceps delivery and episiotomy. If it is administered in this manner, the soda lime circuit on the machine must be disconnected, vasopressors should not be administered, and Pituitrin should not be used. A closed-circuit unit should not be used to administer any type of anesthetic to women who have inhaled Trilene during labor. Small amounts of Trilene that are still present in the system can form phosgene. Trilene alone cannot be used to provide muscle relaxation. When this is attempted, the respirations become rapid and irregular and premature auricular and ventricular beats may be induced.

Ether. Ether is one of the oldest agents and is still widely used. It is safe to administer and relaxes the uterus well for version and extraction or other difficult deliveries. Its disadvantages are that it is unpleasant to take and may irritate the bronchi; it is inflammable; and it may increase bleeding.

Chloroform. Chloroform is a widely used obstetric anesthetic agent that produces good uterine relaxation, is nonexplosive, and is more pleasant to take than ether. It may produce cardiac arrhythmia and liver necrosis and requires a skilled anesthetist. Like ether, its ability to diminish the force of the uterine contractions may increase bleeding.

Cyclopropane. Cyclopropane is pleasant to take, and induction is rapid, but because of the rapid induction it is easy to extend the depth of anesthesia beyond that which is necessary and safe. The oxygen content of the fetal blood after the use of cyclopropane is lower than with the other agents. Cardiac irregularities are common during induction, there may be a slight rise in blood pressure, and bleeding is increased.

Cyclopropane can be administered safely for delivery by an anesthesiologist experienced in its use, but it should not be given by others. It is particularly valuable when it is necessary to provide deep anesthesia and uterine relaxation rapidly and for cesarean section in bleeding, hypovolemic patients. When it is used for either of these purposes, the patient and the obstetrician should be prepared for delivery before the anesthetic is started. Cyclopropane enters the fetal circulation so rapidly that the baby will be seriously depressed unless it is delivered as soon as suitable anesthesia is obtained.

REGIONAL ANESTHESIA

Some sort of nerve block anesthesia usually is preferable because it permits the mother to be awake, and it relieves pain without disturbing fetal oxygenation. Some of the methods, however, have a high potential mortality and must be administered with the greatest caution. The two main types are those that produce loss of pain sensation by blocking the nerve roots and those that block the nerves peripherally.

Nerve root block. For the most part these agents relieve pain completely and paralyze the voluntary muscles but do not interfere with the uterine contractions. There is an associated vasodilatation below the anesthetic level that may be responsible for a fall in blood pressure. These agents do not depress the respiratory center and therefore are beneficial to the fetus unless the maternal blood pressure falls enough to interfere with uterine blood flow, thus decreasing the amount of oxygen available to the fetus. Relaxation of the voluntary pelvic and perineal muscles decreases the pressure on the fetal head, but this loss of resistance may interfere with the normal mechanism of labor, particularly rotation. The relaxation makes delivery easier and less traumatic, but the fact that uterine contractions are not altered makes these techniques unsuitable for intrauterine manipulation.

Caudal or epidural anesthesia may be used for both analgesia during labor and anesthesia for delivery and are particularly advantageous for women in whom the usual methods for relieving pain during labor and delivery are contraindicated. They can be administered only by trained and experienced individuals.

Spinal anesthesia has rightly been considered a dangerous method for producing anesthesia because the mortality is high if it is improperly used. The dangers that are inherent when this technique is used in pregnancy can be obviated by being aware of them and attempting to avoid them. The vasomotor system is unstable in gravid women, and shock may follow ordinary doses of medication given intraspinally.

Spinal anesthesia is of greatest value in primigravidas, to whom it is administered when the head is bulging the perineum. If given to multiparas too early, descent of the head often is prevented, even though uterine contractions continue. It should usually be administered to multiparas when the cervix is 8 or 9 cm. dilated and the head well below the ischial spines. It is only to be used in carefully selected patients in hospitals where there is sufficient help to treat the fall in blood pressure and other complications that may be associated with its administration.

Saddle block, the type of spinal anesthesia most often used for delivery, is given with the patient sitting up. Although it may be given to provide analgesia late in the first stage, it is better used as an agent for delivery because labor is delayed in a substantial number of cases, particularly in multiparas. The agent used is *Pontocaine,* 3 to 5 mg., in 10% dextrose.

Headache often follows the administration of spinal or saddle block anesthesia for delivery. Bumgardner and Burns reduced the incidence substantially by the use of a 26-gauge needle rather than the standard larger sizes. The loss of spinal fluid through the dural defect, which is thought to be a major factor in the production of headache, is minimized when the small needle is used. Other more important complications of spinal anesthesia include *arachnoiditis, nerve root injury* from chemical or direct trauma, and an *overdose of the drug*—any one of which may result in disability or death. Complications can be kept at a minimum by exercising every possible precaution during the preparation of the solution and its administration.

Peripheral nerve block. Local injection of anesthetic agents to block the peripheral nerve endings affords the same advantages to the fetus that nerve root blocks do, but they are less effective in relieving pain and providing muscle relaxation. Since they do not require unusual equipment or the presence of an anesthesiologist, they are excellent for use in the small hospital or at home.

Simple infiltration of the perineum or injection along the line of the proposed episi-

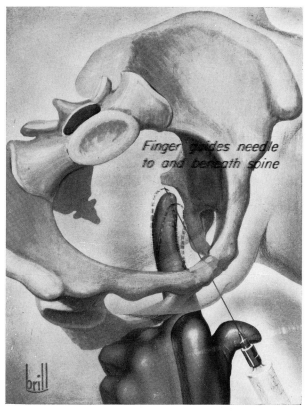

Fig. 30-2. Pudendal nerve block. Needle point is directed behind inferior tip of ischial spine by fingertip. (From Klink, E. W.: Obstet. Gynec. 1:137, 1953.)

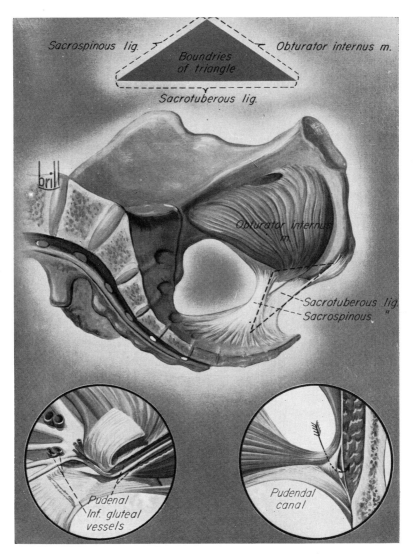

Fig. 30-3. Pudendal nerve block. Localizing landmarks in region of ischial spine and relationship of pudendal nerve to pudendal and inferior gluteal vessels. (From Klink, E. W.: Obstet. Gynec. **1**:137, 1953.)

otomy with 1% procaine or Xylocaine is often sufficient for normal delivery but is inadequate for any other procedure.

Pudendal nerve block by the injection of 10 ml. of 1% Xylocaine around each perineal nerve trunk as it passes behind the ischial spine provides excellent pelvic anesthesia for normal or low forceps delivery and for episiotomy and repair. It is safe, easy to learn, and requires no anesthesiologist or expensive equipment. This procedure, supplemented with nitrous oxide–oxygen or Trilene when necessary, should be suitable for almost all normal deliveries.

A hollow metal guide, such as an Iowa trumpet, is passed along the palmar surface of the index or second finger toward the ischial spine. The tip of the guide is directed to a position just beneath the tip of the spine and is held firmly in place. A 15 cm., 20-gauge needle attached to a syringe containing 1% of Xylocaine is inserted through the guide until its tip reaches the vaginal mucosa. With further pressure the needle is pushed through the triangle formed by the sacrospinous and sacrotuberous ligaments and the obturator internus muscles until the tip is in Alcock's canal, through which the

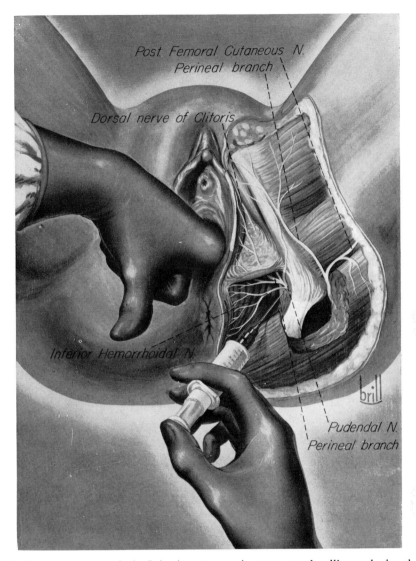

Fig. 30-4. Pudendal nerve block. Injection near main nerve trunk will anesthetize the areas supplied by the hemorrhoidal, perineal, and dorsal clitoral branches. The needle is usually inserted through the vagina rather than through the perineum. (From Klink, E. W.: Obstet. Gynec. **1:**137, 1953.)

pudendal nerve trunk runs. If the needle is properly placed, it can be moved back and forth without resistance. Blood can be aspirated if the pudendal artery or vein has been punctured; in this event the needle should be withdrawn slightly before the anesthetic agent is injected.

Ten millimeters of the solution is deposited in the pudendal canal behind each ischial spine. The anesthetic is in direct contact with the pudendal nerve trunk. The anesthetic effect will be evident within 2 or 3 minutes. Muscular relaxation as well as anesthesia is effected and will last as long as 1 hour.

■ **Special procedures**
PREMATURE DELIVERY

A combination of systemic analgesia during premature labor and inhalation anesthesia for delivery is generally contraindicated because a small infant is more likely to be depressed by these medications than is a mature one. Caudal or peridural analgesia, when available, is the most suitable method. Saddle or pudendal block anesthesia may also be used for delivery. Neither interferes with oxygenation, and both relax voluntary pelvic muscles.

Fifty milligrams of Sparine or Phenergan, alone or combined with 25 to 50 mg. of Demerol, may be given during early labor if caudal analgesia cannot be used. With this medication a regional anesthetic is preferable for delivery. If an inhalation anesthetic must be given, it should be administered with as large a percentage of oxygen and for as short a period of time as is possible.

TOXEMIA

Most patients with toxemia have been well sedated during labor; in fact, they may not even need an anesthetic for delivery. Pudendal block will usually provide adequate anesthesia for vaginal delivery, but caudal anesthesia can be used to control the pain. Caudal, epidural, or local infiltration can be used for cesarean section. Spinal anesthesia usually should be avoided, particularly if the blood pressure is very high and labile. Chloroform may increase liver damage, and all inhalation agents will decrease oxygenation in varying degrees.

MEDICAL COMPLICATIONS

Caudal or epidural techniques are preferable for the delivery of women with *heart disease,* particularly the more advanced grades. Pain and the resultant excessive muscular activity during labor are eliminated without interfering with oxygenation. If caudal anesthesia is not available, morphine, alone or in combination with 25 to 50 mg. of Sparine or Phenergan, can be used during labor with saddle or pudendal block for delivery. Conduction analgesia is also desirable for patients with *tuberculosis or other acute or chronic pulmonary* infections and for those with *diabetes,* unless a severe toxemia also is present.

BLEEDING

Patients who are bleeding profusely from placenta previa or abruptio placentae are best delivered with local infiltration anesthesia: pudendal block for vaginal delivery and local block of the abdominal wall for cesarean section. If inhalation anesthesia seems preferable, as it may for cesarean section, cyclopropane usually is the most appropriate agent because induction is rapid, it can be given with a high concentration of oxygen, and the blood pressure usually is sustained or even rises slightly. If the abdomen is prepared and draped before the anesthetic is started and if the incision is made as soon as possible, the infant can usually be extracted before the cyclopropane concentration in its blood reaches a dangerous level. Spinal anesthesia is generally contraindicated unless the bleeding is slight because it may be accompanied by a fall in blood pressure, which will decrease oxygenation even more than does the bleeding alone.

Conduction anesthesia is preferable for the delivery of women with conditions that may predispose to postpartum hemorrhage. Inhalation anesthetics tend to reduce uterine muscle activity unless minimal amounts are administered, thereby increasing third-stage bleeding.

OPERATIVE DELIVERY

Operations, particularly version and extraction or breech extraction, that require uterine relaxation are most easily and safely performed with open-drop ether or cyclopropane anesthesia. Cyclopropane is more rapid and pleasant, but the degree of uterine relaxation is somewhat less than that which can be achieved with ether. Anesthesia for cesarean section is considered in Chapter 38.

References

Andros, G. J., Dieckmann, W. J., Ouda, P., Priddle, H. D., Smitter, R. C., and Bryan, W. M.: Spinal (saddle block) anesthesia in obstetrics, Amer. J. Obstet. Gynec. 55:806, 1948.

Brown, E. O., Engel, T., and Douglas, R. G.: Paracervical block analgesia in labor, Obstet. Gynec. 26:195, 1965.

Bumgardner, H. D., and Burns, F. D.: Effect of needle size on the incidence of postspinal headache, Amer. J. Obstet. Gynec. 69:135, 1955.

Evans, T. N., Morley, G. W., and Helder, L.: Caudal anesthesia in obstetrics, Obstet. Gynec. 20:726, 1962.

Gordon, H. R.: Fetal bradycardia after paracervical block; correlation with fetal and maternal blood levels of local anesthetic (mepivacaine), New Eng. J. Med. 279:910, 1968.

Hellman, L. M., and Hingson, R. A.: The effect of various methods of obstetric pain relief on infant mortality, New York J. Med. 53:2767, 1953.

Hingson, R. A., and Hellman, L. M.: Anesthesia

for obstetrics, Philadelphia, 1956, J. B. Lippincott Co.

Hingson, R. A., Cull, W. A., and Benzinger, M.: Continuous caudal analgesia in obstetrics; combined experience of a quarter of a century, Anesth. Analg. (Cleveland) **40:**119, 1961.

Klink, E. W.: Perineal nerve block; an anatomic and clinical study in the female, Obstet. Gynec. **1:**137, 1953.

Kobak, A. J., and Sadove, M. S.: Combined paracervical and pudendal nerve blocks, a simple form of transvaginal anesthesia, Amer. J. Obstet. Gynec. **81:**72, 1961.

LaSalvia, L. A., and Steffen, E. A.: Delayed gastric emptying time in labor, Amer. J. Obstet. Gynec. **59:**1075, 1950.

Merrill, R. B., and Hingson, R. A.: Study of incidence of maternal mortality from aspiration of vomitus during anesthesia occurring in major obstetric hospitals in the United States, Anesth. Analg. (Cleveland) **30:**121, 1951.

Morris, L. E., Thornton, M. J., and Harris, J. W.: Comparison of the effect of Pituitrin, oxytocin, and ergonovine on cardiac rhythm during cyclopropane anesthesia for parturition, Amer. J. Obstet. Gynec. **63:**171, 1952.

Rosefsky, J. B., and Petersiel, M. E.: Perinatal deaths associated with mepivacaine paracervical block anesthesia in labor, New Eng. J. Med. **278:**530, 1968.

Taylor, E. S.: Oxygen saturation of the blood of the newborn as affected by maternal anesthetic agents, Amer. J. Obstet. Gynec. **61:**840, 1951.

Taylor, E. S., and Jack, W. W.: A critical analysis of local anesthesia as an agent for the relief of pain in vaginal delivery, Amer. J. Obstet. Gynec. **58:**275, 1949.

Watson, B. P.: Commemoration of the centennial of the introduction of anesthesia in obstetrics by Sir James Y. Simpson, Amer. J. Obstet. Gynec. **56:**205, 1948.

White, R. T.: Apomorphine as an emetic prior to obstetric anesthesia, Obstet. Gynec. **14:**111, 1959.

31

Third stage of labor and postpartum hemorrhage

For the mother the third stage is the most dangerous part of the entire labor because abnormalities in separation and expulsion of the placenta may be accompanied by profuse bleeding. At least 7 of 63 maternal deaths in Michigan in 1967 were due to postpartum hemorrhage. All 7 deaths were attributed by the evaluation committee to the fact that the attending physician failed to recognize that blood loss was excessive and did nothing to find the cause and to correct it until the patient was in irreversible shock. The total mortality from hemorrhage is not always obvious because excessive bleeding may cause death by reducing the patient's ability to cope with other complications, such as infection. Douglas and Davis noted an increase both in incidence of infections and in their severity in women who had lost abnormal amounts of blood at delivery.

The blood loss accompanying the third stage of labor is variable but averages about 250 ml. *Postpartum hemorrhage* can be diagnosed whenever the total blood loss from the genital tract during the first 24 hours after delivery exceeds 500 ml. The incidence of abnormal bleeding can be kept below 5% if labor and delivery are properly managed.

■ Normal third stage

Placental separation. In the past it was thought that the placenta was dissected off the uterine wall during the third stage by the development of a retroplacental hematoma in the spongy layer of the decidua. Warnekros in 1918 and Brandt in 1933, however, by injecting radiopaque material through the umbilical vessels immediately after the baby was delivered, obtained x-ray evidence which indicated that placental separation occurred either during the second stage or with the first contraction or two following the delivery of the infant. Each concluded that that mechanism was primarily mechanical and that retroplacental bleeding played little or no part.

Under normal circumstances the placenta is relatively noncontractile and has only limited ability to alter its size and shape to compensate for changes in the area of the uterine wall over which it is attached. As the uterus becomes smaller, the surface area of its cavity must of necessity diminish after the infant is expelled from the birth canal. As the area of the placental site is reduced, the placenta thickens and its diameter decreases. Since its size cannot be altered enough to equal the change in the uterine wall beneath it, the placenta is partially or completely sheared off as the uterus contracts during the late second stage. The completeness with which the placenta is separated is determined by how much the subplacental area of the uterine wall is reduced. The separation occurs in the spongy portion of the decidua basalis; a thin layer of decidua remains on the uterine wall, and the remainder covers the cotyledons of the maternal surface of the placenta.

After the birth of the baby the uterus continues to contract regularly. At this stage the uterine muscle may be even more active than it was during late labor. The uterus is discoid in shape, being wide transversely but

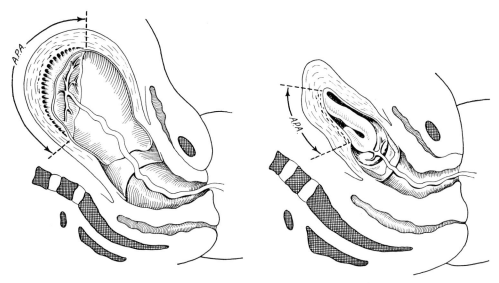

Fig. 31-1. Reduction in size of area of placental attachment (**A.P.A.**) as upper segment contracts, separates placenta, and expels it into the lower uterine segment.

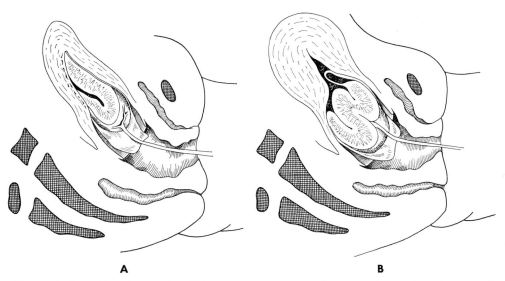

Fig. 31-2. **A,** While placenta is still in the upper segment the uterus is discoid and flattened in anteroposterior diameter. **B,** Uterus becomes globular when placenta is expelled into lower segment.

relatively flattened in its anteroposterior diameter, and lies in the midline with its superior surface below the level of the umbilicus. The placenta has already been partially or completely separated during the expulsion of the baby, but it still is in the upper part of the cavity. The continuing uterine contractions complete the separation of the placenta and force it downward into the flaccid, distended lower segment and

vagina. As the placenta is expelled from the upper segment, this portion of the uterus becomes globular, its cavity is almost obliterated, and the thickness of the wall increases to as much as 5 cm. The bulky placenta distending the relaxed lower segment forces the globular fundus upward and to the right; the superior surface of the uterus can often be felt above the level of the umbilicus. The placenta ultimately is forced from the lower segment and vagina by voluntary bearing-down efforts of the mother or, as is more often the case, is expressed by the attendant.

The duration of the third stage will be from 15 to 30 minutes or even longer if the physician waits for the mother to expel the placenta herself. If the placental phase of labor is properly managed by the medical attendant, its duration can be less than 5 minutes in almost every instance.

Control of bleeding. The branches of the uterine arteries wind between the interlacing smooth-muscle bundles as they traverse the uterine wall, and they eventually open into the large sinuses in the decidua basalis at the placental site. The source of the blood loss after delivery, except that caused by soft-tissue injury, is the sinuses that are left open by separation of the placenta. Excess bleeding is prevented by firm contraction of the uterine muscle bundles, which kink and compress the vessels. This is followed by clot formation and retraction, the usual method by which bleeding from open vessels is controlled.

Placental expulsion. The so-called "signs of separation" of the placenta are more accurately evidences of its expulsion from the firmly contracted uterine fundus into the lower segment and vagina and indicate that it can be delivered. These consist of the following:

1. *A show of blood* as the uterus contracts and the placenta is forced downward. If the placenta is separated completely as the infant is delivered, it usually folds on itself like an inverted umbrella with the fetal surface preceding the periphery through the cervix. With this mechanism of expulsion, the *Schultze method,* the placenta occludes the cervical opening, and there is little obvious bleeding until it is expelled, at which time the blood retained within the uterus gushes out. With the less common *Duncan mechanism* there is a constant trickle of blood because an edge of the placenta, rather than an inverted surface, presents in the cervical opening, and the blood can leave the uterus freely.

2. *The cord advances.* The length of cord visible outside the introitus is increased as the placenta descends into the lower segment and vagina.

3. *The fundus rises* and is deviated toward the right as the placenta, distending the lower segment, elevates the contracted fundal portion.

4. *The shape of the uterus changes.* The fundus becomes globular rather than wide and flat after the placenta has been expelled.

5. *Nontransmission of impulse.* As slight traction is made on the cord while the uterus is pushed downward by suprapubic pressure, the amount of cord outside the vagina increases. If the placenta is still in the upper segment, the cord is withdrawn into the vagina when the suprapubic pressure is released and the fundus is allowed to rise. If the placenta is detached and in the lower segment, the cord is not retracted when the uterus rises.

Management. During the second stage the physician should attempt to empty the uterus slowly, thereby permitting the muscle fibers to retract and decrease the size of the cavity gradually as the infant is being delivered. This encourages prompt and forceful contraction and more complete placental separation. After the head has been born the anterior shoulder is delivered beneath the pubic arch, where it is allowed to remain for 30 to 60 seconds. The head is then elevated and traction is exerted until the posterior shoulder has cleared the perineum. After another 30- to 60-second wait to permit further readjustment of the uterine muscle fibers, the rest of the body is slowly and deliberately extracted. The physician should not try to restrain delivery if the spontaneous uterine contractions are forcing the baby through the birth canal.

After the cord has been clamped and cut, the uterus is gently palpated through the sterile drapes while the cord is held taut but without undue traction. The uterus should not be massaged and manipulated, and no attempt should be made to express the placenta until the uterus contracts. As the fundus becomes firm and globular, placental expulsion can be aided by downward pressure over the superior surface of the uterus with the palmar surfaces of the fingers; it should not be squeezed. Fundal pressure is no longer necessary after the placenta enters the lower segment; therefore, at the moment placental descent can be detected the pressure is transferred from the fundus to the suprapubic area directly over the lower segment. As the contracted uterus

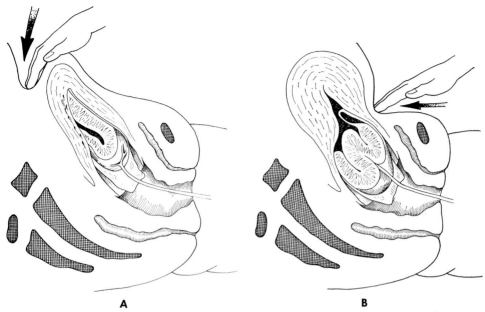

Fig. 31-3. Manual pressure on fundus as the uterus begins to contract, **A,** aids expulsion of placenta into lower segment, from where it can be expressed by upward pressure on the contracted fundus and tension on the cord, **B.**

is pushed upward away from the placenta by firm pressure with the fingertips, the afterbirth, which by now should be visible at the introitus, can be delivered by applying slight traction on the cord. After the placenta has been delivered, the contracted fundus is kept from dropping back into the pelvis by maintaining upward pressure on it through the abdominal wall; this will promote muscular contraction and reduce bleeding. While a nurse or an assistant applies the pressure necessary to hold the uterus up, the physician examines the placenta to make certain it is intact and that none of its cotyledons has been left in the uterine cavity.

Uterotonic drugs stimulate firm uterine contraction and when properly used will reduce the blood loss accompanying placental separation and delivery. Some authorities recommend that one be administered as soon as the anterior shoulder has been delivered and others that it be given at the end of the second stage. Unless they are used with great caution, the placental stage may be prolonged rather than shortened and blood loss may be excessive. It usually is preferable, particularly in smaller hospitals where the number of assistants is limited,

to withhold uterotonic drugs until the uterus is empty.

The oxytocic activity of ergot has long been known, and it has been used extensively in obstetric practice. The purified ergot derivative *Ergotrate* (ergonovine maleate), when administered intravenously or intramuscularly in 1 ml. (0.2 mg.) doses, produces a sustained tetanic contraction of the uterine muscles that reduces the blood loss from the vessels at the placental site. Ordinarily it is given intravenously as soon as the placenta has been delivered. *Methergine* (methylergonovine tartrate), a synthetic preparation, is equally effective and is less likely to elevate the blood pressure. It also is given intravenously or intramuscularly in a dosage of 1 ml. (0.2 mg.).

Oxytocin from which almost all the vasopressor factor has been removed can be administered instead of ergot preparations as an aid in managing the third stage. It is preferable to either Ergotrate or Methergine for women with hypertensive disorders because it is less likely to produce alarming blood pressure elevations. The dosage is 0.5 ml. intramuscularly or 5 ml. dissolved in 1,000 ml. of 5% dextrose solution as an intravenous drip. The latter is more often used to aid in controlling postpartum hemorrhage than in the management of the normal third stage.

■ Postpartum hemorrhage

Postpartum hemorrhage, the loss of more than 500 ml. of blood during the first 24 hours after the completion of the third stage, should occur in less than 5% of all deliveries. In almost every instance excessive bleeding can be controlled, and the blood can be replaced so rapidly that no woman should die as a result of postpartum bleeding.

Etiology. The most important causes are *uterine atony, retention of placental fragments accompanied by atony,* and *soft-tissue injury.* Of these, the first two are by far the most common. The source of the bleeding is either the sinuses of the placental site that remain open after the placenta has separated because the uterus fails to contract properly or blood vessels of the birth canal that are torn during delivery. In either event the amount of bleeding is determined by the size of the involved vessels and the length of time before the blood loss is checked.

Predisposing factors. There are certain factors that increase the possibility that excessive bleeding will occur after delivery. Most of these interfere with the normal mechanism for controlling bleeding.

Overdistention of the uterus. If the uterus has been overdistended by twins, a large infant, or hydramnios, the muscle fibers are stretched to a point at which they cannot contract firmly enough to occlude the open vessels for several minutes after delivery if the uterus is emptied rapidly.

Anesthesia. Deep inhalation anesthesia reduces the effectiveness of uterine contractions and permits more than the normal amount of bleeding.

Dysfunctional or prolonged labor. Ineffective uterine contractions often continue into the third stage.

Improper management of the third stage. Manipulation and massage in an attempt to express the placenta before it has separated completely interfere with the normal mechanism and increase bleeding.

Injury. A considerable amount of blood may be lost from vaginal lacerations, uterine rupture, or even the episiotomy. Odell and Seski state that the average blood loss from an episiotomy is about 250 ml.

Clinical course. Deaths from postpartum bleeding are rarely caused by sudden overwhelming hemorrhage. None of the patients reported by Beecham died in less than 1½ hours, and only 11.5% died within 2 hours. The average time between delivery and death was over 5 hours.

Excessive bleeding may occur while the placenta is still within the uterus or after it has been delivered. As noted previously the excessive blood loss is usually the result of a prolonged trickle of blood rather than massive hemorrhage, but unless the flow is checked the end result is the same. Pregnant women, because of the expanded blood volume, withstand hemorrhage better than nonpregnant women, but the amount any individual woman will tolerate cannot be determined in advance. Those with anemia or chronic debilitating disease and those whose blood volume is decreased because of prolonged labor and dehydration or severe pregnancy toxemia may go into shock with relatively minimal bleeding.

Prevention. Most postpartum hemorrhages can be prevented, but since some cannot, all pregnant women should be considered as potential candidates for excessive bleeding. Predisposing causes should be eliminated, and anemia and nutritional inadequacies should be corrected whenever possible.

The labor should be shortened by recognizing inadequate contractions early and instituting measures that will be helpful in preventing prolonged labor. Early operative delivery during normal labor, on the other hand, may only increase injury and blood loss. Regional anesthesia should be utilized whenever possible, and the second as well as the third stage should be managed in a manner calculated to encourage retraction and firm contraction of uterine muscle fibers.

Treatment. The most important factors in preventing deaths from postpartum hemorrhage are to recognize abnormal bleeding before the blood loss has been excessive, to determine the source of the bleeding and to control it as rapidly as possible, and to replace lost blood promptly. An intravenous infusion of glucose or saline solution should be started through a 15-gauge needle before the delivery of women with conditions that predispose to excessive bleeding, as well as in those women in whom excessive bleeding actually occurs. Blood should be administered to all in whom clinical evidence of blood loss can be detected, even though the amount of bleeding does not seem excessive.

Severe bleeding after the birth of the baby is most often the result of inadequate uterine muscle contraction rather than of injury. The first step in determining the cause, therefore, is to palpate the uterine fundus rather than to search for lacerations in the birth canal. If the uterus is soft and boggy, it is almost always the source of bleeding; this is particularly true if the placenta has not yet been delivered.

At end of second stage. The placenta is expressed if possible or removed manually, and the uterus is pushed upward out of the pelvis and massaged between one hand inserted in the vagina and the other palpating through the abdominal wall to stimulate contraction. Ergotrate or Methergine, 1 ml. (0.2 mg.), is administered intravenously. If the uterus remains relaxed despite these measures, manual exploration to search for an injury or retained placental tissue should be performed promptly.

If the uterus still fails to contract and bleeding continues, an intravenous drip of oxytocin solution (5 ml. oxytocin in 1,000 ml. of 5% dextrose) should be started at a rate of 20 to 30 drops per minute. If bleeding continues, the physician must consider the possibility of a clotting defect and test for it.

The insertion of an intrauterine gauze pack has been used extensively in the past in the treatment of postpartum hemorrhage, but its value is to be questioned. The pack does not exert much pressure on the open sinuses and, by distending the uterus, may actually interfere with normal hemostasis. In most instances the uterus will contract if it is elevated, compressed, and massaged, and further measures are unnecessary.

Hysterectomy may be indicated if all other methods have failed to control bleeding. It should not be delayed until the patient is dying.

At end of third stage. If abnormal bleeding begins after the placenta has been delivered, the treatment is exactly the same as that just outlined. The physician should explore the uterus to make certain that it is intact and empty.

Postpartum hemorrhage from injury. Unless the vagina is extensively lacerated or there are deep cervical tears extending upward into the broad ligament, bleeding from injury is less severe than that from the uterus. The usual cervical lacerations seldom bleed profusely. Injury should be suspected and sought whenever vaginal bleeding continues despite a firmly contracted fundus.

Bleeding from vaginal lacerations can usually be controlled with sutures, which must be placed precisely to make certain that they approximate the entire length of the injured area. An assistant to expose the laceration is essential if bleeding is excessive or if the upper vagina is involved. Continued oozing after the placement of sutures can usually be checked with pressure from a tight vaginal pack.

Cervical lacerations should be repaired whether they are bleeding or not. Deep lacerations that extend upward into the lower uterine segment will often bleed profusely; unless the upper end of the laceration can be identified and sutured, a laparotomy is necessary for adequate repair.

Delayed hemorrhage. Hemorrhage may occur at any time during the first 24 hours after delivery *(early delayed hemorrhage)* or several days later *(late delayed hemorrhage)*.

Early. Hemorrhage during the first 24 hours is most often the result of atony or relaxation accompanying the retention of placental fragments, or it is from the episiotomy or a laceration. Even though the uterus is relaxed and distended with blood, atony may not be the primary factor because blood from a vaginal injury can flow upward and fill the uterus. If simple atony is the cause, the expression of clots and stimulation by abdominal manipulation and the administration of an oxytocic may result in sustained contraction. If bleeding and relaxation recur after an oxytocic has been given, the vagina and uterus must be explored.

Late. Bleeding that begins or becomes profuse several days after delivery is most often caused by retained portions of placenta, although occasionally an injury may be responsible. In most instances the uterovaginal canal should be explored promptly.

Placental tissue can be removed with a large curet.

Another form of late postpartum hemorrhage is that designated as *placental site bleeding.* This usually begins suddenly between the twelfth and twenty-first days and may be profuse. It is presumably the result of separation of the crust of organized fibrin and hyalinized vessels covering the placental site and can usually be controlled by curettage. Blood transfusion may be necessary.

■ Retained placenta

The third stage usually lasts less than 5 minutes, but occasionally it may be prolonged because the placenta fails to separate or because the uterus cannot expel the placenta even though it is partially or completely detached. If the placenta is still completely attached, there can be no bleeding, but if it is partially separated the blood loss from the open placental site sinuses can be profuse. This is a common cause of excessive third-stage bleeding.

Failure of placental separation may be mechanical or a result of abnormal penetration of the trophoblast into the uterine wall *(placenta accreta).* With the former the uterine muscle at the placental site may be relaxed and boggy even though that of the rest of the upper segment is fairly firmly contracted. Because of failure of the muscle at the placental site to contract the usual mechanism for placental separation does not come into play.

With *placenta accreta* all or part of the decidua basalis is absent, and the chorionic tissue grows directly into the muscle, thereby eliminating the normal cleavage plane. The term *placenta accreta* indicates a relatively superficial penetration of the muscle. Deeper penetration is called *placenta increta,* and *placenta percreta* indicates that the trophoblast has grown to or completely through the serosa. Placenta accreta can be *partial,* if only a portion of the placenta is abnormally adherent, or *complete;* with the partial type, bleeding can be profuse when the normal portion of the placenta separates because the uterus cannot complete the separation of the placenta and expel it. Bleeding cannot occur with complete placenta accreta because none of the placenta can separate from its abnormal attachment in the uterine muscle.

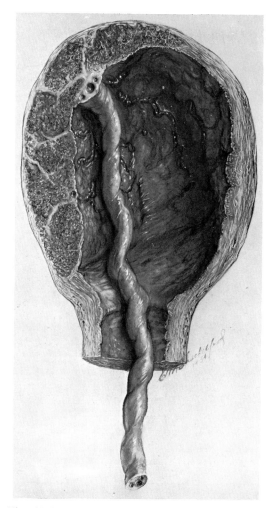

Fig. 31-4. Placenta accreta. Abnormal fusion between placenta and uterine wall with deep invasion of uterine muscle by placental tissue. (Illustration made, by permission, from specimen in Museum of Obstetrics, Johns Hopkins Hospital, Baltimore, Md.; from Willson, J. R.: Management of obstetric difficulties, ed. 6, St. Louis, 1961, The C. V. Mosby Co.)

Management. The management of retained placenta is determined by the amount of bleeding, the surroundings, and the experience of the physician. If bleeding is active and the placenta cannot be expressed in the usual manner, it must be removed immediately by inserting the hand into the uterus, completing the separation, and extracting it. Although manual removal does increase the possibility of infection, the risk is far less than that from hemorrhage.

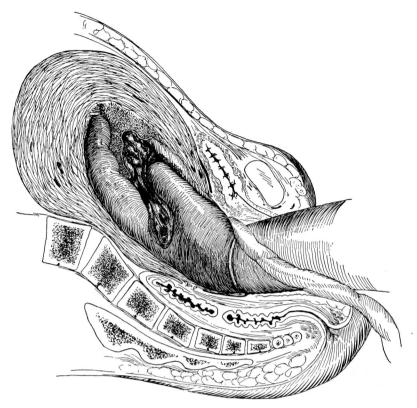

Fig. 31-5. Technique of manual removal of retained placenta. (From Titus, P.: Atlas of obstetric technic, St. Louis, 1949, The C. V. Mosby Co.)

In the absence of bleeding it is safe to wait longer for spontaneous separation and expulsion, but there is no reason to delay more than 5 or 10 minutes.

Hysterectomy usually is necessary for placenta accreta unless the abnormally adherent portion of the placenta involves only a small area. The uterus may be perforated or profuse bleeding may be produced by attempts to dig the cotyledons out of the uterine wall.

■ Inversion of the uterus

Inversion of the uterus occurs rarely, but when it does, the mortality is high unless it is recognized and treated promptly. The inversion may be *partial* or *complete;* those that are discovered at delivery are *acute,* and those that are not detected until days or weeks later are *chronic.*

In most instances the uterine muscles near the placental site, which often is in the fundus, are relaxed, permitting it to prolapse through the dilated cervix. Vigorous attempts to deliver the placenta either by suprapubic pressure or by cord traction are probably important factors in inverting the fundus.

In most instances shock develops promptly when the inversion occurs. The diagnosis can be suspected if the fundus is indented (incomplete inversion) or cannot be felt above the pubis (complete inversion). It can be confirmed by palpating the inverted fundus within the lower uterine segment or the vagina.

The uterus can usually be replaced without difficulty if the diagnosis is made promptly, but if the inversion is not recognized, the constricting collar of muscle may contract and incarcerate the inverted fundus. The entire hand is inserted into the vagina, with the fingertips exerting equal pressure around the collar of uterus just within the cervical opening and the fundus resting on the palmar surface of the hand.

The fundus is gradually replaced, and the cavity of the uterus is packed with gauze to prevent recurrence.

It is usually necessary to perform an operative procedure to correct chronic inversion.

■ Postpartum pituitary necrosis

Partial or complete necrosis of the anterior pituitary gland may follow excessive bleeding during pregnancy. This condition, Sheehan's syndrome, usually cannot be detected in women who die soon after delivery because the necrotic changes have not yet had time to develop. The entire anterior lobe or portions of it may be destroyed.

In the typical patient with severe damage the breasts remain flaccid and no milk is secreted. Pubic hair fails to grow back and axillary hair may fall out. The genital organs atrophy and the menses do not return. The endocrine glands that are under the control of the anterior pituitary cease to function. Complete pituitary necrosis is rarely seen, but the less severe states may be encountered occasionally. There may be enough tissue to carry on normal function, the deficiency only becoming obvious when the gland is subjected to unusual stress, such as another pregnancy, a surgical operation, or a serious infection.

Pituitary necrosis can be avoided by the prevention of excessive bleeding. The prompt replacement of blood may reduce the severity of pituitary damage.

■ Amniotic fluid infusion

The possibility that intravenous infusion of amniotic fluid could cause death was first suggested by Steiner and Lushbaugh. Their theory was questioned by some because many of the patients whose deaths they described had bled profusely. Reid and co-workers have suggested a cause for the bleeding. They postulate that amniotic fluid contains a thromboplastin-like substance that produces intravascular clotting and subsequent defibrination of blood and hemorrhage from the resultant clotting defect.

Amniotic fluid can enter the bloodstream through the vessels at the placental site or those opened by injury. The membranes must be ruptured to permit the escape of amniotic fluid, and the intrauterine pressure must be increased. Rupture of the membranes and the administration of an oxytocic to induce labor increases the possibility of amniotic fluid infusion, as does placenta previa.

Amniotic infusion is most likely to occur in women in labor at or near term, and many patients have been given oxytocin to induce or stimulate labor. Parous women are more often affected than are primigravidas. The symptoms occur suddenly, and the first evidence of the abnormality may be dyspnea and cyanosis or sudden shock. Death may occur promptly or be delayed for several hours. If a coagulation defect occurs, vaginal bleeding usually is evident.

Treatment consists of the administration of oxygen under pressure after endotracheal intubation, phlebotomy if the neck veins are distended or if central venous pressure is elevated, papaverine hydrochloride, 50 to 100 mg. intravenously, to reduce bronchiole artery spasm, atropine, 0.4 mg. intravenously, to relax vagus-induced coronary and pulmonary arteriolar vasoconstriction, and vasopressors. Blood must be administered if the patient is bleeding excessively, and the coagulation defect corrected by appropriate treatment, usually fibrinogen.

This condition can only be diagnosed with certainty by demonstrating the presence of fetal epithelial cells and amniotic debris in the lung capillaries. It can be suspected, however, in a patient in whom a state of collapse develops late in labor or immediately after delivery, and it is essential that treatment be instituted promptly.

References

Anderson, D. G.: Amniotic fluid infusion, Amer. J. Obstet. Gynec. 96:336, 1967.

Beecham, C. T.: An analysis of deaths from postpartum hemorrhage, Amer. J. Obstet. Gynec. 53:422, 1947.

Brandt, M. L.: Mechanism and management of the third stage of labor, Amer. J. Obstet. Gynec. 25:662, 1933.

Bunke, J. W., and Hofmeister, F. J.: Uterine inversion—obstetrical entity or oddity, Amer. J. Obstet. Gynec. 91:934, 1965.

Dieckmann, W. J., Odell, L. D., Williger, V. M., Seski, A. G., and Pottinger, R.: The placental stage and postpartum hemorrhage, Amer. J. Obstet. Gynec. 54:415, 1947.

Douglas, R. G., and Davis, I. F.: Puerperal infection; etiologic, prophylactic, and therapeutic considerations, Amer. J. Obstet. Gynec. 51:352, 1946.

Hendricks, C. H., Eskes, T. K. A. B., and Saameli, K.: Uterine contractility at delivery and in the puerperium, Amer. J. Obstet. Gynec. **83:**890, 1962.

MacPherson, J., and Wilson, J. K.: A radiologic study of the placental stage of labor, J. Obstet. Gynaec. Brit. Comm. **63:**321, 1956.

Odell, L. D., and Seski, A.: Episiotomy blood loss, Amer. J. Obstet. Gynec. **54:**51, 1947.

Reid, D. E., Weiner, A. E., and Roby, C. C.: Intravascular clotting and afibrinogenemia, the presumptive lethal factors in the syndrome of amniotic fluid embolism, Amer. J. Obstet. Gynec. **66:**465, 1953.

Schneeberg, N. G., Perloff, W. H., and Israel, S. L.: Incidence of unsuspected "Sheehan's syndrome"; hypopituitarism after postpartum hemorrhage and/or shock; clinical and laboratory study, J.A.M.A. **172:**20, 1960.

Sheehan, H. L.: Simmonds' disease due to postpartum necrosis of the anterior pituitary, J. Obstet. Gynaec. Brit. Comm. **50:**27, 1943.

Steiner, P. E., and Lushbaugh, C. C.: Maternal pulmonary embolism by amniotic fluid as cause of obstetric shock and unexpected death in obstetrics, J.A.M.A. **117:**1245, 1941.

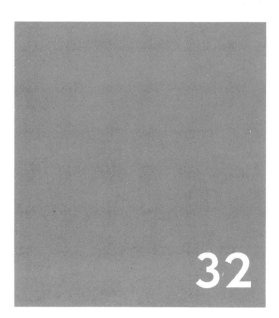

32

Care of the infant during pregnancy, labor, and after delivery

During its intrauterine life the fetus is completely dependent upon the transfer of respiratory gases and the materials essential for its growth from the maternal bloodstream. At birth, however, it must assume responsibility for maintaining all its own necessary functions. The highest mortality occurs during the first 24 hours of life while the infant is attempting to make this change.

The fetus in utero swallows amniotic fluid, which is absorbed from the intestinal tract and ultimately is excreted by the kidneys and returned to the amniotic sac. There is little peristaltic activity in the intestine of the normal infant until birth; the passage of meconium by the unborn infant usually indicates intrauterine anoxia. Respiratory efforts that move amniotic fluid in and out of the nasopharynx and trachea have been demonstrated in human fetuses

as well as in experimental animals. The infant responds to tactile stimuli while it is still in the uterus. It is important that all the necessary functions be developed and in operation by the time the infant is born. Abnormally formed infants may be unable to survive outside the uterus. Those born before 30 weeks' gestation often cannot cope with an independent existence, even though they are otherwise normal.

In order to survive the infant must have developed normally and be born alive and uninjured. The hazards of labor and delivery are increased for the premature infant whose delicate structures may be injured easily and for the excessively large infant who may be damaged during attempts to deliver it.

■ Prenatal influences

From time immemorial people have assumed that the growth of the fetus could be altered by maternal emotional experiences. For example, a baby might be born without an arm if the mother had been frightened by an armless individual during her pregnancy or had witnessed an accident during which an arm of the victim was severed. We know now that in most such instances specific traumatic experiences cannot be correlated with congenital defects because they rarely occur at a time when the involved structure is developing, but we are learning more and more about the influence of drugs, chemicals, and physical and even emotional stimuli on fetal growth and development.

The periods during which organs and tissues develop vary in length and occur at different stages of pregnancy. For each there exists an early stage during which the primordial tissue begins to differentiate; this is followed by a period of cellular growth and beginning development of the structure, and finally the period during which development is completed. Subsequent change is almost entirely one of growth. To produce an anomaly, a stimulus must be applied before development is completed; it will have little effect except to interfere with growth if it is applied after differentiation is completed. Almost all of the important organ systems are developed by the end of the first trimester, but some take longer.

Most pregnant women are regularly exposed to stimuli of one sort or another that may alter fetal development. Fortunately these stimuli are generally either too slight to affect the tissue or occur after the structure already has been formed. Physicians prescribe many medications for their pregnant patients, often with too little thought of their potential effect on the fetus. Most of these drugs have been thoroughly tested on experimental animals, but unfortunately (Thalidomide is an outstanding example) they may be toxic only to human fetal tissue. Physicians and their patients are now aware of the possibilities of disturbing embryonic development, and both are becoming more reasonable about drug therapy during pregnancy—the physician about prescribing it and the patient about demanding it. As a general rule no medication, no matter how innocuous it is presumed to be, should be prescribed during pregnancy unless there is a specific indication for its use and unless the patient may be harmed if it is not used.

Some of the substances that are used frequently during pregnancy and that are known to influence fetal development are listed below.

Hormones. Some of the *progestogens,* particularly the *19-norsteroids,* can cause maldevelopment of the genitalia of the female fetus if they are administered during the first half of pregnancy. Since these medications are used almost exclusively in women who have aborted in previous pregnancies or are now threatening, they are almost always administered when they might interfere with genital development. Fortunately the major anomaly is labial fusion, which can be corrected easily; the ultimate differentiation and function of the rest of the genital organs are usually normal. Since progestogens are of no value in the treatment of threatened abortions, there is no reason to prescribe them.

Cortisone causes cleft palate in certain experimental animals. There is no information suggesting that this occurs in human beings.

Antimicrobial agents. The *tetracyclines* are deposited in the actively growing epiphyses of fetal bones and may cause abnormal bone growth. They also are deposited in the enamel of teeth, producing permanent fluorescent mottling. Since limb buds appear

at about the fifth week and tooth formation begins at about the twelfth week, these drugs should rarely be used during pregnancy.

Sulfonamides may displace bilirubin from its binding sites on serum albumin, and deposition of the free bilirubin in the basal ganglia may cause kernicterus. There is little likelihood of this occurring while the fetus is in utero because the bilirubin is excreted across the placenta into the maternal blood. Sulfonamide therapy during late pregnancy, particularly with long-acting preparations, should be avoided in women who are likely to deliver prematurely.

Chloramphenicol in large doses causes the gray syndrome and death in premature infants. It has no obvious effect on the fetus.

Streptomycin may cause nerve deafness, as it does in adults.

Others of these preparations undoubtedly also affect the fetus, but the problems they cause are not yet clear.

Chemotherapeutic agents. Antifolic acid agents such as *aminopterin* and *methotrexate* produce serious fetal deformities and even death; they should not be administered to pregnant women. *Chlorambucil* may have the same effect. No anomalies have been reported with the use of other agents.

Tranquilizers and sedatives. The information concerning these substances is not entirely clear, but *phenobarbital,* in excess, may cause bleeding in newborn infants. The *phenothiazines* may cause hyperbilirubinemia, and *meprobamate,* mental retardation. Infants of *narcotics addicts* may themselves be addicted and even die after birth. Babies whose mothers receive large amounts of medication during labor are less attentive on second- and fourth-day testing than those whose mothers were less heavily sedated. An increased incidence of chromosome breakage, the most common being chromatid and isochromatid breaks, has been found in *LSD users.* The same defect has been seen in children whose mothers used LSD during pregnancy. The significance of these findings is not yet obvious, but congenital defects occur frequently in the offspring of experimental animals treated with LSD during pregnancy, and anomalous development of human aborted embryos has been observed.

Thiazide diuretics. Neonatal thrombocytopenia has been reported in the new born infants of mothers treated with thiazide diuretics during pregnancy.

X-radiation. During the early days of embryonic development the cells are chemically and structurally similar, but they soon begin to differentiate. Before differentiation the entire mass of cells is either destroyed or completely unaffected by x-radiation. Later, damage and interference with the growth of specific groups of cells may produce anomalies. X-ray examinations, particularly of the abdomen and pelvis, should never be performed until the possibility of an unsuspected pregnancy has been eliminated.

Miscellaneous. Dicumarol and related substances may cause retroplacental hemorrhage and fetal death. Heparin does not cross the placenta, therefore it has no effect on the baby. *Antithyroid substances,* such as propylthiouracil and potassium iodide, may cause goiter in the fetus and even subsequent mental retardation. The babies of mothers who *smoke in excess* may be smaller than those born to nonsmoking mothers.

Infants born of mothers whose *diets have long been deficient in protein* and who themselves are malnourished during the early months of their lives are likely to be retarded in learning, probably because of a decreased number of neurons in the cerebral cortex. Excessive amounts of *intravenous fluids* administered to the mother may disturb fetal fluid and electrolyte balance.

■ Erythroblastosis fetalis resulting from Rh incompatibility

If the fetus's blood group is different from that of its mother, and if the mother has been sensitized to an antigen in the fetal blood cells, her blood will contain an antibody that can cross the placenta and hemolyze fetal red blood cells. Erythroblastosis is most often a result of Rh incompatibility, but differences in the ABO and other blood factors can also cause the disorder.

The fetus is more seriously affected by Rh incompatibilities than by most of the other types. The three most obvious clinical types of erythroblastosis from Rh incompatibility, all of which are part of the same process, are: (1) *hemolytic anemia of the newborn,* (2) *icterus gravis of the newborn,*

and (3) *fetal hydrops.* Each is associated with hemolytic anemia, and all are probably best designated as *hemolytic disease of the newborn.* All are potentially lethal, the mortality with fetal hydrops being 100%. The characteristic fetal manifestations, each of which is related to the hemolytic process, are (1) anemia; (2) erythroblastic hyperplasia of bone marrow; (3) extramedullary centers of erythropoiesis in the liver, spleen, kidneys, and other tissues; (4) erythroblastemia; (5) jaundice, particularly hemolytic but also hepatocellular, appearing soon after birth and with possible resulting kernicterus; (6) tissue damage from anoxia; (7) edema from cardiac failure and hypoproteinemia; and (8) purpura.

Etiology. The blood of about 85% of Caucasians contains the Rh or D factor; these are Rh_0 (D) positive. The blood of the remaining 15% does not contain the factor, and these persons are Rh_0 (D) negative. The factor is inherited as a mendelian characteristic; therefore individuals whose parents are both Rh_0 (D) positive are *homozygous,* and those who had only one Rh_0 (D) positive parent are *heterozygous;* half the sperm or ova of the heterozygous individuals will contain the Rh factor and half will not.

When an Rh_0 (D) negative woman is impregnated by a homozygous Rh_0 (D) postive male, the fetus will be Rh_0 (D) positive. Half the fetuses of heterozygous Rh_0 (D) positive fathers will be Rh_0 (D) positive and half Rh_0 negative. If intact or fragmented Rh_0 (D) positive fetal red blood cells enter the maternal circulation, an antibody against them may be formed. Fetal blood cells may mix with the mother's blood in the intervillous spaces if placental blood vessels are torn during abortion or during late pregnancy; intact cells also may cross the undamaged placenta by pinocytosis, or the products of disintegrated cells containing the antigen may enter the maternal circulation. A final and probably the most frequent method by which fetal red blood cells enter the maternal circulation is by disruption of the fetal placental vessels during the third stage of labor. Maternal antibodies will also be produced in response to blood transfusion with Rh_0 (D) positive donor blood. The Rh_0 (D) factor is the one most often responsible for sensitization, but others may have the same effect. In order of frequency they are: hr′ (c), rh′ (C), rh″ (E), and hr″ (e).

The maternal antibody crosses the placenta and enters the fetal circulation without difficulty; it hemolyzes fetal red blood cells and produces the changes characteristic of erythroblastosis.

Although the potential for the development of erythroblastosis fetalis with an Rh_o (D) negative mother and Rh_o (D) positive father occurs in about 10% of all pregnancies, the actual incidence is about 1 in 250 births, or 1 in 20 in which Rh incompatibility exists. There are several reasons for this:

1. Unless women have been sensitized by blood transfusion or by an early abortion, they have no antibodies during the first pregnancy and the infant is unaffected.

2. Some women never become sensitized because Rh_o (D) positive fetal red blood cells never invade the maternal circulation, or if they do, the number is so small that they stimulate only a weak response.

3. The father may be heterozygous Rh_o (D) positive so that some of the children will be Rh_o (D) negative.

4. The chances of erythroblastosis on an Rh basis are reduced with ABO incompatibilities (if the fetus has A or B factors and the mother lacks them).

Although the first infant born of an Rh_o (D) negative mother and Rh_o (D) positive father almost always is normal, the second or subsequent ones may be affected. After a woman has borne one infant with erythroblastosis the rest of her children are almost certain to have a similar condition if the father is homozygous Rh_o (D) positive. If he is heterozygous, half the sperms will contain Rh factor and half will contain none. As a general rule the disease in the first affected infant is mild, but one cannot predict what will happen during subsequent pregnancies. In some all the babies are only slightly affected, whereas in others the second and all subsequent fetuses develop hydrops or die in utero because of the severity of the hemolytic process.

The two principal types of Rh antibodies are *complete antibodies,* which can be detected in saline suspensions of Rh_o (D) positive red blood cells, and *incomplete* or *blocking antibodies,* which are detected by the indirect Coombs' test. The latter are the ones that enter the fetal circulation and react with Rh-sensitized red blood cells.

Management. An antibody screen should be run during the first trimester in every pregnant woman; if there is a positive response, the exact antibody should be identified. If antibodies against the Rh antigen cannot be detected in the blood of an Rh_o (D) negative woman during early pregnancy, one can presume that she is not sensitized and that the infant will be normal. Another test for Rh antibody should be made at about 28 to 30 weeks of pregnancy. If this also is negative, the physician need not be concerned until delivery, when the baby should be checked for hemolytic disease.

If the initial test is positive, the exact titer should be determined and the blood should be frozen so it will be available for comparison with later specimens. Presumably a rising Rh antibody titer would indicate an advancing process, whereas one that remains the same or increases only slightly would indicate a mildly affected fetus. Unfortunately changes in antibody titer do not accurately reflect the condition. Fetal hydrops and intrauterine death have often been observed with relatively low titers, and slightly affected, or even Rh-negative, babies have been seen when the titer had risen to astronomically high levels. As a consequence one cannot base treatment on Rh antibody titer alone.

A much more accurate evaluation of fetal condition can be made by *spectrophotometric analysis of amniotic fluid.* The spectral absorption curves for amniotic fluid are determined at various wavelengths and plotted with optical density as the ordinate and wavelength as the abscissa. The resultant normal curve is fairly smooth, but the bilirubin-like substance in the amniotic fluid of babies affected by erythroblastosis alters the optical density and produces a broad peak centered at about 450 mμ; the height of the peak is determined by the severity of the hemolytic process. Liley has established three zones for the purpose of evaluating the degree of fetal involvement. Those in the *lower zone* (normal curve or a slight rise) are usually in no difficulty and often need no special treatment. Those in the *middle zone* (a higher peak) are more se-

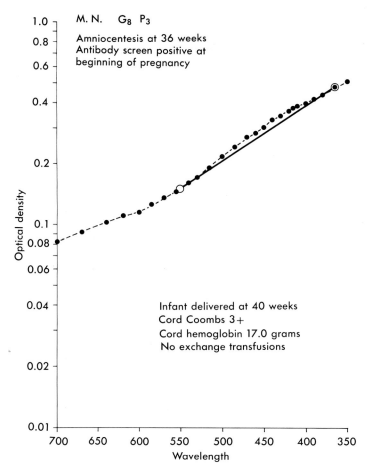

Fig. 32-1. Optical density 450 mμ. There is no elevation, hence no treatment is necessary.

riously involved and should be delivered early; most of these will need exchange transfusions. Those in the *upper zone* (an even higher peak) are seriously involved and are likely to die in utero unless treated.

A more practical method than the use of the zones is to measure the exact height of the peak. The optical density of amniotic fluid is measured at 365, 450, and 550 mμ. and recorded on semilogarithmic paper; a straight line is drawn between the points at 365 mμ and 550 mμ. The height of the 450 mμ peak above this straight line (Δ OD 450 mμ) indicates the amount of bilirubin-like substances in amniotic fluid and, therefore, the severity of the erythroblastosis.

Treatment is based upon this measurement, but a decision cannot be made on the basis of examining a single specimen unless the peak is already so high that there

is little doubt that the baby is seriously affected. The first study is usually made at about the twenty-sixth or twenty-eighth week of pregnancy, or even sooner if early fetal death has occurred in previous pregnancies, and subsequent ones are planned according to the result. If the peak is low, the next amniocentesis may be done at the thirty-second week; if it is higher, the next study may be made at the thirtieth week; if it is even higher, immediate treatment may be indicated. Shulman has divided Rh-sensitized women into four groups, based upon the Δ OD 450 mμ between 28 and 34 weeks. Group A (Δ OD 450 0 to 0.025 mμ) are so mild that they usually can be delivered at term. Group B (Δ OD 450 0.026 to 0.1 mμ) should be restudied in 2 weeks; if the peak is lower, the pregnancy is allowed to continue with delivery planned

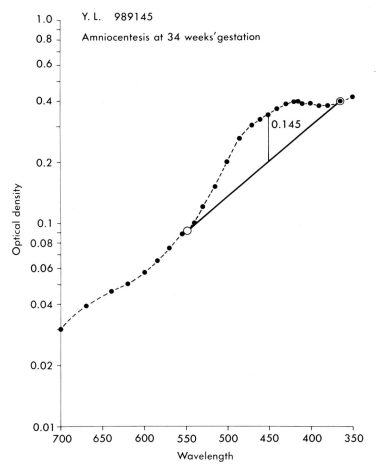

Fig. 32-2. Optical density 450 mμ. Abnormal elevation is at 34 weeks. Repeat amniocentesis in 1 week is indicated.

after the thirty-seventh week. Group C (Δ OD 450 0.11 to 0.23 mμ) should be re-studied weekly; if the peaks are lower, the baby should be delivered between the thirty-fourth and the thirty-seventh weeks. Group D (Δ OD 450 0.25 mμ or higher) should either be treated or delivered at once.

Amniotic fluid should be examined only if the antibody titer is positive because there is a risk of introducing fetal cells into the maternal circulation during needle amnio-centesis.

The babies of mothers who have experienced previous fetal death before the thirty-fifth week of pregnancy or those with a spectrophotometric study in the upper zone during the early part of the third trimester may be saved by *intrauterine intraperitoneal transfusion*. A long needle is inserted into the amniotic cavity through the maternal

abdominal and uterine walls under fluoro-scopic control until it penetrates the fetal abdominal wall. Packed Rh-negative red blood cells are injected into the fetal peritoneal cavity and are absorbed intact into its circulation. Since Rh_o (D) negative cells will not be hemolyzed, they will remain in the fetal circulation. The transfusion can be repeated one or more times during the following few weeks until the fetus is large enough to survive outside the uterus. With adequate transfusion the hematocrit can be increased to a normal level, and almost all the cells in the newborn infant will be of the adult type. Most babies will need one or more exchange transfusions after birth.

Intrauterine transfusions have been performed 120 times, in 69 babies, in the University of Michigan Hospital. Of these, 25 were born alive, survived, and appear to be developing normally. The remaining 44 died either as a direct result of the treatment or because there was not time to transfuse them adequately before intrauterine death or delivery. In each instance we would have anticipated 100% fetal loss without prenatal treatment.

Treatment of the infant. Whenever a patient who probably has an erythroblastotic baby is in labor or her delivery is planned, preparations should be made to examine and treat the baby as soon as it is born. A pediatrician experienced with exchange transfusion should be present at the delivery. A specimen of cord blood is obtained for blood typing, hematocrit, reticulocyte count, bilirubin, and an indirect Coombs' test. Exchange transfusion should be performed promptly if the baby has erythroblastosis and the hematocrit is low. Kernicterus, one of the major causes of death and disability in premature infants with erythroblastosis, can be almost completely prevented by transfusion.

Prevention. Our present management of erythroblastosis is crude and ineffective when compared to what could be achieved by prevention. Rh_o (D) immune globulin (human) when injected intramuscularly into unsensitized Rh_o (D) negative individuals will prevent the development of an antigen against Rh_o (D) positive red blood cells. Ascari and co-workers, reporting on a cooperative study, found that only 1 of 1,081 unsensitized Rh_o (D) negative women who were treated with this material after the delivery of an Rh_o (D) positive infant became sensitized, whereas 51 of 726 control women developed antibodies.

We now give Rh_o (D) immune globulin (human) to all unsensitized Rh_o (D) negative women during the first 72 hours after they have delivered an Rh_o (D) positive infant. Those selected for treatment must be Rh_o (D) negative without identifiable antibodies, and the baby must be Rh_o (D) positive with a negative direct antiglobulin (Coombs') test on cord blood. An Rh_o (D) negative patient who has aborted a pregnancy more than 10 weeks after the onset of the last menstrual period should also be treated if her husband is positive, even though the blood type of the embryo cannot be determined. An antibody study should be obtained 6 weeks after delivery and twice

during subsequent pregnancies. Unsensitized women should be treated after each delivery.

In most instances fetal red blood cells enter the maternal circulation at the time of delivery, and the volume of the feto-maternal transfusion determines whether or not sensitization will occur and even whether or not the gamma globulin will afford protection. Every effort should be made to keep transfusion at a minimum by allowing the blood to drain out of the placenta before it is delivered and by avoiding manual removal and cord traction to reduce the possibility of fetal vessels being torn. Drainage and simple expression of the detached placenta combined with immune globulin will keep sensitization at a minimum.

■ Erythroblastosis fetalis resulting from ABO incompatibility

A fetus of blood group A, AB, or B may develop hemolytic disease from maternal antibodies against any of the antigens not already present in the mother's blood. For instance, if the mother is blood type O, she may become sensitized to either A or B, or if she is A and her fetus is B or AB, she may become sensitized to B.

This situation is similar to Rh sensitization in several ways, but there are differences. Rh sensitization always occurs because of a transfusion of Rh_o (D) positive red blood cells into the maternal blood; ABO sensitization may also develop in this manner, but there are naturally occurring antibodies that may already be present when the patient becomes pregnant for the first time. The antigen responsible for ABO sensitization is secreted in body fluids, as well as being contained in red blood cells. Thus a mother can become sensitized by the antigen "secreted" by the fetus in amniotic fluid that is reabsorbed into the maternal circulation.

There is no reliable way to prognosticate the development of ABO incompatibility during the prenatal period, as there is with Rh erythroblastosis fetalis, but it can be anticipated by comparing the blood group of the mother with that of the child's father. If the mother's blood group is O and the father's is A, B, or AB, the infant is a candidate for ABO incompatibility and a direct antiglobulin (Coombs') test should be run on cord blood. Fortunately the process is almost never as severe as that caused by Rh sensitization. The treatment is exchange transfusion.

■ Fetal hypoxia during labor

The fetus in utero is entirely dependent upon the mother for its supply of oxygen, which it obtains from the maternal blood in the placental sinuses. Circulation of the blood through the sinuses is regulated by the mother's arterial blood pressure and by the activity of the uterine muscle. Maternal blood is injected into the sinuses in spurts from the open ends of spiral arterioles that are scattered, with corresponding venous channels, in the uterine wall beneath the placenta. Some of the blood is forced laterally into the marginal lakes, from which it is returned to the general circulation. Most of it, however, gravitates downward through the branching villi and leaves the intervillous space by way of the venous openings at the base. The pressure within the intervillous space is about the same as, or slightly higher than, the amniotic fluid pressure, being about 5 to 10 mm. Hg when the uterus is at rest and as high as 55 mm. Hg at the peak of a contraction. The intervillous pressure rises during a contraction because the veins are kinked and compressed by the uterine muscle fibers before the caliber of the more resistant arterioles is affected. Thus blood continues to flow into the spaces for some time after its means of egress is closed. Under normal circumstances, during a uterine contraction, the pressure within the intervillous space is lower than the capillary pressure in the placental villi, which is maintained by changes in fetal blood pressure. This prevents the villi from collapsing and impeding the flow of blood through the fetal vessels and permits the exchange of materials back and forth between the fetal and the maternal circulations even during a contraction.

The fetal oxygen supply can be reduced by any of the following:

1. *Reduction in blood flow through the maternal vessels.* The caliber of the arteries may be reduced by spasm in women with hypertensive complications of pregnancy, thus limiting blood flow. It is estimated that arterial blood flow is reduced by 50% in women with hypertensive disease. The flow

of blood will also be impaired whenever the maternal systolic blood pressure is lower than the amniotic fluid pressure. Fetal hypoxia is likely to develop when maternal blood pressure levels fall below 60 mm. Hg. The veins or even the spiral arterioles may be compressed by rapidly recurring or tetanic uterine contractions.

2. *Reduction in blood flow through the uterine sinuses.* This is most often a result of prolonged or tetanic uterine contractions or a reduction in maternal systolic blood pressure.

3. *Reduction of the oxygen content of maternal blood.* The available circulating maternal hemoglobin can be reduced by chronic anemia or hemorrhage, thereby reducing the total oxygen capacity.

4. *Alterations in fetal circulation.* The circulation of blood through the vessels of the infant's body and placenta is maintained by the cardiac action of the baby. Anything that alters its normal function will impair the circulation, as will compression of the umbilical cord. Placental infarction or separation will decrease the total area available for oxygen transfer from the maternal blood, and if a considerable portion of placenta is involved, the infant cannot survive.

The rate and rhythm of the fetal heart provide the only readily available information concerning the condition of the unborn infant. The normal heart rate varies between 120 and 160 beats per minute; rates above and particularly below these extremes suggest the possibility of hypoxia. During each uterine contraction the heart rate decreases 10 or more beats below the previous level. As the uterus relaxes, the heart returns to its original rate. A decrease in the infant's oxygen supply can be suspected when a change in the fetal heart rate or in its rhythm is detected. The early phases of intrauterine hypoxia are more often indicated by a decrease than an increase in fetal heart rate, but terminally the rate may be extremely rapid.

Hon has recorded the heart rate patterns of normally oxygenated infants and those whose oxygen supply was impaired during labor. He described *early deceleration,* which occurs during each contraction and which he considers to be normal. The heart rate begins to decrease a few seconds after the onset of the uterine contraction and returns to its

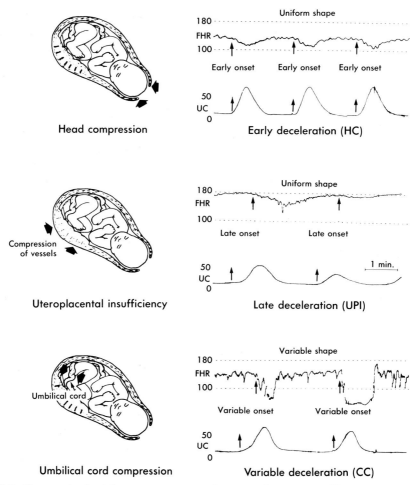

Fig. 32-3. Changes in fetal heart rate patterns due to various causes. (From Hon, E. H.: An atlas of fetal heart rate patterns, New Haven, Conn., 1968, Harty Press, Inc.)

normal level before the uterus is completely relaxed. He attributes this to increased intracranial pressure and vagus nerve stimulation. The pattern associated with umbilical cord compression is described as *variable deceleration*. The onset of the deceleration occurs at any time during the contraction and persists after the uterus has relaxed. The duration of deceleration is variable, and the curve, unlike that of normal labor, does not follow the curve of intrauterine pressure. The variation in heart rate is a result of altered hemodynamics as blood flow through the compressed cord vessels is reduced. The recovery period after each contraction becomes progressively prolonged as labor advances. *Late deceleration* occurs with prolonged forceful contractions and is thought to be indicative of hypoxia from

decreased blood flow through the intervillous spaces. The deceleration begins late in the uterine contraction phase, and the heart rate returns to normal slowly after the uterus relaxes and blood flow is restored.

Although the subtle changes that can be recorded by electronic methods will not usually be detected by clinical examination, the condition of the fetus can be appraised with reasonable accuracy by careful auscultation. *Whenever the fetal heart rate decreases 20 beats per minute or more or falls to less than 100 beats per minute during a uterine contraction, decreased oxygenation should be suspected.* An increase in rate during contractions is of less significance. A decrease in heart rate and the passage of meconium when the vertex is presenting is far more significant than either is alone. A reduction in fetal oxygenation stimulates peristalsis and relaxes the anal sphincter. The passage of meconium in breech positions means little because the meconium is squeezed from the colon by mechanical pressure.

Fetal hypoxia must be detected early if the physician hopes to prevent permanent cerebral damage; consequently the heart tones must be checked at regular intervals. It is well to listen to the heart at least every half hour during the first stage and at least every 5 minutes after cervical dilatation is complete. The rate should be determined during or just after a contraction rather than in the interval between contractions when the uterus is quiescent. Whenever a change in rate or rhythm is detected, pure oxygen should be administered to the mother by mask or catheter, and a vaginal examination should be performed in an attempt to determine the cause.

If no obvious cause is found and if the heart tones remain normal while the mother is inhaling oxygen, labor can be permitted to continue until it is possible to deliver the infant safely, unless the signs of oxygen deficiency recur. It usually is advisable to deliver the infant presumed to be anoxic if the cervix is completely dilated and the presenting part is low in the pelvis, if the extraction can be performed without risk to the baby or the mother. On the other hand, if the cervix is not fully dilated or if the presenting part is high, vaginal delivery may be more dangerous for the infant than the presumed oxygen deficiency. Cesarean section is seldom indicated simply because of possible intrauterine hypoxia, but may be lifesaving in properly selected patients.

A more accurate method for determining the presence of hypoxia in the fetus is to *measure blood pH* and concentrations of oxygen and carbon dioxide. This can be accomplished by obtaining fetal blood by scalp puncture during labor. The fetal blood pH is a more important indicator of hypoxia than is either P_{O_2} or P_{CO_2}, but the pH of the mother's blood must also be measured because the fetus will also be acidotic if the mother is. The techniques are not readily available in general hospitals and are inaccurate unless performed with great care. Single evaluations are of no great value unless they are abnormal because the conditions change as labor advances.

Prolapsed umbilical cord. If a loop of the umbilical cord has prolapsed past the presenting part, it will be compressed against the pelvic wall with every uterine contraction. Each time this occurs, the blood flow through the umbilical vessels ceases, cardiac output is decreased, and the fetal blood pressure falls. The resultant hypoxia is indicated by a fall in the fetal heart rate. Prolapsed cord has no effect upon either the mother or on the course of labor, but unless the obstruction to the fetal circulation is relieved, the infant may die before delivery.

The incidence of prolapse is about 0.5%; it occurs less frequently when the presenting part fits the pelvis snugly, as it does with normal vertex or frank breech positions, than with certain abnormalities. The main etiologic factors are those that prevent the presenting part from occluding the pelvic inlet. These include: (1) complete breech positions; (2) transverse lies, particularly those in which the back lies superiorly; (3) low-lying placenta with marginal insertion of the cord; (4) a long cord; (5) hydramnios; (6) premature rupture of the membranes; and (7) upward displacement of the presenting part during examinations or operations for delivery. The cord can only prolapse after the membranes rupture.

Cord pressure can be suspected whenever the heart rate during a contraction decreases more than 20 beats per minute. The diagnosis can usually be made by vaginal examination. If the membranes have not yet ruptured, the cord may be felt in the intact forebag below the presenting part. This is called a *forelying cord* and is somewhat less serious than a complete prolapse. The forewaters provide a cushion that may impede descent of the infant and thereby reduce the pressure on the umbilical vessels. With *complete prolapse* the cord falls through the cervix and descends into the vagina or even through the introitus. It can be seen or felt without difficulty. An *occult prolapse* is one in which a loop of cord lies alongside the presenting part. The altered heart rate with each contraction is obvious, but the cord is so high that it may be impossible to feel it. Additional information can sometimes be obtained by manipulating the presenting part in the inlet. It is pushed against each lateral pelvic wall, the pubis anteriorly and the sacrum posteriorly, while the heart rate is

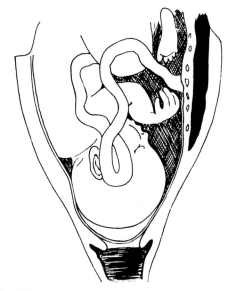

Fig. 32-4. Occult prolapse of the umbilical cord.

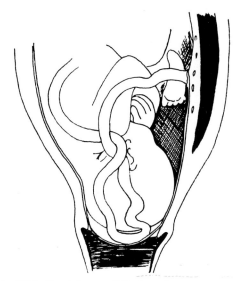

Fig. 32-5. Forelying umbilical cord.

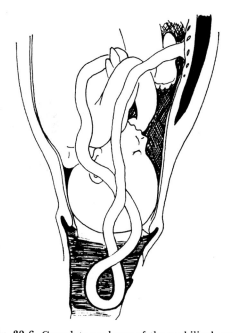

Fig. 32-6. Complete prolapse of the umbilical cord.

counted. A significant decrease in rate when the head is pushed against a specific area of the bony pelvis suggests that it may be compressing a loop of cord.

Treatment of prolapsed cord is unsatisfactory, and infant mortality is high because the cord often is extruded early in labor before the patient has even entered the hospital. By the time the diagnosis is made the infant has already died. No form of treat-

ment will salvage an infant whose heart tones are slow and irregular between contractions; under such circumstances any treatment that adds to the maternal risk is unwarranted.

If a forelying cord is diagnosed during early labor, cesarean section is almost always indicated. If cervical dilatation is almost complete, the presenting part is low in the pelvis, and the baby can be delivered promptly when the membranes rupture, labor may be allowed to continue. The patient should be transported to the delivery room, and the physician should scrub and be prepared to interfere at once if the cord prolapses. Voluntary bearing-down efforts, which may rupture the membranes, can be prevented by the administration of saddle block anesthesia. This is more often applicable to multiparas than to primigravidas.

When an actual prolapse is diagnosed during early labor, cesarean section should be performed if the fetal heart rate is normal. While preparations for the operation are being made, the mother should be placed in Trendelenburg position and given oxygen while an attendant holds the presenting part out of the pelvis with his sterile gloved hand in the vagina to prevent interruption of the fetal circulation. If the heart tones are absent or slow and irregular, any form of operative interference is unwarranted.

If the cord prolapses late in the first stage or during the second stage, it usually is possible to complete delivery by forceps or breech extraction. If the cervix is not yet completely dilated, it can be incised.

It is seldom possible to return the cord to the uterine cavity successfully, but if the conditions are such that labor cannot be terminated, an attempt should be made to replace it. The patient is placed in deep Trendelenburg or knee-chest position, the protruding loop of cord is cleansed, the presenting part is displaced upward, and the cord is returned to the uterine cavity. If the presenting part can then be forced downward to occlude the cervical opening, the cord may remain within the uterus. The Trendelenburg position should be maintained, and a firm abdominal binder applied to keep the presenting part pressed into the pelvis.

Cord entanglement or short cord. If a long cord is looped several times around the neck, body, or extremities of the infant, it may be compressed as the loops are drawn tight during descent. The fetal heart rate decreases during each contraction, but no evidence of prolapse can be detected. Occasionally the physician can suspect this abnormality if he can keep the head from descending during a contraction by pushing upward on it with his hand in the vagina. This prevents the loops from tightening, and the fetal heart rate will remain within normal limits until the manual pressure is released.

If the abnormality first occurs during late labor, it may be possible to complete the delivery without risk. During early labor cesarean section will be effective if cord entanglement is actually producing the change. It is difficult to make an accurate diagnosis because the cord cannot be felt; consequently the physician should consider all the other things that can alter the fetal heart rate before operative delivery is decided upon.

Intracranial hemorrhage. If fetal intracranial hemorrhage occurs during labor, the heart tones may become irregular between as well as during contractions. They usually fail to improve when oxygen is administered.

Head pressure. Occasionally a marked depression in fetal heart rate will be detected late in the second stage when the head is distending the perineum. Since it is impossible to differentiate bradycardia caused by increased intracranial pressure from that caused by hypoxia, it usually is wise to com-

plete the delivery when this can be accomplished without endangering the mother or the baby. Difficult operative extraction may cause more fetal damage than a short period of mild oxygen deprivation.

■ Care of the newborn infant

Most infants make the change from intrauterine to extrauterine existence without difficulty, but some need the help of the physician. The normal infant cries and begins to breathe within 1 minute of its birth without artificial stimulation. Mucus and blood should be aspirated from the mouth and nasopharynx after the head is born or soon after the completion of the delivery. If the infant breathes and seems to be normal, it can be placed in its crib, covered with a light blanket, and watched by a nurse until the placenta has been delivered and necessary repair performed.

Apnea neonatorum. Apnea neonatorum, failure of the newborn infant to breathe spontaneously, can cause extensive damage to the brain and even death if it is not corrected promptly. Although newly born infants are more tolerant of oxygen deprivation than are older children and adults, resuscitative measures should be instituted promptly if respiration is not established within 1 minute.

The causes of apnea neonatorum are varied and not always obvious. The establishment of normal respiration may be prevented by brain damage from intrauterine anoxia. Infants who are narcotized by drugs administered to the mother may be unable to breathe; this is particularly true if inhalation anesthesia is also used. Other causes are injury or malformation such as hypoplasia of the lungs or defects in the diaphragm that permit the bowel to herniate into the chest.

Apnea neonatorum can be diagnosed if the infant does not begin to breathe spontaneously within 1 minute of its birth. The evidences of oxygen lack will be more pronounced in those babies who have suffered intrauterine hypoxia than in those who were well oxygenated until they were born. Apgar has suggested a method for determining the condition of the infant 1 minute after birth based upon five objective signs; each is evaluated and scored as 0, 1, or 2. The highest possible score, 10, indicates an

Table 10. Signs for determining condition of newborn infant*

Sign	0	1	2
Heart rate	Absent	Below 100	Over 100
Respiratory effort	Absent	Slow, irregular	Good, crying
Response to catheter in nostril	None	Grimace	Cough or sneeze
Muscle tone	Limp	Some flexion of extremities	Active motion
Color	Blue, pale	Body pink, extremities blue	Completely pink

*Modified from Apgar, V.: The role of the anesthesiologist in reducing neonatal mortality, New York J. Med. 55:2365, 1955.

optimal condition; most normal infants are scored between 7 and 10. Those who are moderately depressed will usually have scores between 4 and 7. The muscle tone is usually somewhat reduced and the infant is cyanotic, but the heart beats at a rate of 100 beats per minute or more. These infants usually respond to stimuli and can be resuscitated without difficulty. Those with scores below 4 are severely depressed and must be treated promptly if they are to survive. Many of these infants are already suffering from cerebral damage.

The most important factors in treating apnea neonatorum are to clear the air passages and to deliver oxygen to the lungs. Since many infants have aspirated blood, mucus, and debris from the vagina during delivery, the first step in treatment consists of aspirating the nasopharynx and the trachea. The need for tracheal aspiration is obvious if the sternum and rib cage retract each time the infant attempts to take a breath. The tracheal catheter, a woven silk urethral catheter or a small polyethylene tube, can be inserted through the larynx, which has been exposed with an infant laryngoscope, or it can be passed without the use of an instrument. The latter method is entirely satisfactory and can be learned easily.

The shoulders of the infant lying in the dorsal position are elevated on the palm of the nurse's hand; this permits the head to fall backward and straightens the air passages. The index finger of the left hand is inserted into the infant's mouth until it touches the epiglottis, which is pulled forward exposing the larynx. The tip of the catheter is passed along the finger until it lies

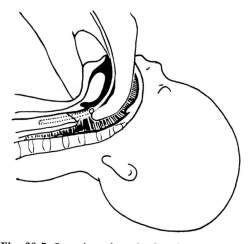

Fig. 32-7. Insertion of tracheal catheter.

over the laryngeal opening. It is directed between the vocal cords by the left index fingertip and is pushed downward into the trachea with a rotary motion. As the catheter is slowly withdrawn, mouth suction is applied to draw the tracheal secretions into a trap at the end of the tube. This is repeated until the trachea is clear.

The infant may begin to breathe spontaneously as the passage is being cleared; if it does not, the next step becomes necessary. With the catheter in the trachea, the lungs are inflated by gently blowing through the tube; only enough pressure to expand the chest cage slightly is necessary. As the pressure is released, the lung can be emptied by gently compressing the chest wall by fingertip pressure. This maneuver, repeated at a rate of about 20 times a minute, will supply air to the lungs; as a result the heart rate will increase and the color will improve.

When the infant begins to breathe by its

own efforts, the catheter can be removed and a mask held above the face to deliver oxygen. An infant who has suffered from apnea neonatorum should remain in an incubator until its respirations are normal.

It is difficult to insert a tracheal cannula in an infant whose muscle tone is good or in one who is gasping, but fortunately it is seldom necessary. In such infants simple measures such as snapping the soles of the feet or rubbing the back or chest may be all that is required to help initiate normal respiration. An oxygen mask should be held over the face until the baby is breathing normally.

All resuscitative maneuvers should be performed gently. There is no place for rough and potentially traumatic procedures such as holding the baby upside down and slapping it, anal dilatation, etc.

Drugs such as pentylenetetrazol (Metrazol) and alpha lobeline are of little value in the treatment of apnea. The infant who has been narcotized by morphine or a similar substance can usually be stimulated by injecting 0.2 mg. of nalorphine HCl (Nalline) into the umbilical vein. This drug is contraindicated if barbiturates have been used and is ineffective in counteracting the depression caused by anesthetic agents.

Ligation of the cord. The blood in the fetal circulation is distributed between the vessels in the infant's body and those in the placenta. At the end of the second trimester about one half of the total blood is in the placenta, but as the baby grows larger, relatively more is contained within the infant itself. The blood volume of the newly born baby is only about 250 to 300 ml. Consequently as much as possible must be preserved.

If clamping and ligation of the cord are delayed for several minutes after the baby is born, as much as 100 ml. of blood will be transferred from the placenta to the baby. The same result can be obtained by stripping the cord from the vulva toward the infant repeatedly until no more blood enters the vessels from the placental end.

The cord is ligated in normal infants with a tie, rubber band, or clamp placed close to the skin edge, and the cord is severed about 1 cm. distal to the ligature. A short length of cord is less likely to serve as a source of infection than a long one. If the mother is Rh negative, the tie is placed 8 to 10 cm.

from the umbilicus to preserve the vessels for exchange transfusion if the infant has erythroblastosis.

The physician should count blood vessels in the umbilical cord because congenital anomalies, many unsuspected, have been reported in from 20% to 47% of newborn infants with a single umbilical artery. Feingold, Fine, and Ingall performed intravenous pyelograms in 24 infants with this defect and found unsuspected anomalies of the urinary tract in 8 (33%) of them. The incidence of absence of one umbilical artery is between 0.5% and 1% in singly born infants and as high as 7% in twins.

The cord mummifies and drops off on about the fifth day of life, leaving a small raw area at the umbilicus, which heals rapidly. Occasionally the stump of the cord becomes infected and edematous and serves as a source of entry for bacteria into the infant's bloodstream.

Treatment of the eyes. Crede in 1884 suggested that a silver nitrate solution be instilled into the eyes of newborn infants as an aid in preventing gonorrheal ophthalmia. Although this did reduce the incidence of eye infections, the development of penicillin and other antibiotic agents has made it less useful than it was in previous years.

Two drops of freshly prepared 1% solution of silver nitrate are dropped into the conjunctival sac, and after 1 minute the chemical is flushed out with warm physiologic salt solution. Some infants develop a mild conjunctivitis from 1% silver nitrate. Stronger solutions may cause permanent blindness. Individual-dose wax ampules especially prepared for newborn infants should be used.

Gonorrheal ophthalmia can be prevented by a single injection of 50,000 units of penicillin, but in many states the law still requires that silver nitrate be used. Penicillin, of course, is far more effective for treating established infections than is silver nitrate or any other chemical.

References

Abramson, H.: Resuscitation of the newborn infant, St. Louis, ed. 2, 1966, The C. V. Mosby Co.

Apgar, V.: Drugs in pregnancy, J.A.M.A. **190:** 840, 1964.

Apgar, V., Holaday, D. A., James, L. S., and Weisbrat, I. M.: Evaluation of the newborn infant; second report, J.A.M.A. **168:**1985, 1958.

Ascari, W. Q., Allen, A. E., Baker, W. J., and

Pollack, W.: Rh$_o$ (D) immune globulin (human). Evaluation in women at risk of Rh immunization, J.A.M.A. **205:**1, 1968.

Cook, C. D., Lucey, J. F., Drorbaugh, J. E., Segal, S., Sutherland, J. M., and Smith, C. A.: Apnea and respiratory distress in the newborn infant, New Eng. J. Med. **254:**562, 1956.

Davidson, H. H., Hill, J. H., and Eastman, N. J.: Penicillin in prophylaxis of opththalmia neonatorum, J.A.M.A. **145:**1052, 1951.

Desmond, M. M., Moore, J., Lindley, J. E., and Brown, C. A.: Meconium staining of the amniotic fluid; a marker of fetal hypoxia, Obstet. Gynec. **9:**91, 1957.

Feingold, M., Fine, R. N., and Ingall, D.: Intravenous pyelography in infants with single umbilical artery, New Eng. J. Med. **270:**1178, 1964.

Kline, A. H., Blattner, R. J., and Lunin, M.: Transplacental effect of tretracyclines on teeth, J.A.M.A. **188:**178, 1964.

Liley, A. W.: Liquor amnii analysis in the management of pregnancy complicated by rhesus sensitization, Amer. J. Obstet. Gynec. **82:**1359, 1961.

McCausland, A. M., Holmes, F., and Schumann, W. R.: I. Management of cord and placental blood and its effect upon the newborn, Part I, Calif. Med. **71:**190, 1949; Part II, Western J. Surg. **58:**591, 1950.

Mengert, W. F., and Longwell, F. H.: Prolapse of the umbilical cord, Amer. J. Obstet. Gynec. **40:**79, 1940.

Nyhan, W. L., and Lampert, F.: Response of the fetus and newborn to drugs, Anesthesiology **26:**487, 1965.

Reynolds, S. M. R.: Regulation of the fetal circulation, Clin. Obstet. Gynec. **3:**834, 1960.

Rodriguez, S. U., Leikin, S. L., and Hiller, M. C.: Neonatal thrombocytopenia associated with antepartum administration of thiazide drugs, New Eng. J. Med. **270:**881, 1964.

Work, B., Jaffe, R. B., Campbell, C., and Whitehouse, W.: A technic of intrauterine transfusion of the fetus, Obstet. Gynec. **27:**319, 1966.

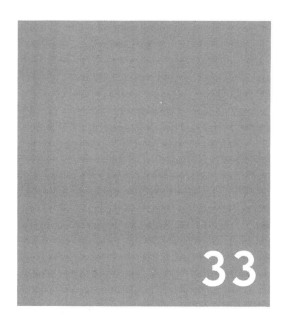

33

Dystocia and prolonged labor

The maximum duration of normal labor has been set at 24 hours; those that extend beyond this period are termed *prolonged*. Some classify multiparous labors of more than 18 hours' duration as prolonged. Long or difficult labors, to which the term *dystocia* is applied, can be caused by ineffective uterine contractions, by abnormalities in the size or position of the fetus, and by alterations in the structure of the birth canal.

■ Dystocia from uterine dysfunction

At the onset of normal labor the uterine contractions last only a few seconds and occur irregularly, but they rapidly increase in frequency, intensity, and duration. Toward the end of labor they may recur at 2-minute intervals and last as long as 90 seconds. The contractions in women with uterine dysfunction recur irregularly every 4 to 8 minutes or more and may last a maximum of 30 to 45 seconds. Although the contractions may be quite uncomfortable, dilatation of the cervix

often does not proceed beyond 4 cm.; this is called a *prolonged latent phase of labor*. When these patients do progress beyond the latent phase, one of three things may happen: (1) the active phase may be normal; (2) the active phase may be slow, the cervix dilating at a rate of less than 1 cm. per hour, and continue this way until delivery (*slow slope active phase*); or (3) an active phase begins, but progress eventually ceases before cervical dilatation is complete (*active phase arrest*).

The gradient of force exerted by the uterine contractions during normal labor is from the fundus to the cervix, and as labor advances the upper segment progressively becomes shorter and its walls thicker as the individual muscle fibers retract. The rising inferior border of the upper segment exerts traction on the lower segment and the effaced cervix, which is pulled upward around the presenting part as the latter is pushed through the gradually enlarging opening. This orderly sequence of events does not occur with uterine dysfunction; either the force of the contractions or the gradient of activity from the fundus downward toward the cervix is altered.

According to Caldeyro and associates there are two kinds of uterine dysfunction that can be distinguished with the tocodynamometer: one characterized by weak contractions but with a normal gradient, and one characterized by incoordinate uterine action. In the latter type, contractions may be initiated by both pacemakers at once rather than by one of them at a time, several areas of myometrium may contract independently and without synchronization, or abnormal contraction waves may spread upward toward the fundus from their sites of origin in the lower part of the uterus (inverted gradient). None of these is effective in retracting and dilating the cervix, even though the amniotic fluid pressure may increase considerably during each contraction.

Although the type of uterine dysfunction cannot be determined precisely without special recording instruments, an abnormal latent or active phase of cervical dilatation can be diagnosed by clinical observation. During normal labor the upper portion of the uterus contracts firmly, whereas the lower segment feels much more relaxed. At the height of a normal contraction the uterus becomes so hard that it cannot be indented with finger pressure. In contrast, with uterine dysfunction the duration of each contraction is less, and the uterus is less firm and can easily be indented with pressure of the fingertips. As a result of the incoordinate activity the muscle fibers of the upper segment fail to retract, development of the lower segment is incomplete, and the cervix remains thick and dilates slowly, or dilatation may cease. The cervix often hangs down ahead of the presenting part instead of being applied tightly against it as in normal labor. Under these circumstances failure of the cervix to dilate in the usual manner is a result of inadequate uterine action rather than of local abnormality in the cervical tissues.

Abnormal progress in either the latent or the active phase can be recognized promptly when cervical dilatation is plotted on a nor-

mal labor curve. The maximum normal latent phase for primigravidas is 17 hours and for multiparas 11.5 hours. *Prolonged latent phase* can be suspected whenever the latent phase extends 2 hours or more beyond the mean of 7.26 hours for primigravidas and 4.14 hours for multiparas. Since the cervix should dilate progressively during the active phase, abnormalities of this part of labor can be recognized early. A *slow slope active phase* can be diagnosed whenever cervical dilatation progresses at a rate less than 0.7 cm./hr. in primigravidas and less than 1.1 cm./hr. in multiparas. An *active phase arrest* can be diagnosed if cervical dilatation does not change during a 2-hour period. By studying the slope of the active-phase curve, the physician does not have to wait until the normal mean duration is exceeded to diagnose dysfunction.

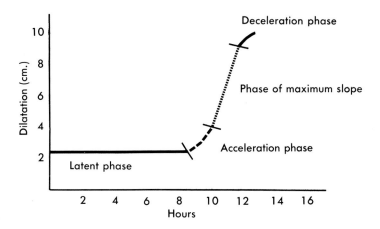

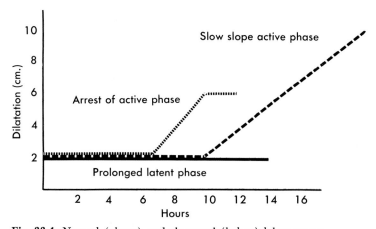

Fig. 33-1. Normal (above) and abnormal (below) labor curves.

Etiology. Uterine dysfunction is almost always encountered in *primigravidas* and rarely recurs during subsequent labors. This fact eliminates structural abnormalities of the uterus or faulty nerve supply as etiologic factors. It is often stated that a prolonged latent phase can be caused by the administration of *analgesic drugs* too early in labor, but this is doubtful. Many women who are given drugs during the latent phase continue to progress at a regular rate, and the quality of the contractions during early normal labor often improves after the patient is relaxed by medication. Analgesics certainly can increase an abnormality already present, but they probably do not cause it. *Overdistention of the uterus* by hydramnios or multiple pregnancy may decrease the efficiency of the uterine contractions, thus delaying progress. A *slow slope active phase,* during which the cervix dilates progressively but at a rate slower than that anticipated, almost always occurs in primigravidas, and no specific cause can be found.

Active phase arrest, in which the cervix fails to dilate over a period of 2 hours, is an ominous sign because it is the most common pattern encountered with cephalopelvic disproportion in primigravidas. Active phase arrest is less likely to occur with cephalopelvic disproportion in multiparas.

Dysfunctional labor may be partly of *emotional origin;* the abnormal labor serves as an attempt to avoid the delivery of an infant that is a threat to the patient, who often is a dependent personality and usually has intense feelings of guilt related to sex and pregnancy. She may express fear that the baby will be abnormal or that she herself will die. These patients show little interest in the pregnancy and only rarely ask questions or evidence any desire to know what is happening or what to expect. It sometimes is possible to predict uterine dysfunction during the prenatal period.

Effect of uterine dysfunction. Prolongation of labor and the consequent multiple orificial examinations increase the incidence of intrauterine infection. The infant may aspirate infected amniotic contents, or the organisms may be disseminated through the infant's bloodstream after invading the placenta. Perinatal mortality is definitely increased by prolonged labor.

The defective uterine contractions usually continue into the third stage, thereby increasing the incidence of postpartum hemorrhage. This is far more serious if labor has been so long that the mother is exhausted and dehydrated and the blood is concentrated. Blood loss may also be increased by injury from operative delivery, which is necessary more often than with normal labor.

Management of uterine dysfunction. Dysfunctional labor can usually be suspected within 6 or 8 hours after the labor begins because the contractions remain irregular and short and produce little change in the cervix or the station of the presenting part. The physician should not wait until he can diagnose dysfunctional latent or active phase on the basis of elapsed time to start his study and treatment.

Although the management of dysfunctional latent phase differs somewhat from that of dysfunctional active phase, these are certain principles that are essential to the proper management of any prolonged labor regardless of the cause. These include evaluation, protection against infection, sedation, and hydration.

Evaluation. A sterile vaginal examination with the patient in dorsal lithotomy position should be performed as soon as dysfunctional labor is suspected. Unanticipated abnormalities in fetal position or cephalopelvic disproportion may be diagnosed, and the consistency and dilatation of the cervix can be determined. X-ray pelvimetry is an important part of the evaluation of women with dysfunctional labor even though cephalopelvic disproportion is seldom a cause.

Protection against infection. Vaginal examinations should be limited because bacteria are carried directly through the cervix on the fingers. Penicillin, 1.2 million units, and streptomycin, 0.5 Gm., may be given every 12 hours if the patient has fever or if it becomes evident that labor will last more than 24 hours.

Sedation. Analgesic drugs administered as during normal labor will usually decrease both the force and the frequency of uterine contractions and prolong labor even more. A phenothiazine preparation such as Phenergan or Sparine, 50 mg., will relax the patient and ease her tension without altering the contraction mechanism. If normal uterine activity can be achieved with oxytocics, any of

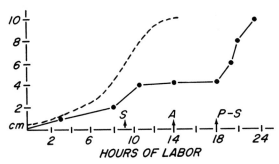

Fig. 33-2. Labor graph of a primigravida with a prolonged latent phase of labor. Sedation was given at 9 hours, and an amniotomy was performed at the fourteenth hour. The latent phase persisted until Pitocin was given. The position was right occiput posterior; the infant weighed 2,405 grams. **S**, Sedation; **P**, Pitocin; **A**, amniotomy.

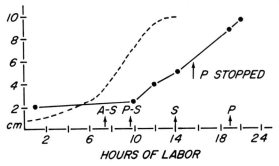

Fig. 33-3. Labor graph of a primigravida with a dysfunctional latent and a slow slope active phase of labor. Notice that amniotomy and sedation did not terminate the latent phase but Pitocin did. Pitocin did not influence the slope of the active phase. Position was left occiput transverse; the infant weighed 3,543 grams. **A**, Amniotomy; **P**, Pitocin; **S**, sedation.

the methods used to control pain during normal labor are applicable.

Fluids. Patients with prolonged labor should be kept well hydrated, particularly during the hot, humid summer months when loss through the skin is excessive. From 2 to 3 L. of fluid are necessary every 24 hours. Since absorption from the stomach is reduced during labor, the fluid should be given intravenously as 10% dextrose.

Dysfunctional latent phase. The frequency with which the diagnosis of latent phase dysfunction is made is in part determined by the obstetrician's decision as to when labor began. To use labor graphs effectively he must make an arbitrary decision when the patient is admitted that labor began at the time she first felt painful uterine contractions. It is true that some of these women will actually be in false labor and will be discharged, but this practice permits early recognition of latent phase abnormalities. A latent phase that extends beyond the normal on a labor graph cannot easily be ignored.

An attempt should be made to correct the abnormality as soon as it becomes evident, by the fact that contractions do not assume a normal pattern and that there is no appreciable change in the cervix, that labor is not progressing at a normal rate. At the end of the sixth or eighth hour of dysfunctional labor a *sterile vaginal examination* is performed to determine fetal position and station and the condition of the cervix. *X-ray pelvimetry* is ordered if there is a question of cephalopelvic disproportion. *Amniotomy* at

this time may be followed by an improvement in uterine contractions and rapid conversion to a normal pattern. If amniotomy is to have no effect upon the pattern, it will be obvious within an hour or two. At that time the uterus should be stimulated with *dilute oxytocin solution.* The method by which this solution is administered is described in the discussion on induction of labor (p. 363). The dosage necessary to stimulate normal contractions may be slightly higher than that required for induction of labor at term, but at the beginning no more than 0.5 to 1 mU./min. of oxytocin should be delivered. If this is not enough to induce a normal contraction pattern, the dosage can be increased gradually. Almost all will enter the active phase with amniotomy and oxytocin stimulation and in some the labor will progress normally without continuing stimulation, but many will develop active phase dysfunction if the oxytocin is stopped.

Slow slope active phase cannot be altered significantly by either amniotomy or oxytocin. If cervical dilatation is progressing at a regular, but reduced, rate and if there is no concern over the adequacy of the pelvis, no active treatment is necessary even though it appears that the total duration of labor will exceed 24 hours. Penicillin and streptomycin may be started after about 12 hours, and intravenous fluids may be administered if an unusually long labor is anticipated. Patients with slow slope active phase need constant emotional support.

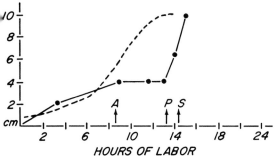

HOURS OF LABOR

Fig. 33-4. Anxious primigravida with a tense, restless latent phase of labor. Amniotomy at 9 hours did not terminate the latent phase. Sparteine sulfate was given at the tenth, eleventh, and twelfth hour, but the latent phase continued. Intravenous Pitocin was started at the thirteenth hour, and a perfectly normal active phase ensued. Position was left occiput anterior; infant weighed 3,293 grams. S, Sedation; **P,** Pitocin; **A,** amniotomy.

Active phase arrest. Arrest during the active phase of labor is cause for concern because it may be an indication of disproportion in primigravidas. If the contractions are irregular and progressive cervical dilatation ceases, vaginal examination and x-ray pelvimetry are imperative. If cephalopelvic disproportion is established, its treatment will depend upon the degree. Cesarean section should be performed promptly if it appears that vaginal delivery is unlikely to occur. If the disproportion is less and vaginal delivery can be anticipated with normal contractions or if there is no obvious disproportion, oxytocin stimulation is indicated. This usually must be continued throughout the rest of the labor. Cesarean section may become necessary if oxytocin-stimulated contractions fail to overcome what is considered to be minor disproportion or if normal progress in labor cannot be established. A decision can almost always be made during the first 4 to 6 hours of stimulation; although delivery may not occur within this period of time, the physician can determine whether it can logically be anticipated.

Delivery. Most women with uterine dysfunction can be delivered vaginally, but at least 10% will require cesarean section. Termination of the labor should not be necessary if progress continues, even though it is slow, but if progress ceases and effective contractions cannot be reestablished, delivery should be considered. The choice between

vaginal and abdominal delivery is made on the basis of pelvic size, position, station, and size of the infant and the amount of difficulty anticipated. In general, vaginal delivery should be possible if the cervix dilates, the presenting part is below station plus 2, and the pelvis is normal. If the presenting part is at station plus 1 or higher or if the cervix is incompletely dilated, cesarean section almost always is preferable.

Spinal or caudal anesthesia, since they do not alter uterine tone but do relax voluntary muscle, is more desirable than inhalation methods. Inhalation methods may be necessary for certain difficult deliveries requiring version or breech extraction.

The incidence of postpartum hemorrhage is increased because the abnormal contractions continue during the third stage and because injury occurs more often than with normal delivery.

Care of the infant. The baby must be handled gently because it may be in shock and sick. Mucus is aspirated from the pharynx and if necessary from the trachea, and resuscitative measures are applied unless normal respirations are established promptly. A source of external heat is provided, and as soon as the infant is breathing normally it is transferred to the nursery.

Postpartum care. During the postpartum period the physician must be on the lookout for uterine relaxation and bleeding. Fluids are given intravenously as necessary, and antimicrobial agents are continued for a day or two. Immediately after delivery a sedative is administered to help the patient sleep, but she should be encouraged to get out of bed on the first day.

■ Constriction ring dystocia

A constriction ring is a tetanic annular contraction of smooth muscle that may occur at any level in the uterine wall. The ring does not change position, and it may be applied so tightly around the infant's body that it prevents descent.

Constriction ring, although rare, should be suspected whenever the uterine contractions are irregular and uncoordinated and is particularly likely to develop with dysfunctional labor. The cervix and lower segment below the ring hang like a cuff ahead of the presenting part and are quiescent when the muscle in the fundus contracts. The infant may actually be pulled up rather than pushed down with each contraction. A depressed area over the ring can occasionally be felt by palpating through the abdominal wall, but the diagnosis can only be made with accuracy by passing the hand upward into the uterine cavity until the band is felt.

If the ring is diagnosed during labor and before cervical dilatation is completed, the intramuscular injection of 5 minims of 1:1,000 Adrenalin chloride may relax it. Although there is no general agreement concerning the efficacy of Adrenalin, it should be tried. When the ring cannot be relaxed, cesarean section is necessary. If the ring is first diagnosed when the cervix is completely dilated, it may be relaxed enough with deep inhalation anesthesia to permit delivery vaginally. The uterus almost never ruptures as a result of constriction ring dystocia.

■ Pathologic retraction ring

A pathologic retraction ring (Bandl's ring) develops during obstructed but otherwise normal labor. The ring forms at the junction of the active upper and the relatively passive lower uterine segments and actually is the lower border of the unusually thick upper segment. Because descent and expulsion of the infant are impeded, the lower segment becomes excessively lengthened and thinned and the upper segment shortened and thickened. Unless the obstruction is overcome, the uterus may rupture. In contrast to constriction ring, a retraction ring does not prevent descent and is a result rather than a cause of obstruction.

The ring can be felt and sometimes even seen as a transverse ridge just below the umbilicus; it becomes more obvious as labor progresses. The treatment consists of delivery by the most expedient method; cesarean section is usually the method of choice because the basic reason for the ring is insurmountable disproportion.

■ Dystocia of fetal origin

Dystocia of fetal origin may be the result of excessive size, abnormal development, or unusual positions in the birth canal.

DYSTOCIA FROM EXCESSIVE DEVELOPMENT

The usual infant at term weighs slightly more than 3,200 grams (7 pounds) and is about 50 cm. (19.5 inches) long. About 10%

weigh at least 4,000 grams (9 pounds), but in no more than 1% or 2% is the birth weight over 4,500 grams (10 pounds).

Multiparity, parental size, and maternal diabetes are the factors most often responsible for overgrowth of the fetus. The birth weight often increases progressively in each pregnancy, so the third or fourth infant may weigh much more than the first. Because of this the physician cannot assume that a multiparous woman will deliver without difficulty as she has before; the present infant may be too large to pass through the pelvis, even though the measurements indicate that it is normal. Approximately 10% of primary cesarean sections in multiparas are performed because of disproportion. Babies whose parents are large usually weigh more than those born to smaller individuals. Fortunately, large women usually have large pelves that will permit the delivery of oversized infants without difficulty. Maternal diabetes is such an important factor that a glucose tolerance test should be performed in any woman who has been delivered of an infant weighing more than 4,000 grams.

Postmaturity has little to do with the development of large infants; in fact, the typical "postmature" baby is likely to be thin and undernourished because of placental insufficiency. Koff and Potter found that the gestational period for oversized infants averaged only 8 days more than for those of average weight.

The mortality for excessively large infants is increased, and many of them are injured during attempts at delivery. Those born of diabetic mothers may also have a metabolic disorder, which if not treated results in their death. The normal-sized pelvis should be adequate for the delivery of infants weighing 4,000 to 4,500 grams if the uterine contractions are forceful enough. If the baby is too large, however, disproportion similar to that encountered with normal infants and contracted pelvis can occur; as a consequence the infant may be injured during difficult extraction.

The physician must be on the lookout for large babies, particularly in women in whom there is a reason for their development. The size cannot always be determined accurately either by palpation or roentgen examination, but an x-ray study should be obtained whenever overgrowth is suspected. During labor

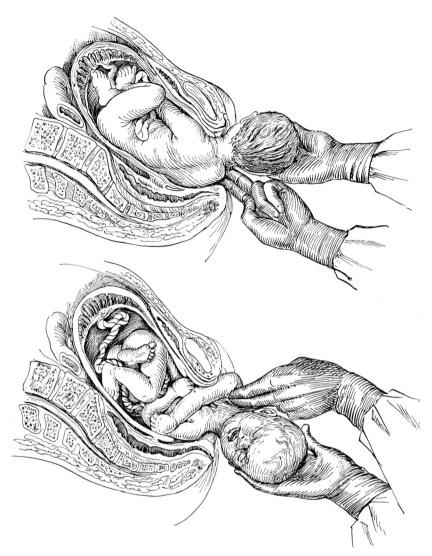

Fig. 33-5. Rotation of impacted shoulders.

the findings are similar to those in disproportion from contracted pelvis, except the latter more often occurs in primigravidas. The head may fail to enter the pelvis, or descent may be slow despite what appear to be normal uterine contractions.

If disproportion is not too great, the head may descend and deliver, but the broad shoulders are not able to pass the inlet *(shoulder dystocia).* When this occurs, the chin will be pulled back tightly against the perineum as soon as the head is delivered through the introitus. Unless the infant is extracted promptly, it will die because its chest is compressed, preventing respiratory efforts, and the circulation through the cord is cut off.

The posterior shoulder usually has descended into the true pelvis below the promontory of the sacrum, but the bisacromial diameter is so long that the anterior shoulder, which lies above the pubis, cannot enter the pelvis. Under such circumstances forceful downward traction on the infant's head not only is ineffectual but may well stretch and injure the brachial plexus or·even fracture the cervical spine. The physician should first attempt to push the anterior shoulder into the pelvis by direct pressure on it through the abdominal wall. If this cannot be accomplished, another maneuver must be tried at once. The hand is inserted into the vagina until the first and second fingers can be hooked in the axilla. The posterior shoulder is rotated anteriorly and pulled downward simultaneously with a corkscrew motion. If this maneuver is successful, the anterior shoulder is rotated into the true pelvis posteriorly while the posterior shoulder is delivered from underneath the symphysis anteriorly. From this point delivery can be completed with little difficulty.

If the shoulders are wedged into the inlet so tightly that they cannot be rotated, the hand is passed over the posterior shoulder and along the chest until the baby's hand can be seized and pulled downward over the chest and through the introitus. This releases the posterior shoulder and will permit its anterior rotation and delivery.

DYSTOCIA FROM DEVELOPMENTAL ABNORMALITIES

Developmental anomalies seldom cause dystocia, but in rare instances they may. This is particularly true of de-

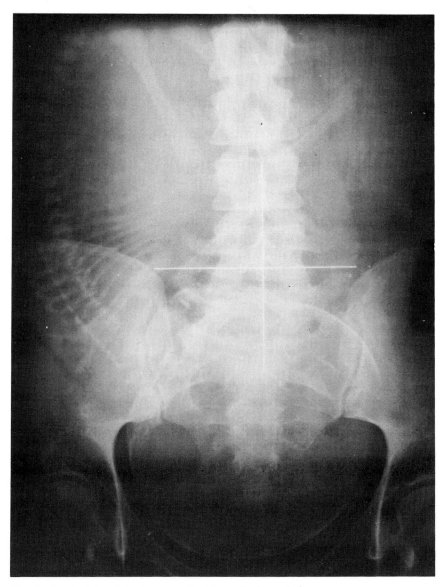

Fig. 33-6. Cephalopelvic disproportion from hydrocephalus.

formities such as hydrocephalus, enlargement of the body or abdomen, or double monsters.

With *hydrocephalus* labor is delayed because the head is too large to enter the inlet. The diagnosis can be suspected if a large mass is felt over the inlet. Upon vaginal palpation the sutures may be wide and the fontanels huge. X-ray examination will provide confirmatory evidence. With breech position, hydrocephalus is sometimes not diagnosed until it is impossible to extract the aftercoming head.

If the head is presenting, vaginal delivery is usually possible if the fluid is withdrawn by puncturing the enlarged ventricle through a suture or fontanel with a small trocar or a spinal puncture needle. This can usually be accomplished with little difficulty after the cervix has reached a dilatation of 3 or 4 cm., even though the head has not yet entered the inlet. Withdrawal of the fluid permits the skull bones to collapse, after which labor usually progresses normally. Cesarean section rarely is necessary and certainly should not be considered unless decompression fails. If hydrocephalus is not recognized and labor is allowed to continue indefinitely, the uterus may rupture. A hydrocephalic aftercoming head usually cannot be extracted unless it is decompressed. The fluid can be evacuated if the needle or trocar is inserted through the foramen magnum or the roof of the mouth. An alternative method is to aspirate the fluid after the needle has been inserted through the abdominal and uterine walls.

The body may be enlarged by *tumors of the liver, abnormal development of the kidneys, urinary retention* from obstruction in the lower urinary tract, or other anomalies. Dystocia from enlargement of the abdomen can be overcome by puncturing the abdominal wall to drain off the fluid or to remove the enlarged organ.

Double monsters are quite rare and present many problems.

■ Dystocia from abnormalities in position and presentation

Abnormalities in position and presentation frequently cause dystocia. If they are recognized promptly and are corrected, the results for both the mother and the infant should be reasonably good.

TRANSVERSE LIE

With transverse lie the long axis of the infant lies at right angles to the longitudinal axis of the mother; its head lies in one flank and its buttocks in the other. One of the shoulders lies over the inlet, the presenting part being the scapula or the achromial process. If the infant's back is directed toward the maternal spine, the presenting part will lie in the right or left posterior quadrant of the pelvis (right or left *scapula posterior position*). If the back is directed anteriorly, the presenting part will lie in the right or left anterior quadrant (right or left *scapula anterior position*). In an *oblique lie* the long axis of the fetus lies obliquely across the abdomen, with either the head or the buttocks directed toward one or the other maternal iliac fossa.

Transverse lie occurs more often in multiparas than in primigravidas, but it actually is relatively uncommon, complicating only about 0.25% to 0.5% of all pregnancies. If the placenta is implanted in the fundus or over the cervix, the infant may be forced to assume a transverse or an oblique position because the length of the uterine cavity is reduced. *In about one third of all transverse lies the placenta occupies the lower segment.* Transverse lie is more frequent in bicornuate or arcuate uteri than in those that have developed normally. It may occur because of hydramnios, which permits the fetus considerable freedom of motion.

Diagnosis. The diagnosis can be suspected if the abdomen looks wider than it does long. If the uterus is relaxed, the head can be felt on one side and the breech on the other; there is no presenting part in the inlet. It may be possible to palpate the shoulder

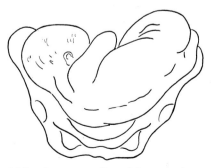

Fig. 33-7. Transverse lie; right scapula anterior position.

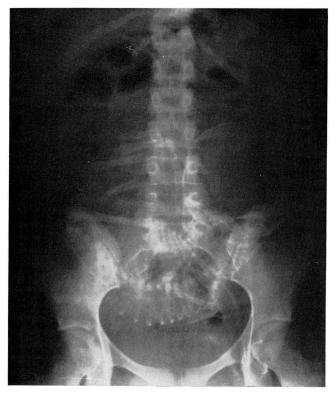

Fig. 33-8. X-ray visualization of transverse lie. The head is directed toward the left and the buttocks toward the right, with the shoulder and thoracic cavity over the pelvic inlet.

through the vagina, but if the membranes are intact, the presenting part is often so high that it cannot be reached. During labor the membranes can be felt bulging through the partially dilated cervix with each contraction. Between contractions the scapula, the clavicle, the axilla, and the rib cage can be palpated. X-ray study will confirm the findings.

Vaginal or rectal examinations should not be performed in the doctor's office on patients suspected of having transverse lies. If placenta previa is present, profuse bleeding may be precipitated.

Course of labor. Spontaneous delivery of a living normal-sized infant should not be anticipated with shoulder presentation. The cervix dilates around the forebag, and the shoulder is forced into the inlet, but it cannot descend. The membranes usually rupture early in the first stage, after which the hand and arm prolapse into the vagina. A small macerated infant may sometimes be forced through the pelvis, but delivery must not be expected. More often descent is impossible,

the lower segment becomes progressively thinner until it ruptures, or labor ceases with the uterus tetanically contracted. The infant is usually dead, and intrauterine infection has developed. This is termed *neglected transverse lie.*

Prognosis. If the abnormality is recognized early and treated properly, the maternal mortality should not be increased. Trauma to soft parts, particularly cervical laceration and rupture of the uterus, may occur as a result of attempt to complete delivery vaginally. Serious puerperal infection occurs less frequently now than in years past, but it still is a hazard.

Infant deaths are caused by anoxia from prolapsed cord, which occurs more often than with normal presentation, by infection, or by injury from prolonged labor or attempts at delivery. The infant mortality rate is as high as 30% to 50% with vaginal delivery, but most babies who are reasonably mature and in good condition should survive if delivered by cesarean section.

Management. If transverse or oblique lie

is recognized during late pregnancy, *external version* to either a breech or a vertex position should be attempted. If this is impossible, an x-ray or isotopic examination for placental site should be obtained and other possible causes of the abnormal lies sought. Many transverse presentations correct themselves spontaneously before labor begins.

During early labor vaginal and x-ray examinations should be performed and external version attempted. If the position cannot be corrected, cesarean section offers the best prognosis for the infant in either primigravidas or multiparas.

Vaginal delivery occasionally is feasible if the diagnosis of transverse lie is made near the end of the first stage. This is particularly true in multiparas or if the duration of pregnancy is less than 32 weeks in either multiparas or primigravidas. The anticipated mortality for infants of less than 32 weeks' gestational development is so high that it is not logical to expose the mother to the immediate and remote complications of cesarean section if delivery by another method is possible. After the cervix has dilated completely the membranes can be ruptured and internal podalic version and extraction performed. Deep ether anesthesia is necessary. Naturally the infant mortality will be high, not only because of injury or anoxia but because the infant is more likely to be premature.

The patient with a neglected transverse lie is usually infected, dehydrated, and tired. Before anything else is done she should be given penicillin and streptomycin, glucose intravenously, and rest. In some patients a small, dead baby can be delivered vaginally by version or by embryotomy if the cervix is completely dilated. If the lower uterine segment is considerably thinned, any intrauterine manipulation may be enough to rupture the wall; consequently cesarean section, often with hysterectomy, usually is the preferable procedure.

OCCIPUT POSTERIOR POSITION

In about one fourth of all vertex deliveries the occiput points toward one of the posterior quadrants during early labor. Almost all infants rotate to an anterior position spontaneously or deliver in the posterior position without difficulty, but in a few patients,

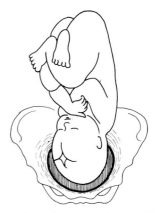

Fig. 33-9. Left occiput posterior position.

particularly those with abnormal pelves, the labor is prolonged and difficult.

One of the most important reasons for occiput posterior position is the shape of the bony pelvic inlet. If the transverse diameter of the inlet is narrowed and if the anteroposterior diameter is lengthened, as in an anthropoid pelvis, the head must descend with its long axis in an anteroposterior diameter. The occiput may be directed either posteriorly or toward the pubis. If the anterior segment of the superior strait is narrow and of the android type, the head is also likely to descend in an oblique posterior position. The forehead fits the anterior segment of the inlet better than does the wider occipital area. In contrast, the infant's head is more likely to enter the gynecoid or the platypelloid pelvis in a transverse diameter, with its long axis in the longest axis of the inlet because it fits better. However, it may also descend through these pelves in a posterior position if they are large enough to accommodate it. If the head flexes as it descends, the uterine contractions are effective, the pelvic size and shape are normal, and the levator muscles are normal, anterior rotation can be anticipated. In primigravidas the second stage may be slightly longer than usual, but in multiparas the head often descends to the pelvic floor in the posterior position and rotates and delivers with one or two contractions.

Failure to rotate may be the result of inadequate uterine contractions that do not provide enough force to push the baby downward, of relaxation and separation of the levator muscles, eliminating the inclined plane up which the occiput is forced, or it may be because the transverse diameter of the bony pelvis is so narrow that the head cannot turn within the birth canal.

The occiput also may fail to rotate anteriorly because the head is slightly deflexed, making some anterior portion rather than the occiput the presenting part. This area will naturally rotate anteriorly, thereby directing the occiput to the hollow of the sacrum, where it stays.

If the head descends to the pelvic floor with the occiput in an oblique posterior position, the patient should be given an opportunity to rotate it herself. As long as rotation is progressing, even though it is slow, and the conditions of the mother and the baby are good, no interference is necessary. If either the maternal or the fetal condition

should change or if no progress is made during a period of 1 hour, delivery should be considered.

If the head descends in a direct occiput posterior position, anterior rotation is less likely to occur because the presenting part lies over the sacrum in the trough formed by the two levator muscles rather than on the inclined plane. If progress ceases, the baby should be delivered, usually by manual or forceps rotation to an occiput anterior position followed by forceps extraction. In many instances, particularly in multiparas with roomy pelves and relaxed soft tissues and in those with anthropoid pelves, spontaneous or low forceps delivery with the occiput in a posterior position is not only possible but may be preferable to operative rotation. The longer diameters of the head may increase

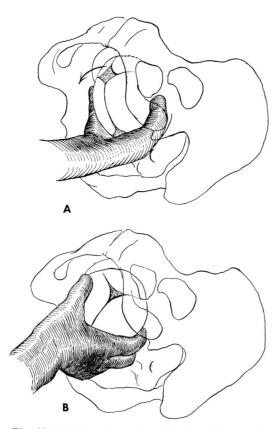

Fig. 33-10. Manual rotation of the head from occiput posterior position. **A,** The right hand is used in left occiput position. **B,** The left hand is used in right occiput position. (From Titus, P.: Atlas of obstetric technic, St. Louis, 1949, The C. V. Mosby Co.)

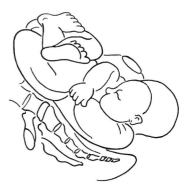

Fig. 33-11. Delivery of the head in occiput posterior position. The area of the anterior fontanel stems beneath the pubic arch.

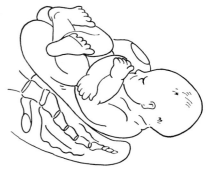

Fig. 33-12. Delivery of the head in occiput posterior position. The area at the root of the base stems beneath the pubic arch. Longer diameters of the head must come through the introitus with this mechanism.

perineal injury slightly, but damage from rotation if the pelvis is abnormal may be even greater.

Cesarean section is rarely indicated for an occiput posterior position in a normal pelvis.

FACE POSITION

When the head is completely deflexed, face position can be diagnosed. The chin (mentum) is the presenting part, and relatively large diameters are presenting. Face positions occur in about 0.25% of all deliveries.

Complete deflexion may be primary, but more often it develops during descent of the head through the inlet; something holds the

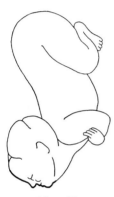

Fig. 33-13. Face position. Note complete deflexion of the head and extension of the fetal spine.

occiput up, thereby encouraging the anterior portion of the head to descend first. Deflexion increases as the head descends. Face positions may develop in women with inlet contraction; the bitemporal diameter is narrower than that of the occiput and fits better in the inlet. The situation with a large baby is comparable. The pendulous uterus in a multiparous woman allows the infant to fall forward or to one side, thereby favoring abnormal positions. Flexion may be prevented by abnormalities of the neck or thorax or by loops of cord around the neck. Anencephalic infants almost all present by the face.

Diagnosis. The fetal spine is extended and the head is deflexed, with the occiput in contact with the back. Upon *abdominal examination* the smooth curve of the flexed spine cannot be felt, but the small parts may be unusually prominent. The cephalic prominence can be felt on the side opposite the small parts. It often is difficult to make a diagnosis by abdominal palpation.

Upon *rectal examination* the face may feel like a breech, but if the cervix is partly dilated, the supraorbital ridges, the nose, eyes, and mouth can be palpated *vaginally*. Great care must be taken not to injure the structures. The abnormal position can be visualized by x-ray examination.

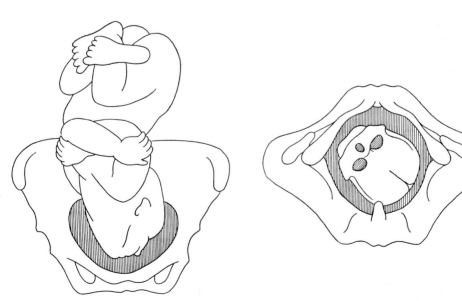

Fig. 33-14. Right mentum anterior position. The cephalic prominence is on the same side as the back and is not easy to feel when the chin is anterior. The bony landmarks as palpated during vaginal examination are indicated on the right.

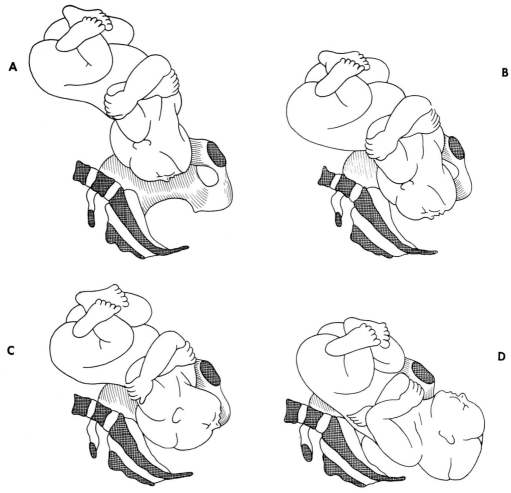

Fig. 33-15. Mechanism of labor in right mentum anterior positions. The head descends in the left oblique diameter, **A,** until the chin reaches the levator sling, **B.** It then rotates anteriorly, **C,** until the submandibular area lies beneath the symphysis. **D,** The head is then delivered by flexion.

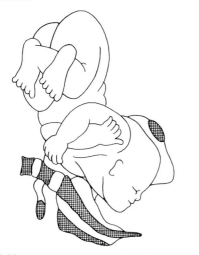

Fig. 33-16. Persistent mentum posterior position.

Course of labor. The mechanism of labor is similar to that in the vertex position, but the chin rather than the occipital portion of the head is the presenting part. As the head descends, extension increases until the head is completely deflexed, with the occiput in contact with the infant's back. The chin is rotated because it is forced downward against the levator sling and the bony side walls of the lower pelvis; as labor continues it gradually rotates anteriorly until it lies beneath the pubic arch, with the occipital portion of the head directed toward the sacrum. The submandibular area stems beneath the pubis, while the occiput is forced upward over the perineum until it is free of the vagina. The head therefore is delivered by flexion. The delivery of the shoulders and body is like that in occiput positions.

If anterior rotation of the chin fails to occur, *persistent mentum posterior position* can be diagnosed. It is almost impossible for a normal-sized infant to deliver in a mentum posterior position because the chin, which lies in the hollow of the sacrum, can only be forced over the perineum by further extension of the head; this is impossible because it already is completely deflexed. Delay from mentum posterior often occurs when the presenting part is relatively high in the pelvis. If the head descends with the chin pointed directly posteriorly, rotation is not likely to occur. If it is directed obliquely posteriorly, rotation can be anticipated, but it usually does not occur until the presenting part begins to bulge the perineum.

It is important to remember that when the face is presenting, the biparietal diameter does not pass the pelvic inlet until the chin reaches the pelvic floor; consequently engagement occurs late in labor.

Management. The management depends upon pelvic size, stage of labor, and the efficiency of the contractions. If an abnormal attitude is suspected by abdominal or rectal palpation, the patient should be examined vaginally. Unless delivery is imminent, x-ray studies should usually be obtained because of the increased incidence of contracted pelvis with face position. If there is no obvious disproportion and particularly if the chin is in an anterior or a transverse position, labor may be allowed to continue. If the chin is directed posteriorly, particularly if the head is wedged into the upper pelvis, the outlook for normal delivery is less favorable. A few hours of labor will usually indicate the outcome. In many instances, particularly in multiparas, face positions are not diagnosed until the patient is delivering.

It may sometimes be possible to flex the head, thereby converting it to an occiput position. Usually, however, this is impossible because the head has already molded considerably and will not fit the pelvis properly in any other position and because the cervix is usually not dilated enough to permit insertion of the entire hand.

If the chin does not rotate spontaneously to an anterior position during the second stage of labor, it may be possible to turn it manually, after which it can be extracted by forceps or allowed to deliver spontaneously. Forceps delivery in the mentum posterior position cannot be performed on normal-sized infants without injuring them and the pelvic structures.

Cesarean section is indicated when progress ceases with the presenting part high in the pelvis or when mentum posterior positions cannot be corrected. It is more often necessary in primigravidas than in multiparas, many of whom deliver rapidly and spontaneously despite the abnormal position.

BROW POSITION

Deflexed attitudes in which the brow is the presenting part occur about once in every 500 to 1,000 deliveries and result from any of the factors that tend to prevent flexion and increase extension. Such causes are a large pelvis or a small infant, contracted pelvis, and abnormalities in the shape of the head.

Spontaneous delivery in the brow position will not always occur even if the pelvis is of normal size because the presenting diameter of the fetal head (occipitomental, 13.5 cm.) is too large to come through the inlet without extensive molding. The brow, however, is frequently a transient position, and enough alteration in position may occur as labor progresses to permit pelvic delivery.

Diagnosis. The diagnosis is made by palpating the anterior fontanel in the middle of the cervical opening with the supraorbital ridges and the root of the nose at one side. Ordinarily the presenting part is well above the spines. Upon abdominal examination the deflexion may be suspected by the straight fetal spine with a cephalic prominence palpable on each side.

Management. The management depends upon the stage of labor, the size of the infant, the size of the pelvis, and the findings upon sterile vaginal examination. Vaginal delivery can be anticipated if the infant is small and if at the time the abnormal position is recognized the presenting part is below the spines. Often the presenting part is unengaged and cannot be depressed into the pelvis. In this event delivery without altering the position is not to be expected. Either flexion of the head to an occiput position or extension to a face position might solve the problem, but neither of these is easy if the head is molded. Cesarean section frequently is the preferable

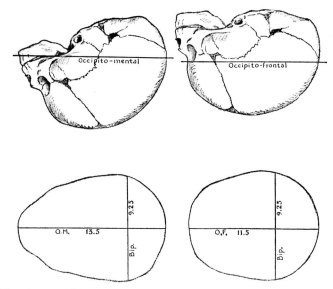

Fig. 33-17. With a brow position the longest anteroposterior diameter of the head, the occipitomental, must pass through the pelvis. (From Beck, A. C.: Obstetrical practice, Baltimore, 1955, The Williams & Wilkins Co.)

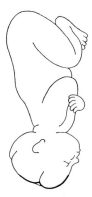

Fig. 33-18. Brow position. The spine is straight, and a cephalic prominence can be felt on each side. The position of the head as it descends through the pelvis is indicated by the heavy black line.

method for delivery, particularly in the primigravida, when progress ceases with incomplete cervical dilatation or if the pelvis is contracted.

COMPOUND PRESENTATION

Compound presentation can be diagnosed whenever one or more of an infant's extremities prolapse alongside the presenting head or breech. This occurs once in 700 to 1,000 deliveries of viable infants. In most instances an upper rather than a lower extremity is involved. Compound presentation occurs most often if the pelvic inlet is contracted or if the infant is premature and so small that it does not occlude the birth canal. It is encountered more often in multiparas than in primigravidas.

Labor usually progresses normally. Occasionally, however, the prolapsed extremity may be responsible for abnormal rotation of the presenting part, or, if large enough, it may even delay descent. Prolapsed cord occurs more frequently with compound presentation.

No treatment is necessary unless labor is delayed. A hand lying beside the infant's head, for example, will usually not prolapse completely because the increasing pressure against it as the head descends will hold it up. If an entire arm or leg has descended through the cervix, it may be necessary to disengage the head and replace the extremity within the uterine cavity. Neither cesarean section nor version and extraction is often warranted.

References

Breen, J. L., and Wiesmeier, E.: Compound presentation; a survey of 131 patients, Obstet. Gynec. 32:419, 1968.

Caldeyro, R., Alvarez, H., and Reynolds, S. R. M.: A better understanding of uterine contractility through simultaneous recording with an internal and a seven channel external method, Surg. Gynec. Obstet. 91:641, 1950.

Calkins, L. A.: Occiput posterior, a normal presentation, Amer. J. Obstet. Gynec. **43:**277, 1943.

Calkins, L. A.: Occiput posterior presentations, Obstet. Gynec. **1:**466, 1953.

Connel, J., and Parsons, M.: Brow presentation, Bull. Margaret Hague Maternity Hosp. **5:**88, 1952.

D'Esopo, D. A.: Dysfunctional labor; recognition and management, Bull. Sloane Hosp. Wom. **14:** 45, 1968.

Feeney, J. K., and Barry, A. P.: Hydrocephaly as a cause of maternal mortality and morbidity, J. Obstet. Gynaec. Brit. Comm. **61:**652, 1954.

Johnson, C. E.: Transverse presentation of fetus, J.A.M.A. **187:**642, 1964.

Johnson, H. W.: The clinical diagnosis of varying degrees of constriction rings, Amer. J. Obstet. Gynec. **52:**74, 1946.

Koff, A. K., and Potter, E. L.: The complications associations with excessive development of the fetus, Amer. J. Obstet. Gynec. **38:**412, 1939.

Ledger, W. J.: Graphic analysis; an aid in the early recognition of labor abnormalities, Univ. Mich. Med. Cent. J. **33:**266, 1967.

Posner, A. C., Friedman, S., and Posner, L. B.: The large fetus; a study of 547 cases, Obstet. Gynec. **5:**268, 1955.

Posner, A. C., Friedman, S., and Posner, L. B.: Modern trends in the management of face and brow presentations, Surg. Gynec. Obstet. **104:** 485, 1957.

Rucker, M. P.: Constriction ring dystocia, Amer. J. Obstet. Gynec. **52:**984, 1946.

Schulman, H., and Ledger, W. J.: Practical applications of the graphic portrayal of labor, Obstet. Gynec. **23:**442, 1964.

Schulman, H., and Ledger, W. J.: Sparteine sulfate; a clinical study of 711 patients, Obstet. Gynec. **25:**542, 1965.

Stevenson, C. S.: Certain concepts in handling of breech and transverse presentations in late pregnacy, Amer. J. Obstet. Gynec. **62:**488, 1951.

Webster, A., and Geittmann, W. F.: Shoulder presentation, Amer. J. Obstet. Gynec. **72:**34, 1956.

Willson, J. R., and Alesbury, R. J.: Prolonged labor; its clinical recognition and management, Amer. J. Obstet. Gynec. **61:**1253, 1951.

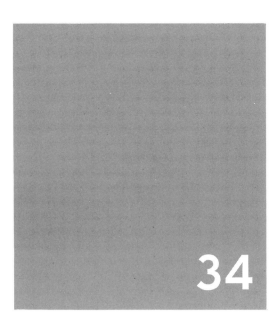

34

Pelvimetry; dystocia from contracted pelvis

One of the important responsibilities of the obstetrician is to determine whether the pelvis is large enough to permit normal delivery. A clinical estimation of pelvic size is usually made at the initial prenatal visit because it is convenient to measure the pelvis at that time. Some physicians prefer to obtain the internal measurements later when the tissues are more supple and relaxed and when the patient is less tense. It makes little difference when the pelvis is measured as long as it is done before labor begins.

Most abnormal pelves can be at least suspected by clinical examination, but x-ray study is necessary to obtain precise measurements and to determine pelvic shape accurately.

■ Normal pelvis

For obstetric purposes the pelvis is divided into the *false pelvis* and the *true pelvis,* or

pelvic cavity, at the level of the sacral promontory, the linea terminalis on each side, and the upper border of the pubis anteriorly. The false pelvis serves no important purpose except to support the enlarging uterus and to direct the presenting part downward. The true pelvis, which is bounded by the sacrum posteriorly, the pelvic bones, muscles, and ligaments laterally, and the posterior surfaces of the rami of the pubis and the ischii anteriorly, is far more significant. Alteration in the size and shape of the pelvis may interfere with the mechanism of labor or even prevent normal delivery.

Pelvic inlet. The pelvic inlet or superior strait, the entrance to the true pelvis, is bounded by the promontory and alae of the sacrum, the lineae terminalis laterally, and the superior surface of the pubic bones anteriorly. It is oval in shape and its *angle of inclination,* the angle the plane of the inlet makes with the horizon with the patient standing, is about 55 degrees. The *conjugata vera,* or *true conjugate,* extends from the midpoint of the sacral promontory to the superior surface of the symphysis and measures 10.5 to 11.5 cm. The *obstetric conjugate* extends from the promontory to the closest point on the convex posterior surface of the symphysis, which is about 0.5 to 1 cm. below the upper margin. This measures about 0.5 cm. less than the true conjugate. The *diagonal conjugate* extends from the promontory to the lower border of the symphysis and measures about 12.5 cm. This is the only anteroposterior measurement that can be obtained clinically. The *transverse diameter* of the inlet represents the greatest distance between each linea terminalis and usually forms a right angle with the true conjugate approximately 5 cm. anterior to the promontory. It measures about 13.5 cm. The *oblique diameters* extend from each sacroiliac synchondrosis to the opposite iliopectineal eminence and measure about 12.5 cm. The right oblique diameter originates at the right sacroiliac synchondrosis and the left oblique diameter on the left side posteriorly.

Pelvic cavity. The *plane of greatest pelvic dimensions,* the roomiest portion of the pelvic cavity, lies above the ischial spines at the level of a line that extends from the junction of the second and third sacral vertebrae to the middle of the posterior surface of the pubis. This measures about 12.75 cm. The

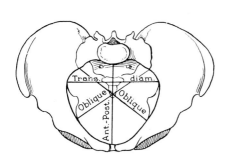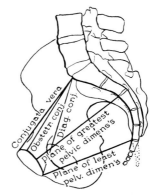

Fig. 34-1. Planes of the pelvic inlet. (From Moloy, H. C.: Evaluation of the pelvis in obstetrics, Philadelphia, 1951, W. B. Saunders Co.)

transverse diameter between the two iliac bones just above the superior surface of each acetabulum measures about 12.5 cm.

The *plane of least pelvic dimensions,* or the *midplane,* extends from the lower border of the pubis anteriorly to the lower sacrum at the level of the ischial spines and measures about 11.5 to 12 cm. The transverse *bispinous diameter* is the smallest in the normal pelvic cavity, measuring about 10.5 cm.

Pelvic outlet. The pelvic outlet or inferior strait is even less a "plane" than is the inlet. Actually it is made up of two triangles sharing a common base at a line joining the two ischial tuberosities. The apex of the anterior triangle is the lower border of the symphysis, and the sides are the descending pubic rami and the ascending ischial rami. The apex of the posterior triangle is the tip of the sacrum, and the sides are the pelvic ligaments. The *bituberous* diameter measures 8 to 11 cm., and the *anteroposterior diameter,* or the distance between the lower border of the symphysis and the tip of the sacrum, is 11.5 cm.

There are many variations in the normal pelvis that are produced by heredity, variations in hormone stimulation, pressure, and disease. Most pelves are quite adequate for childbearing, but in some the deviation may be sufficient to disturb the mechanism of labor.

Classification. Caldwell and Moloy have suggested a classification of normal pelves based upon the configuration of the inlet and the corresponding changes in the midpelvis and lower pelvis as demonstrated by x-ray examination. This provides an accurate method for visualizing pelvic contour and for

predicting the mechanism of labor and its outcome.

The pelvic inlet is divided into a *posterior segment,* behind the line representing the widest transverse diameter, and an *anterior segment* in front of it (Fig. 34-1). The information necessary to classify the inlet includes the length of the transverse diameter and the anteroposterior length of each segment. The sacrosciatic notch is visualized by a lateral film: A wide notch means that the sacrum is displaced posteriorly or that the curve is deep, thus increasing the antero-posterior diameter at the midpelvis. A narrow notch indicates a reduced anteroposterior diameter because the sacrum lies farther forward than usual.

Evaluation of the midpelvis and outlet includes measurement of the bispinous diameter and observation of the shape of the spinous processes, and the length, width, and curve of the sacrum. The subpubic angle is estimated and the contour of the arch is noted. The degree of convergence or divergence of the lateral walls (splay) is also of importance; with considerable convergence toward the outlet, delay may be anticipated.

Female pelves are grouped into four pure and ten mixed types on the basis of morphology as determined by stereoscopic x-ray study.

Gynecoid pelvis. Gynecoid pelvis occurs in 40% to 45% of women. The inlet of the typical female pelvis is rounded or slightly oval with both anterior and posterior segments rounded and spacious. The sacrum is well curved and of average length, and the sacrosciatic notch is of medium width. The

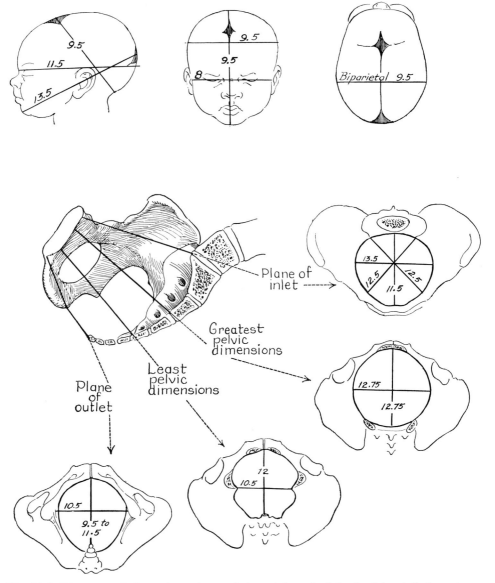

Fig. 34-2. Diameters of the various planes of the pelvis and of the fetal head that must pass through it.

subpubic angle is wide, and the sides of the arch are curved. The bispinous and bituberous diameters are wide and the side walls are straight.

Android pelvis. Android pelvis occurs in 25% to 35% of white women and 10% to 15% of black women. This is a masculine type of pelvis with a wedge-shaped inlet. The posterior segment is wide and relatively flat, and the anterior segment is narrow with a narrow retropubic angle. The sacrum is straight and inclined forward, and the sacro-

sciatic notch is narrow. The subpubic angle is narrow and the bones of the arch are straight. The side walls converge, reducing the bispinous and bituberous diameters. This is the typical *funnel pelvis.*

Anthropoid pelvis. Anthropoid pelvis occurs in 20% to 30% of white women and 40% to 45% of black women. The transverse diameter of the inlet is reduced, making it a long narrow oval with an increase in the lengths of both the anterior and posterior segments. The sacrosciatic notch is wide and

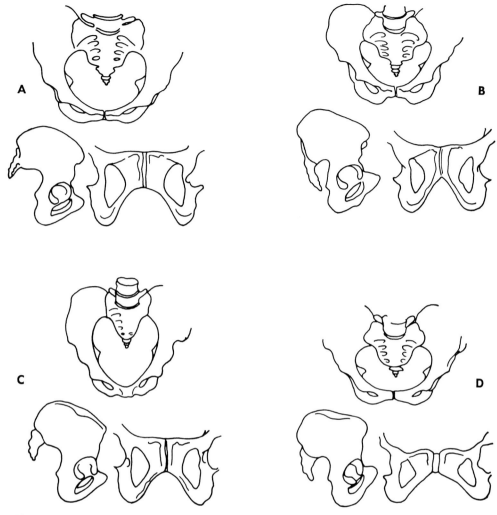

Fig. 34-3. The female pelvis showing normal growth types. **A,** Gynecoid. **B,** Android. **C,** Anthropoid. **D,** Platypelloid.

shallow, and the sacrum has an average curvature but is long and narrow. The subpubic arch is narrowed. The side walls of the pelvis are straight, but both the bispinous and the bituberous diameters are shortened.

Platypelloid pelvis. Platypelloid pelvis occurs in 2% to 5% of white women and only occasionally in black women. The transverse diameter of the inlet is lengthened and the anteroposterior diameter is reduced. Both segments are rounded but flat, and the retropubic angle is rounded. The sacrum is normal, but the sacrosciatic notch is narrowed. The subpubic angle is wide. The side walls are straight, but the bispinous and bituberous diameters are increased.

Mixed types. Pelves in which the anterior and posterior segments are of different types are frequently encountered. They are named by mentioning first the shape of the posterior segment and then that of the anterior segment.

■ Estimation of pelvic capacity
CLINICAL PELVIMETRY

Clinical measurements are less accurate than those obtained by x-ray examination, but they are quite adequate for almost all patients. In the past a ritual was made of measuring the external diameters, but these are of little clinical significance and give no information concerning the size of the cavity.

PURE TYPES   MIXED TYPES   MIXED TYPES

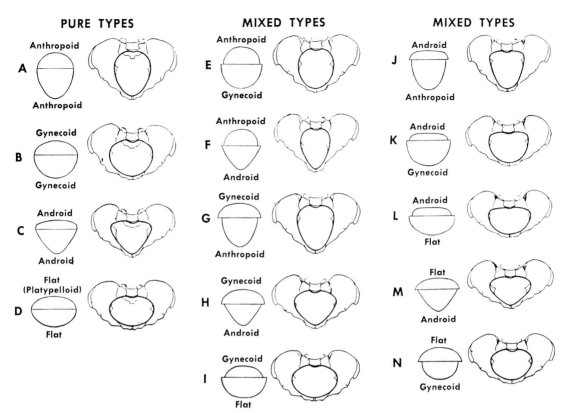

Fig. 34-4. The female pelvis showing pure and mixed types. (From Moloy, H. C.: Amer. J. Obstet. Gynec. **48:**149, 1944.)

Internal measurements can be made at any period of normal pregnancy and if carefully performed will provide a considerable amount of information concerning the pelvis.

Pelvic inlet. The only diameter of the inlet that can be measured with even reasonable accuracy is the *diagonal conjugate.* From this the length of the conjugata vera can then be estimated.

With the patient in lithotomy position, legs abducted, and the buttocks slightly over the edge of the table, the examiner's index and second fingers are inserted through the introitus until the sacrum is reached. His elbow is depressed until it rests against his hip, with which he exerts firm pressure, pushing the palpating fingers upward along the sacrum toward the promontory as the flexed third and fourth fingers flatten the perineum. When the tip of the second finger touches the promontory or can be inserted no farther, the entire hand is pivoted forward until the radial surface of the index finger or its metacarpal presses against the

apex of the pubic arch. The index finger of the opposite hand marks the point on the examining hand that touches the inferior border of the pubis, and the fingers are withdrawn from the vagina. The depth of insertion can be determined by measuring the distance between the tip of the second finger and the point at which the symphysis was contacted. If the promontory is touched, this represents the length of the diagonal conjugate. If the promontory is not reached, the measurement should be recorded as the distance the fingers were inserted plus (CD = 10 cm. plus), which will indicate that the greatest distance is greater than that noted.

The *conjugata vera* is estimated by subtracting 1.5 to 2 cm. from the diagonal conjugate. If the pubic depth is short, 1.5 cm. is subtracted, and if long, 2 cm. The physician cannot even estimate the true conjugate if he fails to touch the promontory, but if the fingers can be inserted at least 11.5 cm., the anteroposterior diameter probably is normal.

The *transverse diameter* cannot be mea-

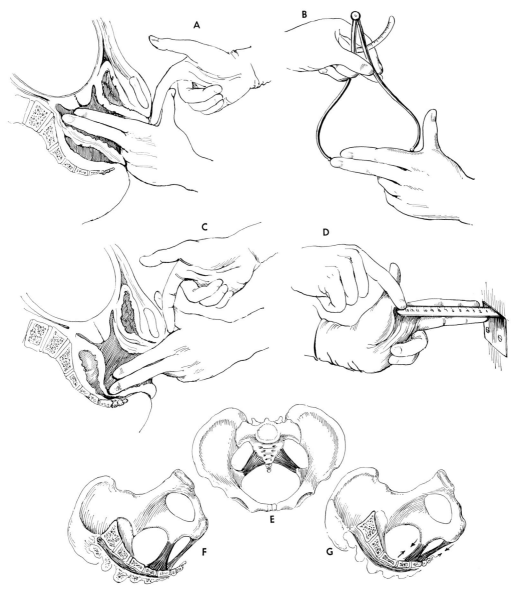

Fig. 34-5. Manual measurement of inlet and midpelvis. **A,** Estimation of diagonal conjugate diameter. **B** and **D,** Methods for measuring anteroposterior diameters. **C,** Estimation of anteroposterior diameter of outlet. **E** to **G,** Differences in length of sacrospinous and sacrotuberous ligaments estimated by sweeping the examining finger along them. (From Willson, J. R.: Management of obstetric difficulties, ed. 6, St. Louis, 1961, The C. V. Mosby Co.)

sured, but the width of the inlet can be estimated by attempting to palpate the linea terminalis. If the entire lateral border of the inlet can be touched on each side, the transverse diameter probably is shortened.

Midpelvis. The *bispinous diameter* cannot be measured clinically, but an impression as to the adequacy of the midpelvis can be ob-

tained. The normal ischial spine projects only slightly into the cavity, but it can be located by identifying the sacrospinous ligament and following it laterally. If the spines are long, sharp, and heavy and project into the pelvis, the physician should suspect that the midpelvis is small. This is more likely to be true if the subpubic arch is narrow and

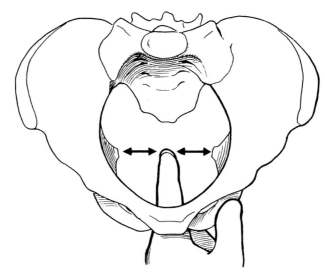

Fig. 34-6. Estimation of bispinous diameter. (From Moloy, H. C.: Evaluation of the pelvis in obstetrics, Philadelphia, 1951, W. B. Saunders Co.)

if there is considerable resistance as the fingers are swept from one side of the pelvis to the other.

If the sacral curvature is flattened or if the sacrum is rotated farther anteriorly than usual, the anteroposterior diameter at the midpelvis and the outlet will be reduced. This is associated with shortening of the sacrospinous ligaments, which ordinarily are about 4 cm. long. Posterior rotation of the sacrum increases both the anteroposterior diameter and the length of the sacrospinous ligaments (Fig. 34-6). The sacrum, the ischial spines, and the ligaments can be felt most accurately by rectal palpation.

Pelvic outlet. The *angle of the pubic arch* can be estimated by laying a thumb or forefinger along the inner aspect of each ramus with their tips meeting at the symphysis. The normal subpubic angle is at least 85 degrees. The angle probably is reduced if it is impossible to separate the index and second fingers placed side by side beneath the symphysis. The curvature of the pubic rami should also be studied.

The length of the *bituberous diameter* alone does not determine the adequacy of the outlet because the distance between the tuberosities varies with the depth of the pelvis and the subpubic angle. If the true pelvis is deep, the bituberous diameter may be of normal length even though the subpubic angle is considerably below normal

(Fig. 34-9). The bituberous diameter can be measured with a suitable pelvimeter, but the measurement is not particularly accurate. The amount of fat overlying the bone varies, and it may be difficult to determine exactly where the most widely separated points on the tuberosities are located. The measurement will be short if taken too far anteriorly. The physician can also estimate the adequacy of the outlet by attempting to insert his clenched fist between the tuberosities. If the average-sized fist can be pushed through the outlet, it should be of ample size.

The *anteroposterior diameter* of the outlet is obtained in much the same manner as the diagonal conjugate. The fingers are inserted until the sacrococcygeal junction can be palpated, and the distance between the fingertip and the point at which the index finger contacted the lower border of the symphysis is measured.

Although each of these measurements is described individually and the pelvis is divided into the three main areas, variations rarely affect only one portion. For instance, if the sacrum is straight and the bispinous diameter is reduced, the side walls usually converge and the subpubic angle and the bituberous diameter are reduced.

ROENTGEN PELVIMETRY

There are many methods for measuring the pelvis by x-ray examination, and most of

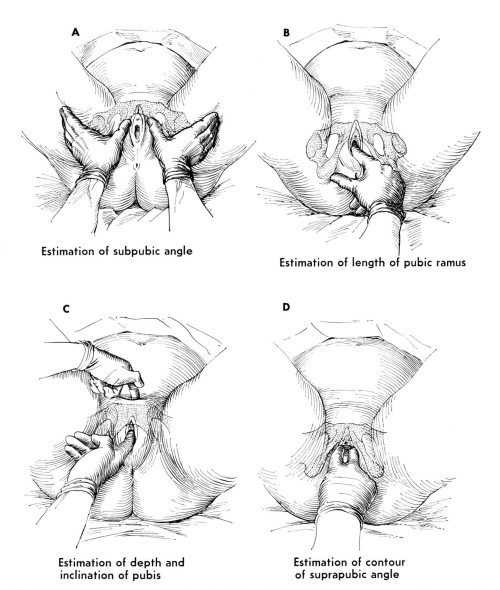

A

Estimation of subpubic angle

B

Estimation of length of pubic ramus

C

Estimation of depth and
inclination of pubis

D

Estimation of contour
of suprapubic angle

Fig. 34-7. Manual measurement of outlet. (From Willson, J. R.: Management of obstetric difficulties, ed. 6, St. Louis, 1961, The C. V. Mosby Co.)

them provide more precise information than
does clinical evaluation. Some physicians
recommend x-ray pelvimetry for every primigravida, but from a practical point of view
this does not seem necessary because most
deliver uneventfully. There is little reason to
obtain an x-ray study during early pregnancy
because at this time the physician cannot determine whether vaginal delivery is possible.
The most important information to be obtained from an x-ray study is a comparison
between the size of the infant and the ca-

pacity of the pelvis; this is possible only late
in pregnancy or during labor.

The radiologist should measure and
classify the pelvis, but unless disproportion
is obvious, he usually cannot prognosticate
the outcome with accuracy. The physician
who orders the x-ray films should examine
them with the radiologist and not simply receive the report by the telephone. He not
only is familiar with the clinical course that
may influence the opinion of the consultant,
but by examining the films he may be able

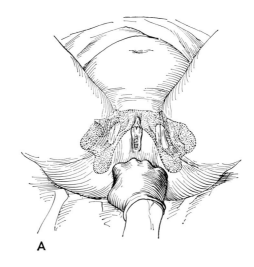

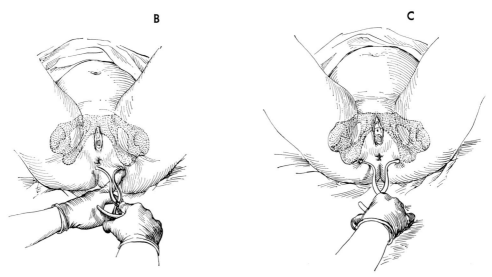

Fig. 34-8. Manual measurement of bituberous diameter. **A,** Bituberous diameter is probably normal if an average-sized clenched fist can be inserted between tuberosities. **B** and **C,** Measurement with DeLee pelvimeter taken between inner surfaces of tuberosities as far posterior as possible. (From Willson, J. R.: Management of obstetric difficulties, ed. 6, St. Louis, 1961, The C. V. Mosby Co.)

to determine why labor is delayed and how it can be corrected. The size of the pelvis alone does not determine the outcome.

Indications for roentgen pelvimetry. X-ray pelvimetry is indicated in the following circumstances:

1. During most *dysfunctional labors,* particularly if the physician is considering using oxytocin
2. In patients with *abnormal clinical measurements* if there is any question as to

pelvic adequacy after a vaginal examination has been performed during early labor

3. During a *trial labor for contracted pelvis* before a decision to administer oxytocin or to perform cesarean section is made
4. In many *breech positions* during labor at term or whenever an *abnormal fetal position* is suspected
5. In patients who have had *disease or*

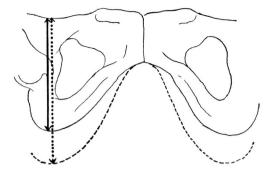

Fig. 34-9. Variations in width of bituberous diameter with differences in length of pubic rami. With deep pelvis the bituberous diameter may be normal even though the angle is narrow. (From Caldwell, W. E., and Moloy, H. C.: Amer. J. Obstet. Gynec. 26:479, 1933.)

injury involving the bony pelvis or hips

6. In patients who have had *difficult labors or large infants previously*
7. Whenever there is *suggestive evidence of disproportion,* such as a floating head during early labor in a primigravida

■ **Contracted pelvis**

Any pelvis that is reduced in size or distorted enough to interfere with normal labor can be considered as contracted.

Classification. The classification of Caldwell and Moloy, although designed to indicate the configuration of all pelves, can be used to describe those that are contracted. The shape may conform to one of the standard types, but at least one of the essential measurements is reduced.

1. *Normal growth types:* Gynecoid, android, anthropoid, and platypelloid
2. *Abnormal growth types:* Infantile and dwarf
3. *Types caused by disease of the pelvic bones and joints:* Rachitic, congenital, inflammatory, atypical, and traumatic
4. *Types secondary to abnormalities of the spinal column:* Kyphotic, scoliotic, kyphoscoliotic, spondylolisthetic, etc.
5. *Types secondary to abnormalities of the lower extremities:* Femoral luxation, atrophy, or loss of extremity

Other common terms used to indicate abnormal pelves are *generally contracted,* which is equivalent to a gynecoid type with reduced measurements; *funnel* or *masculine,* which is equivalent to the android type; and

simple flat, which is equivalent to the platypelloid type. The configuration of each is like that of its normal parent growth type, but the measurements are reduced.

The *classic rachitic pelvis,* which is included in the Caldwell-Moloy classification under the types caused by metabolic disorders, is less common than it was before the widespread administration of vitamin D, but minor rachitic changes are often encountered in black women. In the typical rachitic pelvis the anteroposterior diameter of the inlet may be greatly shortened: If the true conjugate measures less than 8 cm., the pelvis is almost always of the rachitic type, but it does not necessarily have to be so short. The body of the first sacral segment may be displaced forward, forming a *false promontory* between the first and second sacral segments, and the sacral vertebrae are concave. The sacrum itself is usually broad and flat and shorter than normal, and its lower third is acutely angulated anteriorly. The outlet is large because the pubic arch is wide and the bituberous diameter is increased. Most rachitic pelves do not demonstrate all these changes; the most frequently encountered deviations are the shortening of the inlet and the angulation of the sacrum.

Effect of contracted pelvis on pregnancy. There usually is no change during pregnancy except in those patients with pronounced contractions of the pelvic inlet. Because of the reduced measurements the fetus is more likely to be carried high, and lightening is less likely to occur.

Effect of contracted pelvis on labor and delivery. Since lightening may not occur in women with inlet contraction, the head is likely to be unengaged or even above the pelvic brim when labor begins. Abnormal positions and presentations occur more frequently in women with contracted pelvis; deflexed attitudes of the head, shoulder presentation, and compound presentations are encountered two or three times as often. The labor is likely to be prolonged and more difficult, and the incidence of operative delivery is increased. As a result, soft-tissue injury, postpartum hemorrhage, infection, and fetal injury occur frequently.

Mechanism of labor in contracted pelvis. Significant alterations in the size or shape of the bony pelvis naturally affect the course of labor, but since the shapes of many contracted pelves are like those of the normal growth types, the mechanism is often similar to that which occurs normally.

Gynecoid pelvis. The mechanism in the small gynecoid pelvis is like that in the normal pelvis except that the head must flex at a higher level and mold more to descend through the inlet. Because all the diameters are reduced, resistance to descent is encountered at all levels of the birth canal.

Platypelloid pelvis. The main alteration in shape and size in the platypelloid pelvis involves the anteroposterior diameter of the inlet; consequently delay occurs during the first and the early second stages of labor. The head must engage in the transverse diameter; therefore descent will be impeded if the anteroposterior measurement of the inlet is less than the biparietal diameter of the fetal skull (9.5 cm.). Under these circumstances the mechanism by which the head enters the inlet is an exaggeration of the normal. The head assumes an attitude of exaggerated asynclitism, with the anterior parietal bone presenting over the inlet (*anterior parietal bone presentation*) and the sagittal structure in the transverse diameter just anterior to the promontory. With each contraction the parietal bones are forced against the sacrum posteriorly and the pubis anteriorly, gradually causing their edges to overlap at the sagittal suture. This is called *molding* and serves to decrease the biparietal diameter. While the head is being molded, the anterior parietal bone is forced downward behind the pubis where it remains fixed, acting as a fulcrum on which lateral flexion takes place as the uterine contractions force the posterior parietal eminence past the promontory. As this occurs, the sagittal suture gradually approaches the anterior segment of the inlet. As soon as the biparietal diameter has passed the inlet, the head descends through the pelvis in the transverse diameter, usually not rotating until it reaches the pelvic floor.

The mechanism with *posterior parietal bone presentation,* which occurs somewhat less frequently, is the reverse of that just described.

If the parietal bosses ride above the promontory posteriorly and the pubis anteriorly with the sagittal suture near the center of the pelvis (synclitism), another mechanism may occur. Since the head cannot descend, it extends slightly with each contraction until the relatively short bitemporal diameter is forced into the inlet. This is one of the mechanisms by which deflexed attitudes are produced.

The primary effect of inlet contraction is upon engagement, but it may also interfere with normal termination of labor. If much molding, elongation of the head, and caput formation occur, the lowest portion of the head can descend well down into the pelvis before the biparietal diameter passes through the inlet. The conjugata vera is so short and the head fits the inlet so tightly that it can neither rotate to an anterior position nor follow the curve of the sacrum anteriorly while it remains in the transverse position; consequently descent ceases even though the capacity of the lower pelvis is ample. This is called *transverse arrest* of the head. *Deep* transverse arrest occurs with the lowest portion of the head at about station plus 2, and *high* transverse arrest with the head near the spines.

Android pelvis. In the android pelvis the anterior segment of the inlet is wedge shaped and the posterior segment is flattened; consequently the head often descends in an oblique occiput posterior position. In this position the relatively narrow frontal portion of the head fits better into the forepelvis than does the broad occipital area. The occiput usually descends without great difficulty to a point just below the ischial spines, but progress may cease at this level if convergence of the bony side walls is pronounced and if forward displacement of the sacrum considerably reduces the posterior sagittal diameter at the midpelvis. If the head can descend farther, the narrow lower pelvis may prevent anterior rotation of the occiput, but unless the diameters are too small, delivery in an occiput posterior position usually is possible.

Anthropoid pelvis. In the anthropoid pelvis occiput posterior positions are common; in fact it may be impossible for the head to enter the pelvic inlet except in an occiput posterior or an occiput anterior position. Because the transverse diameter is reduced throughout the entire length of the pelvis, the head usually descends and delivers without rotating. Occasionally the head fails to enter the inlet, either because of extreme transverse narrowing or because it lies in a transverse or oblique position rather than an occiput anterior or posterior position, which is more favorable in transversely contracted pelves.

Management of labor in contracted pelvis. For purposes of treatment, abnormal pelves can be divided into those in which the primary contraction is at the inlet and those in which the primary contraction involves the midpelvis and outlet.

Abnormal labor can be anticipated in women with reduced pelvic measurements or those in whom dystocia has occurred during previous labors. An unusual fetal position or a floating head at term should suggest the possibility of inlet disproportion, even though the measurements are normal.

A sterile vaginal examination with the patient in lithotomy position should be performed during early labor in any woman whose pelvic measurements are reduced or in whom there is any suggestion of disproportion. X-ray pelvimetry should be obtained unless the vaginal examination indicates conclusively that the pelvis is adequate and fetal position is normal.

Inlet contraction. Inlet contraction can be diagnosed if the true conjugate is 10 cm. or less in length or if the diagonal conjugate measures 11.5 cm. or less. The outcome of labor is in part dependent upon the length of the true conjugate, but other important factors are pelvic configuration, size and position of the infant, and the effectiveness of the uterine contractions. Although it may not always be possible to prognosticate the eventual outcome, inlet contractions are usually relatively easy to manage as compared to the abnormalities involving the lower pelvis.

A reasonably accurate evaluation of whether the head will pass the inlet can be obtained at vaginal examination. Disproportion can be diagnosed if it is impossible to insert the first two fingers between the head in the inlet and the posterior surface of the pubis or if the head is overriding the pubis and cannot be forced into the inlet by downward pressure on the uterine fundus or on the suprapubic portion of the head. If the head can be pushed down to station minus 1 or 0, the size of the inlet probably is adequate.

Although the inability to impress the head into the pelvis does not prove that there is significant disproportion, it does indicate the need for x-ray study. Roentgen pelvimetry should be obtained whenever there is any question of disproportion. The attending physician ought to examine the films with the radiologist because in almost every instance the visual image of the relationship between the head and the pelvic cavity provides more valuable information than do pelvic measurements alone.

ELECTIVE CESAREAN SECTION. An elective cesarean section is usually indicated in women at least 38 weeks pregnant if the conjugata vera is 10 cm. or less with the breech presenting or 8 cm. or less with vertex presentation. Elective abdominal delivery may also be considered at the same stage of pregnancy with a relatively minor contraction if the membranes rupture prematurely while the cervix is firm and uneffaced and the head is floating and cannot be depressed into the inlet. X-ray examination for more exact evaluation is indicated before cesarean section is performed.

TRIAL LABOR. Since most women with mild inlet contractions and some of those with more pronounced deformities will deliver vaginally if the uterine contractions are forceful enough, they should be given an opportunity to do so by means of a trial labor. If the uterine contractions are of normal quality and recur every 3 to 5 minutes, the physician can ordinarily decide within 10 to 12 hours whether vaginal delivery is possible. If the inlet contraction can be overcome, the cervix will dilate and the head will descend through the superior strait. If this occurs, labor can be permitted to continue with the expectation that it will terminate normally even though it may take longer than usual. The physician must make certain that descent and engagement actually are occurring. In some instances the lower portion of the head descends into the pelvis because of extreme molding and caput formation, whereas the biparietal area remains relatively stationary above the inlet. If there is any question concerning descent, a lateral x-ray study should be repeated for comparison with the original study during early labor. If descent does not occur, cesarean section can be performed safely after an adequate trial labor.

The membranes usually rupture spontaneously during the course of labor, but if they do not, they should be ruptured artificially.

Intact membranes will sometimes prevent the head from descending even though the pelvic capacity is perfectly adequate for delivery. The head often descends and delivers after amniotomy. There is some danger of the cord prolapsing if the amniotic sac is perforated while the presenting part is high. If this should occur, it is immediately obvious and the infant can be delivered alive by cesarean section.

Unfortunately a good trial labor is not always possible. Many women with contracted pelves also have dysfunctional labors with irregular, ineffective uterine contractions. Others will begin what appears to be a normal labor, cervical dilatation progressing to 6 or 7 cm. after which the contractions become irregular and ineffective—an *active phase arrest*. This is a common response to cephalopelvic disproportion in primigravidas. Oxytocin stimulation is justifiable if the physician determines by vaginal and x-ray examinations that the disproportion is minor. If it seems obvious that vaginal delivery will not occur, even with forceful uterine con-

tractions, cesarean section should be performed. In contrast to primigravidas, multiparous women with contracted pelves often have tumultuous labors. If the disproportion is insurmountable, the uterus will rupture.

Sedatives may be administered if the labor is normal, but they must be withheld is there is any question concerning the adequacy of uterine activity. Orificial examinations should be kept at a minimum to reduce the chance of infection; descent can be followed by palpating the anterior shoulder and measuring its distance above the pubis. If a long labor is anticipated, it often is wise to administer penicillin, 1.2 million units, and streptomycin, 0.25 to 0.5 Gm., intramuscularly every 12 hours.

Midpelvic and outlet contraction. There is no reliable method for evaluating the adequacy of the lower pelvis, and a trial labor is much less satisfactory than with inlet contractions. Sterile vaginal examination should be performed early in the course of labor; if the head has already reached the level of the spines and can be depressed farther, it

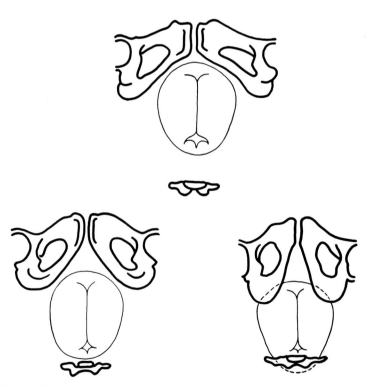

Fig. 34-10. Reduced bituberous diameter showing effect of length of posterior sagittal diameter on outcome. (From Willson, J. R.: Management of obstetric difficulties, ed. 6, St. Louis, 1961, The C. V. Mosby Co.)

probably will continue to descend and will deliver unless the outlet is too small. On the other hand, if the head is high, in a posterior position, and cannot be depressed past the long spines and the anteriorly projecting sacrum, the outlook is less favorable. X-ray pelvimetry is indicated unless it is obvious that vaginal delivery can occur.

Cesarean section is not usually necessary for midpelvic and outlet contractions, but it almost always is preferable to a traumatic forceps extraction. It has been suggested that vaginal delivery is possible if the sum of the bituberous and the posterior sagittal diameters at the outlet equals 15 cm. Obviously this is an oversimplification because the adequacy of the outlet is determined by its shape as well as by the length of these two diameters, but it is helpful in evaluating the outlet (Fig. 34-10). If the presenting part fails to descend or if previous labors have been difficult and traumatic, abdominal delivery should be considered.

If the head descends to station plus 2 or more, vaginal delivery usually is possible. The head can be turned to an anterior position by manual or forceps rotation. With either method the head must usually be dislodged and pushed upward to a roomier part of the cavity. A generous episiotomy usually is necessary. Saddle block, caudal, or deep inhalation anesthesia will relax the pelvic muscles, making delivery easier and safer.

Complications. Infant mortality and morbidity are increased. The main fetal complications are from injury incident to the long labor or the operations for delivery, anoxia, and infection.

Maternal morbidity is caused mainly by soft tissue injury, hemorrhage, and infection.

References

Auer, E. S., and Simmons, J. M.: The floating fetal head in the primipara at term, Amer. J. Obstet. Gynec. 58:291, 1949.

Bishop, P. A.: Radiologic studies of the gravid uterus, New York, 1965, Paul B. Hoeber, Inc., Medical Book Department, Harper & Row, Publishers.

Brown, W. E.: The management of the borderline pelvis, Southern Med. J. 44:1046, 1951.

Caldwell, W. E., and Moloy, H. C.: Anatomical variations in the female pelvis and their effect on labor with a suggested classification, Amer. J. Obstet. Gynec. 26:479, 1933.

Caldwell, W. E., and Swenson, P. C.: The use of the roentgen ray in obstetrics. III. The mechanism of labor, Amer. J. Roentgen. 41:719, 1939.

Eller, W. C., and Mengert, W. F.: Recognition of midpelvic contraction, Amer. J. Obstet. Gynec. 53:252, 1947.

Javert, C. T., and Steele, K. B.: The transverse position and the mechanism of labor, Int. Abstr. Surg. 75:507, 1942.

Kaltreider, D. F.: Pelvic shape and its relation to mid-plane prognosis, Amer. J. Obstet. Gynec. 63:116, 1952.

Snow, W.: Roentgenology in obstetrics and gynecology, Springfield, Ill., 1952, Charles C Thomas, Publisher.

Steer, C. M.: Evaluation of the pelvis in obstetrics, Philadelphia, 1959, W. B. Saunders Co.

Tancer, M. L., and Vandenberg, W.: Disproportion in the multipara, Obstet. Gynec. 14:753, 1959.

Thoms, H.: The clinical application of roentgen pelvimetry and a study of the results in 1100 white women, Amer. J. Obstet. Gynec. 42:957, 1941.

Thoms, H.: Precision methods in cephalometry and pelvimetry, Amer. J. Obstet. Gynec. 46:753, 1943.

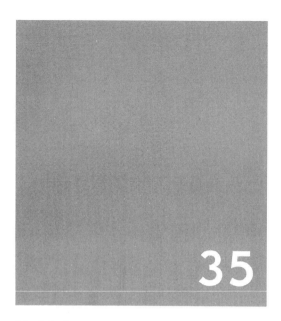

Multiple pregnancy

Multiple pregnancy, one in which more than one fetus is produced, occurs relatively frequently in human beings but is probably not normal. Greulich reported the following incidences in over 121 million births: twins, 1:85; triplets, 1:7,629; quadruplets, 1:670,734; and quintuplets, 1:41,600,000 single births. According to Guttmacher multiple pregnancy of all varieties occurs more often in blacks than in whites; the lowest incidence is found in Mongoloid races. Twins occur in a ratio of 1:73.8 and triplets in a ratio of 1:5,631 single births in nonwhites as contrasted to 1:92.4 and 1:9,828, respectively, in whites. The difference is due to a variation in the incidence of dizygotic twins; the occurrence of monozygotic types is similar in all. The infants are of the same sex in about two thirds of all twin deliveries, but the proportion of males to females is less than in single births.

It is well known that there is a genetic factor in twinning as evidenced by the fact that multiple pregnancies occur frequently in some family lines and rarely in others. An inherited tendency influences only the rate of dizygotic twinning; monozygotic twins appear to develop by chance. It has been assumed that a familial tendency in either the maternal or the paternal line will influence the number of multiple births for a particular couple. White and Wyshak, however, found that the father actually has little influence on twinning. Women who themselves are dizygotic twins produce twins at a rate of 17.1 per thousand deliveries, whereas the rate for wives of husbands who are dizygotic twins is only 7.9 per thousand. Female siblings of dizygotic twins behave like female twins in this regard, but the male siblings behave like male twins.

Twins are either *dizygotic* (double ovum or fraternal) or *monozygotic* (single ovum or identical). In dizygotic twins two separate ova produced during the same period of ovulation are fertilized by two spermatozoa. The twins need not be of the same sex, and often they do not resemble each other any more than singly born siblings. There are two separate placentas with no communication between the two circulatory systems, even though the placentas may be so completely fused that they look like a single structure. The infants are separated from each other by two layers of amnion and two of chorion.

Theoretically, *superfecundation* and *superfetation* are possible in human beings although either is hard to prove. The term superfecundation indicates that two ova produced during the same period of ovulation are fertilized by two separate acts of coitus. This can be proved definitely only if individuals of three different races are involved. With superfetation two ova produced during different ovulation periods are fertilized. This might possibly occur before the cervix is occluded by the mucous plug, but since ovulation is suspended during pregnancy it must be extremely rare if it ever happens.

Monozygotic twins occur in about one third of all double pregnancies. The individuals are always of the same sex and are either almost identical in appearance or mirror images. Both infants come from a single fertilized ovum and usually share a single placenta; the circulations communicate with each other through the placental vessels. Each infant usually is enclosed within its own

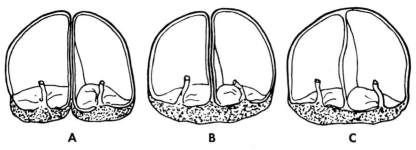

Fig. 35-1. Placenta and membranes in twin pregnancy. **A,** Dizygotic twins with two complete placentas and membranes. **B,** Dizygotic twins with double membranes and fused placenta. **C,** Monozygotic twins with double amniotic cavities enclosed within one chorion. (Modified from Eastman, N. J., and Hellman, L. M.: Obstetrics, New York, 1961, Appleton-Century-Crofts.)

amniotic sac; both of these are surrounded by a single chorion. The infants therefore are separated from each other only by two layers of amnion. In about 25% of monozygotic twins the two daughter cells separate immediately after fertilization; as a consequence each twin has its own complete placenta and membranes. Much less often the separation into two distinct embryos occurs 7 to 13 days after fertilization and after the amniotic cavity has formed. In this type, *monoamniotic twins,* there is a single placenta, and both infants develop in a common amniotic cavity.

Identical twins can be produced experimentally by applying an abnormal stimulus that retards the growth of a fertilized ovum at some special stage of its development. Double embryonic areas, each of which eventually develops into a separate infant, appear when the stimulus is removed. If separation is incomplete, a double monster may be produced. Newman has suggested that inadequate spermatozoa, delayed nidation, and heredity may retard growth in the human being.

■ Fetal development

Each twin at birth is usually smaller than a single infant of the same gestational age, but the combined weights of the babies are likely to be much more. One fetus may be larger than the other. Small differences in size are usually unimportant, but if one twin is much larger than the other, the physician should consider the possibility of *transfusion syndrome.* The larger twin is plethoric, edematous, and polycythemic and has cardiac and renal hypertrophy. There also is an accompanying hydramnios due to increased urine production. The smaller twin is pale, anemic, and dehydrated and has less than the usual amount of amniotic fluid. The basic cause is an inequality in placental circulation resulting from anastomoses between the placental arteries of one twin and the placental veins of the other. The degree of change is determined by the number and size of anastomoses. Although a certain number of anastomoses between the vessels of twins are to be expected, they usually produce no difficulty; this is particularly true if the connections are artery to artery or vein to vein. With uncompensated arteriovenous anastomoses, however, the recipient twin is constantly perfused by blood entering its circulation under high pressure from the donor twin's arteries. The recipient twin becomes plethoric and the donor becomes hypovolemic and anemic.

In some instances one of the infants fails to develop and is deformed; *acardius acephalus* is a condition in which only the pelvis and lower extremities can be identified, and *acardius amorphus* is that in which the infant has almost no recognizable form. One infant may die early and become compressed, whereas the other grows normally. This is called a *fetus papyraceus.* Occasionally one of a set of double ovum twins will be aborted while the other continues to develop.

■ Clinical course

Early nausea and vomiting may be more severe and last longer. The amount of fluid in the combined amniotic sacs is greater than that with a single pregnancy. This cannot

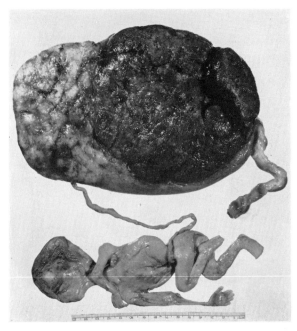

Fig. 35-2. Fetus papyraceus. The infarcted nonfunctioning placenta to which the degenerated fetus is attached can be seen at the left. The other infant was normal.

be considered as true hydramnios, however, because the volume in each sac is usually not excessive. Preeclampsia develops more often than with single pregnancy. Patients with twins are uncomfortable because the uterus is larger than with a single pregnancy and because varicosities, backache, pelvic pressure, hemorrhoids, and edema all occur more frequently.

Labor begins early, usually 2 or 3 weeks before term. Behrman reported that labor began before the thirty-seventh week of pregnancy in 39% of 248 twin pregnancies delivered in the University of Michigan Hospital. Uterine dysfunction may occur if the uterus is greatly overdistended, and as a consequence postpartum blood loss is often excessive. Cephalopelvic disproportion is seldom encountered because each baby is relatively small. The position of the infants is variable, but in at least 90% both lie parallel to the longitudinal axis of their mother's body. Both heads may present, or one presentation may be a vertex and the other a breech. Occasionally both present as breeches, or one may lie longitudinally and the other transversely. Abnormal position, particularly of the second twin, occurs more often than in single pregnancies.

■ Diagnosis

The diagnosis should be suspected whenever the uterus seems larger than it should for the calculated period of gestation, in the presence of an excessive amount of fluid, or if a profusion of small parts, or more than one head or more than two fetal poles can be felt.

The circumference of the abdomen at the umbilicus usually measures less than 100 cm. in normal women at term; with multiple pregnancy it is usually larger. If two separate sets of fetal heart sounds that are widely separated and of different rates when counted simultaneously are heard, the diagnosis is certain.

If the physician exerts downward pressure on the superior pole of a single fetus, the presenting part will descend slightly into the pelvis. This can be detected by vaginal palpation as the pressure is applied. With a twin pregnancy pressure over one pole will produce the same effect, but when the maneuver is performed on the second superior pole, there may be no change in the station of the presenting part because it belongs to the other infant.

Twins can also be diagnosed by electrocardiographic evidence of two fetal hearts or

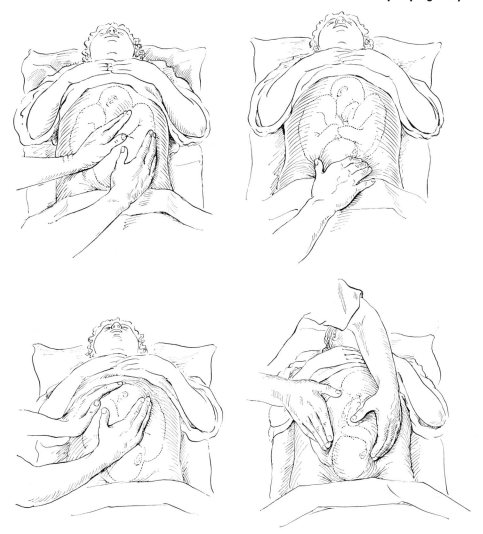

Fig. 35-3. Twin pregnancy showing abdominal palpation.

by the use of ultrasound. With these methods the diagnosis can sometimes be made before the middle of pregnancy.

The most accurate method of diagnosis is by x-ray examination. This examination should be performed at some time during the last trimester to confirm the presence of twins and to determine the fetal positions so that the physician can anticipate any problems that may arise during labor or at delivery.

All the evidences of twin pregnancy are exaggerated when three or more infants develop. An exact count can be made only by x-ray examination.

■ Management

Most women with multiple pregnancy will be more comfortable with a maternity gar-ment to support the large abdomen. Salt intake should be limited in an effort to reduce the incidence of preeclampsia and the amount of edema. Cervical effacement occurs earlier than with a single pregnancy, and labor usually begins before term; consequently women with multiple pregnancy ought not to travel during the last trimester. Bed rest will delay the onset of labor; consequently a woman with multiple pregnancy should be encouraged to spend as much time as possible in bed after the thirty-second week. Actually, a week or two of complete bed rest at about the thirty-second week of pregnancy has been recommended. This is difficult for most women with children, but it should be encouraged. It may be particularly important for primigravidas because the incidence of prematurity is much higher than for multiparas. Rest before the thirty-second week has no effect upon the rate of premature delivery. She should refrain from coitus during most of the last trimester to prevent the possibility of traumatic rupture of the membranes.

Labor and delivery. Compatible blood should be available to use if postpartum bleeding is excessive, and an intravenous infusion should be started through an 18-gauge needle when delivery is imminent. Twin pregnancy has little effect upon the length of labor in either primigravidas or multiparas, but dysfunctional labor occurs more often than with single pregnancies. Artificial rupture of the presenting sac to reduce distention will usually improve labor.

If labor begins several weeks before term, sedation must be used with caution, but when the pregnancy has progressed to 37 weeks or more, analgesic drugs ought not to harm the infants. Paracervical block or caudal or epidural techniques are appropriate for controlling pain during labor, particularly if it has started prematurely.

The physician should attempt to make an exact diagnosis of position by vaginal and, if not already done, by x-ray examinations.

The first child may be allowed to deliver spontaneously, or the head may be extracted by outlet forceps. With breech positions partial extraction is usually preferable to either spontaneous expulsion or complete extraction. The cord should be doubly clamped before it is cut to prevent exsanguination of the second of uniovular twins.

The position or even the lie of the second twin may change as the first baby leaves the uterus; consequently the presenting part of the second infant should be identified soon after the first is delivered so that plans can be made for its delivery. If the second infant is lying transversely, the physician should attempt, by combined external and internal manipulation, to bring either the head or the buttocks over the inlet while the uterus is still relatively relaxed and before the membranes rupture. This will make its delivery easier and safer. As a general rule the membranes should be ruptured artificially and a breech extraction performed if the buttocks present. If the head presents, it often will descend after amniotomy and may deliver spontaneously. If this does not occur, it can be extracted with forceps. If the second twin lies transversely over the inlet and it cannot be rotated into a more favorable position, or if the cord prolapses, version and extraction are necessary.

There have been numerous reports of hours or even days between the births of twins, but unnecessary delay subjects the second baby to an undue hazard. The placenta may separate as the uterine muscle contracts, and cord prolapse is favored by the fact that the second presenting part is usually high or because the infant lies transversely. The results are best when the second twin is delivered within 5 to 10 minutes of the first.

Regional anesthesia usually is preferable to inhalation anesthesia because pregnancy often terminates prematurely and because the distended uterus tends to contract poorly. Pudendal block alone or supplemented by nitrous oxide–oxygen during the delivery may be adequate. Intrauterine manipulation for delivery of the second twin usually cannot be performed with pudendal or local block alone, but the addition of a small amount of an inhalation anesthetic will usually permit any procedure that may be necessary for delivery. Operative extraction of the second twin can be performed without difficulty if the patient already has been given a caudal or saddle block anesthetic.

Occasionally the placenta of the first infant will deliver while the second twin is still in the uterus, but more often both placentas are extruded simultaneously. If the placenta cannot be expressed by the usual maneuvers, it must be removed manually. The placenta may separate partially after the first child is born. When this occurs, the second infant must be delivered promptly or it will die of anoxia.

Complications. *Prolapsed cord* occurs more often than in single pregnancies and is more likely to complicate the delivery of the second infant than the first. Behrman reported six prolapsed cords in 248 second twins, but only one in first twins.

Collision between two fetal poles attempting to enter the inlet simultaneously may delay descent. If the higher presenting part is pushed upward, the lower one usually will descend. A tight abdominal binder may help to hold it in place. If the first infant presents as a breech and the second as a vertex, *the heads may lock at the inlet* after the body of the presenting twin has been delivered. According to Cohen, Kohl, and Rosenthal, locking occurs once in 817 twin deliveries and once in 87 with breech-vertex presentations. This is a grave complication, particularly for the first infant, who will usually die of anoxia during the manipulations neces-sary to free the heads. The physician can anticipate the possibility of locking if x-ray examination demonstrates the necessary breech-vertex combination.

Prognosis. The perinatal mortality is higher than for single births, principally because of prematurity, prolapsed cord, and

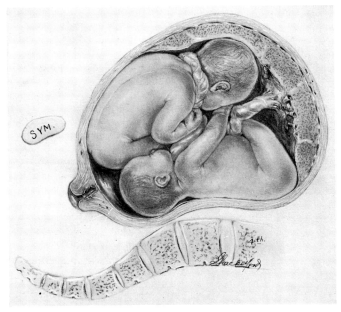

Fig. 35-4. Collision of twins at superior strait, preventing engagement of either. (From Willson, J. R.: Management of obstetric difficulties, ed. 6, St. Louis, 1961, The C. V. Mosby Co.)

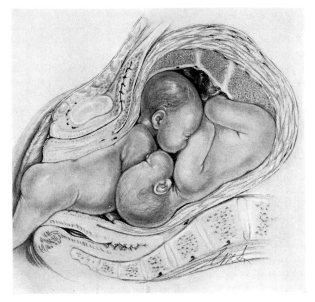

Fig. 35-5. Locking of twins. (From Willson, J. R.: Management of obstetric difficulties, ed. 6, St. Louis, 1961, The C. V. Mosby Co.)

anoxia in the second twin. Many of these complications can be prevented by complete evaluation of the patient early in labor, by careful observation during labor, and by intelligent management of the delivery. Since the mortality for second infants is higher than for first, it is essential that its position be determined immediately after the delivery of the first baby in order that it may be corrected if necessary. The second infant should be delivered without too much delay, and version and extraction should be performed only when an abnormal position cannot be corrected or if the operation is necessary for rapid delivery because of placental separation.

An important way to reduce infant mortality is to recognize the *transfusion syndrome* promptly and treat the babies properly. The plethoric infant may develop cardiac failure; the dangers from this can be reduced by phlebotomy. The anemic baby needs blood and should be transfused. The blood withdrawn from the plethoric twin can be administered.

The maternal risk is somewhat increased because of the relatively high incidence of postpartum hemorrhage.

References

Aaron, J. B., Silverman, S. H., and Halperin, J.: Fetal survival in twin delivery, Amer. J. Obstet. Gynec. 81:331, 1961.

Behrman, S. J.: Hazards of twin pregnancies, Postgrad. Med. 38:72, 1965.

Benirschke, K.: Accurate recording of twin placentation, Obstet. Gynec. 18:334, 1961.

Cohen, M., Kohl, S. G., and Rosenthal, A. H.: Fetal interlocking complicating twin gestation, Amer. J. Obstet. Gynec. 91:407, 1965.

Conway, C. F.: Transfusion syndrome in twin pregnancy, Obstet. Gynec. 23:745, 1964.

Dafoe, A. R.: Dionne quintuplets, J.A.M.A. 103:673, 1934.

Greulich, W. W.: The incidence of human multiple births, Amer. Natur. 64:142, 1930.

Guttmacher, A. F.: The incidence of multiple births in man and some of the other unipara, Obstet. Gynec. 2:22, 1953.

Jonas, E. G.: The value of prenatal bedrest in multiple pregnancy, J. Obstet. Gynaec. Brit. Comm. 70:461, 1963.

Kurtz, G. R., Keating, W. J., and Loftus, J. B.: Twin pregnancy and delivery; analysis of 500 twin pregnancies, Obstet. Gynec. 6:370, 1955.

Newman, H. H.: Multiple human births, New York, 1940, Doubleday & Co., Inc.

Nichols, J. B.: Plural births in the United States, Western J. Surg. 61:229, 1953.

Raphael, S. I.: Monoamniotic twin pregnancy, Amer. J. Obstet. Gynec. 81:323, 1961.

Strandskov, H. H.: Plural birth frequencies in total, "white" and "colored" U. S. populations, Amer. J. Phys. Anthrop. 3:49, 1945.

White, C., and Wyshak, G.: Inheritance in human dizygotic twinning, New Eng. J. Med. 271:1003, 1964.

36

Breech delivery

Breech positions, which occur in about 3% of all deliveries of infants weighing more than 2,500 grams (5½ pounds), are longitudinal lies in which the buttocks alone or the buttocks and some portion of one or both lower extremities descend through the birth canal first. The sacrum is the guiding point; therefore the possible positions in the maternal pelvis are sacrum anterior (S.A.), left and right sacrum anterior (L.S.A.-R.S.A.), left and right sacrum transverse (L.S.T.-R.S.T.), left and right sacrum posterior (L.S.P.-R.S.P.), and sacrum directly posterior (S.P.).

■ Varieties of fetal attitude

In the *frank,* or *single, breech,* which is present in about two thirds of all breech deliveries, the infant's hips are flexed on the abdomen and the knees are extended so that the feet lie in front of the face or the head.

In a *double,* or *complete, breech,* which makes up about one third of the total, the attitude is one of complete flexion; both the hips and knees are flexed and the feet present with the buttocks. With the less common *incomplete breech* attitudes one foot *(single footling)* or both feet *(double footling)* descend through the cervix ahead of the buttocks because the hips and knees are partially extended. In the other type of incomplete breech one or both *knees present* because of partial or complete extension of the hips, whereas the knees remain flexed.

■ Etiology

There undoubtedly are many reasons why an infant assumes a breech position in utero. The buttocks are more likely to present in the relaxed multiparaus uterus where motion is relatively free, especially during the second trimester and the early weeks of the third trimester when the amount of amniotic fluid is relatively greater than at any other stage of pregnancy. When breech position occurs repeatedly in successive pregnancies, the physician should consider the possibility of a developmental uterine anomaly such as a bicornuate or double uterus as a cause.

Stevenson found the placenta to be implanted in one of the uterine cornua in the majority of patients with breech positions that persisted during late pregnancy. The buttocks, feet, and legs are larger than the head and can accommodate themselves more comfortably in the lower segment than in the fundus of the uterus when the wide transverse diameter of the latter is reduced by the placental mass. When the placenta is in its usual site on either the anterior or the posterior wall, the available space in the fundus is less limited.

The reduced capacity of the fundus with high lateral placental implantation does not account for the position in frank breech, in which the buttocks alone occupy the lower segment and the larger head occupies the fundus. Fetal motion undoubtedly plays an important part in spontaneous conversion to a cephalic position; therefore if the knees are extended, the ability of the fetus to make crawling motions is eliminated, and the breech remains as the presenting part. This may well account for many instances of the frank breech attitude.

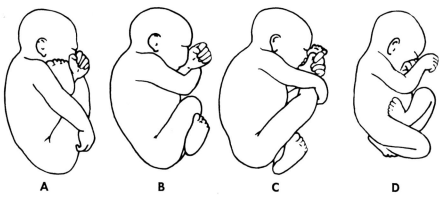

Fig. 36-1. Breech attitudes. **A,** Frank breech. **B,** Complete breech. **C,** Single footling. **D,** Knee. (From Titus, P.: Atlas of obstetric technic, St. Louis, 1949, The C. V. Mosby Co.)

■ Prognosis

The *maternal mortality* should not be significantly altered from normal rates if breech positions are managed properly. *Maternal morbidity* may be increased by the manipulation and the deep anesthesia sometimes necessary for delivery. Cervical and vaginal lacerations and uterine rupture are often produced during attempts to extract the infant before the cervix is completely dilated, and these, of course, cause bleeding and predispose to infection.

The gross uncorrected *perinatal mortality* may be as high as 20% to 30%, but this should be reducible to 5% or less with good care. The most important causes of infant mortality are as follows:

1. *Anoxia,* resulting from delay in delivery of the aftercoming head and from prolapsed cord, which occurs about ten times more often than in vertex positions. Morley, studying 538 term breech deliveries conducted in the University of Michigan Hospital found a 5% incidence of prolapsed cord with complete breech presentations, 15.7% with double footling, and 14.5% with single footling. No instance of prolapsed cord occurred in 345 patients with frank breech positions, presumably because the presenting part occluded the cervix completely, as does a well-applied head. Three of the babies whose cords prolapsed died, and 3 others developed incapacitating neurologic deficiencies.

2. *Injuries,* the most serious of which are intracranial hemorrhage and fractures of the spine.

3. *Complications of prematurity.*

4. *Developmental anomalies.*

■ Diagnosis

If the abdominal wall is not too thick and if the fetus is large enough to permit accurate palpation, the diagnosis of breech position can usually be made by abdominal examination alone, unless the uterus is tense, irritable, or tender. It may, however, be necessary to perform other studies to confirm the impression obtained by palpation.

Abdominal examination. The firm, round, ballotable head can be felt in the fundus of the uterus and the irregular, softer breech over the pelvic inlet. The cephalic prominence cannot be palpated over the pubis. The smooth, firm, curved back is directed laterally with the small parts on the opposite side. The fetal heart is usually best heard on the side of the abdomen toward which the back is directed and above the level of the umbilicus, unless the breech lies deep in the pelvis.

Orificial examination. If the cervix is partly dilated and if the presenting part has descended far enough to permit adequate palpation, the bony irregularities of the lower fetal pelvis can be identified fairly accurately by vaginal examination. Rectal examination is considerably less accurate, but it certainly should lead the physician to suspect the possibility that the breech is presenting.

The physician can feel the triangular sacrum and coccyx with an ischial tuberosity on either side. One or both feet can be palpated in the incomplete or complete breech attitudes, and if the circumstances are favorable, the genitals can be identified. If the membranes are ruptured, fresh meco-

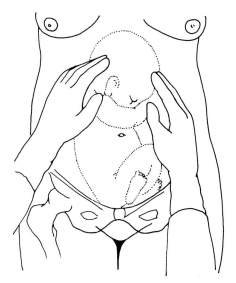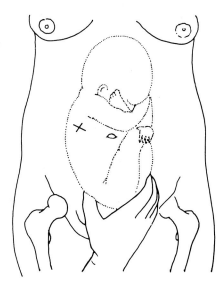

Fig. 36-2. Abdominal palpation, showing breech position.

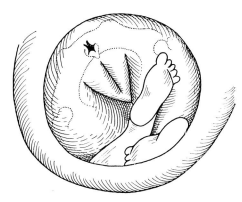

Fig. 36-3. Vaginal examination of complete breech. The bony prominences of the fetal pelvis, the anus, the external genitals, and the feet can be felt.

nium may be present on the examining finger. Unless the manipulations are performed gently, the anus or the genitals may be injured.

The most frequent error is mistaking the breech for a face or a shoulder. If the face is presenting, the bony orbits can be outlined, the sucking action of the mouth can be recognized, and there is no fresh meconium. With a shoulder presentation the scapula and ribs can be identified.

X-ray examination. It is seldom necessary to resort to x-ray examination only for diagnosis during the prenatal period, but if there is any question as to the position during early labor, roentgen examination should be obtained.

■ Mechanism of labor

Labor usually progresses at a normal rate, but a slight prolongation is not unusual. The cervix dilates at the usual rate in both primigravidas and multiparas if the uterine contractions are normal, but the presenting part may remain at or just above the level of the ischial spines until cervical dilatation is complete, after which it descends. The fact that the breech does not descend much during the first stage does not indicate disproportion. The breech is smaller than the head and will usually come down rapidly during the second stage, even though the pelvis is too small to permit delivery of the head.

In a complete breech the presenting part usually enters the inlet with its widest diameter, the bitrochanteric, in the transverse or in one of the oblique diameters of the pelvis. It descends in this diameter until the anterior hip meets the resistance of the muscular pelvic floor. As descent continues, the increasing pressure of the anterior hip against the levator sling causes the hip to rotate 45 degrees anteriorly to a position beneath the pubic arch; the opposite hip is now directed toward the maternal sacrum, and the infant's spine is directed toward the lateral pelvic wall. With further descent the anterior hip becomes visible in the introitus, at which

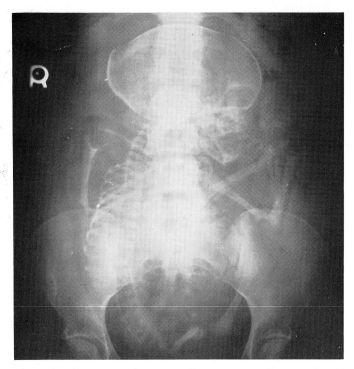

Fig. 36-4. X-ray examination of breech. (From Titus, P., and Willson, J. R.: The management of obstetric difficulties, St. Louis, 1955, The C. V. Mosby Co.)

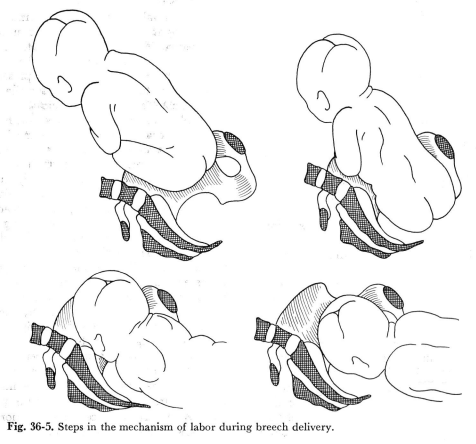

Fig. 36-5. Steps in the mechanism of labor during breech delivery.

time it impinges beneath the symphysis and remains relatively stationary while the posterior hip is forced upward and anteriorly over the perineum as the infant's spine bends laterally. After the posterior hip clears the perineum it falls backward, permitting the expulsion of the anterior hip from the vagina.

With a few more contractions the shoulders enter the inlet in the same oblique diameter that was occupied by the bitrochanteric diameter of the presenting part or in the transverse. They too descend until the more anterior of the shoulders strikes the levator sling and rotates 45 degrees or more to a position beneath the pubic arch with the axilla visible; the posterior shoulder now lies in the hollow of the sacrum. The continuing uterine contractions force the posterior shoulder anteriorly over the perineum until it and the arm are delivered, after which it falls backward, permitting the anterior shoulder and arm to emerge from beneath the symphysis.

The head is usually slightly deflexed and enters the inlet with its long axis in either the transverse or in an oblique diameter, with the occiput directed obliquely anteriorly. The head descends and the occiput is rotated anteriorly until the the neck impinges beneath the pubis, after which the head becomes progressively more flexed as it descends, and as a result the chin, nose, forehead, vertex, and occiput are forced over the perineum.

Variations in mechanism. The previous description applies to most breech deliveries in women with normal pelves. Variations can be expected if the pelvis is small or with frank or incomplete varieties.

Frank breech. The extended legs may act as splints and prevent the lateral flexion of the spine that is necessary to allow the breech to descend through the curving pelvic canal and slide anteriorly over the perineum. Descent may stop at station 0 to plus 1; in this event operative extraction becomes necessary.

Incomplete breech. If one foot or knee is prolapsed ahead of the buttocks while the other remains high, the prolapsed extremity rather than the breech itself will usually

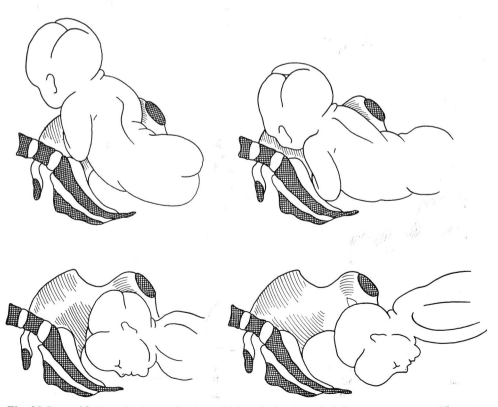

Fig. 36-5, cont'd. Steps in the mechanism of labor during breech delivery.

serve as a presenting part. If the anterior leg is prolapsed, the labor will probably progress as usual, with the anterior extremity and its hip rotating 45 degrees up the levator sling to a position beneath the pubis. If the posterior extremity is prolapsed, it will meet the levator sling posteriorly and usually rotates posteriorly.

Deflexed head. If the head extends after the shoulders deliver, the diameters that present may be too long to permit its passage through the inlet. If the head passes the inlet but deflexes as it descends, the occiput may rotate posteriorly into the hollow of the sacrum rather than anteriorly. This may complicate extraction of the head, particularly if the chin becomes impinged behind the pubis.

Extension of the arms. If the pelvic inlet is contracted or if an attempt is made to extract the shoulders through an incompletely dilated cervix, one or both arms may be swept upward alongside the head *(extended arms)* or even wrapped around the neck

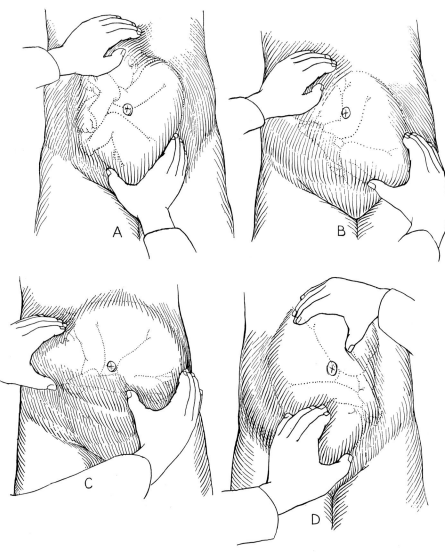

Fig. 36-6. External cephalic version. **A,** Buttocks are dislodged and head is flexed. **B,** Buttocks are pushed upward and head downward until infant lies in transverse position. **C** and **D,** Version is completed by further manipulation. (From Titus, P.: Atlas of obstetric technic, St. Louis, 1949, The C. V. Mosby Co.)

posteriorly *(nuchal arms).* This interferes with delivery of the head.

■ Management

Breech positions cannot be regarded lightly because, even if the patients are managed by experts, the fetal mortality is greater than if the vertex presents. All breech labors should be conducted in the hospital, and general practitioners and inexperienced house staff should ask for consultation as soon as the position is recognized.

During pregnancy. If the breech can be converted to a vertex by *external version,* the danger to the infant will be reduced. This maneuver should be attempted at about the thirty-fourth week when most spontaneous versions will already have occurred, but it may also be possible to change the position at a later stage of pregnancy or even during early labor. Cephalic version cannot always be performed successfully, but if it fails, no harm is done.

The patient is placed in slight Trendelenburg position to allow the fetus to gravitate upward away from the pelvic inlet, and its exact position is determined. One hand manipulates the head toward the pelvis while the other attempts to mobilize the buttocks in the lower segment and push the breech toward the fundus of the uterus. The head is rotated in the direction that provides the shortest course to the pelvis. The fetal heart must be checked frequently during attempted version because cord entanglement or pressure or anything else interfering with fetal oxygen supply will be reflected in an alteration of cardiac rhythm. If the manipulations produce pain, the physician should desist. Even though it is possible to rotate the baby successfully, it may return to the original position. Abdominal binders, pressure pads, or the like, which are sometimes applied in an effort to hold the infant in the vertex position, are unnecessary because they will not prevent the baby from resuming its previous position if there was an anatomic reason for the breech originally.

During labor. When labor begins, the physician must make certain that the pelvis is large enough to permit delivery of the infant. If the pelvic capacity is reduced, the physician cannot rely upon a trial labor, as he can when the vertex presents, because the buttocks and the body will descend through a pelvis too small to permit passage of the unmolded aftercoming head. If the head is too large and is extracted forcibly, the baby will undoubtedly be injured; if it is allowed to mold and deliver gradually, the infant will die of anoxia because the cord is compressed between the head and the pelvic brim and the baby cannot breathe until its head is free.

A sterile vaginal examination should be performed on all patients with breech positions soon after labor begins, and in most instances roentgen pelvimetry should also be obtained. It is difficult to determine by either vaginal or x-ray examination whether the pelvis will permit the head to pass because it is in the uterine fundus, and the usual maneuvers designed to detect cephalopelvic disproportion cannot be performed. The biparietal diameter of the fetal skull can be measured precisely by ultrasonic methods, but necessary facilities are available in only a few centers. Zatuchni and Andros have developed a scoring system based upon *parity* (primigravida 0, multipara 1); *gestational age* (39 weeks or more 0, 38 weeks 1, and 37 weeks or less 2); *estimated fetal weight* (over 3,630 grams 0, 3,629 to 3,176 grams 1, and less than 3,176 grams 2); *previous breech delivery* (none 0, one 1, and two or more 2); *cervical dilatation* (2 cm. 0, 3 cm. 1, and 4 cm. or more 2); and *station* (above minus three 0, minus two 1, and below minus one 2). In patients with breech positions of normally developed single infants weighing more than 2,500 grams, the complications of labor and delivery occur with much greater frequency in those who score 3 or less. Of 139 breech deliveries of normal term infants, 37% were nulliparous and 63% multiparous. The duration of labor for low-score nulliparas was about 12 hours, and for those with high scores it was about 8½ hours. Comparable figures for multiparas were about 9 and 6 hours. Labor was abnormal in 23 of 30 low-score patients and in only 12 of the 109 patients with high scores. Twenty-three of the low-score patients were eventually delivered by cesarean section, whereas all but one of those with high scores were delivered vaginally. Six of the 7 vaginal deliveries in low-score patients were complicated, whereas all but 1 of the 109 high-score patients were delivered without difficulty. The only infant death occurred in a low-score patient, but 5 of the 29 surviving infants of mothers with low scores had nerve palsy, convulsions, or other complications.

The membranes should not be ruptured artificially in normal labors because this may permit the cord to prolapse past the irregular presenting part, which occludes the cervix less completely than does the firm, round head. This is more likely to occur with complete breech than with the frank variety.

There has been considerable concern over the use of *oxytocin to stimulate labor* when the breech presents. Neimand and Rosenthal found no difference in fetal survival of infants weighing more than 1,500 grams in 105 labors during which oxytocin was used and 115 that were unstimulated. Zatuchni and Andros believe that oxytocin is contraindicated in patients with low scores but may be given when necessary if normal delivery can be anticipated.

Sedation may be administered as necessary to control pain, and the fetal heart tones should be recorded regularly. The *passage of meconium* is of no significance during breech labors, but an attempt must be made to determine a cause for abnormal fetal heart tones whenever they are detected.

Progressive cervical dilatation usually

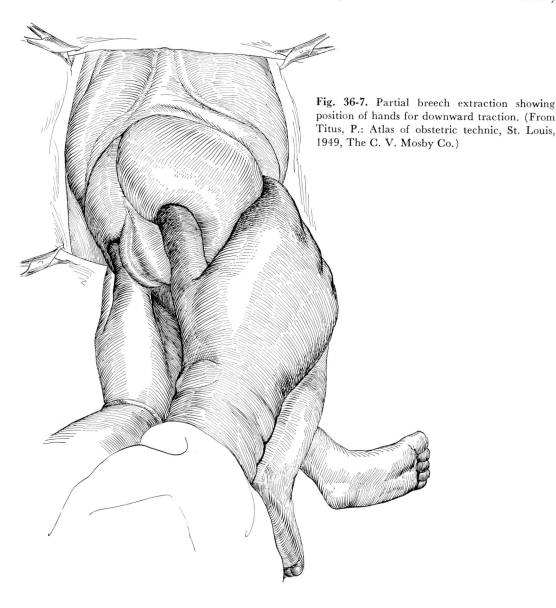

Fig. 36-7. Partial breech extraction showing position of hands for downward traction. (From Titus, P.: Atlas of obstetric technic, St. Louis, 1949, The C. V. Mosby Co.)

occurs, but the presenting part often remains at or only slightly below the level of the ischial spines throughout the first stage. If descent fails to occur during the second stage, another vaginal examination should be performed in an effort to determine the reason for the delay.

Delivery. The delivery should be supervised by a physician who is familiar with the problems of breech delivery and who has had enough experience to prevent complications whenever possible and to solve those that occur.

The physician must be certain that the cervix is completely dilated before attempting breech delivery. The buttocks, the body, and even the shoulders can descend through a cervix that is not sufficiently dilated to

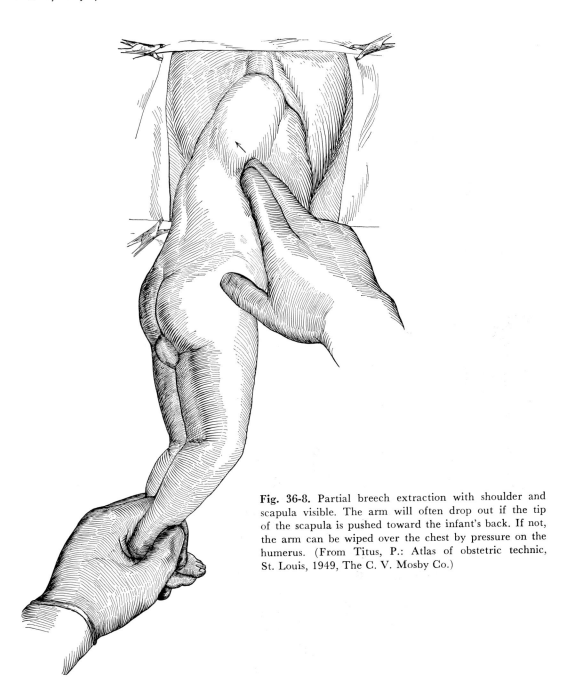

Fig. 36-8. Partial breech extraction with shoulder and scapula visible. The arm will often drop out if the tip of the scapula is pushed toward the infant's back. If not, the arm can be wiped over the chest by pressure on the humerus. (From Titus, P.: Atlas of obstetric technic, St. Louis, 1949, The C. V. Mosby Co.)

permit passage of the head. This is particularly true with premature infants whose heads are larger than their shoulders. With a frank breech the presenting part is smaller than the buttocks, feet, and legs of an infant in the complete breech attitude and will pass through a cervical opening much smaller than that required for the complete variety.

Spontaneous delivery. With spontaneous delivery the entire delivery is completed without manipulation by the attendant. This most often occurs with small premature infants and in multiparas with large pelves and rapid labors.

Partial breech extraction. Partial breech extraction, also known as *assisted breech delivery,* consists of spontaneous, controlled expulsion as far as the umbilicus, after which the shoulders and the head are extracted by the physician. When the breech reaches the pelvic floor in a primigravida and sooner in a multipara, the patient is taken to the delivery room. When the breech begins to distend the introitus and about 4 to 5 cm.

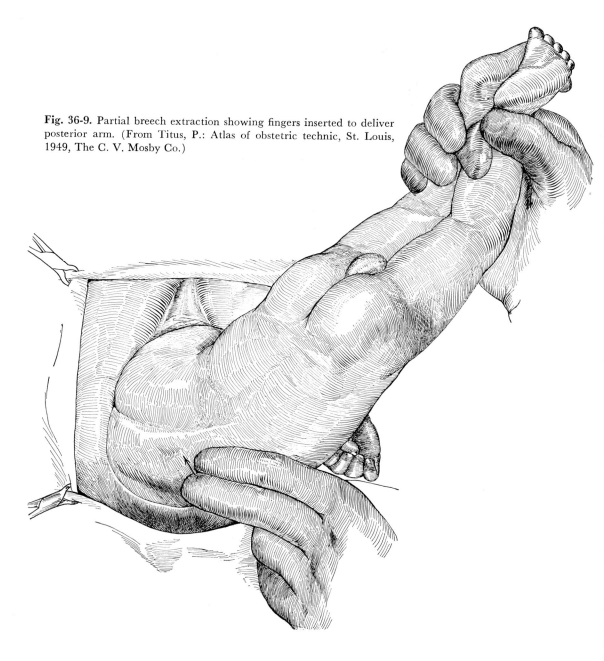

Fig. 36-9. Partial breech extraction showing fingers inserted to deliver posterior arm. (From Titus, P.: Atlas of obstetric technic, St. Louis, 1949, The C. V. Mosby Co.)

of the presenting part is visible during a contraction, an episiotomy is performed if necessary. If this is done at the proper time, the next few contractions will force the buttocks and the abdomen through the introitus, after which the rest of the body is extracted.

Downward traction is applied to the pelvic girdle with the thumbs placed parallel to each other over the sacrum or along the femurs, and the index fingers encircling the iliac crest. The body is gradually pulled downward, keeping the back directed anteriorly until the anterior axilla comes into view and the scapula emerges from beneath the pubic arch. Two fingers are introduced beneath the arch to a position along the humerus, and the arm is wiped down over the infant's chest and delivered. The body is then lifted upward and the posterior arm is delivered in the same manner.

The head can usually be delivered by manual manipulation alone with the Celsus-Wigand-Martin maneuver, by which it can be brought through the inlet in the trans-

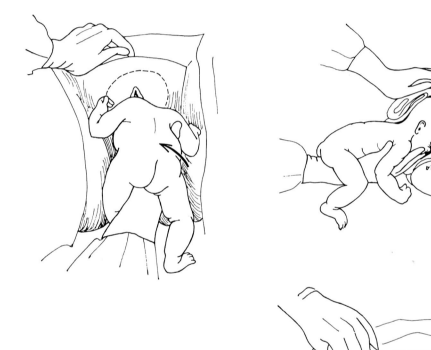

Fig. 36-10. Delivery of head with Celsus-Wigand-Martin maneuver showing exposure and aspiration of mouth and nose when head delivery is delayed.

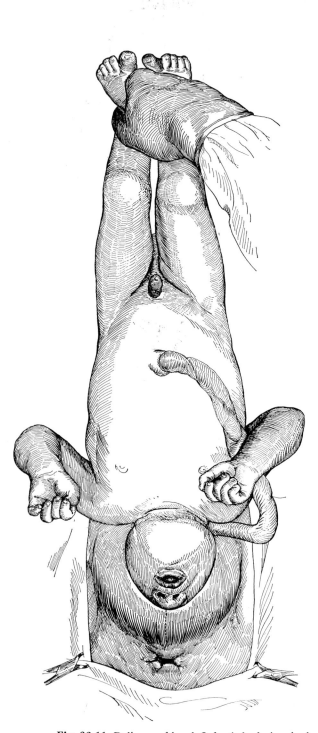

Fig. 36-11. Delivery of head. Infant's body is raised to deliver the head over the perineum. (From Titus, P.: Atlas of obstetric technic, St. Louis, 1949, The C. V. Mosby Co.)

verse or oblique diameter and then rotated to the anteroposterior diameter of the lower pelvis and delivered over the perineum by flexion.

It is usually stated that the head must be delivered within 8 minutes after the umbilicus appears at the introitus to prevent fatal anoxia, but this is not necessarily true. The maneuvers for delivery should be performed rapidly but deliberately; undue haste and forceful traction at this stage may cause more serious damage than a brief period of oxygen deprivation. If the head cannot be delivered easily from the lower pelvis, the infant will be able to breathe if its nose and mouth are exposed by forcible retractor depression of the perineum and posterior vaginal wall.

Complete breech extraction. In complete breech extraction the entire infant is extracted from the birth canal. This is one of the most difficult and potentially traumatic of all the obstetric operations and should be performed by an expert. The main indications for complete breech extraction are cessation of progress for 2 hours or more during the second stage, despite regular normal uterine contractions, and signs of fetal hypoxia during the second stage. Extraction is much easier with complete than with frank breech attitudes because in the complete breech the feet lie in the vagina with the buttocks, whereas in the frank breech they must be brought out from within the uterus.

Cesarean section. Abdominal delivery is seldom indicated simply because of breech position, but it probably has been used too infrequently in the past. It is likely that 15% to 20% of patients with breech presentations should be delivered abdominally. Cesarean section is more often indicated in primigravidas, particularly those over 30 years of age, than in multiparas. If the true conjugate measures less than 10 cm. and the pregnancy is of 38 or more weeks' duration, cesarean section should be considered because the unmolded aftercoming head may be too large to pass the small inlet. Cesarean section also is justifiable in women with dysfunctional labors that cannot be improved with intravenous oxytocin and whenever the physician suspects that the infant is unusually large or that a difficult extraction will be necessary.

Forceps extraction. Forceps are frequently applied to the aftercoming head but only after it has rotated to an anterior position and is well down in the pelvis. This procedure is comparable to low forceps extraction in vertex positions. Forceps should never be used in an attempt to bring the head through the inlet or through an incompletely dilated cervix.

Extended and nuchal arms. The arms usually remain in their normal position as the body descends unless the pelvis is contracted, in which event they may be swept upward beside the head. The same effect is produced by attempting to pull the baby through the pelvis, particularly if the cervix is not yet completely dilated. This complication can usually be prevented, but if it does occur, each arm must be freed individually by manually rotating the infant's body away from the locked arm until it lies beside the head near the face and then by sweeping it down over the ventral surface of the infant to deliver it.

Anesthesia. Most breech deliveries in multiparas can be completed with local perineal infiltration or pudendal block supplemented with nitrous oxide–oxygen mixtures. Saddle block anesthesia can be used in primigravidas whose labors have been normal and in whom the breech is crowning

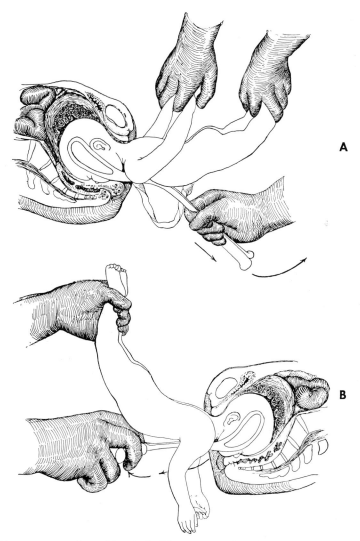

Fig. 36-12. Forceps extraction of head. **A,** Piper forceps. **B,** Simpson forceps. (From Titus, P.: Atlas of obstetric technic, St. Louis, 1949, The C. V. Mosby Co.)

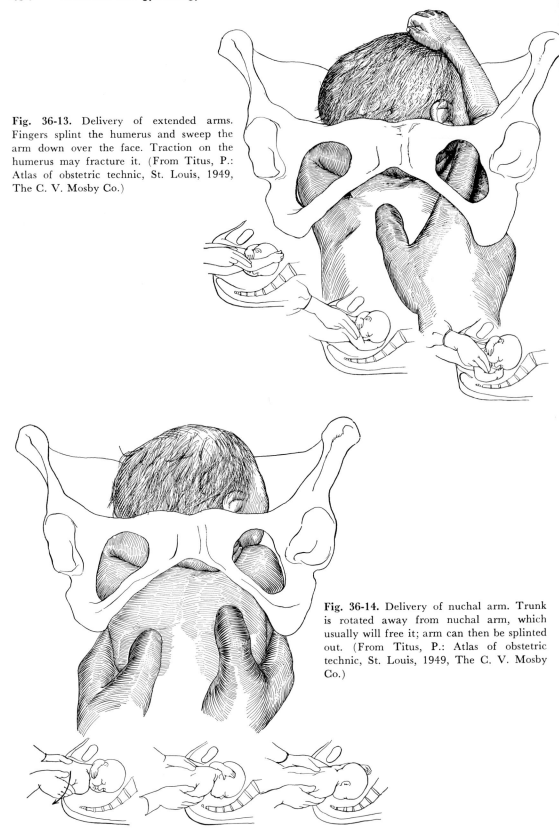

Fig. 36-13. Delivery of extended arms. Fingers splint the humerus and sweep the arm down over the face. Traction on the humerus may fracture it. (From Titus, P.: Atlas of obstetric technic, St. Louis, 1949, The C. V. Mosby Co.)

Fig. 36-14. Delivery of nuchal arm. Trunk is rotated away from nuchal arm, which usually will free it; arm can then be splinted out. (From Titus, P.: Atlas of obstetric technic, St. Louis, 1949, The C. V. Mosby Co.)

well when the anesthetic is administered. For breech extraction the uterus must be relaxed with ether or chloroform if it is necessary to splint the feet and legs out of the uterus, but with a complete breech the extraction can be performed with caudal, saddle block, or even pudendal block and nitrous oxide–oxygen if the feet can be grasped at the introitus. Unless the uterine muscle is completely relaxed, the manipulation necessary to flex the knees and to bring the feet down may rupture the wall.

References

Cox, L. W.: Breech delivery; the foetal risk, J. Obstet. Gynaec. Brit. Comm. 57:197, 1950.

Daley, D., and Michael, A. M.: The foetal risk in breech presentations, J. Obstet. Gynaec. Brit. Comm. 40:492, 1953.

Dieckmann, W. J.: Breech delivery at the Chicago Lying-in Hospital 1945-1952, Amer. J. Obstet. Gynec. 70:252, 1955.

Morley, G. W.: Breech presentation—a 15-year review, Obstet. Gynec. 30:745, 1967.

Neimand, K. M., and Rosenthal, A. H.: Oxytocin in breech presentation, Amer. J. Obstet. Gynec. 93:230, 1965.

Randall, C. L., Baetz, R. W., and Brandy, J. R.: Risks in breech delivery associated with fetal size and the induction of labor, Amer. J. Obstet. Gynec. 82:27, 1961.

Ryder, C. H.: Breech presentations treated by cephalic versions in the consecutive versions of 1,700 women, Amer. J. Obstet. Gynec. 45:1004, 1943.

Stevenson, C. S.: Certain concepts in handling of breech and transverse presentations in late pregnancy, Amer. J. Obstet. Gynec. 62:488, 1951.

Tompkins, P.: An inquiry into the causes of breech presentation, Amer. J. Obstet. Gynec. 51:595, 1946.

Zatuchni, G. I., and Andros, G. J.: Prognostic index for vaginal delivery in breech presentation at term, Amer. J. Obstet. Gynec. 98:854, 1967.

Forceps delivery

37

Obstetric forceps are instruments designed to *extract* the infant from the birth canal or to *rotate* its head within the vagina. They are never used to compress the head or to aid in dilating the cervix. Forceps are applied only to the head of the infant and never to any other part of its body.

More than 600 types of forceps have been designed, many of them for a specific purpose such as extraction of the aftercoming head in breech delivery or for rotation of the head from certain abnormal positions. All forceps are alike in that they consist of two blades that articulate at the point where the shafts cross and lead into the handles. The blades have two curves, the *cephalic curve,* which conforms to the contours of the infant's head, and the *pelvic curve,* which approximates the curve of the pelvic canal. The blades may be fenestrated or solid. The left blade is the one that is inserted into the left half of the pelvis, the handle being held in the operator's left hand. This blade artic-

ulates with the right one by means of a flanged lock on the shafts of the instrument.

■ Types of forceps application

Forceps operations are classified according to the station and position of the presenting part at the time the forceps are applied.

Low forceps application. The term *low forceps* indicates that the skull has reached the pelvic floor, the position is direct occiput anterior, and the scalp can be seen in the introitus during each contraction. After the patient has been anesthetized for delivery, particularly with spinal or pudendal block anesthesia which eliminates perineal sensation and the urge to bear down, the head may retract slightly in the birth canal. One would still classify the extraction as low forceps if the criteria had been met before the anesthetic was administered.

Midforceps application. The term *midforceps* indicates that the head is engaged but the criteria for low forceps have not yet been met. In some classifications midforceps deliveries are further subdivided into *high* and *low.* A *high midforceps application* is one in which the presenting part lies between the level of the ischial spines and station plus 2. The sagittal suture is usually in an oblique or a transverse diameter of the pelvis. With a *low midforceps application* the presenting part is below station plus 2 but is not yet visible, or if it can be seen, it has not yet rotated to a direct occiput anterior position.

High forceps application. The presenting part lies between the plane of the inlet and that of the ischial spines in high forceps application.

It is not sufficient merely to name the type of forceps delivery because some midforceps extractions are easy and atraumatic, whereas others are most difficult. Much more information is made available if an exact description of the station and position of the head and the difficulties encountered during the application of the forceps and the delivery of the infant is recorded in the hospital record.

The *position* of the forceps in the pelvis is determined by the pelvic diameter that passes at a right angle through the center of the fenestra. If each blade is applied to the lateral pelvic wall with its pelvic curve directed anteriorly, the forceps are in the

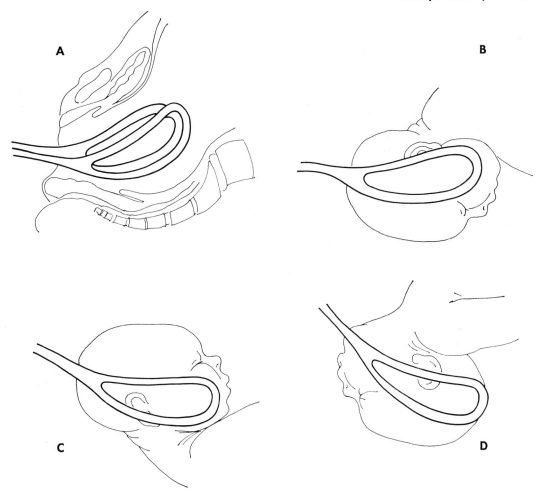

Fig. 37-1. Cephalic application of forceps. **A,** Forceps in transverse position in pelvis with pelvic curve corresponding to curve of birth canal. **B,** Occiput anterior. **C,** Occiput posterior. **D,** Breech, or mentum anterior.

transverse diameter of the pelvis. If the blades are then rotated 45 degrees, they lie in an oblique diameter. If they are rotated another 45 degrees, the pelvic curve is directed toward the lateral pelvic wall with one blade overlying the sacrum and the other beneath the pubic arch; they are now in the anteroposterior diameter.

The blades are said to be in the *cephalic,* or *ideal, application* if they have been applied to the head in the occipitomental diameter and equidistant from the sagittal suture. If the blades are applied to the sides of the pelvis with the front of the forceps directed anteriorly without regard to the position of the fetal head, they are in *pelvic application.*

■ Indications

The use of forceps is indicated whenever it is necessary to terminate labor in the interest of either the mother or the infant and when forceps extraction is the easiest and safest method for delivering the baby.

Maternal indications. Maternal indication for forceps delivery are cessation of progress because of inadequate uterine contractions during the second stage of labor, abnormal position, or minor degrees of pelvic contraction; to eliminate the perineal phase of labor in certain patients with heart disease and tuberculosis; and to shorten labor in others with toxemia of pregnancy or complications resulting in hemorrhage.

Fetal indications. Fetal indications for

forceps delivery are fetal distress caused by prolapsed cord, pressure on the head, placental separation, or maternal anoxia.

Elective low forceps application. The elective low forceps operation is usually combined with episiotomy to eliminate the last 15 to 30 minutes of labor, during which the pressure of the fetal head on the distending perineum may injure both structures. This usually does not constitute a definite indication for the use of forceps, but it accounts for the majority of such deliveries. It can only be done in a suitable hospital by a physician experienced in forceps delivery if it is to remain as safe as spontaneous delivery.

Incidence. The incidence of forceps delivery varies from 1% to 2% in some hospitals to almost 100% in others. Forceps are necessary in less than 10% of all deliveries, and of these, 2% to 4% are midforceps and the remainder are low forceps deliveries.

■ Contraindications

The use of forceps is contraindicated in certain abnormalities of position, such as impacted mentum posterior and brow, and breech delivery (except on the aftercoming head). They are not to be used if labor is delayed by serious contraction of the bony pelvis or by an incompletely dilated cervix. If the head is not yet engaged when delivery becomes necessary, forceps are contraindicated. Forceps delivery should only be performed in the hospital.

■ Requirements

Although a true indication for forceps delivery may be present, such an operation is dangerous both to mother and baby unless the following requirements or conditions are met.

The operator must be familiar with the mechanism of labor and trained in the application and use of forceps. The doctor who has not had special training in operative obstetrics should usually refrain from the use of forceps, particularly the difficult midpelvic types. The midpelvic deliveries include those that are among the more difficult of obstetric procedures. Consultation should be sought for all such problems.

The cervix must be completely dilated. No one can forcibly extract an infant through an undilated cervix without producing a laceration that may extend into the lower uterine segment. In addition, the presenting part usually remains relatively high in the pelvis until the cervix is completely dilated. Forceps extraction from a high station, particularly in primigravidas, often results in deep soft-tissue lacerations as the head is drawn through the unprepared vagina.

There can be *no marked disproportion* between the size of the baby and the size of the pelvis.

The head must be engaged. The lower the head is in the pelvis the safer and easier will be the delivery. The physician must make certain by pelvic and x-ray examination that the head actually is engaged before he attempts the operation. If a huge caput has formed or if the head is molded and greatly elongated, its most dependent part may be deep in the vagina while the biparietal diameter is still above the plane of the inlet.

The vertex or the face must be presenting in a position that will permit delivery, and the head must be large enough to be grasped by the blades.

Anesthesia must be adequate for the procedure. For most low forceps deliveries, pudendal block provides satisfactory anesthesia. For the more difficult varieties, particularly when it is necessary to rotate the head, it is essential that the voluntary muscles be relaxed. For these operations low spinal, caudal, or deep inhalation anesthesia is required.

The membranes must be ruptured.

■ Selection of patients

The best obstetrician is not necessarily the one who can do the most perfect midforceps delivery but is more likely to be an individual who knows when to interfere and when to wait for the mother to bring the head to a point from which it can be delivered by an easy forceps extraction. The dangers to both mother and infant must always be kept in mind when considering forceps delivery because a reduction in the incidence of unindicated and traumatic deliveries will increase fetal and maternal survival.

Low forceps extraction. Low forceps extraction, when properly executed, does not add to the risk for either the mother or the

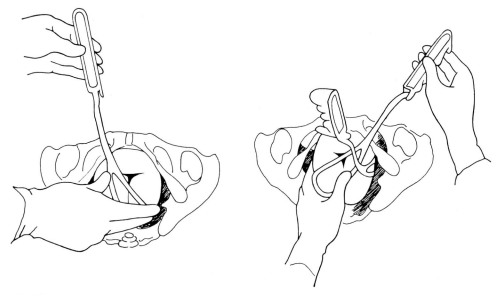

Fig. 37-2. Low forceps extraction showing application of blades.

infant. Many obstetricians perform episiotomy and low forceps extraction electively in most primigravidas and many multiparas. This operation may become necessary if the patient is unable to utilize her secondary powers to aid in the expulsion of the infant or if the uterine contractions become ineffectual late in the second stage. Under such circumstances forceps delivery may be preferable to oxytocic stimulation.

Technique. The patient, in litotomy position and properly anesthetized, is examined to determine the exact position of the fetal head. Episiotomy usually is performed at this time. The left blade of the forceps is introduced between the head and the guiding fingers of the physician's right hand until it lies in proper cephalic and pelvic application. The right blade is then introduced into the right side of the pelvis. The forceps are locked after any necessary adjustments in their position have been made. If the physician cannot lock the forceps easily, he should suspect that the blades are not properly applied.

After a final examination to make certain that the application is correct, the head is extracted. Traction at first is directed toward the floor in order to pull the head through the proper axis of the birth canal. As soon as the occiput appears beneath the pubic arch, the handles of the forceps are elevated each time traction is applied. This tends to extend the head as it descends, a duplication of the sequence of events during normal labor. The forceps are removed in the reverse order of their application, the right one first and then the left.

Midforceps extraction. Midforceps extraction is generally contraindicated unless there is a clear-cut reason to terminate labor. Most midforceps deliveries are performed because the orderly progress of the second stage of labor ceases. Forceps delivery should be considered whenever the head fails to descend and rotate during a 2-hour period in the second stage if the uterine contractions are normal and if there is no significant disproportion. Under such circumstances an unfavorable fetal position combined with mild disproportion often are the factors that interfere with labor and make the operation necessary. When the delay in labor is a result of uterine inertia, however, a trial of oxytocin stimulation usually is preferable to immediate forceps extraction. If effective uterine activity can be restored, the labor may terminate spontaneously or at least progress until an easy low forceps extraction is possible.

When midforceps delivery becomes necessary, the head has usually not yet rotated to an anterior position. Although a transverse or even a posterior position does not contraindicate forceps delivery, it makes the application of the blades and the subsequent extraction more difficult. The head can be

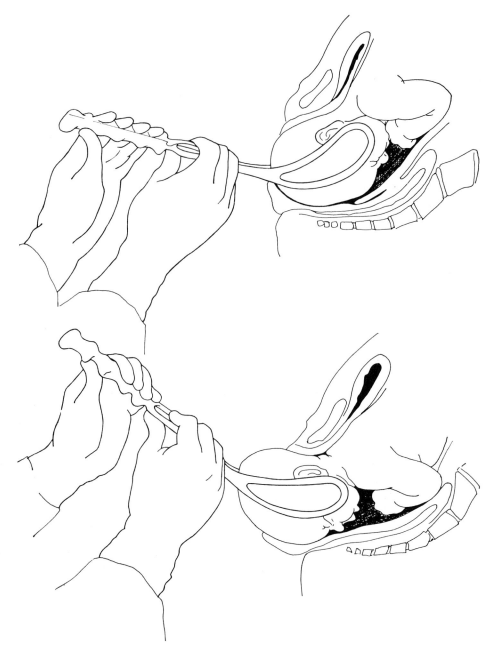

Fig. 37-3. Low forceps extraction of the head. The traction force is downward as well as outward until the occiput appears beneath the pubic arch. The handles are then raised to extend the head over the perineum.

rotated to a more favorable position by manual manipulation. This can also be accomplished with the forceps, and many obstetricians prefer this to manual rotation. In any event the physician must be completely familiar with the normal mechanism of labor and attempt to duplicate it during the manipulations for delivery.

Cesarean section often is preferable to a difficult midforceps delivery. This is particularly true if the presenting part has not descended below station plus 1, if it cannot be rotated to a favorable position for extraction, or if there is definite cephalopelvic disproportion. If, on the other hand, the presenting part is at station plus 2 or lower

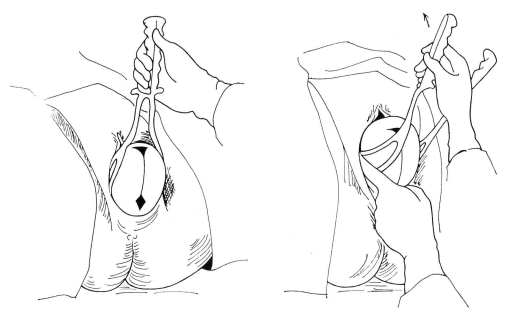

Fig. 37-4. Low forceps extraction showing completion of delivery of the head and removal of forceps.

and if there is no significant disproportion, vaginal delivery may well be possible.

High forceps extraction. For all practical purposes high forceps deliveries can rarely be justified. Cesarean section is almost always preferable when the need for delivery arises before the head is engaged.

Trial forceps application. On rare occasions the physician may be able to apply forceps with reasonable accuracy but may not be able to extract the head. This is usually a result of disproportion or of an unfavorable position. If the position can be corrected or the disproportion can be overcome without using an undue amount of force, the delivery can be completed successfully. Forceful traction, which may result in serious injury to the infant or the maternal soft tissues, is contraindicated. When forceps extraction is impossible or is thought to be too hazardous, cesarean section should be performed immediately. Bacteria are inevitably introduced during the manipulations necessary to apply forceps, and cesarean section after several hours is much more hazardous.

■ Results

The mortality and morbidity rates for both mother and infant should be reduced if forceps are properly utilized, since it is to be assumed that if their use is indicated the mother or the child is in danger. Low forceps extraction, when properly performed, does not increase morbidity, but the more difficult the procedure is the more dangerous it is. Mortality and morbidity will be increased if forceps deliveries are carelessly done or carried out in the face of contraindications or failure to meet the requirements. Steer reported that the infant mortality attributed to midforceps extractions was 4%, whereas that caused by spontaneous expulsion was zero, and that by cesarean section 0.1%. The only maternal death in 1,295 patients studied occurred after midforceps extraction.

The main immediate danger to the mother is from hemorrhage from lacerations, which may also become infected. If the pelvic supporting structures are injured, cystocele, rectocele, and even uterine prolapse may develop later. Traumatic lesions in the infants from forceps delivery include skull fracture, intracranial hemorrhage, seventh nerve palsy, and soft-tissue laceration.

■ The Malmström vacuum extractor

In 1954 Malmström reported his experiences with the vacuum extractor as a substitute for the conventional obstetric forceps. The instrument is basically a suction cup attached to a traction handle. The cup is placed against the fetal scalp, and a vacuum of 0.6 to 0.8 kg./sq.cm. is produced. This permits the operator to exert traction on the fetal head and even to rotate it within the birth canal. Although the purpose of the extractor was to reduce the damage produced by forceps manipulation, it is far from safe when it is used carelessly. Agüero and Alvarez reported that almost every infant suffered some damage, from superficial ecchymosis to avulsion of the skin, after delivery with the instrument.

References

Agüero, O., and Alvarez, H.: Fetal surgery due to the vacuum extractor, Obstet. Gynec. **19:**212, 1962.

Aveling, J. H.: The Chamberlens and the midwifery forceps, London, 1882.

Das, K.: The obstetric forceps; its history and evaluation, St. Louis, 1929, The C. V. Mosby Co.

Delee, J. B.: The prophylactic forceps operation, Amer. J. Obstet. Gynec. **1:**34, 1920.

Dennen, E. H.: Forceps deliveries, Philadelphia, 1955, F. A. Davis Co.

Dill, L. Y.: The obstetrical forceps, Springfield, Ill., 1953, Charles C Thomas, Publisher.

Malmström, T.: Vacuum extractor—obstetrical instrument, Acta Obstet. Gynec. Scand. (supp. 4) **33:**1, 1954.

Steer, C. M.: The effect of type of delivery on future childbearing, Amer. J. Obstet. Gynec. **60:**395, 1950.

Taylor, E. S.: Can midforceps operations be eliminated? Obstet. Gynec. **2:**302, 1953.

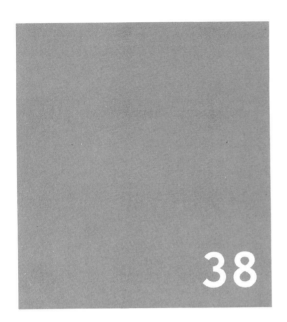

38

Cesarean section

Cesarean section is an operative procedure by which the infant is delivered through incisions in the abdominal and uterine walls. This term should not be applied to the removal of an extrauterine abdominal pregnancy or to delivery through the birth canal following vaginal hysterotomy.

In ancient times these operations were performed only after the death of the mother; during the eighth century Roman law made burial of an undelivered pregnant woman illegal. Cesarean section in living women is more recent. Early in the sixteenth century a Swiss swine gelder named Nufer presumably performed a successful operation upon his own wife after many attempts at delivery through the vagina had failed. Many authorities believe that this woman had an abdominal rather than an intrauterine pregnancy. Trautman of Wittenberg reported the performance of cesarean section in 1610,

and from then on it was done more frequently, but the high maternal mortality made it an almost useless procedure. The modern era began in 1882 when Sänger described a procedure similar to the classic operation used today. He also was the first to close the uterine incision, thereby limiting the amount of infected intrauterine material that would drain into the peritoneal cavity. Application of the principles of aseptic surgery, the development of safe anesthetic methods, blood transfusion, and advances in operative technique have made cesarean section a safe procedure for the management of certain obstetric complications.

Cesarean section, safe as it may be, cannot replace normal methods for delivery, nor is it a means of solving all complications. The *incidence* varies from hospital to hospital, but in most well-organized institutions it averages between 5% and 10%. The incidence figure is not important if all the operations are indicated and if patients are properly selected for abdominal delivery.

Before any section is performed the physician should make certain that there is not only a well-defined indication but no contraindication. The individual doing the first cesarean section on any patient assumes responsibility for the rest of her childbearing career. Should the first operation have been unnecessary and should she die in a subsequent pregnancy as the result of that section, the original physician ought to be held accountable for her death.

■ Indications

Mechanical dystocia. Disproportion, which is one of the most frequent reasons for cesarean section, can be caused by either soft-tissue or bony obstruction. If the conjugata vera is less than 8 cm. or the bituberous diameter less than 7 cm., it is unlikely that an average-sized term infant will pass through the birth canal.

In such patients cesarean section should be performed soon after the onset of labor unless the pregnancy is of less than 36 to 37 weeks' duration, when the baby should weigh 2,500 grams or less, or unless x-ray and pelvic examination indicate that normal delivery may occur. If the pelvic measurements are only slightly reduced, cesarean section should not be performed until disproportion has been verified by a trial labor.

Ovarian cysts, uterine fibroids, and other tumors that lie in the pelvis below the presenting part may produce the same effect as a contracted pelvis. Ovarian cysts or pedunculated uterine myomas that are diagnosed during early pregnancy should usually be removed before the sixteenth week. The patient can then be permitted to deliver normally. Cesarean section is almost always necessary if a tumor low in the posterior uterine wall or the posterior cul-de-sac is first discovered after the twenty-fourth week of pregnancy. By this time the uterus is usually so large that it is almost impossible to remove a cul-de-sac mass without disturbing the pregnancy.

Unverified disproportion. Certain patients with unverified disproportion may be delivered by cesarean section. These include women with borderline pelves in whom a trial labor would ordinarily be given but in whom the membranes have ruptured prematurely and labor has not yet begun and cannot be established. Bacteria invade the uterus rapidly, and cesarean section after the membranes have been ruptured for 24 hours becomes progressively more hazardous. A full-scale trial labor may well be contraindicated in women with serious heart lesions or other medical complications. Elective cesarean section is less dangerous than the same operation after several hours of labor.

Placenta previa. Almost all patients with complete placenta previa and most of those with incomplete varieties can be delivered more safely by cesarean section than through the vagina.

Abruptio placentae. With severe bleeding from premature placental separation when vaginal delivery is not feasible, abdominal delivery may be necessary. Cesarean section solely in an attempt to save the infant is contraindicated if the fetal heart rate is slow and irregular. The fetus is already hypoxic and undoubtedly will either die before it can be delivered or will be severely damaged.

Malposition of fetus. Cesarean section is indicated for most transverse lies, unless the baby already is dead or is so small that it is unlikely to survive, and for abnormal vertex positions that cannot be corrected and delivered vaginally.

Toxemia of pregnancy. Toxemia is seldom an indication for cesarean section, but if labor cannot be induced in women with ad-

vancing severe preeclampsia or temporarily controlled preeclampsia or eclampsia, cesarean section is warranted. Certain women with severe chronic hypertension or glomerulonephritis whose infants have died in utero during previous pregnancies may be delivered by elective cesarean section if labor cannot be induced at the appropriate time.

Previous cesarean section. The pregnancies of most women who have previously been delivered abdominally should be terminated by elective cesarean section.

Fetal indications. Fetal indications alone do not often warrant cesarean section, but occasionally when the *cord prolapses* through an incompletely dilated cervix and the infant's condition is good, abdominal delivery may be selected. The physician would rarely perform cesarean section simply because of *abnormal fetal heart tones* alone, but if the change in heart rate is accompanied by the passage of meconium, a diagnosis of fetal distress is more tenable and cesarean section may well be justified. The passage of meconium has no significance when the breech is presenting. If the infant has *died in utero* in more than one previous pregnancy, early cesarean section may be indicated if labor cannot be induced. Serial urinary estriol determinations may help in timing the delivery in women with diabetes or toxemia, and spectrophotometric examination of amniotic fluid may indicate the optimum time for termination with Rh isoimmunization.

Breech. Breech position in a woman with contracted pelvis may be an indication if the pregnancy is of at least 37 weeks' duration.

Elderly primigravida. The primigravida over 35 years of age need not be delivered by cesarean section simply because of her age, but the operation is generally used a bit more liberally for the management of complications, particularly dysfunctional labor, disproportion, and abnormal positions.

Medical conditions. Women with *diabetes mellitus* are frequently delivered by cesarean section because it is wise to terminate the pregnancy several weeks before term, at which time it may be difficult to induce labor successfully. *Advanced tuberculosis* or other lesions with which pulmonary function is greatly reduced make cesarean section justifiable. This is particularly true if prolonged or abnormal labor is anticipated.

Abnormal labor. Cesarean section may

occasionally become necessary in women with *dysfunctional labor* that cannot be corrected by oxytocic stimulation or other medical treatment.

■ Contraindications to transperitoneal section

Dead baby. Unless there is some other indication (severe abruptio placentae, absolute pelvic contraction, etc.), cesarean section should not be done only to remove a dead baby. It will leave a scar in the uterus, and rupture and death may occur in a subsequent pregnancy.

Repeated attempts at vaginal delivery. If labor has been prolonged and forceps have been applied unsuccessfully several times, the uterine cavity is almost certain to be infected. Under these circumstances transperitoneal cesarean section is dangerous. In certain patients, however, cesarean section may be performed after an attempted forceps delivery has failed because disproportion or an abnormal fetal position prevents extraction *(trial forceps)*. The cesarean operation must be performed immediately after the attempted forceps delivery before the bacteria, which inevitably are deposited in the uterine cavity during the manipulations, have had a chance to multiply.

Prolonged labor or prolonged rupture of membranes. The mortality associated with cesarean section rises as the period of labor or of time elapsed after rupture of the membranes increases. It is important that a decision as to the need for abdominal delivery be made early, preferably during the first 24 hours. In elective procedures cultures taken from the uterus at the time of operation are sterile in almost all patients, but as the hours of labor increase, so does the incidence of positive cultures. After 24 hours of labor with ruptured membranes the anaerobic *Streptococcus* has been cultured from 50% and an aerobic *Streptococcus* from 25% of patients.

Mild disproportion. Unless proved by a trial labor, disproportion of a minor degree does not justify cesarean section.

Heart disease. Most patients with heart disease, except those in whom there is an obstetric indication for cesarean section, can be permitted to deliver vaginally.

Bleeding. Most women with mild abruptio placentae in labor can be delivered promptly and safely vaginally. If there is evidence of fetal damage and the bleeding can be controlled, cesarean section is definitely contraindicated. The same is true of *marginal placenta previa* if bleeding can be controlled and delivery can be accomplished vaginally with minimal risk to the baby.

Fetal monstrosities. Fortunately fetal abnormalities that interfere with delivery do not occur often, and when they do, delivery can usually be accomplished through the vagina. For example, aspiration of the fluid from a huge hydrocephalic head will permit it to collapse and pass through the birth canal. Cesarean section should be utilized only when other methods are inappropriate.

■ Conditions necessary for performance of cesarean section

Cesarean section can be performed successfully only if it is done in the proper environment by the proper people. The following requirements must be met.

1. *Adequate facilities*—A clean hospital, a reliable supply of blood, a capable anesthesiologist, and assistants are basic essentials.

2. *A capable operator*—The surgeon must be able to do any of the types of cesarean section and not have to fit the patient to his one operation.

3. *Mother and baby should be in the best possible condition*—This is easier to accomplish with an elective section than for some of the emergency procedures. The mother should be rested and in a good state of hydration; she should be transfused prior to operation if bleeding has been pronounced.

4. *A good indication and no contraindication.*

■ Choice of operation

Classic section. In classic cesarean section the uterine incision is made through the upper contractile portion of the fundus above the dome of the bladder. It is easy to perform but has certain disadvantages that make it undesirable. The incision in the thick, active upper segment bleeds more and may not heal as well as the low segment incision. It also cannot be peritonealized, and thus there is more chance for infected uterine contents to seep into the peritoneal cavity, producing infection, ileus and distention, and adhesions. The mortality from infection is high after this operation if the membranes have been ruptured or if the patient has been in labor.

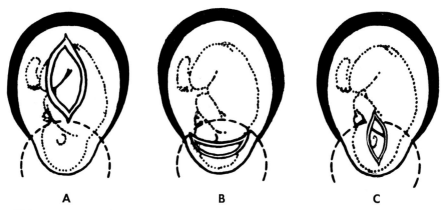

Fig. 38-1. Cesarean section showing position of uterine incision. The dotted line indicates the approximate position of the bladder. **A,** Classic incision. **B,** Low segment transverse incision. **C,** Low segment longitudinal incision. (Modified from Tenny, B., and Little, B.: Clinical obstetrics, Philadelphia, 1961, W. B. Saunders Co.)

Rupture of the uterine scar in subsequent pregnancies occurs more often after the classic than the lower segment operations. This operation may be preferable to the lower segment operations if the bladder is firmly adherent to the uterus, for transverse lie, for anterior wall placenta previa, in the occasional patient with carcinoma of the cervix, and when it is necessary to empty the uterus rapidly.

Low segment section. In low segment cesarean section the uterine incision is made in the thin lower segment after the visceral peritoneum over the uterus has been cut and the bladder has been separated and pushed downward from its attachment to the anterior uterine wall. The low segment operation may take a little longer and be a bit more difficult to perform, but anyone who is qualified to perform cesarean section can master the technique. The primary advantage is that since the incision is behind the bladder, it can be completely covered by peritoneum; thus the seepage from the uterus is reduced and postpartum peritoneal infection is less likely to occur than with the classic method. It can be used more safely after the membranes have been ruptured or labor has been in progress for some hours.

Extraperitoneal section. In extraperitoneal cesarean section the uterine incision is in the lower segment behind the bladder, but the peritoneum has been dissected off the dome of the bladder without entering the peritoneal cavity. The bladder is then pushed downward to expose the uterine wall. The extra-

peritoneal section is more difficult to perform, requiring a skilled operator, and bladder and ureteral injuries are more common than with the other operations. It does not solve the problem in the severely infected patient and probably is not necessary in the potentially infected patient; therefore its value is limited.

Cesarean hysterectomy. Cesarean section followed by removal of the uterus is indicated if there is a definite reason for hysterectomy, for example, multiple fibroid tumors, partial rupture, etc. Its value in the infected patient is greatest if the uterine wall is deeply and heavily infected and contains multiple small abscesses that may produce a constant source of infected emboli.

■ **Anesthesia**

There should be no increase in maternal or fetal mortality from the anesthetic. The same factors that influence the administration of medication and anesthesia in vaginal delivery hold true with cesarean section. The fetus is narcotized or anesthetized by all the medication given the mother.

Preoperative sedation. Morphine or a barbiturate usually is given prior to an abdominal operation. This type of premedication cannot be used in patients scheduled for cesarean section because of the potential adverse effects on the fetus. Atropine or scopolamine should be administered 1 to ½ hour preoperatively to reduce bronchial secretions. Sparine, 50 mg., or Phenergan, 50 mg., can be given for its sedative effect.

These drugs reduce apprehension and provide relaxation without affecting the baby.

Anesthetic agents. Regional or inhalation anesthetic agents may be used.

Conduction techniques. Conduction techniques provide adequate anesthesia for the performance of cesarean section without influencing uterine activity. They have no direct effect upon the infant. One of the following methods should be suitable for most normal women and for many with complications that make the operation necessary.

Local infiltration of the abdominal wall and peritoneum with 0.5% Xylocaine or procaine is associated with almost no increase in maternal mortality, and there is no effect upon the fetus. Although this is by far the safest anesthetic for cesarean section, it provides the least complete relief from pain. The abdominal wall can be anesthetized completely, but it is almost impossible to eliminate the pain associated with the peritoneal manipulation during the actual delivery of the baby. Best results are achieved if patients are carefully selected and prepared in advance for the technique.

Spinal anesthesia completely relieves the pain without interfering with uterine contractions or fetal oxygenation unless the blood pressure falls. It should not be used in patients in shock, those who are bleeding profusely, or those with hypertension or labile blood pressures. It must be given by an experienced anesthetist.

Epidural anesthesia provides the same advantages as does spinal anesthesia, and at the same time the blood pressure variations are less.

Inhalation agents. Inhalation agents are usually less satisfactory than the conduction techniques for the average patient. The anesthetic level must be fairly deep to permit opening the abdomen; hence narcosis in the infant frequently occurs. The maternal complications of aspiration, postoperative vomiting, and distention make all such anesthetics undesirable. However, an inhalation agent such as cyclopropane, which will induce unconsciousness promptly, may be the drug of choice when rapid delivery is essential, as in prolapsed cord, hemorrhage from complete placental separation, etc. In order to save the infant from prolonged exposure to the anesthetic agent the mother is catheterized, and

her abdomen is prepared and draped by the surgeon before the anesthetic is started. The baby can usually be delivered within 6 or 8 minutes, before its blood level of anesthetic is greatly increased.

■ Repeat cesarean section

A patient who has been delivered by cesarean section in one or more previous pregnancies must be managed somewhat differently from one with an intact uterus. There is always a question as to whether she should be delivered by elective cesarean section or whether she should be permitted to go into labor and deliver vaginally. A major factor in arriving at a logical decision is the integrity of the uterine scar. If it is strong and well healed, labor will undoubtedly terminate uneventfully, but if it is weak, it may rupture late in pregnancy or after contractions begin. Unfortunately there is no accurate method for evaluating the strength of the scar during pregnancy.

The uterine incision heals, as does any wound, by the proliferation of fibroblasts and scar formation. The integrity of the scar depends upon how the healing was accomplished. An uneventful postoperative course does not necessarily guarantee a strong scar, nor does a complicated recovery indicate poor healing. The wound may separate at any time during pregnancy or labor, but approximately two thirds of those that rupture do so during the last few weeks or after labor has started. The placenta often implants over an upper segment scar, and even though there is a defect in the old wound the pregnancy will progress normally until labor begins. After the contractions start both the placenta and the fetus may be pushed through the defect into the peritoneal cavity. Separation of a lower segment incision is less dramatic and may even go unnoticed because the baby is propelled through the birth canal rather than through the opening in the uterine wall. The scar is above the level of the presenting part and covered by the bladder.

Pedowitz and Schwartz found 48 persons with *silent ruptures* of scars at repeat cesarean section: 8.3% of 266 transverse lower segment incisions, 12.9% of 155 longitudinal lower segment incisions and 18.2% of 33 classic incisions. This is higher than the usually reported incidence of rupture of 2% to

4%; most of the latter reports concern only the symptomatic separations not the total number, many of which go undiagnosed.

Since the physician cannot tell in advance how well the uterine scar will tolerate the stress of labor, I believe that an *elective repeat operation* is advisable for most women who have once been delivered by cesarean section. This is particularly true of those in whom the initial procedure was made necessary by pelvic contraction that will always be present. Although this practice will not prevent all ruptures, it will reduce the incidence of late catastrophic separations considerably. Repeat section should be considered even for patients who have delivered normally in one or more pregnancies after the original operation. Five of Feeney and Barry's 16 patients with ruptured scars had previously been delivered without event.

Patients are admitted to the hospital for repeat cesarean section some time after the thirty-eighth week of pregnancy. The exact time is selected on the basis of the date of the last menstrual period, a comparison between the size of the uterus and the history at the first and subsequent examinations, the date at which fetal motion was first felt, the estimated size of the infant, the condition of the cervix, and fetal age as estimated by x-ray study. If the due date is uncertain or if the infant seems smaller than it should be for the duration of pregnancy, it is wise to delay the operation even though the pregnancy presumably has progressed to 38 weeks. When the cervix becomes soft and patulous and the roentgenographic signs of fetal maturity are present, the physician can proceed. Occasionally it may be necessary to delay until labor actually begins. Since repeat cesarean section is performed primarily in the interests of the infant, the physician must be as certain as possible that he delivers a mature infant and not one who cannot survive because of prematurity.

Some authorities recommend vaginal delivery for selected women in pregnancies subsequent to cesarean section. This is certainly safe for the majority, whose scars will be intact, but it may be catastrophic for those with weak or open ones. If the physician chooses to deliver such patients vaginally, he must be prepared to interfere immediately if the uterus should rupture during the labor. An operating room and a surgical team must be available constantly, and 2,000 ml. of compatible blood should be prepared in advance. After the patient has been delivered the physician ought to explore the uterus to make certain that it actually is intact. Vaginal delivery subsequent to cesarean section is contraindicated in patients with cephalopelvic disproportion, twins, or an abnormal fetal position and in those who previously have been delivered by classic cesarean section. Repeat section is preferable in general hospitals in which the requirements for safe vaginal delivery cannot be met.

Occasionally women on whom repeat cesarean section is planned will enter the hospital already in labor. If the presenting part has descended below the ischial spines and if the cervix is 5 cm. or more dilated, prompt delivery can be anticipated. Under such circumstances the physician may usually permit labor to continue but should be prepared to treat the patient promptly if the scar should rupture.

■ Sterilization

The fact that a woman must be delivered by cesarean section does not necessarily limit her reproductive career, but repeated abdominal operations are far more dangerous than an equal number of vaginal deliveries. A tubal ligation may be performed in conjunction with cesarean section if the patient and her husband request it, but there is no reason to insist upon the operation for normal women. Tubal ligation may be recommended if a serious medical complication such as severe cardiovascular disease is present or if the scar has repeatedly failed to heal properly. Some authorities recommend hysterectomy rather than tubal ligation as a means of terminating fertility.

It is not easy for a woman to give up her reproductive capacity, even though she really does not want more children. A decision to perform an operation for sterilization should not be made until the attitudes of the patient and her husband toward it have been explored and until the physician is certain that she really wants to be sterile and that she understands the procedure. Many women equate sterilization with castration and fear that they will lose their sexual attractiveness and ability but agree to the operation because it will prevent pregnancy. Such fears can usually be eliminated by encouraging the patient to discuss her concerns with you, by asking pertinent questions, and by explaining the procedure and its results in some detail. If this cannot be accomplished, it is questionable whether the physician should agree to perform the operation.

■ Complications

The mortality associated with cesarean section even under the most favorable conditions is greater than for normal delivery. This is not entirely from the operation itself but is in part from the complications that made the procedure necessary. Cesarean section need not be as dangerous as it has been in the past. Several series of more than 1,000 consecutive sections without a maternal death have been reported.

Infection. Infection, which is one of the major causes of death, can be prevented. It is caused by the spill of infected uterine contents into the peritoneal cavity during the operation or from leakage through the wound. This can be prevented by early decision to do a cesarean section and by more use of the low segment operation. Antibiotics to treat infection cannot compare in any way with prevention, and although they are of great value, they do not cure every patient.

Bleeding. Cesarean section is not a blood-conserving procedure; the blood loss averages about 1 L., and many patients lose much more. Adequate replacement in those who bleed abnormally will reduce deaths from bleeding. Since many cesarean sections are made necessary by hemorrhagic pregnancy complications, the combined blood loss from the lesion and the operation may be lethal unless the blood is replaced. The average patient upon whom cesarean section is performed need not be transfused, but replacement is desirable if the initial blood count is low or if blood loss is excessive.

Anesthesia. Unless the anesthesia is carefully controlled, it may contribute substantially to the mortality.

Infant mortality. Cesarean section delivery does not guarantee infant survival. In fact, the infant mortality with cesarean section is higher than the average rate for pregnancy in general. Many of the deaths occur because of the complication that necessitated the operation (hypertensive disease, diabetes, abruptio placentae, etc.) or because delivery becomes necessary several weeks before term. More premature infants survive after vaginal delivery than cesarean section; hence cesarean section should be selected for the termination of pregnancy before 36 weeks only if it is safer for the mother.

Many mature infants seem to do less well for the first few days of life after cesarean section than do those that were delivered vaginally. Most should be given special care, often in the premature nursery, for the first day or two.

References

Cavanagh, D., Membery, J. H., and McLeod, A. G. W.: Rupture of the gravid uterus; an appraisal, Obstet. Gynec. 26:157, 1965.

Feeney, J. K., and Barry, A. P.: Rupture and perforation of the uterus in association with pregnancy, labor and the puerperium, Brit. Med. J. 1:65, 1956.

Gordon, C. A.: The maternal and perinatal mortality with cesarean section, Amer. J. Obstet. Gynec. 73:65, 1957.

Grossman, M., and Benson, R. C.: Fetal mortality in cesarean sections, J.A.M.A. 162:1289, 1956.

Kobak, A. J., Fields, C., and Fitzgerald, J. E.: Antibiotics and low cervical cesarean section in dystocia and intrapartum sepsis, J.A.M.A. 148:1478, 1952.

McNally, H., and Fitzpatrick, V. deP.: Patients with four or more cesarean sections, J.A.M.A. 160:1005, 1956.

Pedowitz, P., and Schwartz, R.: The true incidence of silent rupture of cesarean section scars, Amer. J. Obstet. Gynec. 74:1071, 1957.

Pedowitz, P., Schwartz, R. M., and Goldberg, M.: The perinatal mortality in primary cesarean section, Obstet. Gynec. 14:764, 1959.

Schwartz, O. H., Paddock, R., and Bortnick, A. R.: The cesarean scar; an experimental study, Amer. J. Obstet. Gynec. 36:962, 1938.

Schwartz, R. M., Pedowitz, P., and Goldberg, M.: Perinatal mortality in repeat cesarean section, Obstet. Gynec. 14:773, 1959.

Van Praagh, I. G. L., and Tovell, H. M. M.: Cesarean section for fetal distress, Obstet. Gynec. 31:674, 1968.

Van Praagh, I. G. L., and Tovell, H. M. M.: Primary cesarean section in the multipara, Obstet. Gynec. 32:813, 1968.

Waters, E. G.: Supravesical extraperitoneal cesarean section, Amer. J. Obstet. Gynec. 39:423, 1940.

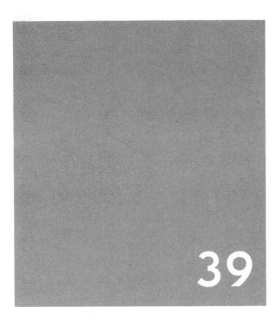

39

Immediate and remote effects of childbirth injury; uterine retrodisplacement

Some damage to the soft-tissue structures of the birth canal and adjacent organs occurs during every delivery. It usually is more pronounced in primigravidas, whose relatively firm tissues offer more resistance to the descent of the baby than do those of multiparas. Damage to the pelvic supports is usually caused by an injury that is obvious at delivery, but in some instances the skin and vaginal mucosa remain intact even though there are numerous small tears in the underlying fascia and muscle. In some women, notably blacks, the soft tissues are so readily distensible that they stretch without tearing to permit expulsion of the infant. In such persons the supports remain intact even after several pregnancies. In contrast, extensive damage may occur in other persons, even though every effort is made to preserve the

structures; such women may also develop varicose veins and diastasis recti, suggesting that they may have a generalized supporting-tissue deficiency that is basically responsible for the failure to heal properly.

All obvious injuries incurred during delivery should be repaired immediately unless there is a good reason for delay. Approximation of the injured tissues will permit them to heal and will limit the extent of interference with their normal function. Repair also reduces the possibility of infection. The cervix, vagina, and perineum should be carefully inspected after each hospital delivery.

The primary support of the uterus and the upper vagina is offered by the *cardinal ligaments* (Mackenrodt's ligaments), which are made up of connective tissue and extend laterally and posteriorly from the endopelvic fascia surrounding the cervix to fuse with the fascia overlying the obturator and levator muscles. The round ligaments and the broad ligaments have relatively little supporting function.

The muscles making up each levator ani sweep downward from their attachments along the ileopectineal line and form the pelvic diaphragm, the superior surface of which is covered by a strong layer of endopelvic fascia. The pubococcygeus portion of the levator surrounds the rectum, the vagina, and the urethra and is intimately connected to each. The levator bundles are held together between the rectum and the vagina by the fascia which, with the tissues in the lower portion of the rectovaginal septum, make up the perineal body. The bladder and the rectum are supported by the muscle in the wall of each of the organs and the extensions of the endopelvic fascia in the rectovaginal and vesicovaginal septa.

■ Perineal lacerations

Perineal lacerations are divided into four types, depending on their depth. In a *first-degree laceration* the tear extends through the skin and the superficial structures above the muscles. In a *second-degree laceration* the tear extends through the muscles of the perineum but does not involve the sphincter ani. A *third-degree laceration* severs the sphincter, and with a *fourth-degree laceration* the anterior rectal wall is also torn. At least the lower vagina is involved whenever the perineum is injured. The vaginal portion

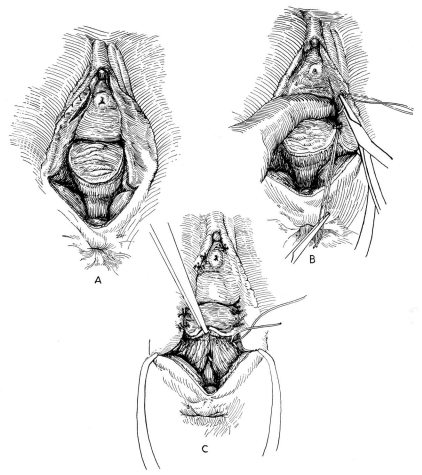

Fig. 39-1. Repair of second-degree laceration with sulcus tears. **A,** Note separation of muscle structures in the midline, intact anal sphincter, and lateral involvement of vaginal mucosa. **B,** Sulcus tears are closed with interrupted sutures. **C,** Levator muscle bundles are approximated in midline. (From Titus, P.: Atlas of obstetric technic, St. Louis, 1949, The C. V. Mosby Co.)

of the tear usually extends up one or both lateral sulci rather than up the midline; the depth depends upon the extent of the perineal injury. The levator fascia is injured in all but the most superficial perineal lacerations.

In addition to the perineal injury small tears may be produced in the mucosa below the pubic rami and lateral to the urethra and clitoris. These often bleed profusely because there are many large venous channels in the area.

TREATMENT

Perineal lacerations should be repaired immediately with chromic No. 3-0 catgut. The more superficial ones can be closed with one layer of interrupted sutures, but two or more layers may be necessary for the more extensive injuries. It often is advantageous to use No. 4-0 catgut on an atraumatic needle to close the wounds near the clitoris, since the small needle and suture will provoke less bleeding.

It is particularly important to repair third-degree and fourth-degree lacerations in order that the patient retain fecal continence. The rectal defect is closed by inverting the torn edges with two layers of interrupted catgut sutures carefully placed in the submucosal tissues but not through the mucosa itself. The cut ends of the sphincter muscle are located and approximated with two or three interrupted catgut sutures. The separated levator

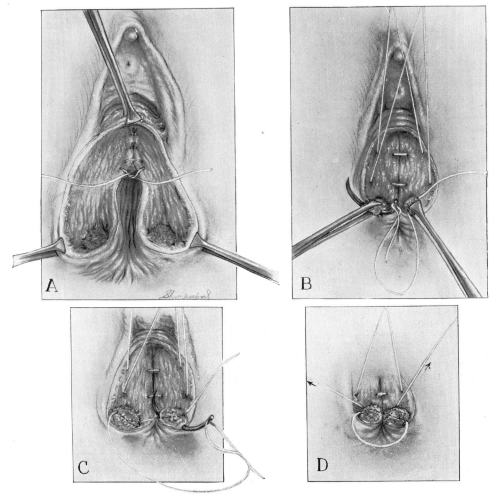

Fig. 39-2. Repair of fourth-degree laceration. **A,** Repair of rectal mucosa; inverting sutures are buried in muscles of rectal wall. **B,** Sutures of levator muscle to be buried; ends of sphincter are drawn forward, which is first step of sphincter suture. **C,** Second step of sphincter suture, beginning figure-of-eight suture. **D,** Sphincter suture is completed and ready for tying. Remainder of perineal repair is carried out in usual manner. (From Willson, J. R.: Management of obstetric difficulties, ed. 6, St. Louis, 1961, The C. V. Mosby Co.)

bundles and the more superficial muscles, which are also involved in the injury, are next approximated to complete the repair. No special postpartum care is required, but it usually is wise to keep the stools soft for several days. It is not necessary to prescribe antimicrobial drugs.

LATE RESULTS

Simple perineal injuries that do not involve the levator ani usually produce no permanent disability even though they are not repaired. If the severed ends of the superficial perineal muscles, particularly the bulbocavernosus, are not approximated, the vaginal introitus may gape.

If a sphincter tear is overlooked, the patient will probably be incontinent of feces unless the levator ani muscles are strong enough to take the place of the torn sphincter. Since the levators as well as the sphincter are involved in the injury, this usually does not occur. It is easier to repair a fresh laceration than a chronic one, and the results are generally better. If a third-degree laceration has been overlooked and if the patient plans on having more children, the defect can be repaired quite satisfactorily at the next de-

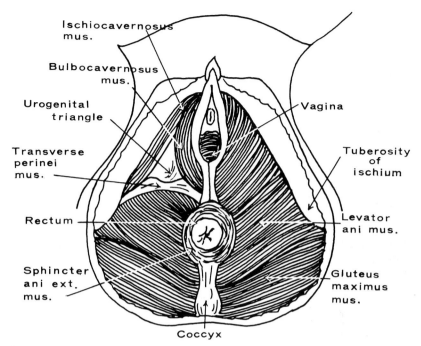

Fig. 39-3. Pelvic musculature. The superficial structures have been omitted on the right side of the diagram.

livery. If she is past the childbearing age or desires no more children, the lesion can be corrected at her convenience by an experienced gynecologic surgeon.

■ Vaginal lacerations

As was mentioned previously, perineal injuries usually extend up the lateral vaginal sulci and, if deep enough, will also involve the levator ani. The vaginal mucosa may also be injured at the level of the ischial spines or in the vault of the vagina. The tears in the vault of the vagina are often circular and may be the result of forceps rotation, particularly if there is some degree of cephalopelvic disproportion.

Vaginal lacerations may bleed profusely, and as a consequence it is difficult to expose and repair them, particularly if the physician does not have adequate assistance.

■ Injuries to the levator sling

Perineal and vaginal lacerations may be relatively superficial, leaving the important deep supporting structures intact, or they may extend more deeply and interrupt the integrity of the levator sling and the endopelvic fascia. Lacerations in the deep structures are usually obvious, but extensive damage to the deep supporting structures can occur even though there is no visible injury involving the skin or the vaginal mucosa.

As the presenting part descends through the birth canal and distends the lower vagina, the levator bundles are separated and the levator fascia is stretched. If the fascial layer is unusually resilient, it can stretch enough to permit the birth of the baby and then return to normal, but more often it tears, permitting the levator muscles to separate and retract laterally.

This is usually accompanied by perineal and vaginal lacerations that disrupt the endopelvic fascial layer in the rectovaginal septum, destroying the support of the rectum anteriorly. The levator pillars may also be detached from the lateral walls of the rectum, further reducing its support. The lacerations are usually irregular, and the involved tissue is often badly bruised.

Frequently, serious lacerations occur because labor terminates so forcibly and rapidly that the structures are torn apart rather than stretched slowly and because there is disproportion between the size of the infant and that of the pelvis. Another common cause is a narrow pubic arch. As the head is delivering, it cannot fit snugly beneath the

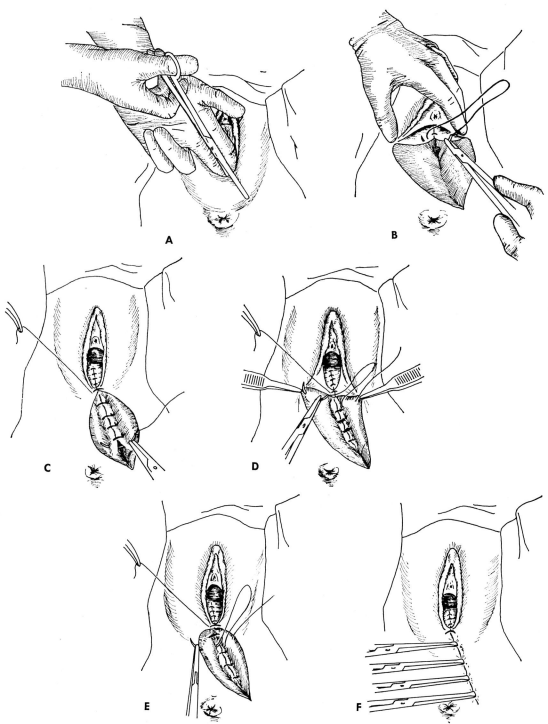

Fig. 39-4. Left mediolateral episiotomy. **A,** The perineum is incised from the midline of the fourchette toward the ischial tuberosity. **B,** Repair of mucosa. The submucosal muscle and fascia are included; continuous suture ends just outside the hymenal ring. **C,** Approximation of levator muscle and fascia. **D,** Approximation of cut ends of bulbocavernosus muscle to close introitus. **E,** Closure of superficial muscles and fascia. **F,** Allis clamps to seal skin edges; no skin sutures are necessary.

symphysis but is forced backward toward the posterior pelvis, putting undue strain on the soft tissues as it passes through the introitus. Other less frequent causes are edema, extensive perineal scarring from past deliveries, and unskillful attempts at operative delivery.

TREATMENT OF POSTERIOR WALL INJURY

Immediate approximation of the torn levator structures and of the vaginal and perineal injuries will permit the tissues to heal and will reduce subsequent deformity. There may be a considerable amount of permanent relaxation of the structures, however, because they usually have been rather seriously injured by the extreme distention that preceded their final bursting.

PREVENTION OF POSTERIOR WALL INJURY

Even though the physician makes every possible effort to eliminate unusually traumatic deliveries, the supporting structures will be injured unless special precautions are taken. The most important measure for preventing serious posterior wall injury is episiotomy, or incision of the perineum and the underlying supporting structures. A clean surgical incision is less traumatizing, can be repaired more satisfactorily, and heals better than a jagged, bruised muscle tear. Episiotomy should be performed on almost on almost every primigravida and on most multiparas with intact pelvic supports.

If episiotomy is to offer maximum protection, the perineum must be incised before the tissues have already been stretched and injured by the advancing presenting part. The incision, which must be long enough to cut all the tissues holding the levator bundles together in the midline, is made when the perineum is flattened and bulging and when the vaginal opening is dilated about 4 cm. during a contraction. A median or a mediolateral episiotomy will produce equally good results if the incision is made properly and at the right time and if it is carefully repaired. With an adequate mediolateral incision the fat in the ischiorectal fossa usually is visible in the lower angle, and a median incision usually exposes the sphincter ani.

Regional or general anesthesia is essential for the performance of an adequate episiotomy because it must be made before the tissues have been injured. The practice of making a small incision without anesthesia

in the overstretched and blanched perineum offers relatively little protection and should be eliminated.

The entire episiotomy is repaired with chromic No. 3-0 or 4-0 catgut, which produces relatively little local reaction. It is not necessary to take great sweeping bites of tissue with each stitch, nor must the physician tie the sutures tightly except when it is necessary to control bleeding. The repair should not be started until the placenta has been delivered and the uterus is well contracted. It will be difficult to explore the uterus after the wound is closed unless the sutures are removed. The blood loss with episiotomy averages about 150 ml.

LATE RESULTS OF POSTERIOR WALL INJURY

If injuries are left unrepaired or are improperly sutured, permanent defects in support may result. Occasionally, however, the same lesions develop in women whose injuries have been carefully repaired, in those in whom an attempt has been made to prevent lacerations, and even in those who have never been pregnant.

Rectocele. Unrepaired posterior lacerations disrupt the endopelvic fascial support of the rectal wall, permit the levator bundles to retract laterally, and destroy the perineal body, thereby eliminating the normal support of the rectum. This permits the rectum and the posterior vaginal wall to sag anteriorly. When the patient is on her feet, the weight of the abdominal contents produces an increase in descent of the rectal wall. Each time she strains in an attempt to evacuate her rectum, the fecal mass is forced downward against the relatively thin rectovaginal wall, stretching it a little more. The rectum gradually protrudes more and more into the vagina until eventually a large pouch may be visible through the relaxed introitus. This lesion, which is called *rectocele,* is the most common late result of childbirth injury. Most are small and produce few symptoms, but some are huge and bulge outside the vaginal canal whenever the patient stands up.

The relaxation often remains relatively small and produces few symptoms until after the patient has gone through the menopause. When tissue atrophy develops because of withdrawal of the estrogenic hormones, the size of the rectocele increases rapidly.

Symptoms. The symptoms produced by

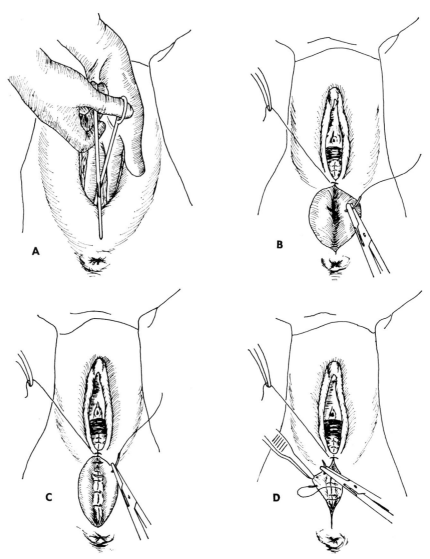

Fig. 39-5. **A,** The perineum is incised in the midline from the posterior fourchette toward the anus until the sphincter is visible. **B,** Approximation of levator fascia. The mucosa has been closed. **C,** Approximation of superficial muscle and fascia. The cut ends of the bulbocavernosus muscle have been approximated. **D,** Subcuticular plain catgut skin closure. Allis clamps may also be used.

rectocele are related to the loss of muscular and fascial support and the consequent disturbance of bowel function. If the lesion is large, most women will experience "bearing down" and a sensation of lack of support when on their feet. They feel as though all the pelvic organs were going to fall out through the introitus. They may also complain of the protrusion of a mass. Those with large rectoceles find it difficult to evacuate the rectum because the fecal material is pushed into the rectal pouch instead of being

deflected toward the anal opening by the structures of the perineal body that has been destroyed. If questioned, these women will usually state that they must hold the mass up with the fingers in the vagina to permit evacuation of fecal material. The symptoms disappear when they lie down.

Diagnosis. The diagnosis is made by observing the mass protruding from the vagina and identifying it as a rectocele by performing rectal as well as vaginal examination.

Treatment. Symptom-producing rectoceles

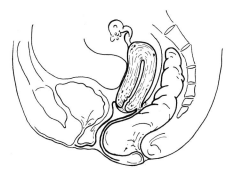

Fig. 39-6. Rectocele. Note destruction of perineal body and bulge of rectum into vagina.

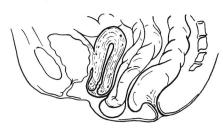

Fig. 39-7. Enterocele. Note small bowel in hernial sac between vagina and rectum.

can only be corrected by an operative procedure by which the separated levator muscles and their fascia and the structures of the perineal body are approximated in the midline between the anterior rectal and the posterior vaginal walls, thereby restoring the continuity of the supports. This procedure is performed with a vaginal approach and is called *perineorrhaphy, posterior colpoplasty,* or more simply *posterior vaginal repair.*

Enterocele. Enterocele, also called *posterior vaginal hernia* or *cul-de-sac hernia,* consists of herniation of the peritoneum of the posterior cul-de-sac downward between the uterosacral ligaments into the rectovaginal septum. The cul-de-sac in women who develop this defect probably is lower than usual, and when its support is destroyed by childbirth injury, the weight of the intestine and omentum and the intra-abdominal pressure gradually enlarge the sac and force it downward between the rectum and the vagina. This lesion occurs frequently in association with prolapse of the uterus and with rectocele.

Symptoms. Enterocele produces few symptoms except pressure and a bearing-down sensation, which may be caused primarily by the relaxation of the other structures.

Diagnosis. Upon superficial inspection enterocele may resemble a rectocele, and in fact both lesions often are present in the same patient. Unless it is recognized and repaired, the first indication of its presence may be a persistent posterior wall bulge after posterior vaginal plastic surgery or a herniation of the vaginal vault after vaginal hysterectomy.

The herniation can usually be recognized by performing a rectovaginal examination and feeling the increased thickness of the rectovaginal wall above the thin rectocele and by asking the patient to cough while palpating the bulge. If an enterocele is present, the increased intra-abdominal pressure will be transmitted to the fingertip as through the usual type of hernia. In many patients the sac is discovered during an operation for vaginal repair.

Treatment. The hernia is usually treated by vaginal operation because rectocele and uterine prolapse are almost always present. The sac is opened, its contents are reduced, the opening is closed, and the cul-de-sac defect is obliterated by approximating the uterosacral ligaments and the levators in the midline. An abdominal operation that accomplishes the same thing can also be performed but is not usually necessary.

■ Injury to the anterior vaginal wall

In nulliparous women the bladder is supported by the integrity of the vesical and vaginal walls and by an extension of the endopelvic fascia between the inferior vesical wall and the anterior vaginal wall. During labor the bladder, which is attached to the anterior surface of the uterus, is pulled up out of the pelvis as the lower uterine segment elongates. As a consequence only the urethra, the vesical neck, and a portion of the bladder floor are vulnerable to injury. As the presenting part descends and dilates the vagina, the structures in the vesicovaginal septum are stretched or even torn in multiple areas beneath the mucosa. If the infant is unusually large, the delivery precipitous, or the bony pelvis small, more damage occurs than from the usual delivery. If there is some degree of disproportion, there may be so little room between the head and the bony walls of the pelvis that the soft-tissue structures are pushed down ahead of the presenting part each time the uterus contracts. This will eventually stretch and injure the supports unduly. The same effect is produced if the soft tissues are relatively rigid and do not dilate properly as labor progresses. Injury to the bladder itself usually occurs while the presenting part is relatively high because the bladder is pulled upward out of the pelvis fairly early in labor.

The bladder neck and the urethral wall may be injured if they are compressed against the posterior surface of the pubic bones or pushed down ahead of the presenting part. If the muscular structures of the posterior vaginal wall are strong and heavy, the presenting part is forced anteriorly and compresses the bladder neck and urethra against the pubis; descent also is delayed because it takes longer to overcome the soft-tissue resistance. The combination of slight prolongation of the expulsive phase and increased pressure against the bladder neck and urethra increases the chance of injuring these structures.

TREATMENT

The vaginal mucosa covering the anterior wall is seldom torn; consequently there is little obvious soft-tissue damage and nothing that can be repaired. Tears in the lateral or posterior vagina and those in the vault do not affect the bladder.

PREVENTION

Injuries to the anterior wall can be minimized by a few simple procedures. The physician should not allow the bladder to become distended during labor. If the patient cannot void, she must be catheterized. The performance of episiotomy will eliminate the resistance offered by the muscle and fascia posteriorly and will permit the head to descend through the posterior portion of the outlet, thereby reducing injury to the latter structures, it offers little protection to the bladder wall itself; injury to the bladder occurs higher in the birth canal. Low forceps extraction, if the delivery of the head is delayed, will also reduce anterior soft-tissue trauma, but difficult forceps operations may increase it.

LATE RESULTS

Relaxation of bladder and urethral supports can develop as a result of pregnancy even though there was no obvious soft-tissue damage at the time of delivery.

Cystocele. A cystocele, the protrusion of the bladder downward into the vaginal canal, develops because the supporting structures in the vesicovaginal septum have lost their integrity. As with rectocele, anterior wall relaxation is not present immediately after delivery but develops over a period of time and often after the patient has had several babies. When she stands up, the weight of the urine in the bladder forces the vesicovaginal septum downward. This stretches the injured bladder wall and increases its capacity, thereby permitting more urine to accumulate in the pouch. As time goes by, the cystocele becomes larger and larger, until it protrudes through the introitus. Urine may be retained in the cystocele because it hangs below the bladder neck and cannot be emptied completely. The stagnant urine often becomes infected. A rectocele is usually present in women with relaxation of the anterior wall, and the bladder descends when the uterus prolapses.

Symptoms. Small cystoceles and even some huge ones produce few symptoms. Some women complain only of a bearing-down sensation or of protrusion of a mass through the introitus. Urinary control is retained unless the bladder neck and urethra are damaged; in fact, women with large cystoceles often find it difficult to void at all unless the sagging bladder is pushed upward with the fingers. Most women with relaxation of the anterior wall of any extent experience recurrent attacks of cystitis.

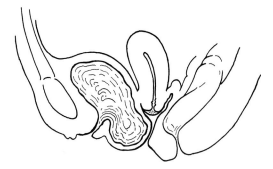

Fig. 39-8. Cystocele. The urethra is normal and the area of the bladder neck is intact. Note the narrow urethrovesical angle.

Diagnosis. The diagnosis of cystocele is made by identifying the vaginal bulge as involving the anterior wall. Unless there is an associated urethral injury, the urethra and bladder neck may be well supported behind the pubis even when the patient strains and the cystocele is pushed downward. The size of the pouch and the degree of protrusion can often be better appreciated by examining the patient while she stands upright.

Treatment. The bulge of the cystocele is obliterated by plicating the bladder wall with interrupted chromic catgut sutures after it has been exposed by deflecting the vaginal mucosa off it. This can only be accomplished by a vaginal approach because the involved area cannot be reached through an abdominal incision. The fact that a cystocele is present does not mean that treatment is necessary; only those that produce symptoms should be operated upon.

Urethrocele and stress urinary incontinence. Urethrocele is similar to cystocele except that it involves the urethra rather than the bladder itself. In most women urethrocele is accompanied by relaxation of the structures that support the bladder neck and the bladder wall; thus a lesion known as *cystourethrocele* is produced.

Symptoms. A urethrocele alone causes few if any symptoms, but if the bladder neck structures have also been injured, urinary control may be disturbed. The most frequent

symptom produced by such an injury is *stress urinary incontinence;* the patient loses urine whenever the intra-abdominal pressure is increased as she coughs, laughs, or sneezes. Many multiparous women have slight stress incontinence in conjunction with menstruation but maintain good control at other times. If the dysfunction is more pronounced, incontinence is present throughout the month and gradually increases in severity. In some women the initial symptoms are experienced after the birth of the first baby, whereas in others it does not appear until after they have had several. Many women first notice the incontinence after the menopause, and in most women the symptoms become more annoying as the tissues atrophy.

The mechanism for urinary control is not completely understood, but there is a sphincter mechanism at the bladder neck that compresses the upper urethra and pulls it upward behind the symphysis, thereby forming an acute angle at the junction of the posterior urethral wall and the base of the bladder. In this position the urine is retained within the bladder even when the intravesical pressure is increased over the normal. When the patient wishes to void, the sphincter complex relaxes, and the internal urethral orifice is opened by the muscles of the trigone, which contract and expand the opening and pull it upward as the bladder wall contracts and forces the urine out.

Simultaneous measurements of intravesicle and intraurethral pressures indicate that the latter always exceeds the former in continent women. If the sphincter mechanism is intact, an increase in intravesicle pressure is compensated for by a simultaneous increase in

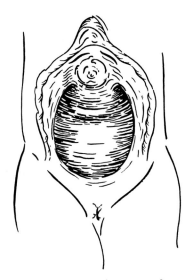

Fig. 39-9. Cystourethrocele, external appearance.

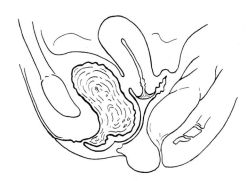

Fig. 39-10. Cystourethrocele. Note double bulge of urethra and bladder and funneling at bladder neck. The urethrovesical angle is wide.

intraurethral pressure, which prevents leakage of urine. In incontinent women the mechanism for increasing intraurethral pressure is disturbed, and it cannot change rapidly enough to compensate for the sudden increases in intravesicle pressure that occur during coughing and sneezing. As a consequence, urine will spurt from the urethra.

The mechanism for urinary control can be disturbed if the muscles do not function properly and in unison. The sphincter mechanism may be damaged so that it is strong enough to occlude the urethra under normal circumstances but too weak to prevent leakage of urine when the intra-abdominal, and as a result the intravesical, pressure is suddenly elevated. If the bladder neck sags and the supporting pubococcygeus muscle is injured, the normal angle between the urethra and the base of the bladder may be increased or even obliterated; this, coupled with failure of urethra compression, produces severe incontinence. Muscles in the lower urethra have little to do with urinary control. The entire distal two thirds of the urethra can be amputated without disturbing urinary function.

Women with large cystoceles or advanced stages of uterine prolapse may be completely continent because the bladder pouch hangs below the urethral opening and the urine cannot spill, even though the sphincter muscles are weak. If the cystocele alone is corrected, women who previously controlled the urine well may be totally incontinent postoperatively because the pouch in which the urine collected has been obliterated but the urethral orifice is relaxed and wide open.

Diagnosis. The diagnosis of urethrocele can be made by observing the pouching and by inserting a probe into the urethra and palpating its tip through the thin posterior wall. Occasionally a *urethral diverticulum* will resemble urethrocele. With this lesion, which lies between the urethral mucosa and the anterior vaginal wall, the tip of a sound cannot be felt from the vaginal side.

Relaxation of the structures that support the urethra and bladder neck can be demonstrated by asking the patient to bear down. If the bladder neck and urethra remain elevated behind the pubis when the patient strains, the area is reasonably well supported even though a cystocele descends. If the patient can constrict her pubococcygeus mus-

cle strongly and pull the bladder neck and urethra well up behind the pubis, she should usually be able to control the urine.

The integrity of the bladder neck mechanism can be tested by having the patient cough or hold her breath and bear down while in lithotomy position. Urine will usually spurt from the meatus in those with defective muscles. The bladder must contain urine to test for incontinence; consequently, if the patient has voided shortly before the examination, 200 to 300 ml. of water should be instilled into the bladder through a catheter. If she does not lose urine in the lithotomy position, the test should be repeated with the patient standing.

The physician must not assume that incontinence is a result of muscle relaxation alone without considering other possible causes such as neurogenic bladder dysfunction, which may evidence itself as overflow incontinence. Urinary tract fistulas may also lead to loss of urine. Perhaps the most common causes of incontinence are urinary tract infections and urethral strictures, both of which should be eliminated before treatment is prescribed. Urgency of urination and urge incontinence are more likely to be caused by bladder or urethral disease than by muscle relaxation. A complete examination is essential before operating upon a patient with urge incontinence.

Treatment. In some women, particularly those with relatively little descent of the bladder and urethra, stress incontinence can be corrected by *systematic muscle exercise.* The patient is taught how to contract the pubococcygeus muscles that pull the bladder neck upward and angulate it and constrict the distal urethra. If she contracts the muscles 80 or 100 times a day and attempts to check the flow of urine suddenly while she is voiding, the pubococcygeus may become strong enough to prevent leakage. The administration of *estrogen* may improve urinary control in postmenopausal women with a good bit of local atrophic change but little obvious tissue relaxation.

Surgical treatment should be selected for those with more serious relaxation and for the ones whose incontinence is not improved by muscle exercises. Most surgical procedures are directed toward restoring the integrity of the lost supports and particularly toward improving the function of the sphincter mechanism. This can usually be accomplished by plicating the bladder and urethra through a vaginal incision. This elevates the bladder neck, restores the urethrovesical angle, and narrows the urethral orifice. For some women an abdominal approach is preferable. In the Marshall-Marchetti-Krantz or retropubic vesical neck suspension operation the urethra and bladder neck are sutured to the posterior border of the pubis and the rectus fascia; this also restores the urethrovesical angle and prevents the bladder neck from descending. More complicated procedures in which slings of rectus fascia are used to support the bladder neck are seldom necessary.

■ Injuries to the uterus
CERVICAL LACERATIONS

The cervix often is torn during delivery, but the lacerations are usually shallow and bleed little; consequently they rarely constitute a major cause of postpartum hemorrhage. More extensive lacerations that extend upward and involve the lower segment may produce serious bleeding. These are most often caused by precipitous delivery or by ill-advised attempts to "dilate" the cervix artificially or to extract the infant before dilatation is complete.

The cervix may also be injured if the anterior lip is caught and incarcerated between the descending head and the pubic bone. This occurs most often with some degree of cephalopelvic disproportion. Since the trapped cervix cannot be retracted up-

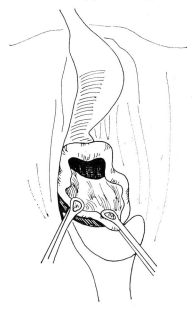

Fig. 39-11. Exposure and inspection of the cervix after delivery.

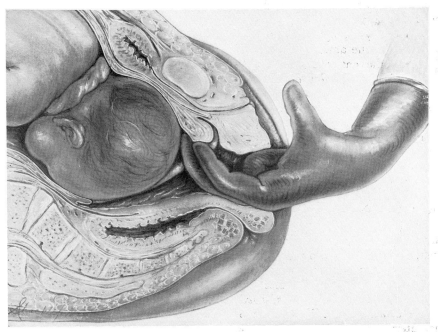

Fig. 39-12. Incarcerated edematous anterior cervical lip. (From Willson, J. R.: Management of obstetric difficulties, ed. 6, St. Louis, 1961, The C. V. Mosby Co.)

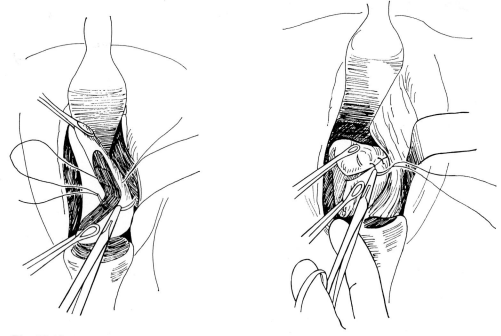

Fig. 39-13. Exposure and repair of cervical laceration. Interrupted sutures are placed through entire thickness of cervix.

ward around the presenting part, the lower segment becomes excessively thinned and may even rupture. The anterior lip of the cervix becomes edematous and diffused with blood and may be almost black in color. Unless it is freed by disengaging the head slightly and pushing the anterior lip upward with the fingers, the entire cervix may be torn loose, a so-called *annular amputation.*

The cervix should be exposed and inspected after each hospital delivery, even those that terminate spontaneously. If a laceration is found, the defect should be closed with interrupted chromic No. 3-0 catgut sutures.

RUPTURE OF THE UTERUS

Rupture of the uterus is the most serious of the childbirth injuries, but fortunately it occurs only once in 1,500 to 2,000 deliveries. The uterus may rupture during pregnancy, but usually the wall gives way during labor.

Etiology. During pregnancy the most frequent cause of rupture is *separation of a scar* from previous cesarean section. Rupture of the normal uterus except by direct trauma seldom occurs. The ruptures that occur during labor also may involve a scar. Injuries

to the lower segment are frequently the result of *obstructed labor* from cephalopelvic disproportion or malposition. The presenting part cannot descend through the pelvis, and the continuing contraction and retraction of the muscle fibers in the upper segment stretch and thin the lower segment to a point at which separation occurs. Other traumatic causes are the *administration of oxytocin* in doses that are too large or to a patient in whom stimulation is contraindicated (obstructed labor, abnormal positions, etc.) and *operative deliveries* such as version and breech extraction. Rupture is particularly likely to occur when operative delivery is attempted after labor has been prolonged and the lower segment is overstretched or as a result of failure to relax the uterus and abolish its contractions by adequate anesthesia before such procedures are attempted. The uterus almost never ruptures during dysfunctional labor.

Pathologic anatomy. Traumatic ruptures during labor and delivery more often occur in the thin lower segment, but they may extend upward and involve the upper segment or downward into the cervix. They usually run transversely or obliquely unless they are extensions of a deep cervical laceration, in which event the tear is usually a longitudinal one in the lateral wall.

A *complete rupture* is one that extends through the entire uterine wall into the peritoneal cavity or the broad ligament; with an *incomplete rupture* the visceral peritoneum remains intact. With either type, hemorrhage is severe. The blood is lost directly into the peritoneal cavity if the rupture is complete, or into the broad ligament with a lateral wall defect. There may be some external bleeding, but the major hemorrhage is usually concealed within the broad ligament or the abdominal cavity.

Diagnosis. The diagnosis should be suspected when a pregnant woman or one in labor has sudden abdominal pain followed by clinical evidence of blood loss. If these symptoms occur during a labor that has been abnormally long or obstructed or if a pathologic retraction ring has been detected, the diagnosis is more likely. When the uterus ruptures under such circumstances, the patient usually experiences a sharp agonizing pain, uterine contractions cease, and evidences of bleeding develop rapidly. If the baby has been extruded into the peritoneal cavity, it may be possible to palpate it outside the uterus, and the presenting part can no longer be felt through the cervix.

"Threatened rupture" of the uterus is difficult or impossible to diagnose.

Treatment. The possibility that the uterus may rupture during abnormal labor should always be considered, and necessary precautions should be taken to prevent its occurrence. Since about two thirds of the ruptures of cesarean section scars occur after the thirty-eighth week of pregnancy or during labor, *elective repeat cesarean section* will reduce the incidence of ruptures at this time. Recognition of the cause and proper management of *prolonged labor,* adequate *anesthesia* for operative deliveries, and the judicious use of *oxytocic drugs* will also serve as preventive measures.

If rupture does occur in spite of these precautions, the active treatment is determined somewhat by the surroundings and the condition of the patient. Expectancy is almost never warranted. Prompt transfusion with whole blood and laparotomy are usually indicated; it is almost always necessary to perform hysterectomy unless the laceration is small, in which event it may be possible to repair it and leave the uterus intact.

If the rupture occurs when the patient is ready for delivery, the infant should usually be extracted. This procedure may save its life and will permit the uterus to contract, thereby helping to control bleeding until the abdomen can be opened. If the infant lies in the peritoneal cavity, no attempt should be made to extract it through the vagina.

Prognosis. The *infant mortality* is almost 100% if the fetus is extruded from the uterus into the peritoneal cavity. If labor is well advanced and the presenting part is deep in the pelvis at the time of the rupture, the infant may remain within the birth canal and prompt delivery can save its life. The *maternal mortality* is primarily from hemorrhage and can be kept at a minimum by prompt and adequate treatment, but it may be as high as 20% to 50%. Rupture of cesarean scars is less lethal for the mother since they are relatively avascular.

■ **Injuries involving uterine support**

The major support for the uterus and vagina is provided by the thickenings of the endopelvic fascia known as the cardinal or Mackenrodt's ligaments. They extend from about the level of the internal os upward and laterally to blend with the fascia covering the obturator internus muscle. The round ligaments, broad ligaments, and uterosacral ligaments are more concerned with maintaining uterine position than with supporting it.

Tearing of the cardinal ligaments during labor and delivery must be rare, but they can be unduly stretched if the baby is large or if attempts are made to complete delivery forcibly before the cervix is completely dilated.

LATE RESULTS

If the cardinal ligaments are injured or stretched during labor and do not return to normal, they can no longer support the uterus, and it will sag backward and downward into the vagina. The axis of the uterus ordinarily forms an acute angle with the axis of the vagina, which in itself tends to prevent prolapse. Descent of the uterus can only occur when the other supporting structures as well as the cardinal ligaments relax, thereby altering the relationship of the

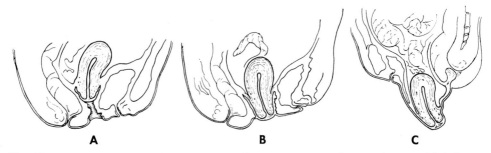

Fig. 39-14. Uterine prolapse. **A,** First degree. **B,** Second degree. **C,** Complete, or third degree.

uterus to the vaginal axis and permitting it to descend.

Descensus, or *prolapse,* of the uterus may occur in infants and nulliparous women as well as in multiparas. Defects in innervation and in the basic integrity of the supporting structures account for descensus in the first two and childbirth trauma for the latter. The uterus often prolapses in children with spina bifida and with congenital extrophy of the bladder. The uterus seldom descends immediately after delivery, but the defect develops gradually. Cystocele and rectocele, which almost always accompany prolapse, enlarge and pull down on the uterus and cervix. The cervix usually elongates because the weight of the sagging vaginal tissues pulls it downward, whereas the attached but weak cardinal ligaments tend to support it. As the cystocele enlarges and the cervix elongates, the ligaments become weaker until they can no longer hold the uterus in place. The more advanced stages of uterine prolapse are most often encountered in women past the menopause. Atrophy of the tissues eliminates whatever support was left.

A *first-degree prolapse* is one in which the cervix lies between the level of the ischial spines and the vaginal introitus. In *second-degree prolapse* the cervix protrudes through the introitus whereas the corpus remains within the vagina. In *third-degree,* or *complete, prolapse* both the cervix and the body of the uterus have passed through the introitus, and the entire vaginal canal is inverted.

Symptoms. The symptoms are primarily those related to the weight of the descending organs and their protrusion through the introitus. If the prolapsed cervix becomes ulcerated, it may bleed.

Diagnosis. The diagnosis is made by pelvic examination. The prolapse may reduce itself spontaneously when the patient lies down. Consequently to determine the extent of the lesion it often is necessary to have her strain and push the cervix down, to exert traction on it with a tenaculum, or even to examine her in an upright position. Prolapse must be differentiated from simple hypertrophy and elongation of the cervix that does not involve loss of uterine support.

Treatment. The treatment of prolapse usually is operative, but in certain poor-risk patients or those who are very old a pessary may be inserted to hold the uterus in place. The physician should be certain that the patient actually is a poor operative risk before advising pessary support. Advanced age alone does not necessarily contraindicate surgical treatment.

Operative correction of prolapse rarely requires an abdominal operation. The faulty supporting structures can only be approached vaginally; hence procedures such as abdominal suspension of the uterus often fail because they do not correct the fundamental pathologic change. An adequate, effective operative procedure must correct the cystocele and rectocele, return the uterus to a forward position, shorten the elongated cervix, and shorten the cardinal ligaments. An alternate method is to remove the uterus. Operative procedures that will accomplish these aims are: *Manchester-Fothergill operation* (cervical amputation and shortening of the cardinal ligaments and vaginal plastic repair), *vaginal hysterectomy* and plastic repair, and *colpocleisis* (Le Fort operation) in which the vagina is obliterated by denuding and approximating the anterior and posterior vaginal walls.

■ Genital fistulas

Fistulous openings between the bladder and the genital tract (vesicovaginal, vesico-cervical, or vesicouterine), between the ureter and the vagina (ureterovaginal), and between the rectum and the vagina (recto-vaginal) are caused by radiation, operative trauma, or injuries during labor and delivery.

URINARY TRACT FISTULAS

The most common urinary tract fistula is that which forms in the anterior vaginal wall, a *vesicovaginal fistula*. In past years almost all such fistulas were caused by necrosis of the vesicovaginal septum from pressure during delayed labor, but today the majority follow hysterectomy. These may result from necrosis at the site of a suture in the bladder wall, from operative injury, or from interference with blood supply. They most often follow total hysterectomy. As a result of the abnormal opening, the patient is partially or completely incontinent of urine, and the constant flow of urine from the vagina excoriates the vulva and thighs. If the defect is large, all the urine will be passed through the vagina, but if it is small, the patient may void normally even though some of the urine seeps through the fistulous opening.

Ureterovaginal fistulas are being produced more and more frequently as the number of radical operations for cancer is increasing. The defect in the ureter develops near the ureterovesical junction, and the seepage of urine is usually first noted during the third week after the operation.

Diagnosis. The diagnosis of vesicovaginal fistula is confirmed by demonstrating the opening between the bladder and the vagina by vaginal and cystoscopic examination. If a small pack is placed in the vagina and methylene blue is instilled into the bladder, the dye will seep through the opening and discolor the pack.

Ureterovaginal fistula can usually be suspected when the physician attempts to pass ureteral catheters. It often is impossible to insert the catheter beyond the constricted site of the fistula. Indigo-carmine, when injected intravenously, will be excreted in the urine, and if there is a ureterovaginal fistula, some of the dye will enter the vagina and stain a pack. Since this will also occur, of course, with a vesicovaginal fistula, one more test is necessary to differentiate the two lesions: Methylene blue instilled into the bladder will enter the vagina through a vesicovaginal fistula, but this will not occur if the defect is in the ureter. These tests combined with cystoscopy and pyelography should localize any urinary tract fistula quite accurately.

Treatment. Most vesicovaginal fistulas can be closed satisfactorily by an experienced gynecologist through a vaginal approach. The treatment of a ureterovaginal fistula is determined by its location. For those near the ureterovesical junction the ureter can be severed above the defect and implanted into the bladder. If the fistulous opening is several centimeters away from the bladder, the severed ends can usually be anastomosed. Occasionally it is necessary to remove the kidney on the involved side.

RECTOVAGINAL FISTULAS

Rectovaginal fistulas are caused by infection in an episiotomy, a suture placed through the rectal wall during repair, or an unrecognized rectal injury during delivery or vaginal repair. They may also be caused by extension of cervical cancer or from radiation necrosis following its treatment. Most of the traumatic lesions are found near the vaginal opening, whereas those caused by cancer are higher. All result in fecal incontinence and passage of fecal material from the vagina. These lesions can be differentiated from incontinence due to complete perineal laceration by the fact that with a fistula the sphincter ani is intact.

Treatment. These lesions can almost always be corrected by a surgical procedure, but since the operative field is infected, the repair may break down. The bowel should be prepared for several days preoperatively by reducing the diet to liquids for a day or two before operation, giving enemas, and prescribing neomycin, 0.5 Gm. every 4 hours during the 24-hour period before operation. Colostomy may be necessary preceding operation for complicated rectovaginal fistulas.

■ Injuries to the pelvic joints

The *symphysis pubis* always separates to some extent during delivery, but if the baby is forcibly extracted or is unusually large, a serious injury can be produced. When the patient attempts to move or stand on her feet after delivery, she experiences severe pain in the region of the symphysis and in the sacroiliac joints. The symphysial area is tender and the ends of the pubic bones are widely separated. The bone ends are unusually mobile and can be felt to shift several centimeters when the patient shifts her weight from one foot to the other. The bladder neck and the urethra may be injured, and as a result the urine may be bloody.

Treatment of separation of the symphysis consists of immobilization of the pelvic girdle by a tight binder or adhesive strapping until the pubis heals. The symptoms improve rapidly.

If the *coccyx is dislocated,* the patient may complain of pain localized to the area and radiating down both legs. The dislocated coccyx can be felt overriding the end of the sacrum and can often be reduced by digital manipulation. Soreness and tenderness may persist for several weeks.

■ Hematoma formation

A hematoma may form in the rectovaginal septum, in the episiotomy, or in the base of the broad ligament after delivery. A large amount of blood can accumulate in the loose subcutaneous tissue of the labium without any evidence of external bleeding. Evidence of shock may be one of the first signs of blood loss.

An enlarging hematoma causes pelvic pain and rectal pressure soon after delivery. Unfortunately this often is attributed to the episiotomy and is treated symptomatically without examination. Inspection of the perineum usually reveals it to be distended and ecchymotic, and when rectal examination is performed, it is easy to feel the tender mass. Women who have been delivered under spinal or saddle block anesthesia will usually be unable to appreciate perineal pain for several hours after delivery; consequently a large hematoma may form without their being aware of the symptoms.

A hematoma in the episiotomy must be evacuated at once. If the bleeding vessel can be demonstrated, it should be ligated. Occasionally it is necessary to pack the cavity to check diffuse oozing, but the bleeding can almost always be controlled by resuturing the episiotomy. Small hematomas in the vaginal wall usually need no treatment.

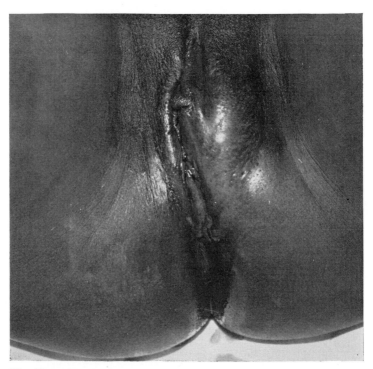

Fig. 39-15. Hematoma in episiotomy.

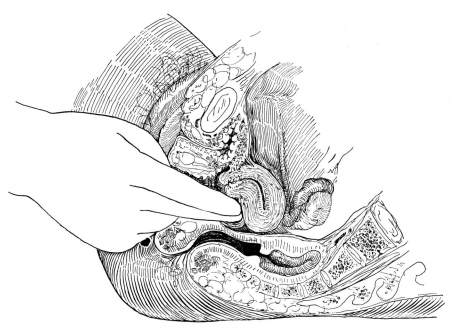

Fig. 39-16. Retrodisplacement of uterus. The cervix points in the axis of the vaginal canal, and the fundus can be felt in the posterior cul-de-sac. (From Titus, P.: Atlas of obstetric technic, St. Louis, 1949, The C. V. Mosby Co.)

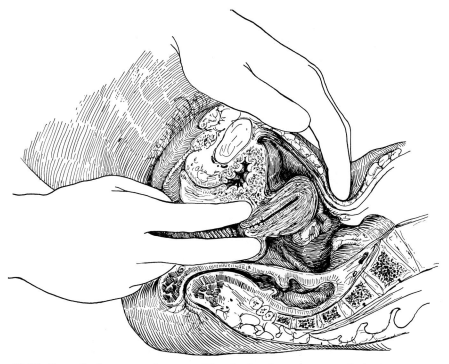

Fig. 39-17. Retrodisplacement of uterus. The fundus is pushed anteriorly by the fingers in the vagina until it can be held forward by the fingers pressing the abdominal wall inward. (From Titus, P.: Atlas of obstetric technic, St. Louis, 1949, The C. V. Mosby Co.)

■ Retrodisplacement of the uterus

The term *retrodisplacement* includes several situations in each of which the body of the uterus is displaced from its usual location overlying the bladder and occupies a position in the posterior pelvis. With *retroflexion* the fundus lies posteriorly, whereas the cervix retains its usual position in the vagina; the uterus is flexed in the region of the isthmus, the axis of the body forming an angle with the cervix. A *retroverted* uterus is one in which the fundus rotates posteriorly and the cervix anteriorly around an axis at the level of the internal os. *Retrocession* indicates that the entire uterus has sagged backward into the posterior pelvis.

Retrodisplacement, which can be detected in 20% to 30% of all women, is caused by an alteration in the supporting structures of the pelvis. The uterus rotates in an anteroposterior plane around an axis situated about at the level of the internal os. Anterior traction on the corpus or posterior traction on the cervix therefore will tend to rotate the uterus into its normal position, with the fundus overlying the pubis and the cervix pointing toward the rectum, the long axis of the uterus forming an acute angle with the axis of the vagina. The anterior position of the uterus is maintained by a number of forces: The *uterosacral ligaments* pull the cervix backward and upward, and the *round ligaments* help to return the fundus to an anterior position if for some reason it is rotated poste-

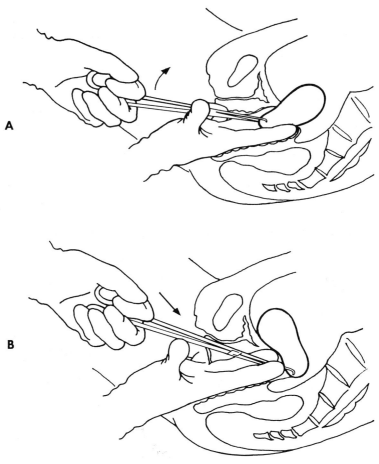

Fig. 39-18. Replacement of uterus with tenaculum. **A,** The cervix is grasped with a tenaculum and pulled downward in the axis of the vagina until it is straight. The two fingers in the vagina push upward on the fundus. **B,** The cervix is pushed posteriorly between the two fingers. The uterus can be held anteriorly by pressure against the cervix while the tenaculum is removed and the pessary is inserted. (Modified from Tauber, R.: Gynecologic diagnosis, New York, 1949, Thomas Nelson & Sons.)

riorly. When a woman assumes an erect posture, the *intra-abdominal pressure* and the loops of *intestine* pressing on the posterior surface of the uterus force the fundus toward the pubis, thereby rotating the cervix backward and upward until it lies above the level of the corpus. With the patient lying on her back the fundus is directed toward the ceiling and may fall either anteriorly or posteriorly; thus its position may vary from one examination to the next. If the bladder is distended, the fundus will be pushed posteriorly.

In some women the uterus is congenitally displaced and can be found lying posteriorly throughout their entire lives. In others retrodisplacement develops after childbirth when the supporting structures are injured. Retrodisplacement must occur before the uterus can prolapse. The chronically displaced uterus may be enlarged, boggy, and congested, and the tubes and ovaries often prolapse behind into the cul-de-sac.

Symptoms. In the past, backache, dysmenorrhea, infertility, abortion, nervousness, disorders of menstrual flow, and a host of other symptoms were attributed to retrodisplacement, and thousands of operative procedures were performed to correct this "abnormality." A retrodisplaced uterus may produce symptoms, but when groups of women with retrodisplacements are compared with those whose uteri are in an anterior position, the same symptoms occur in about the same ratio in each group.

If the body of the retrodisplaced uterus is enlarged, boggy, heavy, and tender, it may cause pelvic pressure, low backache, and dyspareunia, and it may interfere with evacuation of the rectum. The uterus can be bound down in the posterior pelvis by the adhesions of endometriosis or those of chronic pelvic inflammation, in which event symptoms are more often caused by the disease process itself than by the position of the uterus. A

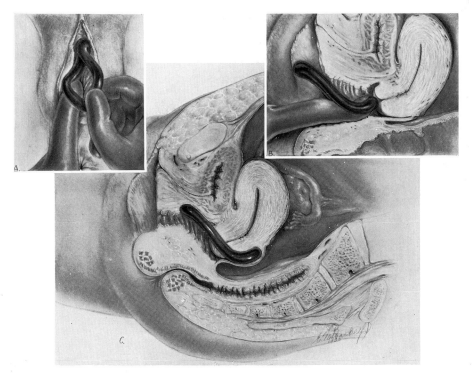

Fig. 39-19. Pessary support for retrodisplacement of uterus. **A,** Insertion while introitus is enlarged by downward traction on vaginal floor. **B,** Transverse bar of pessary is pressed downward and backward behind cervix. **C,** Some degree of descensus of uterus is always found in acquired retrodisplacements; anteflexion is maintained chiefly by pressure of pessary on uterosacral ligaments, drawing cervix backward. (From Willson, J. R.: Management of obstetric difficulties, ed. 6, St. Louis, 1961, The C. V. Mosby Co.)

normal-sized, freely movable, retrodisplaced uterus rarely produces symptoms.

Diagnosis. The diagnosis is made by bimanual examination and by rectovaginal palpation. Either the axis of the cervix lies parallel with the axis of the vagina, or the tip of the cervix may point anteriorly toward the bladder. The body of the uterus can be felt lying in the posterior cul-de-sac by palpating behind the cervix through the posterior fornix.

It sometimes is difficult to differentiate a retrodisplaced uterus from one in normal position with a fibroid arising from the posterior wall and occupying the cul-de-sac or from an enlarged ovary prolapsed behind the uterus. If the physician inserts a sound into the uterine cavity, he can usually tell which way the fundus points.

Treatment. There is no need to suggest treatment for a retrodisplacement unless the patient has symptoms such as pelvic pain, dysmenorrhea, pressure, infertility, etc., which could possibly be related to the position of the uterus. If the symptom is relieved after the uterus has been replaced and held in an anterior position by a proper pessary and recurs when it is permitted to fall posteriorly, the physician can suspect that there is a relationship between the position of the uterus and the symptom. If, on the other hand, the symptom is still present after the retrodisplacement has been corrected, no such relationship can be assumed.

The initial therapeutic step in studying a patient with a retrodisplaced uterus and a pelvic symptom is actually diagnostic. The fundus is elevated by combined vaginal and abdominal manipulation, and a suitable pessary is inserted into the vagina to maintain the anterior position. The manipulations can usually be performed with the patient in lithotomy position, but it sometimes is easier in the knee-chest position. The pessary is left in place for 2 or 3 months, during which time it must be removed and cleaned every 4 weeks. At the same time the vagina is examined for evidence of pressure necrosis or infection.

If the symptoms are not eliminated by elevating the uterus, they obviously are not caused by its posterior position. If they are relieved while the pessary is in place and recur when the uterus falls backward after it is removed, it can be assumed that the symptoms are caused by the retrodisplacement, and surgical correction can be considered. Operation to correct retrodisplaced but otherwise normal uteri should rarely be necessary. In many instances the uterus falls back without the support of the pessary, but the symptoms do not recur. In such patients no further treatment is necessary. Long-continued pessary treatment is generally unwarranted.

Uteri that are fixed in the cul-de-sac by endometriosis or chronic tubo-ovarian inflammation are not suitable for pessary treatment because the uterus usually is so firmly bound down that it cannot be moved without an operation.

References

Falk, H. C., and Kaufman, S. A.: Partial colpocleisis; the Le Fort procedure, Obstet. Gynec. 5:617, 1955.

Feeney, J. K., and Barry, A.: Rupture and perforations of uterus in association with pregnancy, labor, and the puerperium, Brit. Med. J. 1:65, 1956.

Fothergill, W.: Anterior colporrhaphy and amputation of the cervix combined as a single operation for use in the treatment of genital prolapse, Amer. J. Surg. 29:161, 1915.

Gainey, H. L.: Postpartum observation of tissue damage, Amer. J. Obstet. Gynec. 70:800, 1955.

Green, T. H., Jr.: The problem of urinary stress incontinence in the female; an appraisal of its current status, Obstet. Gynec. Survey 23:603, 1968.

Kegel, A.: Progressive resistance exercise in functional restoration of perineal muscles, Amer. J. Obstet. Gynec. 56:238, 1948.

McElin, T. W., and Scott, R.: Rupture of the symphysis pubis during spontaneous labor, Obstet. Gynec. 25:401, 1965.

Mengert, W. F.: Mechanics of uterine support and position, Amer. J. Obstet. Gynec. 31:755, 1936.

Miller, N. F.: Treatment of vesicovaginal fistulas, Amer. J. Obstet. Gynec. 30:675, 1935.

Miller, N. F., and George, H.: Lower urinary tract fistulas in women, Amer. J. Obstet. Gynec. 68:436, 1954.

Zacharin, R. F.: The anatomic supports of the female urethra, Obstet. Gynec. 32:754, 1968.

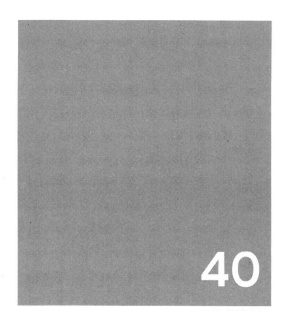

40

Pelvic infection

Acute illness caused by pelvic infection and pain and disturbances of normal function from chronic inflammatory changes account for many of the problems that confront the obstetrician-gynecologist. The infections are of two broad types: those that follow pregnancy and those that develop in nonpregnant women. Although there are many similarities between the two, the infecting organisms and the manner in which they are introduced into the body, the paths of extension from the point of entry, and the end results are all quite different.

■ Puerperal infection

Any infection developing in the genital tract as a consequence of abortion, labor, or delivery, is called puerperal infection. Synonyms are *puerperal sepsis* and *puerperal septicemia*. A patient whose temperature is elevated to at least 100.4° F. on any two of the first 10 postpartum days, exclusive of the first 24 hours after delivery, is described as having *puerperal morbidity*. All patients with puerperal infection are not necessarily included in this classification because in some the temperature may exceed 100.4° F. on only 1 day, whereas in others it may be elevated for several days but never reach 100.4° F. These patients should be included in the morbidity figures as examples of *1-day fever* or *low-level fever*. Although those with fevers from urinary tract infections and other extragenital sources should be included in total morbidity figures, they cannot be considered as instances of true puerperal infection.

The incidence of febrile morbidity depends in part upon the frequency with which temperatures are recorded. More infections will be diagnosed if temperatures are taken four or five times daily than if they are taken only once or twice. The actual incidence is less than 5%, being higher in ward than in private patients and in black than in white patients.

Bacteriology. Any organism that is pathogenic for human beings can cause puerperal infections, but the current spectrum of bacteria is different from that encountered during the fourth and fifth decades of this century. Some potentially pathogenic bacteria inhabit the normal vagina (endogenous), whereas others do not, infection occurring because they were introduced during labor and delivery (exogenous).

Douglas and Davis cultured anaerobic nonhemolytic streptococci from 36.7% of patients with puerperal infections, aerobic nonhemolytic streptococci from 11%, staphylococcus albus from 10.8%, and nineteen other organisms including *Escherichia coli* in smaller numbers. Other investigators reported similar distributions of bacteria. Quite in contrast is the recent experience of Sellner at the Sloane Hospital for Women. During the years 1961 to 1965, cultures were obtained from 464 women with puerperal endometritis. The distribution of bacteria was as follows: *E. coli* 37%, enterococcus 15.7%, *Klebsiella* 15.1%, and other strains each accounting for less than 10%. White and Koontz obtained cultures from the cervix during pregnancy, labor, and delivery and identified alpha hemolytic streptococci, *Streptococcus faecalis,* and *E. coli* as the most frequent pathogenic bacteria. Other pathogens, even *Clostridium welchii,* are occasionally grown from the cervix of seemingly healthy women.

Pathologic changes. Puerperal infection is for all practical purposes a wound infection. The severity depends upon the original site of the infection, the organisms, and the ability of the tissues to resist its invasion.

The bacteria invade from the point of entry in the uterus or vagina to the parametrium by way of the veins (phlebitis) and the lymphatics (lymphangitis). Since the blood vessels and the lymphatic channels tend to extend laterally from the vagina and the uterus, the predominant change with puerperal infection occurs in the parametrial areas rather than in the posterior pelvis. The source of entry, the placental site or a cervical laceration, is often at the side of the uterus or cervix rather than on the anterior or posterior wall; therefore, the principal site of extension may be unilateral rather than bilateral, as is characteristic of tubal infections, especially those caused by gonococci. Fluid pours into the loose areolar tissue in the parametrial area in response to the progressing infection, and a *cellulitis* develops. This is the characteristic response in postabortal or postpartum infections. The localized edema and induration reduce the blood supply further, and a *pelvic abscess* may develop in the center of the area of cellulitis. Other structures in the area or in distant parts of the body may eventually be involved.

Traumatic or incised vaginal and perineal wounds. Traumatic vaginal and perineal wounds will become infected if they are not repaired. A carefully made and repaired episiotomy and properly sutured lacerations almost always heal primarily. If a laceration high in the vagina, particularly one in the lateral fornix, becomes infected, the infection may extend along the lymphatics into the parametrium, producing a typical cellulitis. Those lower in the canal cause local inflammation, which is evidenced by erythema and tenderness along the suture line and induration or fluctuation in the wound.

Endomyometritis. Endomyometritis is the most common type of puerperal infection. It involves the endometrium and the superficial muscle layer of the uterine wall. The uterine cavity usually is sterile during and immediately after normal labor, but it is soon invaded by organisms; by the third day almost all cultures should be positive. Bacteria can be cultured from the uterine cavity in many women during prolonged or difficult labor

and in those with prolonged rupture of the membranes. Adherent bits of placenta in the area of the placental site, the shaggy decidua, and blood clots in the uterus serve as excellent media for the growth of bacteria, and as a consequence almost every recently delivered woman has a mild and inconsequential endometritis.

The clinically important infections are more obvious. The temperature is usually slightly elevated from the day of delivery on, but by the third day it may be as high as 101° to 102° F. The patient has few symptoms other than malaise and perhaps slight abdominal tenderness. The lochia may be profuse, purulent, and malodorous or almost completely absent. The latter condition accompanies the unusual infections caused by the *beta hemolytic Streptococcus,* in which systemic invasion occurs rapidly without much local involvement.

Absence of the lochia is more often an evidence of *lochial block.* This is produced by an obstruction to drainage of the uterine cavity by a sheet of retained membrane, a blood clot, or an abnormal position of the uterus. With this condition the temperature rises abruptly when the drainage is impeded. It often is preceded by slight daily temperature rises.

The uterus is usually boggy, larger, and less well contracted than it should be. It is tender, but the parametrial areas can be palpated without producing any great amount of discomfort. Unless the symptoms are caused by lochial block, the vagina may be filled with purulent discharge.

In the more serious cases of endomyometritis the entire thickness of the uterine wall is involved and may even be the site of multiple small abscesses. This type of infection usually follows poorly managed, excessively prolonged labor. All the symptoms and the findings that characterize endomyometritis are exaggerated, and there usually is parametrial tenderness as well.

Parametritis. Further extension of the organisms along the blood vessels and lymphatics produces cellulitis within the peritoneal folds of one or occasionally both broad ligaments. The signs are similar to those with endomyometritis but are much more severe. The temperature may reach 103° to 104° F. The pulse is elevated and the white blood cell count may be 30,000 or more. The

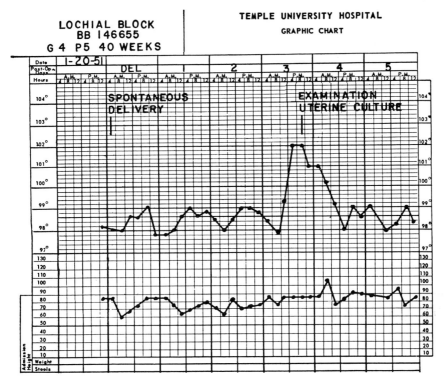

Fig. 40-1. Lochial block. Profuse discharge and lysis of fever followed examination without other treatment. (From Willson, J. R.: Management of obstetric difficulties, ed. 6, St. Louis, 1961, The C. V. Mosby Co.)

uterus is boggy and tender, limited in mobility, and sometimes pushed to one side by tender induration filling one half of the pelvis; the other side may be relatively normal. An *abscess* may develop in the center of the area of cellulitis. As it enlarges, it may eventually dissect downward to point in the posterior cul-de-sac, or it may extend upward until it can be felt above the inguinal ligament. In either event as an abscess develops, the evidences of pelvic infection become more pronounced.

The patient with postabortal cellulitis may be even more seriously ill than one with postpartum involvement. The findings are similar, but the uterus usually is smaller and fixed by the cellulitis, which may fill the entire pelvis. The cervical os is patulous, and bloody fluid can be seen exuding from it.

Peritonitis. Peritonitis almost always accompanies parametritis and pelvic cellulitis. It is more likely to occur after septic abortion than delivery and varies in severity from relatively mild involvement of the peritoneal covering of the broad ligaments to widespread generalized infection. Because the extension of the infection is primarily along blood vessels and lymphatics rather than upward over the mucosa of the uterus and oviducts, the infection in the tubes is of a type called *perisalpingitis.* This infection involves the peritoneal covering and the tubal wall rather than the mucosal surface. Because the mucosa is not involved, permanent tubal closure occurs less often than with gonorrhea. Bacterial contamination of the tubal mucosa occurs regularly during the normal puerperium. This is the result of upward extension of bacteria from the uterine cavity. It is seldom obvious clinically.

Bacteremia. Since phlebitis in the pelvic and the ovarian veins occurs as part of every serious puerperal infection, hematogenous spread of the offending bacteria can occur readily. Septic emboli carried through the bloodstream lodge in distant parts of the body, producing multiple abscesses, which are often found in the brain, lungs, liver, spleen, kidneys, and other abdominal organs.

Sources of infection. Some of the bacteria that cause puerperal infection are introduced from the outside. Such *exogenous sources* include droplet infection from doctor to patient or patient to patient, instruments or equipment, introduction of organisms from infected skin areas or even normal skin, self-examination either voluntarily or involuntarily during labor, and other similar sources. Intercourse is seldom a cause of infection, but pathogenic organisms on the penis could possibly be introduced into the open cervix late in pregnancy or during early labor.

If a pathogenic organism, such as the beta hemolytic streptococcus is introduced from an exogenous source, serious puerperal infection can result. The remarkable change in the spectrum of organisms responsible for puerperal infection is largely due to the sensitivity of the streptococcus to antibiotics and the failure of this organism to develop significant antibiotic resistance. This has lowered the prevalence of both streptococcal infections and streptococcal carriers in the population at large and has contributed to the general relaxation of the strict standards of asepsis in labor and delivery rooms. The problem of puerperal sepsis due to the hemolytic streptococcus has not been eliminated because in the past few years obstetric services in Boston and New York City have reported such infections in two separate epidemics.

Endogenous sources account for the majority of the puerperal infections today. Most of the organisms responsible for puerperal morbidity are normal inhabitants of the vagina and may be introduced into the uterus through the cervix during even the most careful rectal or vaginal examination during labor. The final outcome of the repeated introduction of bacteria into the upper genital tract depends upon the integrity of the defense mechanisms of the uterus.

Predisposing causes. The resistance of normal tissues overcomes the bacteria that invade the uterus during almost every labor and delivery, thereby preventing the development of clinically obvious puerperal infection. Serious infection may develop if an overwhelming number of bacteria are introduced or if tissue resistance is weakened. The possibility of infection is much greater in women who are exhausted and dehydrated from prolonged labor. Other predisposing causes include excessive unreplaced blood loss, particularly in patients who already are anemic, traumatic deliveries during which the soft tissues are damaged excessively, retention of placental fragments, an excessive number of vaginal examinations during labor, and intrauterine manipulation without due regard for sterility. Sellner noted nulliparity, maternal age less than 20 years, and ruptured membranes for more than 5 hours as significant factors in the genesis of puerperal infection.

Prophylaxis. Prevention of infection is far more satisfactory than treatment. Although there has been a remarkable reduction in maternal mortality from infection in recent years, at least as much credit must be given to prevention as to the use of antimicrobial drugs, since the decline began before the drugs were introduced.

Prophylaxis includes treatment and eradication of pelvic and distant sources of infection during the prenatal period. Malnutrition and anemia should be corrected. The patient should be delivered in a clean, well-equipped, and well-staffed maternity unit that is separate from the rest of the hospital. Personnel with infections of any sort should be excluded from the care of patients in labor or those recently delivered. Masks that cover the mouth and nose and sterile gowns and gloves should be worn in the delivery rooms. All vaginal examinations should be performed with sterile gloves, using aseptic technique. Prolonged labor, injury, excessive bleeding, and dehydration should be prevented whenever possible. Incised wounds and injuries should be repaired in order that they may heal primarily. Placental tissue should be removed completely. Excessive blood loss should be replaced.

Treatment. An expectant attitude toward any febrile patient is unwise. The physician must consider each temperature elevation to be an indication of infection, and he must make an attempt to determine the cause before therapy is begun. The indiscriminate prescription of antibiotic and chemotherapeutic agents without complete examination of the patient is dangerous and deplorable.

Evaluation of the postpartum patient who has a fever should begin at the time of the initial temperature elevation; a careful general examination is made to eliminate extragenital sources, and the patient is questioned to elicit any suggestive symptoms. Should the temperature continue to rise during the first 24 hours of its presence or recur on the following day, a more complete investigation is necessary and includes a repeat general examination, white blood cell count, examination of a catheterized urine specimen, and a sterile pelvic examination. The pelvic examination is made to detect evidence of episiotomy, uterine, or parametrial infection, to check for a sponge inadvertently left in the vagina at delivery, and to obtain cultures for identification of the organisms and antibiotic sensitivity from within the uterine cavity. At the time the swab is inserted into the uterus for culture, a lochial block may be released.

Endomyometritis. In endomyometritis the most important measure is to establish adequate uterine drainage; this is far more important than any other therapy and in almost every patient is the only treatment necessary. This may be accomplished by having the patient assume an upright posture and by examination. Dislodging a blood clot or removing membranes occluding the cervix will permit more adequate drainage, after which the temperature may promptly fall to normal. Methergine or Ergotrate, 0.4 mg. orally three times daily, may promote drainage by stimulating uterine contractions, but they should only be administered after a complete examination.

Antibiotics are ordinarily not necessary for the patient with an uncomplicated endometritis, but if the temperature does not fall promptly when drainage is established or if there is definite parametrial tenderness, they may be prescribed. A Gram stain of the lochia may be a useful guide to initial therapy while awaiting results of cultures for aerobic and anaerobic organisms. Penicillin is the drug of choice for suspected streptococcal infections. It can be administered intramuscularly in doses of 1.2 million units every 6 hours, or if the patient requires intravenous fluids, 2 million units can be administered every 6 hours by this route. If enterococci are suspected, streptomycin, 0.5 Gm. intramuscularly every 6 hours, may be added to the regimen. If gram-negative organisms are found in the smear, larger doses of penicillin and an antibiotic other than streptomycin may be indicated. Antibiotics particularly effective against gram-negative organisms include kanamycin, poly-

myxin, and chloramphenicol. An alteration in dosage or the use of other antibiotic combinations may be necessary if the responsible bacteria are found to be resistant to the drugs originally used. For example, tetracycline is clearly the drug of choice if *Bacteroides* is suspected as the offending organism.

Parametritis. Parametritis, particularly that which accompanies septic abortion, presents a much more serious problem and requires more definite and active treatment. Lost blood should be replaced by blood transfusion; this is particularly important in abortions, since a profound anemia may be present. Because most women with parametritis have some degree of peritonitis it usually is wise to withhold food and fluids by mouth and to maintain hydration by the use of intravenous dextrose. Gastric suction should be used in patients who are vomiting. As the peritoneal signs disappear, food, fluids, and medications may be taken orally.

Antibiotic therapy should be started at once without waiting for a report on the intrauterine culture. Here again, a Gram stain of the lochia obtained from the endocervical canal may be a valuable aid in the selection of antibiotics. If gram-positive cocci predominate on the smear, penicillin may be administered in the intravenous fluids, 4 million to 8 million units per day, with streptomycin, 0.5 Gm. given every 6 hours intramuscularly. If gram-negative organisms predominate on the smear, the penicillin dosage should be increased to 50 million units daily, and kanamycin given intramuscularly, 1 Gm. initially and then 0.5 Gm. every 12 hours. The total dosage of kanamycin to any patient should probably not exceed 12 Gm. If the patient is allergic to penicillin, a cephalosporin may be substituted. A failure of clinical response or the discovery of resistant organisms on culture should be used as a guide for changing the antibiotic regimen.

As the general condition of the patient improves, the dosages of the drugs can be reduced. The temperature should begin to fall and the evidence of peritonitis should decrease in 48 to 72 hours. If this does not occur, the development of a *pelvic abscess* is to be considered. Pelvic examination every 3 to 4 days in patients not responding to treatment is necessarily to detect this complication. When an abscess is found, it must be drained; this should be done through the vagina if possible, but if it points upward, an abdominal extraperitoneal approach will be necessary.

In all types of infection adequate replacement of blood, sufficient fluids, and drainage of collections of pus are important parts of therapy. Patients can be managed successfully only by careful hour-to-hour evaluation and examination to follow the course of the disease. Prevention, early recognition of infection, and proper therapy will keep mortality at a minimum. Severe puerperal sepsis following delivery is uncommon today because it is being prevented. The mortality is still high but definitely can be reduced by prompt and adequate therapy.

■ Puerperal thrombophlebitis

Although thrombophlebitis is present in all patients with uterine infection, it is usually confined to the blood vessels in the uterine wall. If the process extends laterally and involves the large vessels along the lateral pelvic wall, the prognosis becomes worse. *Pelvic thrombophlebitis* often is first suspected during the latter part of the first postpartum week, although in most instances the temperature has never been normal after delivery.

The patient may complain of discomfort in the abdomen and pelvis, and tenderness may be elicited upon deep pressure. There usually is no evidence of peritonitis. There is tenderness, often localized to one side of the pelvis, the uterus may be limited in mobility, and motion produces pain on the affected side. Occasionally the involved veins may be palpated.

The most serious involvement of the veins of the extremities is that of the femoral vein, which produces the process known as "milk-leg." This usually appears at the end of the second week or later, and the patient experiences edema and pain in the affected leg and chills and fever. It seems likely that most postpartum involvements of the leg veins represent retrograde extensions from a pelvic thrombophlebitis.

Diagnosis. The diagnosis of pelvic thrombophlebitis is difficult since the stage of phlebothrombosis is seldom detected and since involvement of the pelvic veins is difficult to discern. The physician should suspect the diagnosis in any postpartum patient with persistent unexplained fever, particularly if it is associated with pelvic pain and tenderness. If the veins of the lower extremities are involved, the signs and symptoms are like those produced by the same infection in nonpregnant patients.

Treatment. The treatment of postpartum thrombophlebitis is like that for nonpregnant women. Since the most common infecting organisms are the anaerobic streptococcus or *Bacteroides*, the initial choice of antibiotics may depend upon the findings of a Gram stain of the lochia or a culture. If gram-positive organisms are identified, penicillin should be given, but if a *Bacteroides* infection is suspected, tetracycline is preferable. The anticoagulant preparations should also be utilized. During the prenatal period Dicumarol should not be administered because in both human beings and experimental animals retroplacental bleeding and placental separation have followed its use. Heparin may be administered if indicated.

Ligation of veins is of questionable value unless both the iliac or vena cava and the ovarian vessels are tied. Femoral or saphenous ligations will not prevent embolism from pelvic veins.

Pulmonary embolism has been estimated to be responsible for about 1 death in 30,000 deliveries (1:8,000 complicated deliveries), but it occurs somewhat more frequently. It is usually found in patients in whom vein disease has not been suspected and may often come from the pelvic vessels. It can only be prevented by reducing the incidence of infection and recognizing and treating phlebothrombosis. The treatment of the actual embolism is the same as in postoperative or medical patients. Vein ligation is only necessary for those who have repeated emboli despite anticoagulant therapy, in which event the vena cava and the ovarian veins must usually be tied.

■ Mastitis

Postpartum mastitis usually begins at least 2 weeks after delivery and is most common in women who are nursing or have attempted to nurse their infants. The bacteria are usually introduced through the nipples, and the incidence is not influenced by elaborate breast care. Infection is far more common in white than in black patients.

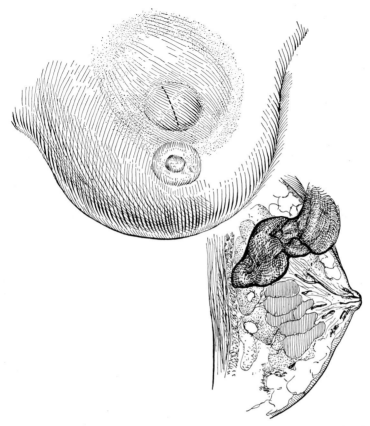

Fig. 40-2. Breast abscess treated by incision. A gauze pack is left in the cavity for 24 hours. (From Titus, P.: Atlas of obstetric technic, St. Louis, 1949, The C. V. Mosby Co.)

The patient may note pain in one quadrant of the breast, followed by fever, chills, and enlargement of the affected gland. The reaction to a small area of infection may be pronounced. Upon examination the breast is erythematous, indurated, and tender, and if the process is far enough advanced, fluctuation may be detected.

Treatment consists first of prevention, by prohibiting nursing by those women whose nipples are inverted and abnormal, those in whom cracks and fissures do not heal promptly, those who have bleeding from the nipples, and those whose nipples are injured by the baby. Curative treatment must be started early to be effective. Nursing is immediately stopped, the breast is immobilized with a tight binder, and ice is applied. Chloramphenicol, 500 mg. every 6 hours for 24 to 48 hours and then 250 mg. every 6 hours, is administered starting as early as possible. Penicillin in doses of 2 million to 3 million units daily also is effective unless the responsible organism is a penicillin-resistant *Staphylococcus.*

Such treatment usually aborts or cures the infection, but if the temperature remains elevated and fluctuation appears, incision and drainage become necessary. Extensive destruction of breast tissue may result from unrecognized abscess formation. The sulfonamide drugs are usually valueless and occasionally dangerous, since they may delay the advance of the infection while they are being administered but allow the process to become reactivated after they are stopped.

■ Gonorrhea

Gonorrhea is seldom encountered in private patients, but it is seen regularly in those who are treated in clinics. In such patients the changes produced by recurrent infections with the gonococcus are common causes of pain, disability, and infertility. The infection is transmitted from person to person almost entirely by sexual intercourse, and although modern methods of treatment could eliminate it, its dissemination is difficult to control.

Gonorrheal infections are divided into those affecting the *lower genital tract* and the urethra and those involving the *upper genital tract*. In those of the lower genital tract, the urethra, Skene's glands, Bartholin's glands, and the cervical glands are involved, and those of the upper genital tract affect the mucosal lining of the fallopian tubes and the pelvic peritoneum. The adult vaginal mucosa is resistant to infection with the gonococcus, but in prepubertal girls and postmenopausal women infection of the smooth, thin, unstimulated vagina occurs regularly.

Acute lower tract infection. The initial symptoms are most often related to the urinary tract and appear from 3 to 5 days after exposure. The patient first notices frequency of urination and dysuria and some discomfort in the vagina; this is soon followed by a profuse purulent discharge from the infected cervical glands. Bartholin's glands are not always involved, but those that are infected are indurated, erythematous, and tender, and pus can be seen exuding from the duct openings. The urethra is reddened and pouting, and pus can be expressed by stripping it from above downward by finger pressure through the anterior vaginal wall. The vagina is reddened, and the thick greenish yellow discharge it contains can be seen pouring from the inflamed and everted cervical canal.

The diagnosis can be confirmed by culturing the secretions from the urethra and the cervical canal. Although gonococci can often be demonstrated by Gram stain, culture provides a more accurate method of diagnosis and will more often be positive than will the staining techniques. The material must be collected from the surfaces of the urethal and cervical canals because the pus in the urethra, the cervical canal, the vagina, or the vestibule may contain only dead bacteria. If the material to be cultured is obtained by scraping the cervical canal gently with a dry cotton swab, a wire loop, or a tiny sharp curet, the culture is more likely to be positive. It is important that an accurate diagnosis be made before a patient is told she has gonorrhea. Untold difficulties have been caused because nonspecific cervicitis, trichomoniasis, and other innocuous infections have been diagnosed as gonorrhea.

It has been easy until recently to cure gonorrhea because the gonococci were so susceptible to moderate doses of penicillin. Unfortunately, this susceptibility is decreasing and there are many penicillin-resistant strains. It is important therefore, that adequate treatment be administered when the diagnosis is first made and that each patient be followed to make certain that the infection actually has been eradicated. There are alternative methods of treatment. For example, *tetracycline* may be given; 1 Gm. orally and 0.5 Gm. intramuscularly is usually adequate. When *penicillin* is used, it is important that high dosages of a relatively short-acting compound be administered. Shapiro and Lentz obtained the best cure rate (94.2%) with a total dosage of 4.8 million units of penicillin; 2.4 million units of aqueous penicillin G, and 2.4 million units of procaine penicillin G in oil. Despite the increasing resistance, penicillin remains the drug of choice for initial treatment because many patients have acquired syphilis as well as gonorrhea, and the spirochete responsible for the former remains highly susceptible to penicillin. Benzathine penicillin (Bicillin) should probably not be given to these patients because the release of low levels of penicillin over low periods of time may contribute to the development of penicillin-resistant gonococci. If this long-acting penicillin is utilized for therapy against syphilis, its administration should follow the initial dosage of at least 4.8 million units of procaine penicillin.

Cultures should be obtained shortly after the completion of treatment and after the next three menstrual periods. If they remain positive, another course of penicillin in larger dosage may prove effective, but if this does not eliminate the infection, tetracycline, 500 mg. every 6 hours for 5 days, may.

The blood serologic reaction should also be tested after enough time has elapsed to permit it to become positive, to see if the patient also acquired syphilis. General treatment measures include advising the patient of the contagiousness of the infection and warning her specifically of the possibility that the disease can be transmitted to others.

Acute upper tract infections. The cervix acts as a barrier against upward extension of the infection, and the disease often is

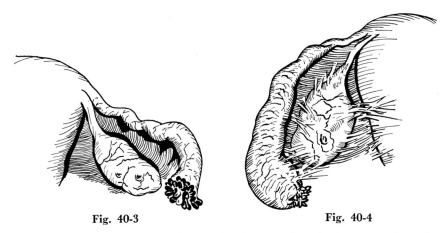

Fig. 40-3   Fig. 40-4

Fig. 40-3. Acute endosalpingitis. The fimbriated end of the tube is open, and pus is escaping from it.

Fig. 40-4. Pyosalpinx. The fimbria are agglutinated, confining the pus within the distended, inflamed tube.

limited to the lower tract and is eventually overcome even though no treatment is given. In many persons, however, the infection involves the fallopian tubes and the adjacent structures in the peritoneal cavity. Upward extension most often occurs during or just after a menstrual period.

The spread of gonococcal infection is almost entirely by way of mucosal surfaces; consequently there occurs a transient *endometritis,* which is soon followed by *endosalpingitis,* the characteristic tubal lesion of gonorrhea. The acute infection of the tubes produces an outpouring of purulent exudate from the tubal mucosa. In an effort to confine the infection to the tube itself, the fimbria become agglutinated, thereby sealing off the lumen from the peritoneal cavity and producing a distended, inflamed structure known as *pyosalpinx,* or a "pus tube." Before the tubal opening is closed, however, leakage of pus from its fimbriated end infects the pelvic peritoneum, producing *peritonitis* and *oophoritis.* The inflamed, heavy, pus-filled tube coils around the ovary and prolapses behind the uterus into the cul-de-sac, where it becomes adherent. The bowel and omentum adhere to the inflamed structures, attempting to restrict the infection to the pelvis and prevent its spead throughout the rest of the peritoneal cavity.

Examination reveals evidence of peritonitis, with the most distinct signs below the umbilicus over the entire lower abdomen.

Point tenderness is absent. There is exquisite tenderness throughout the whole pelvis. The mobility of the uterus is limited, and attempts to change its position produce severe pain. The tenderness often makes it impossible to outline the abnormal adnexa, but the bilaterality aids in eliminating lesions such as tubal pregnancy, twisted ovarian neoplasms, and appendicitis. The white cell count is usually between 20,000 and 30,000, and there is no clinical or laboratory evidence of blood loss. The temperature may peak at 103° to 104° F., and the elevation is sustained.

The course of such an acute infection is quite characteristic. After about 72 hours the temperature begins to fall and the symptoms improve. The patient usually feels much more comfortable within about 5 days, but the pelvic structures are still tender, indurated, and fixed. The tubes are enlarged and retort shaped and may be adherent to the posterior wall of the uterus and the broad ligament. The tissue reaction gradually regresses during the subacute phase, which lasts for several weeks after the temperature becomes normal.

The treatment of acute gonorrheal salpingo-oophoritis is similar to that for other conditions that cause pelvic peritonitis. Penicillin, 1.2 million units every 6 hours, will bring the infection under control rapidly and will reduce tubal damage if given early. Unless treatment is started during the first 24 hours, it is unlikely that the tubes will escape serious damage. Penicillin treatment that is started 3 or 4 days after the onset of symptoms appears to alter the acute stage of the disease only slightly. The temperature response and the initial regression of the infection are almost identical in treated and untreated patients, but total recovery is more rapid in those who are treated with penicillin. Oral feedings are withheld as long as there is evidence of peritonitis, and hydration is maintained by administering fluids intravenously. Usually within 48 hours food and fluid can be taken by mouth. There is no need to examine a patient whose infection is responding to treatment because pelvic manipulation may cause an exacerbation.

Operative intervention for acute lesions is contraindicated because most of them will become quiescent without any form of treatment, and in some the structures may even return to normal. If, as so often happens, the physician cannot differentiate between acute salpingo-oophoritis and appendicitis, ectopic pregnancy, or some other acute surgical condtion, an operation must be performed. If nothing but inflamed tubes is found, however, the abdomen should be closed without disturbing them more than is necessary to make a diagnosis.

Chronic and recurrent upper tract infection. Recurrent acute exacerbations of upper tract infections occur frequently in tubes that have been damaged by gonorrhea. With each acute attack the symptoms, the physical findings, and the course of the disease are similar to those during the first episode, but it is seldom possible to culture gonococci either from the cervix or the involved tubes. Recurrent infections are caused by organisms such as anaerobic streptococci and others, as well as by the gonococcus. Each attack damages the pelvic structures more, and eventually the patient may experience constant or recurrent pain, which prevents her from working or managing a household, or menstrual disturbance from interference with ovarian function. These may be present even though the infection is inactive.

Surgical treatment of chronic pelvic inflammatory disease may become necessary because of severe pain, incapacitating dysmenorrhea, or abnormal bleeding. In each instance a reasonable attempt must be made to control the symptoms by nonsurgical therapy consisting of pelvic diathermy, the use of analgesics during menses, and the elimination of sources of reinfection. If the patient is disabled in spite of these measures, operation become necessary. Such operations should usually be delayed until the acute infection has become quiescent and pelvic induration has regressed as completely as it will. This may require from 4 to 6 months.

Since most women who must be operated upon are young, it is desirable to preserve ovarian function whenever possible. Unfortunately, however, the symptoms are not always relieved by incomplete operations, and subsequent surgical procedures may be necessary. The physician should not hesitate to perform *hysterectomy* and *bilateral salpingo-oophorectomy* if the damage from repeated attacks is extensive, if there is already a disturbance in ovarian function, if a more conservative operation has already been performed, or in women in their late thirties or forties, regardless of the evident involvement. In younger women *cornual resection* severs the tubes from their uterine connections, thereby preventing reinfection from below. This procedure is best used in those who have had repeated infections and in whom the tubes are adherent and bound down but not greatly distended. Unilateral *salpingectomy* or *salpingo-oophorectomy* may be considered if the opposite tube seems reasonably normal; in some patients one adnexus can be removed and a cornual resection performed on the more normal side. When the surgeon contemplates such procedures, he should be aware that more than one half of the women treated this way will require a subsequent operation.

Tubo-ovarian abscess. A pyosalpinx is actually an abscess, but the term *tubo-ovarian abscess* has a different connotation. After repeated episodes of infection the tube and ovary are so intimately attached to each other that it is impossible to identify them individually in the inflammatory mass. The tubal portion may be thin walled and distended with clear fluid, a *hydrosalpinx,* between the acute attacks. At this stage the patient may be completely free from pelvic symptoms, and no systemic evidence of infection can be detected, even though bilateral tubo-ovarian masses can be felt. With the recurrence of an acute episode, pus once more forms within the lumen, and the tubo-ovarian structure may enlarge to several times its usual size with the purulent material under great pressure. Unless the advance of the infection is halted, the tube will burst and pus will be disseminated throughout the abdomen. The mortality from ruptured tubo-ovarian abscess is almost 100% unless treatment is instituted promptly.

The development of a tubo-ovarian abscess can be suspected whenever a large fluctuant

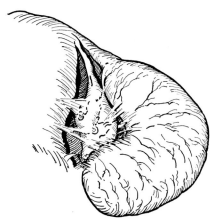

Fig. 40-5. Hydrosalpinx. Note that the fimbria are no longer present and the tube is closed.

tender mass is palpated during an episode of acute recurrent pelvic inflammation. It rarely occurs until the tubes have been extensively damaged by repeated attacks. If the temperature falls, the symptoms regress, and the size of the mass decreases under antibiotic treatment, there is little danger. If, on the other hand, the symptoms increase, the temperature remains elevated, the patient appears more and more toxic, and the size of the fluctuant mass is increasing, rupture may be imminent. Such a patient should be operated upon promptly before the abscess bursts.

The operative procedure is determined by the degree of involvement of the pelvic organs and the general condition of the patient. In most women with extensive bilateral tubo-ovarian disease there is little hope of salvaging reproductive, or even ovarian, function; under such circumstances the uterus and the adnexa should be removed. Occasionally the major involvement is of only one adnexus, the other appearing reasonably normal. In young women the physician might consider removing the tubo-ovarian abscess only and performing a cornual resection on the opposite side, but complete removal of the pelvic structures usually is preferable. An

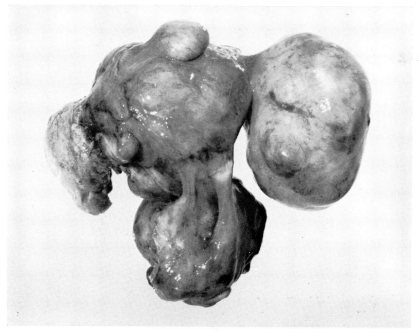

Fig. 40-6. Chronic tubo-ovarian abscess. The tube and ovary cannot be identified as individual structures.

operation should be performed when the abscess already has ruptured, even though the patient's condition is precarious, but under these circumstances it usually is wise to excise only the abscessed adnexa. The uterus can be removed later if necessary. Women with large tubo-ovarian abscesses that repeatedly become infected should be operated upon between attacks. The structures are usually damaged beyond salvage, and removal will prevent their rupturing during an acute episode.

■ Pelvic tuberculosis

Tuberculosis of the pelvic organs usually is secondary to tuberculous infection in some other part of the body, but the primary source is often quiescent at the time the pelvic involvement is discovered. The infection reaches the tube by hematogenous transmission or, less often, from an infection involving the pelvic peritoneum. It spreads downward along the tubal mucosa to the endometrium and then to the cervix and vagina. Since the extension is from above downward, the structures in the lower genital tract are not often involved. It is possible, however, that lesions on the external genitals, vagina, and cervix can come from an extrinsic source such as tuberculous epididymitis. Tuberculous peritonitis may originate from a tubal focus.

Tuberculous pelvic inflammatory disease is encountered less often in the United States than in other parts of the world, where it is said to account for about 5% of all cases of salpingitis. Tuberculosis is found in from 5% to 10% of all women studied for infertility in Israel, Scotland, and some other countries but much less often here.

The most characteristic lesions involve the tubes and the endometrium. There may be many small tubercles over the peritoneal surface, and the tube may be enlarged, thickened, and adherent. The lumen often contains cheesy, necrotic material, but in contrast to the findings in gonorrheal salpingo-oophoritis, the fimbriated end is open. Tubercles may be seen in any of the layers of the tubal wall. Usually there are many of them, but occasionally they are difficult to find. The ovarian involvement is usually superficial.

Endometrial tuberculosis is almost always secondary to infection in the tubes and can usually be diagnosed microscopically without difficulty, particularly when the infection is advanced.

Diagnosis. The symptoms are variable and are determined by what structures are involved. Extensive tubal tuberculosis with distortion and fixation usually causes dysmenorrhea and dyspareunia and may interfere with descent of the ovum. If the endometrium is involved, the menstrual cycle often is altered, but there is no characteristic change. The flow is increased and irregular at least as often as it is decreased. Most of the patients are infertile. Lesions of the vagina and cervix may resemble cancer and can be differentiated from it only by biopsy.

The diagnosis should be suspected in any person without a history of an acute inflam-

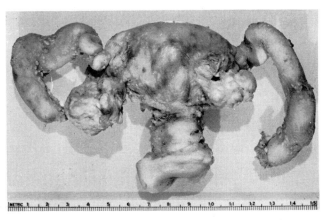

Fig. 40-7. Pelvic tuberculosis. Note the tubercles over the walls of the tubes and the fimbria on the right.

matory episode who has pelvic pain and enlarged adherent adnexa. This is particularly true in virgins. In such a patient *endometrial biopsy* or *curettage* may demonstrate the lesion. If the endometrium is involved, the tubes are almost certain to be infected also, but since the transmission is from above downward, tuberculous salpingitis can be present even though the endometrium is normal. Failure to demonstrate tubercles in the endometrium, therefore, does not eliminate the diagnosis. The lesion at this stage can sometimes be detected by *culture* of uterine discharge, particularly that collected during the first day or two of a menstrual period. A contraceptive diaphragm can be used to collect menstrual blood or discharge. Cultures may also be made from material obtained from aspiration of the endometrial cavity. Another satisfactory method is to submit half the endometrium obtained at curettage for histologic examination and the rest for culture.

Treatment. Most authorities agree that antibiotic therapy is beneficial, but there is considerable controversy concerning how long it should be continued and the advisability of following it with operation.

Active and prolonged antibiotic treatment, often combined with a surgical operation, is usually indicated for lesions that cause enlargement and distortion of the adnexal structures. Streptomycin is given intramuscularly in daily doses of 1 Gm. for 4 to 6 weeks and then 1 Gm. twice weekly. Isonicontinic acid (Isoniazid), 5 mg./kg. of body weight, and para-aminosalicylic acid (PAS), 12 Gm., are taken orally each day in 3 or 4 divided doses. After 3 or 4 months of medical treatment total hysterectomy and bilateral salpingo-oophorectomy should be performed. Some authorities have recommended less radical surgical procedures, such as retention of one or both ovaries or even the uterus. There seems to be little need for this, particularly if the patient is in her late thirties or forties. Normal pregnancy almost never occurs after medical treatment for pelvic tuberculosis, but tubal pregnancy is encountered relatively frequently. Medical treatment should be continued for 18 to 24 months after operation.

Minimal lesions, those in which there is no obvious tubal enlargement, the diagnosis having been made by endometrial biopsy or curettage, must also be treated vigorously. Schaefer calculated the relapse rates within 3 years of short-term therapy (6 weeks to 3 months) to be from 15% to 40%. Medical treatment is the same as that for more advanced lesions, but operation is less important because the infection can usually be eradicated by the medications alone. It may be necessary to continue treatment for 2 or 3 years. Operation need not be considered if endometrial tuberculosis disappears, cultures remain normal, menstruation is regular, and there is no clinical evidence of tubal disease. Surgery is necessary when medical treatment fails.

Many women will not take streptomycin week after week, and occasionally one will react unfavorably to it. The main complication is nerve deafness, which usually does not progress if the drug is stopped at the onset of the symptoms. PAS often causes nausea and vomiting.

■ Rare infections

Other forms of pelvic inflammatory disease, such as those due to actinomycosis, should be considered if the symptoms do not fit the usual pattern or if treatment is ineffective, but they are too rare to consider here in detail.

References
Puerperal infection

Burns, T.: The value of early diagnosis and adequate treatment in thromboembolic disease in obstetrics and gynecology, Amer. J. Obstet. Gynec. **71**:260, 1956.

Douglas, R. G., and Davis, I. F.: Puerperal infection; etiologic, prophylactic and therapeutic considerations, Amer. J. Obstet. Gynec. **51**:352, 1946.

Gopelrud, C. P., and White, C. A.: Postpartum infection; a comparative study for the period 1926 through 1961, Obstet. Gynec. **25**:227, 1965.

Holmes, O. W.: Puerperal fever as a private pestilence, Boston, 1855.

Schwartz, O. H., and Dieckmann, W. J.: Puerperal infection due to anaerobic streptococci, Amer. J. Obstet. Gynec. **13**:467, 1927.

Sellner, H. A.: The current complexion of puerperal infection, Bull. Sloane Hosp. Wom. **14**:22, 1968.

Semmelweis, I. P. (Trans. F. P. Murphy): The etiology, concept, and prophylaxis of childbed fever, Baltimore, 1941, The Williams & Wilkins Co.

Villa Santa, U.: Thromboembolic disease and pregnancy, Amer. J. Obstet. Gynec. **93**:142, 1965.

White, C.: Treatise on the management of pregnant and lying-in women, London, 1773.

White, C. A., and Koontz, F. P.: Bacterial flora of the cervix during pregnancy, Obstet. Gynec. **32:**402, 1968.

Gonorrhea

Curtis, A. H.: Gonorrheal disease of female genitalia. In Curtis, A. H., editor: Obstetrics and gynecology, vol. 2, chap. 52, Philadelphia, 1933, W. B. Saunders Co.

Shapiro, L. H., and Lentz, J. W.: Clinical evaluation of treatment of gonorrhea in the female, Amer. J. Obstet. Gynec. **97:**968, 1967.

Tuberculosis

Barns, T.: The natural history of pelvic tuberculosis, J. Obstet. Gynaec. Brit. Comm. **62:**162, 1955.

Schaefer, G.: Tuberculosis in obstetrics and gynecology, Boston, 1956, Little, Brown & Co.

Schaefer, G.: Antimicrobial treatment of tuberculous salpingitis, Amer. J. Obstet. Gynec. **77:** 996, 1959.

Sutherland, A. M.: The treatment of tuberculosis endometritis with streptomycin and PAS, J. Obstet. Gynaec. Brit. Comm. **61:**614, 1954.

Townsend, L.: The diagnosis of pelvic tuberculosis, J. Obstet. Gynaec. Brit. Comm. **62:**404, 1955.

41

The puerperium

The puerperium is the period from 6 to 8 weeks after delivery during which the physical and physiologic changes produced by pregnancy regress.

■ Normal changes

Uterus. The uterus, which at term weighs about 1,000 grams, returns to its nonpregnant weight of 40 to 60 grams by a process known as *involution*. Normal pregnant women are in positive nitrogen balance during pregnancy, retaining an average of about 1.8 grams daily. The retained nitrogen is utilized for the development of the fetus and placenta and for the growth of the uterus, the breasts, and other protein-containing structures. After delivery the excess protein in the uterine muscle cells is broken down by autolysis and is used, at least partially, if the patient is lactating, or it is excreted in the urine. The increase in urinary nitrogen that is expected after vaginal delivery is considerably reduced if the uterus is removed at or shortly after delivery.

After the lower segment has regained its tone during the first few hours after delivery, the superior surface of the fundus can be felt at about the level of the umbilicus and to the right of the midline. The size of the uterus decreases rapidly so that at the tenth to twelfth day it is at the level of the upper border of the pubis, and by the sixth week it usually has returned to normal size.

The more superficial layers of the decidua become necrotic and slough, but the bases of the glands that dip into the muscularis remain intact and active. The new endometrium, which eventually will line the entire cavity, regenerates from the remaining glandular epithelium. Epithelization, except at the placental site, usually is complete within 3 weeks. Immediately after delivery the placental site diameter is reduced to about half that of the placenta. The decidual tissue at the base of the placental site is covered by fresh blood clot. The decidua and the superficial layer of the myometrium beneath the placental site are soon infiltrated with white blood cells, and tissue necrosis begins on the second day. By the end of the first week placental site necrosis is complete and the surface crust, composed of decidua, vessels, glands, and myometrium, separates from the normal myometrium. The placental site is reepithelized by endometrium growing in from the edges and from the bases of glands in the myometrium.

The discharge from the uterus, which is made up of blood from the vessels of the placental site and debris from decidual necrosis, is called *lochia*. The discharge of pure blood from the open vessels soon changes to the *lochia rubra,* which is made up of necrotic decidua and blood. It gradually becomes less red as the vessels thrombose, but in some women bloody discharge persists for 4 or 5 weeks. The *serosanguineous lochia,* which is tan in color, contains less blood and finally changes to the serous *lochia alba.* Bloody discharge may persist if placental fragments remain in the uterus or if for some reason involution does not proceed at its usual rate.

The endometrial cavity is sterile from 6 to 24 hours after normal delivery but then becomes contaminated from the upward migration of vaginal bacteria. Infection of the shaggy necrotic decidua contributes to the discharge. The infective process may extend farther upward into the tubes, producing an endosalpingitis. This process usually produces no symptoms.

Ovarian function and menstruation. During pregnancy the ovaries are inactive, estrogen and progesterone being elaborated in the placenta. Ovarian activity remains suspended for varying periods of time after delivery. Most women who do not nurse their babies will have a period of bleeding within 4 to 6 weeks of the baby's birth, whereas those who are lactating often, but not invariably, are amenorrheic as long as they nurse. Sharman reported the return of menstrual function in 91% of nonlactating primiparas and in one third of lactating primiparas within 3 months after delivery. Multiparas more often started to menstruate earlier, even though lactating.

In most instances the first period of bleeding is heavier than a normal menstrual period and is anovulatory. By the third or fourth period bleeding and ovulation should have returned to normal. Lactating women usually are amenorrheic, but ovulation can occur, as is evidenced by the frequency with which women who assume they are protected against pregnancy while nursing do conceive. Sharman, studying postdelivery endometrial regeneration by biopsy, first found secretory endometrium, presumably due to ovulation, on the forty-fourth postpartum day. Kava and co-workers obtained secretory endometrium from 15 women between the thirty-third and forty-seventh postpartum days and on the ninety-third day in another patient.

Cervix. Immediately after delivery the cervix is relaxed and flabby, but it regains its tone fairly rapidly. Within a few days the canal re-forms as both the internal and the external os contract; by the end of 10 to 14 days the canal is well formed and narrow. Cervical lacerations heal by proliferation of fibroblasts.

Vagina. The vagina never returns completely to the pregravid state, and sometimes there may even be some relaxation following cesarean section. The tags of tissue that represent the hymenal ring are called *carunculae myrtiformes.* The vaginal mucosa looks thin and smooth like that of postmenopausal women until the ovaries again begin to function and produce estrogen. If the mother does not nurse her baby, ovarian estrogen production may begin in 3 or 4 weeks, but

if she is lactating, it may not begin until the baby is weaned.

Urinary tract. The bladder may be edematous and hyperemic, and there may even be areas of submucosal hemorrhage from the trauma of delivery. The hydronephrosis and hydroureter regress rapidly if the urinary tract is normal and within 2 or 3 weeks may have disappeared completely. Diagnostic urography should be delayed for about 6 weeks to make certain that the gestational changes have regressed. A marked diuresis begins within the first 12 hours after delivery in normal women; this is the mechanism by which the excess tissue fluid is eliminated. Naturally the diuresis is more pronounced in women who have been edematous than in those whose pregnancies have been more normal.

Breasts. During pregnancy the ductal as well as the glandular tissue proliferates under the stimulus of the placental hormones. Estrogen promotes growth of the ducts, and progesterone promotes that of the alveoli. The high levels of placental estrogen and progesterone also inhibit the anterior pituitary production of luteinizing hormone (LH), which is responsible for initiating milk production after delivery. *Colostrum,* a thin, yellow, alkaline fluid containing a large amount of protein, particularly serum albumin, but less fat than milk, is secreted during late pregnancy and during the first few days after delivery. It has been stated that the child obtains immunity against certain infectious diseases from the euglobulin fraction of the albumin in colostrum.

When the pituitary-inhibiting effect of placental estrogen-progesterone is removed by delivery, the secretion of LH, the anterior-lobe prolactin or milk-secreting hormone, is initiated. On the third or fourth day after delivery the breasts become *engorged,* and are distended, firm, tender, and warm, and milk can be expressed from the nipples. Engorgement may involve axillary breast tissue or even that in the area of accessory nipples along the milk line. The breast distention is primarily from engorgement of blood vessels and lymphatics rather than from an accumulation of milk.

There is no large supply of ready-made milk; much of it is produced in response to the stimulus of nursing. The activity of the suckling infant initiates a nervous stimulus from the nipple that releases oxytocin from the posterior lobe of the pituitary gland. Oxytocin stimulates the myoepithelial cells surrounding the mammary glands and ducts to contract and force the milk from the nipples. This is called milk ejection, or "let-down." In some instances the sight of the baby or even the thought of nursing will initiate the reflex.

Both quality and quantity of milk can be altered by diet, activity, and emotional disturbances. A normal pregnancy diet supplemented with an additional pint of milk each day will usually replace the materials secreted in breast milk. The milk production can be halted almost overnight by serious emotional shocks.

Vital signs. There should be no great change in *body temperature* during the puerperium. A rise usually indicates infection. The *pulse rate* often is low. A rapid pulse should suggest the possibility of undue blood loss. *Blood pressure* should be altered only slightly in normal women.

Blood. The white blood cell count increases during labor and in the early puerperium. It may reach 20,000 or 30,000 if the labor has been prolonged. This usually returns to normal within a few days.

As the plasma volume diminishes during the puerperium, the hemoglobin reading and the red blood cell count will rise. The patient who has had an adequate iron intake during pregnancy and who has not bled excessively at delivery should not be anemic.

Body weight. There is an immediate weight loss at delivery of 10 to 12 pounds. During the first few days of the puerperium the weight will decrease by 4 or 5 pounds more as the excess tissue fluid is eliminated. If the patient has been edematous, the loss will be greater. A further decrease will occur as the uterus involutes and plasma volume contracts.

Endocrine status. The major sources of hormone production during pregnancy are the placenta, the adrenal, the thyroid, and the anterior pituitary gland. Hormone production changes considerably after delivery.

The hormones that are produced by the trophoblastic cells are of necessity all reduced after delivery. Only a small amount of *chorionic gonadotropin* can be detected in the urine after the first day. *Estrogen* metabolism is a function of the fetoplacental unit

and ceases with delivery. The concentrations of estrone and estradiol reach the nonpregnant range within a week, but the estriol concentration decreases more slowly, this hormone being present for 2 or 3 weeks. *Progesterone,* as evidenced by pregnanediol, can no longer be detected in the urine after the first week.

Adrenal function is increased during pregnancy and returns to normal rather rapidly after delivery. *Aldosterone* production ceases promptly after delivery, and the excretion of *corticoids, 17-ketosteroids,* and *11-oxycorticosteroids* usually returns to normal levels during the first week.

The changes in *thyroid function,* as evidenced by elevations in protein-bound iodine, butyl-extractable iodine, and iodine uptake are reversed by delivery and slowly return to the normal level.

Pituitary function, except for the productions of LH *(prolactin)* and of *oxytocin* which are increased by suckling, appears to be unchanged by delivery. The production of anterior pituitary gonadotropic hormones is gradually resumed.

■ Care following delivery

The patient should remain in the delivery or recovery room for at least 1 hour after delivery. During this time her pulse and blood pressure should be checked every 15 minutes. The uterus is palpated frequently to make certain that it remains well contracted, and the vulvar pad is inspected for evidences of bleeding. The physician should not have to manipulate and massage the uterus to prevent relaxation; if this is necessary, something is wrong. The patient may be returned to her room at the end of 1 hour if the pulse is below 100, the blood pressure is stable, the uterus remains contracted, there is no bleeding, and she is awake. She must be checked frequently in her room for several hours.

Puerperal care is directed toward returning the patient to normal as rapidly as possible. In general the patients are not ill and need not be treated like those who have undergone major surgical procedures. The normal woman may be out of bed within 6 to 12 hours and may walk about and become completely ambulatory as rapidly as she is able. Those who have had spinal anesthesia for delivery should not be allowed up until both sensation and voluntary muscle control have returned.

Ideally visitors should be limited to the husband and the patient's parents during the entire hospital stay. No more than two persons should visit at a time. Too many visitors tire the patient unduly.

During the first 24 hours the patient may have either liquid or solid food, depending upon her wishes. A general diet may be ordered as soon as the patient wants it. The diet is similar to that during pregnancy, but mothers who are nursing their babies should have at least an additional pint of milk. This will supply the protein, calcium, and other ingredients to replace those secreted in breast milk.

Lactation. Breast milk is clean, inexpensive, and readily available, and mothers should be encouraged to nurse their babies. Involution progresses more rapidly in lactating mothers because breast stimulation causes the uterus to contract. Many mothers will notice painful contractions and an increase in vaginal discharge while the infant is at breast.

The baby remains in the nursery for about 12 hours after delivery to permit it and the mother to rest. It is then brought to the mother by a nurse experienced in the care of infants, who shows her how to hold the infant and to help it grasp the nipple and suck. Both mother and infant must usually be taught the technique of nursing. The nursing time at the beginning should be limited to conserve the mother's strength. At the first feedings the infant remains at the breast for only a few minutes, but nursing time is gradually increased to a 15- to 20-minute feeding period, which usually is adequate for an active baby. Suckling should not be limited too much because nursing success may depend upon how frequently the infant nurses and is more likely if infants are fed on demand rather than by the clock. Usually the baby nurses at one breast at each feeding, but when the milk supply is somewhat limited or the nipples are tender, both may be used each time. If the nipples are flattened because of engorgement, they can be pulled out with a breast pump to permit the baby to grasp them. The intramuscular injection of 1 unit of oxytocin or the use of a nasal spray of the same material just before the infant is put to breast will stimulate the "letdown" reflex and initiate lactation. This tends to reduce breast distention, making the nipples easier to grasp.

The nipples should be kept clean and as dry as possible between feedings. They are washed with soap and water daily and cleansed with water before each nursing period. Antiseptics are unnecessary. The breasts are supported with a snugly fitting nursing brassiere that is changed at least daily.

If the nipples are sore or cracked, nursing on the affected side should be discontinued for 24 to 48 hours. During this time a bland ointment such as lanolin is applied, and the nipples are exposed to the air to help prevent maceration. When the tissues are healed, the baby may again nurse, starting with 1 to 2 minutes and gradually increasing. The baby should usually be taken from the breast if fissures cannot be healed or if they recur, if the nipples bleed, or if nursing causes severe pain. Inverted nipples are abnormal, and the epithelium often does not stand up under nursing.

Engorgement is temporary, the acute symptoms lasting only a day or two. The discomfort is mostly due to lymphatic and venous engorgement rather than to distention with milk; pumping the breasts may not be particularly helpful and may even increase the symptoms after relieving them temporarily. The periodic injection of 1 unit of oxytocin or the use of an oxytocin nasal spray may relieve the discomfort by stimulating the milk ejection reflex. Ice bags may be applied, and aspirin, 0.65 Gm., and codeine, 0.065 Gm., can be taken every 3 hours as needed. Both estrogen and the male hormone, when given early enough, will reduce the initial engorgement, but neither is particularly effective after the symptoms are already present.

Bladder care. The renal excretion of urine is increased during the early puerperium, but the patient may have difficulty in voiding because of perineal pain or local edema from trauma. The bladder may be atonic and can become remarkably distended without producing discomfort. If the patient voids spontaneously after delivery, no particular care is necessary except to check for the adequacy of urinary output and to palpate the abdomen frequently to make certain the bladder is not distended.

The patient who has not voided during the first 6 hours after delivery should be encouraged to try. If she is unsuccessful, the administration of codeine and aspirin orally or of a belladonna and opium suppository by rectum to relieve perineal pain may relax muscle spasm and aid in voiding. If she cannot use a bedpan, she may be assisted to the bathroom or to a bedside commode. If she still is unable to void, she should be catheterized. This may be repeated every 4 to 6 hours, more often if she is uncomfortable or if the distended bladder can be felt above the pubis, until she can urinate voluntarily. An indwelling catheter can be left in place for 24 to 48 hours if it is neces-

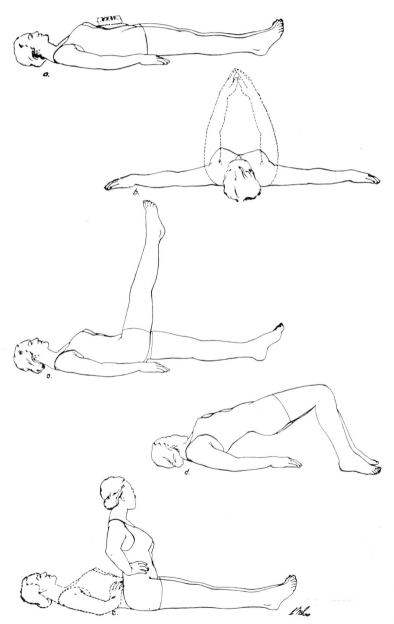

Fig. 41-1. Exercises to restore muscular tone after delivery. (From Willson, J. R.: Management of obstetric difficulties, ed. 6, St. Louis, 1961, The C. V. Mosby Co.)

sary to empty the bladder more than two or three times. Drugs are of little value in promoting bladder function.

Bowel. Many women are constipated during the puerperium. Food intake has been limited, and many have had an enema during labor. Thirty milliliters of milk of magnesia or another laxative may be taken daily as needed. If the bowels have not moved by the third postpartum day, an enema may be given.

Perineal care. While the patient remains in bed, the vulva should be cleansed by the nurse two or three times daily and after each bowel movement. When she becomes ambulatory, she can cleanse the vulva herself after voiding and bowel movements with soft tissue and soap and water or a hexachlorophene solution; no antiseptics are necessary. The perineum should be wiped from its anterior aspect toward the anus; the paper is discarded at the end of each stroke.

Tenderness in the episiotomy is usually caused by edema from too much suture material or sutures that have been tied too tightly. The discomfort can be relieved by the use of a heat lamp for 20 to 30 minutes three times daily or by the administration of aspirin and codeine or the insertion of a belladonna and opium rectal suppository three or four times daily. Hot sitz baths can be taken as soon as the patient can get into the tub.

Perineal pads should be changed frequently, at least each time the patient voids and more often if the discharge is profuse.

Afterpains. Multiparas often are troubled by painful uterine contractions during the first 48 hours after delivery. These usually are stronger while the baby is nursing. They almost never occur after the first delivery. They can be relieved with aspirin and codeine.

Exercises. Exercises such as leg or body raising to strengthen the abdominal muscles can be started any time the patient can perform them comfortably. Knee-chest exercises and other similar ones that are assumed to prevent retrodisplacement of the uterus are unnecessary.

The *pubococcygeus muscles* should be exercised systematically by contracting them slowly six or eight times in succession four or five times daily. This will help to prevent relaxation and urinary stress incontinence.

Blood count. The hematocrit level should be determined on the fourth or fifth day. An iron preparation should be prescribed for all postpartum patients.

Bathing. Postpartum patients may shower on the second day if they are strong enough. Tub bathing may be resumed after the first week.

■ Rooming-in

The development of large central nurseries was necessary because the mother was confined to her hospital bed for 9 or 10 days and was unable to care for herself, much less her baby. With early ambulation the postpartum patient is perfectly able to assume increasing responsibility for her infant after the first 24 hours and should be encouraged to do so by having the baby with her in her room or an adjoining small nursery. The primary advantage of the rooming-in plan is that it permits the mother to carry out, under supervision, all the details of infant care that were formerly the responsibility of the nurses, thereby making her transition from hospital to home far simpler than had the infant remained in the nursery except during the brief nursing periods. Other advantages are that the incidence of breast-feeding is increased and that the father as well as the mother is given an opportunity to participate in the early care of the child.

As pointed out by Montgomery and associates, rooming-in does not require elaborate equipment or specially constructed nurseries but may be instituted in any hospital in which the patients' rooms are of adequate size. The nursing staff can instruct the mother in the care of her infant and supervise her early efforts. Rooming-in does not decrease the required amount of nursing care and should not be instituted with this as its primary goal.

The infant may remain with the mother constantly, or the plan can be modified to include daytime care at the bedside, returning the baby to a central nursery or smaller peripheral nursery during the night. With the modified program the baby is brought to the mother's bedside early each morning. During the day she assumes responsibility for its care under the supervision of the nurses, but before midnight the infant is returned to the nursery in order that the mother may have a period of uninterrupted sleep. Visitors are permitted to visit the mother, but the baby should be removed while they are in the room. The father should be encouraged to hold the baby and to change and feed it. He should wash his hands and don a clean hospital gown before handling the infant. Although this method does not provide round-the-clock maternal care, it has the advantage of permitting long periods of contact between the mother and her baby and of allowing the father to become acquainted with the infant. At the same time it gives the mother an opportunity for uninterrupted sleep during the night. We know of no instance of cross infection or other harm to the infant as a result of this practice.

■ Discharge from the hospital

Unfortunately the need for obstetric beds and increasing costs have reduced the postpartum stay to 4 or 5 or even fewer days. Although patients who are out of bed early are much stronger than those who get up after several days, a period of hospitalization of at least 5 days is desirable, particularly if the patient has no help at home.

Before the patient is discharged, the breasts, abdomen, perineum, and uterus should be inspected and palpated. The physician should be sure that she is voiding normally, that her blood pressure is stabilized, and that she is physically able to cope with her responsibilities at home. Each patient should be instructed specifically as to what she may and may not do after leaving the hospital.

It usually is preferable that she limit her activity for a week or two after delivery. She may go up and down stairs at the end of the first week and may gradually increase activity as she feels able. Intercourse should be avoided until the episiotomy has healed and the pelvis is reasonably normal. Douches are not ordinarily necessary.

■ Subsequent examinations

Normal patients return to the office for examination when the infant is 6 weeks old. Those with abnormalities must, of course, be seen earlier. At the first visit the patient is weighed and her blood pressure, breasts, abdomen, and pelvis are examined. A clean-voided urine specimen should be examined if she has had one of the toxemias, a urine culture should be ordered if she has had a urinary tract infection, and a blood count should be obtained if she was anemic when she left the hospital or has been bleeding. This is also a good time to obtain material for a cytologic examination.

If involution is complete and if she appears normal physically, she should be instructed in some form of contraception if she wishes it and asked to return in 6 months. Any abnormalities present at this time should be corrected before the patient is discharged.

■ Postpartum complications

Bleeding. Abnormal bleeding can occur at any stage of the puerperium. Its management is discussed in Chapter 31.

Hemorrhoids. During labor and delivery, pressure from the presenting part impedes the flow of blood through the hemorrhoidal veins, and the resultant distention of the vessels may produce permanent injury to their walls. The hemorrhoids usually decrease in size rapidly and cause little discomfort, but some may produce severe pain, particularly if they thrombose.

The local application of witch-hazel packs or ice will reduce the distention and relieve discomfort. Belladonna and opium rectal suppositories will provide relief for those that are more painful. The clot should be evacuated from those that thrombose, and prolapsed hemorrhoids should be replaced within the anorectal canal. Hot sitz baths may also be ordered.

Backache. Backache occurs frequently in puerperal women and is most often caused by the unusual activity necessary for the care of the new baby. A suitable support, rest, and heat will usually control it.

Pubic separation. The symphysis may be unusually mobile, and there may be considerable separation of the pubic bones. This causes severe pain when the patient attempts to walk. The area is tender to palpation and the defect can be palpated readily. The only treatment necessary is adhesive strapping or a tight supporting garment and rest in bed. Recovery usually is rapid.

Subinvolution. Involution of the uterus may be delayed by endometritis, inadequate uterine drainage, retention of placental fragments, uterine fibroids, and other less obvious causes. It occurs most often in multiparas.

With delayed involution, bloody discharge

is more profuse and lasts longer than usual. The uterus is large, soft, boggy, and may be retrodisplaced. It usually is freely movable and there is no evidence of infection.

Normal involution can be aided by promoting adequate uterine drainage during the early puerperium. This is best accomplished by ambulation and upright posture. The course of involution is influenced only slightly by oxytocic drugs, and they ordinarily need not be prescribed during the puerperium.

If the uterus has not yet reached normal size and if bloody discharge is still present 6 weeks after delivery, subinvolution can be diagnosed. Unless the delay in involution is a result of retained placental fragments or a far more serious but unusual complication such as choriocarcinoma, hot vaginal douches taken twice daily for a week or two will usually hasten the return to normal.

Amenorrhea. Return of menstruation may be delayed after delivery because of minor and easily correctable dysfunctions of the endocrine organs. Other disorders such as anterior pituitary necrosis (Sheehan's syndrome) are more difficult to treat. The postpartum *galactorrhea-amenorrhea (Chiari-Frommel) syndrome,* which is characterized by amenorrhea and persistent lactation, is probably of hypothalamic origin, but an occasional one may be caused by a pituitary tumor. Anterior pituitary gonadotropin production ceases, and as a consequence ovarian activity is suspended. The resulting estrogen deficiency causes atrophy of the uterus, vagina, and external genitals, but lactation continues because pituitary lactogenic hormone production is preserved. Uterine bleeding may be precipitated by the administration of estrogen, but the effect is temporary. Most cases will correct themselves spontaneously with time, but recurrence following a subsequent pregnancy is to be anticipated. It may be possible to stimulate ovulation and pregnancy by the use of human menopausal gonadotropin-chorionic gonadotropin therapy.

Uterine retrodisplacement. During the early puerperium the large, heavy uterus will often fall posteriorly, particularly when the patient lies on her back. As involution progresses, the uterus will assume its normal prepregnancy position unless the pelvic supports have been extensively damaged.

Most retrodisplaced uteri produce no symptoms and need no treatment, but if the uterus is large, boggy, subinvoluted, and retrodisplaced at the first postpartum visit, it can be replaced and held forward with a pessary. This may aid drainage and promote involution. When involution is complete, the pessary should be removed. If the uterus again assumes a retrodisplaced position, it can be managed as described in Chapter 39.

Cervicitis. The cervix is almost always injured during labor and delivery, and most multiparous women have some sort of cervical lesion, of which cervicitis is the most common. One of the most important duties of the physician is to detect and eradicate the common benign cervical lesions since this may aid in preventing the later development of carcinoma. This can best be accomplished during the puerperium.

An unepithelized area is often noted around the external os of recently delivered women, particularly if involution is not yet complete. If such a lesion is found at the first postpartum office visit, it can be cauterized if the pelvic organs have already returned to their normal nonpregnant state. If the uterus is still enlarged and boggy, the cervical lesion may well heal spontaneously as involution progresses. Such patients should be advised to return for examination in 4 to 6 weeks. If the lesion is still present, it can be treated at that time; if it has healed, no therapy is necessary.

References

Anderson, W. R., and Davis, J.: Placental site involution, Amer. J. Obstet. Gynec. **102:**23, 1968.

Callahan, J. T.: Separation of the symphysis pubis, Amer. J. Obstet. Gynec. **66:**281, 1953.

Kava, H. W., Klinger, H. P., Molnar, J. J., and Romney, S. L.: Resumption of ovulation postpartum, Amer. J. Obstet. Gynec. **102:**122, 1968.

Montgomery, T. L., Steward, R. E., and Shenk, E. P.: Observations on rooming-in program of baby with mother in ward and private service, Amer. J. Obstet. Gynec. **57:**176, 1949.

Newton, M., and Newton, N.: The normal course and management of lactation, Clin. Obstet. Gynec. **5:**44, 1962.

Newton, N., and Newton, M.: Psychologic aspects of lactation, New Eng. J. Med. **277:**1179, 1967.

Rankin, J. S., Goldfarb, A. F., and Rakoff, A. E.: Galactorrhea-amenorrhea syndromes; postpartum galactorrhea-amenorrhea in the absence of intracranial neoplasm, Obstet. Gynec. **33:**1, 1969.

Schwarz, O. H.: The pathology of chronic metritis and subinvolution, Amer. J. Obstet. **76:**69, 1919.

Sharman, A.: Postpartum regeneration of the human endometrium, J. Anat. **87:**1, 1953.

Sharman, A.: Menstruation after childbirth, J. Obstet. Gynaec. Brit. Comm. **58:**440, 1951.

Slemmons, J. M.: Involution of the uterus and its effect upon the nitrogen output of the urine, Bull. Hopkins Hosp. **21:**195, 1914.

Williams, J. W.: Regeneration of the uterine mucosa after delivery with especial reference to the placental site, Amer. J. Obstet. Gynec. **22:**664, 1931.

Zuspan, F. P., and Goodrich, S.: Metabolic studies in normal pregnancy. I. Nitrogen metabolism, Amer. J. Obstet. Gynec. **100:**7, 1968.

42

Benign cervical lesions

The relative ease with which the cervix can be examined has assisted materially in the study of the wide variety of pathologic lesions that may arise in it. Infection, injuries, and neoplasia occur in the cervix uteri with a frequency that makes them commonplace. To appreciate cervical disease fully some basic knowledge of the histology is essential.

■ The normal cervix

The portio vaginalis of the normal, nulliparous cervix is completely covered with pink, smooth, squamous epithelium. It is similar in appearance to the epithelial lining of the vagina. The small, round opening of the cervical canal (*external cervical os*) is centrally placed in the vaginal face of the nulliparous cervix. The external os in the multipara is usually a transverse slit. Columnar (mucus-secreting) epithelium lines the cervical canal, and its connection with the squamous epithelial covering of the

portio is referred to as the *squamocolumnar junction*. This union of two different cellular structures is a critical zone. It is here that cervical pathology, for the most part, has its inception.

■ Squamocolumnar junction

Microscopically, the union of columnar and squamous cells may be so abrupt as to present a distinctive line (Fig. 42-2). This, however, is not the general rule because about two thirds of sections examined show a zone of labile, shifting cells between the lining of the cervical canal and the covering of the portio vaginalis. This area is referred to as the *transitional zone* and consists of basal or reserve cells. These reserve cells have the inherent ability to differentiate into either columnar or squamous cells. The inconstant cellular picture created by cells disintegrating and regenerating within the transitional zone is one of a microscopic area of cellular unrest. Considerable variations are to be found in the width and location of the zone at different age levels. The narrowest transitional zone will be found in the newborn infant, the widest during pregnancy. The transitional zone is situated high within the cervical canal in postmenopausal women and near the external os during the reproductive age.

■ Cervicitis and erosion

Cervicitis in one form or another is the most frequently encountered gynecologic lesion. It may be associated with other lesions in the vagina, the corpus uteri, or the cervix per se.

Acute cervicitis. An acute inflammation of the cervix is not as common as might be expected. It is seen in the first stages of gonorrhea but not with the same frequency as in preantibiotic days.

Foreign bodies such as forgotten tampons or lost condoms that lie against the cervix create a surprising amount of softening and severe, acute infection. Acute cervicitis is most often encountered as part of a vaginitis whose etiology is *Trichomonas vaginalis*, *Candida albicans*, or both. Almost every pathogenic bacterial agent and many viruses have been known to cause acute cervical infection.

The pathologic changes with acute cervicitis are similar to those of inflammation else-

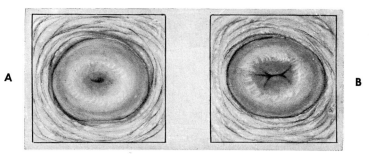

Fig. 42-1. Normal cervix. **A,** Nulliparous. **B,** Parous. (From Titus, P., and Willson, J. R.: The management of obstetric difficulties, St. Louis, 1955, The C. V. Mosby Co.)

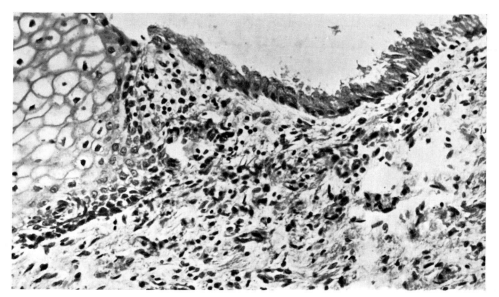

Fig. 42-2. Section through the squamocolumnar junction, the usual site of origin for carcinoma in situ. Note in this instance the abrupt transition between the squamous epithelium on the left and the tall columnar epithelium of the endocervix. (×279.)

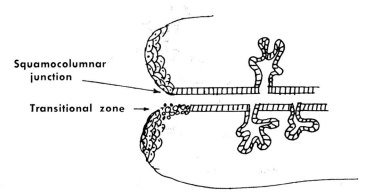

Fig. 42-3. Diagrammatic sketch of the squamocolumnar junction and the transitional zone.

where. The cervix is fiery red in appearance and markedly edematous. Leukocytic infiltration in stroma and lymphatics is evident in histologic sections.

A red and inflamed cervix, often with a copious, thin, grayish or yellow purulent discharge exuding from the external os, suggests a diagnosis of acute cervicitis. Cultures of cervical secretions for bacterial identification and sensitivity studies must be taken.

Chronic cervicitis. Nearly all women demonstrate some evidence (at least microscopic) of long-standing infection in the cervix. Not only does chronic cervicitis generally follow the acute stage, but it seems naturally to follow the trauma of cervical dilatation during abortion or delivery. Even without the traumatic effects of childbirth or an attack of acute cervicitis, the virgin cervix may demonstrate chronic infection.

As the acute stage subsides, the normal pink color of the portio returns. If recovery is complete, the endocervical secretions again become clear and mucoid. As a rule, however, residual infection of a mixed variety remains in the cervical glands, and a persistent gray-yellow mucoid leukorrhea results. The portio vaginalis of the cervix is rough and granular because of persistence of granulation tissue.

Although the gross appearance of chronic infection of the portio is distinctive, the histologic change encountered is almost a subject unto itself. Inflammation has a disturbing effect on the labile transformation zone of undifferentiated basal or reserve cells. Many cellular changes undoubtedly represent nature's attempt at healing, such as metaplasia and epidermization (Fig. 42-4). These changes are benign and should in no sense be worrisome to the pathologist.

Other cellular changes such as hyperplasia of the basal epithelial cells may appear. Several atypical cellular features are created in this manner, and their presence is disturbing to the pathologist. Among these associated epithelial changes are to be found potentially malignant alterations. These will be considered in more detail later. The gross appearance counts for little in this most common of cervical diseases since *cancer* and *benign* lesions are similar in appearance.

Symptoms. A *mucopurulent discharge* is generally the only symptom produced by most of the benign lesions, whereas some cause none. *Pain,* although not common in cervicitis, is occasionally noted in paracervical areas. It probably is caused by involvement of the lymphatics that drain the infected cervix. *Abnormal bleeding* of the post-

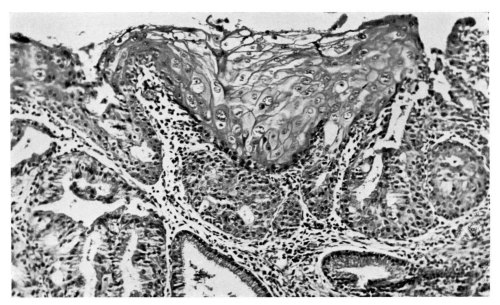

Fig. 42-4. Section showing squamous metaplasia of the endocervical mucosa and the contiguous glands. Note the complete maturation and the orderly arrangement of the metaplastic epithelium. A minimal degree of dysplasia is manifest by increase in nuclear size and slight variability in size and shape. (×164.)

traumatic variety occurs in some cases but is more characteristic of carcinoma than of benign lesions.

Erosion. An erosion uncomplicated by infection has a clear mucous discharge, somewhat in excess of the usual cervical gland secretion. With superimposed infection the mucoid material will become yellow, tenacious, profuse, and annoying.

Grossly, the portio vaginalis of the cervix is covered by varying amounts of reddish proliferating tissue extending into the cervical os. The granular-appearing areas are commonly referred to as an *erosion*. Since there is usually no ulcer the term *erosion* is not entirely accurate in a pathologic sense, but usage has made it acceptable. Erosions are formed by columnar epithelium growing down from the canal and creating a new squamocolumnar junction on the portio instead of within the external os.

Histologically, the picture is often confused, and rarely do we find pure columnar epithelium covering the surface. Squamous epithelium will be seen in patches, often overlying columnar cells. In addition the squamous epithelium may form lips for the cervical glands in this area and may extend into them, displacing columnar epithelium. This tissue change, referred to as *squamous metaplasia*, is one of the most common alterations noted. Background for this change is provided by the incompletely differentiated cells in the transitional zone, proliferating into squamouslike cells. These cellular changes are thought to be due to the combined effects of trauma, infection, and estrogen. The role of each is not clear.

The orifices of the cervical mucus-secreting glands become obstructed by regenerating squamous epithelium, and the glands dilate to form *nabothian cysts*. Since the columnar cells continue to function, these cysts are filled with normal-appearing cervical mucus. Proliferating squamous cells that extend the transformation zone into the cervical canal produce *epidermization* of the endocervix.

What appears as an eroded cervix may upon closer inspection prove to be an *eversion*. This lesion results from bilateral lacerations deforming the cervix. When a vaginal speculum is opened to inspect the cervix, it causes the anterior and posterior lips to separate, exposing the endocervical canal. The canal may or may not be infected. It should

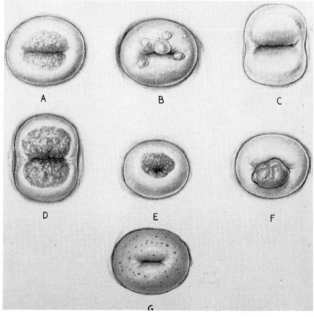

Fig. 42-5. Common lesions of the cervix. **A,** Cervicitis in a multiparous cervix. **B,** Nabothian cysts. **C,** Bilateral healed lacerations. **D,** Bilateral lacerations with eversion and endocervicitis. **E,** "Erosion" in a nulliparous cervix. **F,** Cervical polyp. **G,** "Strawberry" spots with vaginal trichomoniasis. (From Kleegman, S. J.: Amer. J. Surg. 48:294, 1940.)

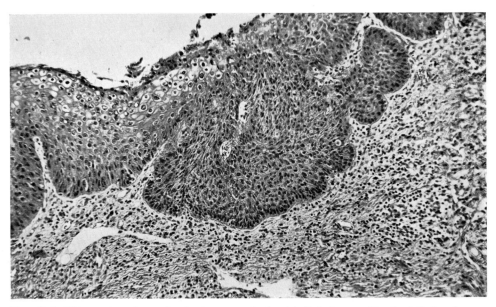

Fig. 42-6. This section shows dysplastic or atypical epithelial change. On the left the changes are those of koilocytotic atypia, whereas on the right the proliferating cells have a squamous morphology and pattern when the basal layer is prominent. Rete peg formation and proliferation may be noted at the center. (×255.)

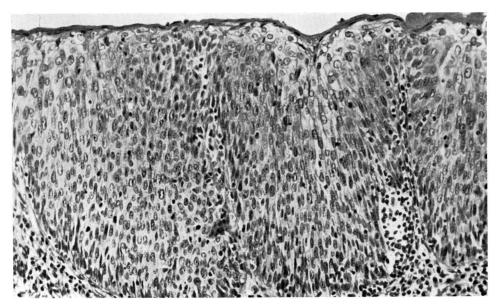

Fig. 42-7. This section demonstrates cellular surface layer. When the cells are closely packed, there is a fairly orderly arrangement. Maturation is to be noted in roughly the upper half of the epithelial surface to the point of keratin production in the surface. This is the picture of severe dysplasia. (×255.)

be understood that the endocervix is closed when the speculum is withdrawn.

Diagnosis. Satisfactory diagnostic procedures are relatively simple. A properly taken cervical smear, stained by the Papanicolaou method and read in a reliable laboratory, provides the first step in *screening* any cervical lesion. The study of exfoliated cells from the transitional zone of the squamocolumnar junction will generally reveal atypical cellular findings if cell growth is

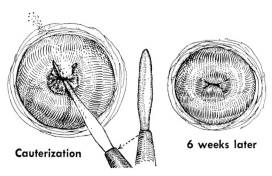

Cauterization   **6 weeks later**

Fig. 42-8. Cauterization. The lesion can be cauterized with radiating strokes as shown, or the entire lesion can be coagulated. (From Titus, P.: Atlas of obstetric technic, St. Louis, 1949, The C. V. Mosby Co.)

anaplastic. Since an accurate diagnosis of cancer cannot be made by cytology alone, a suspicious smear clearly indicates the need for further study. On the other hand, treatment of a cervicitis may proceed without further diagnostic work if the smear is normal.

If the area of chronic cervicitis under scrutiny is too large for local treatment or if the cytologic smear is abnormal, a *conization operation* should be done. This procedure not only provides the pathologist with adequate tissue for necessary study but will doubtless cure the cervicitis at the same time.

Various cellular pictures may be found in chronic cervicitis. Again, in the transitional zone the undifferentiated cells above the basement membrane may show abnormal growth patterns. This abnormal cellular activity, when confined to the basal cell layer, is called *basal cell hyperplasia*. This represents the first recognizable step in a series of *dysplastic* histologic events that may eventuate in carcinoma. A wide variety of anaplastic changes can be identified between basal cell hyperplasia on the one hand and carcinoma in situ on the other. The various degrees of *dysplasia (anaplasia, atypism)*

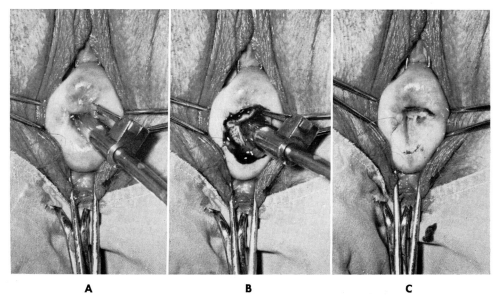

      A   **B**   **C**

Fig. 42-9. Cold-knife conization with Seiger cervitome. **A,** The cervix is stabilized with four tenaculums while the knife blade is inserted into the cervix. **B,** The cone of tissue including the entire cervical canal and the squamocolumnar junction has been cut free. **C,** The cervix immediately after conization. Sutures are usually necessary to control bleeding but were not needed in this patient.

create borderline lesions, histopathologic interpretation of which is difficult. These lesions are potentially malignant, but the ultimate fate of various degrees of dysplasia is by no means certain, and every patient with such a lesion must be followed indefinitely. McKay and co-workers, following up patients for 10 years, found 26.4% of the lesions unchanged, whereas 3.8% progressed to carcinoma in situ or invasive cancer.

Treatment. The treatment of acute cervicitis is determined by identifying the causative organism. Culture and sensitivity studies will indicate the appropriate medication.

Before any treatment of chronic cervicitis is undertaken, malignancy of the cervix should be ruled out. This is accomplished by a Papanicolaou smear from both the endocervix and the squamocolumnar junction. Although cytologic examination is to be considered as only a screening test, it is reasonably safe to perform *electrocauterization* when the cytology is normal. Cauterization is particularly suitable for lesions that are not accompanied by marked edema of the portio vaginalis. Cautery should be used over the entire affected vaginal face of the cervix, as well as into the lower 1 cm. of the endocervical canal. Nabothian cysts should be emptied of their contents by the cautery tip, and their base should be cauterized. Daily instillations of an antibiotic cream by the patient for approximately 1 week after this procedure will materially shorten the treatment period. Since about 2 months are required for complete sloughing and tissue

regeneration, inspection or further cauterization should be delayed until then.

If the cervix is not completely healed 2 months after it has been cauterized, a tissue study is in order at once. Characteristically, with an early carcinoma the cervical tissue will not regenerate and heal as it does after cauterization of a benign lesion.

Large, cystic, infected cervices are best treated by *conization*. The procedure is therapeutically effective because the infected material is removed; at the same time it provides the pathologist with an adequate block of tissue for study. In such a study it is possible for the pathologist to rule out the presence of malignancy with reasonable certainty.

■ Polyps

Cervical polyps are next in frequency of occurrence to chronic cervicitis and its associated epithelial changes. These small, pedunculated lesions stem from the endocervical canal and consist almost entirely of columnar epithelium with or without squamous metaplasia. They vary in size from a few millimeters up to 2 and 3 cm. They are soft, red, and friable. Bleeding may be induced by the slightest trauma. Presumably polyps have little to do with the development of malignancy in the cervix, and they rarely undergo carcinomatous change.

Cervical polyps are often responsible for episodes of slight vaginal bleeding. The physician must be cautioned concerning the patient who experiences some unexplained

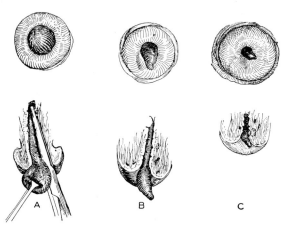

Fig. 42-10. Cervical polyps. **A,** Method for twisting a polyp off at its base. **B** and **C,** Usual appearance of endocervical polyps. (From Titus, P.: Atlas of obstetric technic, St. Louis, 1949, The C. V. Mosby Co.)

vaginal bleeding and has a cervical polyp. If he assumes the polyp is responsible for the bleeding and does not perform an endometrial and endocervical curettage, a corpus carcinoma may go undetected. This is particularly true in postmenopausal women.

Cervical polyps should be excised at their base. If a polyp is asymptomatic, the cervix well epithelized, and the cytologic smear normal, it is safe simply to excise the growth. On the other hand, polyps accompanied by obvious lesions are best treated by conization.

■ Hypertrophy of the cervix

Both the diameter and the length of the cervix may increase severalfold. Usually the increase in diameter results from edema that accompanies a long-standing chronic infection. Vaginal relaxation and prolapse of the uterus, however, are frequently associated with hypertrophy and lengthening of the cervix. The weight of the cystocele and rectocele pulling on the cervix gradually stretches this portion of the uterus to several times its normal length (Fig. 42-11).

At such times the cervix takes on a hyperkeratotic or leukoplakic appearance when seen protruding from the vulvar orifice. If the uterine supports remain reasonably intact, the cervix may elongate so that it protrudes far beyond the introitus, even though the uterus descends only slightly.

The treatment of hypertrophy alone depends a great deal upon the accompanying pathology and the age and physical condition of the patient. A high cervical amputation with an accompanying vaginal plastic operation may be all that is necessary. Usually a vaginal hysterectomy and vaginal plastic repair are the procedures of choice.

■ Cervical stenosis

Stenosis of the cervical canal is caused by scar tissue contracting and by the agglutination of raw surfaces within the endocervix. This has been known to follow cauterization, conization operations, cervical amputations, and intrauterine radium applications. Troublesome alterations in the menstrual pattern may occur with stenosis. The flow may be scant, painful, and prolonged because of the stricture of the cervical canal. An acquired dysmenorrhea after cervical operations strongly suggests cervical stenosis. Obstruction may be complete in rare instances, with hematometra resulting. Severe cervical stenosis has caused complete cervical dystocia in labor, making cesarean section mandatory for the undilatable cervix.

In the postmenopausal individual atrophy of the cervix and corpus uteri is the rule. Contraction and stenosis may so completely close the endocervix that secretions from the atrophic endometrial cavity have no escape. These secretions and cellular debris accumulating within the body of the uterus may eventually become infected, and *pyometra* results. Pyometra may also occur with endo-

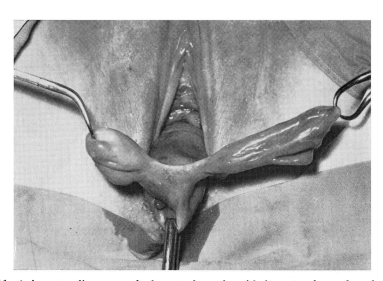

Fig. 42-11. A long-standing, severely lacerated cervix with hypertrophy and prolapse.

metrial carcinoma or with cancer of the cervix that obliterates the cervical canal. Treatment consists in dilatation of the cervix and culture of the escaping purulent material. Appropriate antibiotics may be needed, although this is usually unnecessary. The cervix must be kept open by the passage of a 3 or 4 mm. dilator once a week until the point of stricture remains open without force. This takes about four to six dilatations. In rare instances patency cannot be maintained, and hysterectomy is indicated if the infection recurs. Diagnostic curettage is essential in women with pyometra.

■ Benign new growths

In addition to the common polyp previously discussed, *myomas* often involve the cervix. These are considered in Chapter 46. Likewise, *endometriosis*, although infrequent in the cervix, does occur and is discussed in Chapter 9.

References

Auerbach, S. H., and Pund, E. R.: Squamous metaplasia of the cervix uteri, Amer. J. Obstet. Gynec. **49**:207, 1945.

Beecham, C. T., and Andros, G. J.: Cervical conization in pregnancy, Obstet. Gynec. **16**:521, 1960.

Fluhmann, C. F.: The histogenesis of squamous cell metaplasia of the cervix and endometrium, Surg. Gynec. Obstet. **97**:45, 1953.

Fluhmann, C. F.: The squamocolumnar transitional zone of the cervix uteri, Obstet. Gynec. **14**:133, 1959.

Hellman, L. M., Rosenthal, A. H., Kistner, R. W., and Gordon, R.: Some factors influencing the proliferation of the reserve cells in the human cervix, Amer. J. Obstet. Gynec. **67**:899, 1954.

McKay, D. G., Terjanian, B., Poschyachinda, D., Younge, P. A., and Hertig, A. T.: Clinical and pathologic significance of anaplasia (atypical hyperplasia) of the cervix uteri, Obstet. Gynec. **13**:2, 1959.

Stoddard, L. D.: The problem of carcinoma in situ with reference to the human cervix uteri. In McManus, J. F. A., editor: Progress in fundamental medicine, Philadelphia, 1952, Lea & Febiger.

TeLinde, R. W.: Cancer-like lesions of the uterine cervix, J.A.M.A. **101**:1211, 1933.

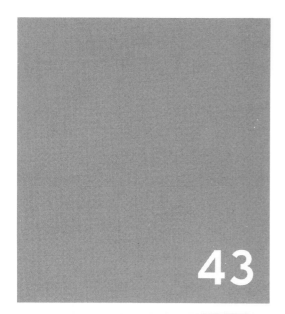

43

Malignant cervical lesions

Invasive carcinoma of the cervix is a *preventable* disease. Preventability is predicated on the basis of cooperative women being observed regularly by alert physicians making thorough use of the diagnostic tools at hand today.

From birth on there is a probability that 2.3% of our female population will develop cervical malignancy; the disease makes up 15% of all cancers in women. Over the past 25 years the mortality from uterine cancer has declined from 34.9 to 15.7 per 100,000 population.

Although no age group is free of cervical carcinoma, the greatest incidence occurs between the ages of 35 and 55 years, the average being 49.9 years.

Epidemiologic data reveal a significant relationship between early and continuing coitus and the development of cervical malignancy. The incidence of cervical cancer is increased in all women of low socioeconomic status, but it is particularly high in blacks.

It is in these classes of people that cohabitation is likely to start in the early teens and to continue for many years. Cancer of the cervix is diagnosed more often in women of high parity than in nulligravidas, but it seems likely that the age of first coitus and its frequency and duration play a more important role in the genesis of carcinoma of the cervix than does the number of pregnancies and births.

The highest incidence rate so far published is 28.3 cervical cancers per 1,000 population in a women's corrective institution. A more representative figure was arrived at by the large-scale screening program in Floyd County, Georgia, where an incidence of 4.7 per 1,000 was obtained. The significant difference in these figures suggests that cervical malignancy is an occupational hazard of promiscuity.

Jewish women rarely have cervical carcinoma. This has led to much etiologic speculation as to the role of the uncircumcised male and the effect of poor penile hygiene upon non-Jewish women. The inference is that bacteria or viruses, greatest in the uncircumcised man, are transmitted by coitus and are factors in developing cervical carcinoma.

■ Types

It is well established that most cervical cancers begin in the labile transitional zone of the squamocolumnar junction. There the reserve cells are capable of differentiating to either squamous or columnar cells. Since microscopic cancer seems to grow up the canal first, it is surprising to find that 95% of cervical cancer is of the squamous cell variety and only 5% adenocarcinoma. Rarely, sarcoma, mixed mesodermal tumors, or malignancies of the lymphoid series (reticulum cell sarcoma, malignant lymphoma, etc.) may be primary in the cervix.

■ Pathology

Chronic cervicitis with associated *basal cell hyperplasia* in the purest sense is evidence of minimal cellular unrest. Although this is considered a benign tissue change, it is the earliest recognizable cellular alteration that *may* be a forerunner of invasive cancer. Basal or reserve cell hyperplasia may extend toward the surface of the epithelial layer, taking on added *dysplastic (anaplastic)* fea-

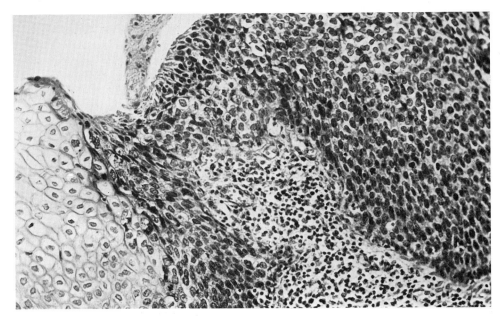

Fig. 43-1. Carcinoma in situ of the cervix. Note the mature cells on the left with an abrupt change to complete loss of maturation on the right, with an intact basement membrane.

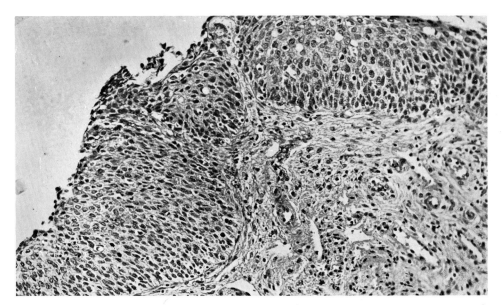

Fig. 43-2. Carcinoma in situ on the left side with very cellular surface epithelium. The cells are closely packed and disarrayed with numerous and dark nuclei. On the right there is some attempt at maturation as seen in severe dysplasia. (×186.)

tures. Disorderly cellular arrangement with mitoses, multinucleated cells, enlarged nuclei having coarse chromatin, or varying amounts of irregular hyperchromatic changes prevail. What started as an "innocent" basal cell hyperplasia will in some women progress slowly through degrees of dysplasia until there is no longer evidence of cellular maturation. When the full epithelial layer is made up of anaplastic cells, the diagnosis changes from dysplasia to *carcinoma in situ*.

Dysplasia is thought to progress to carci-

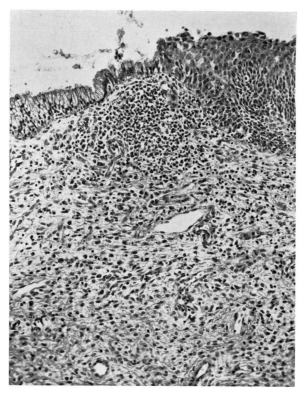

Fig. 43-3. Normal endocervical mucosa is seen on the left with an abrupt change on the right where proliferation of the reserve cells in the transitional zone to incomplete maturation and carcinoma in situ is found. (×186.)

noma in situ in about 3 years. Atypical cellular changes often do not progress to malignancy and may be cured by cone biopsy or even by cautery, but this cannot be relied upon.

Carcinoma in situ is the earliest stage at which cancer of the cervix can be diagnosed. Except for *invasion* this lesion possesses all the cellular changes to be found in invasive carcinoma. The length of time required for carcinoma in situ to become invasive is thought to be between 3 and 10 years.

Pathologic interpretation of dysplastic lesions and carcinoma in situ is not always easy. Pathologists are often in disagreement on specific instances of severe dysplasia and carcinoma in situ with or without microscopic invasion. The basic minimum requirements for the adequate study of cervical tissues are (1) that we provide the pathologist with ample material by taking a cone biopsy, and (2) that the pathologist examine multiple sections of the material submitted. Such studies repeatedly point out the *existence of*

dysplasia with and without carcinoma in situ on the periphery of an invasive cancer. Punch biopsies would hardly provide an adequate sample for pathologic interpretation.

Invasive carcinoma has degrees of undifferentiation, and this is the foundation for Broder's classification, in which grade I shows the most and grade IV the least cellular differentiation. Classic studies by Reagan and associates on the size of cancer cells have provided us with further fundamental knowledge now being used in an attempt to predict the behavior of cervical carcinoma.

Chromosomal alterations. Labeling nuclear chromosomal DNA with tritiated thymidine (H^3-thymidine) has shown fundamental changes as normal cervical epithelium becomes dysplastic and finally malignant. H^3-thymidine in vitro uptake is confined to about 5% of the basal or parabasal cells in normal cervical tissue. Richart has shown "altered labelling indices that increase logarithmically" as this tissue develops carcinoma in situ. Jones and co-workers in their cyto-

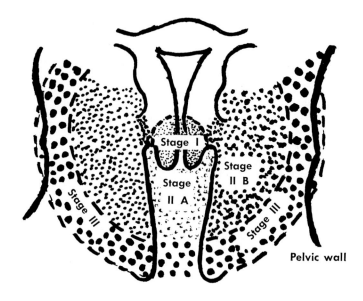

Fig. 43-4

Preinvasive carcinoma of the cervix.

    Stage 0 —Carcinoma in situ, intraepithelial carcinoma. Cases of stage 0 should not be included in total therapeutic statistics.

Invasive carcinoma of the cervix.

    Stage I —Carcinoma strictly confined to the cervix (extension to the corpus should be disregarded).

    Stage IA—Cases of early stromal invasion (preclinical carcinoma).

    Stage IB—All other cases of stage I.

    Stage II —The carcinoma extends beyond the cervix but has not extended on to the pelvic wall. The carcinoma involves the vagina, but not the lower third.

    Stage IIA—Vaginal but no parametrial extension.

    Stage IIB—Parametrial extension but not to the wall.

    Stage III—The carcinoma has extended on to the pelvic wall. On rectal examination there is no cancer-free space between the tumor and the pelvic wall. The tumor involves the lower third of the vagina.

    Stage IV—The carcinoma has extended beyond the true pelvis or has involved the mucosa of the bladder or rectum. A bullous edema as such does not permit allotment of a case to stage IV.

(From Kottmeier, H. L.: J. Int. Fed. Gynec. Obstet. 1:86, 1963.)

genetic investigations of dysplasia, carcinoma in situ, and invasive carcinoma consistently find an aneuploid chromosome number. There is no consistent range to the aneuploidy, however, using Feulgen cytophotometry. Wilbanks and co-workers noted a "highly variable population of cells whose range of DNA content is similar" in carcinoma in situ and invasive carcinoma.

■ Clinical stage

The extent to which the cervix and surrounding structures are involved with cancer is referred to as the *clinical stage* of the disease. This factor definitely influences prognosis or cancer salvage. The small early lesions have the best prognosis, whereas the

carcinoma extending beyond the cervix has far less chance of a cure.

It is futile to attempt a description of an early cervical cancer. Every practicing physician has found cancer by routine use of the Papanicolaou smear or chance cervical biopsy in women with grossly normal, well-epithelized cervices. If there is any visible change in the squamocolumnar junction, it will resemble a simple cervicitis with a reddish, tufted, granular appearance. Rarely, it might resemble a tiny ulcer. Gentle sponging with cotton usually produces bleeding. On the other hand, red granular cervical lesions that bleed to the slightest trauma and strongly suggest cancer may prove to be severe chronic cervicitis on biopsy study. The safest rule to

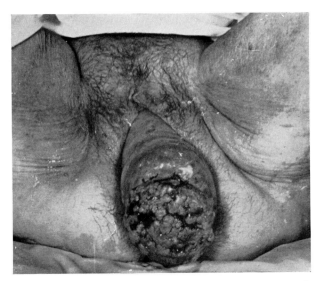

Fig. 43-5. Large carcinoma of the cervix in a patient with complete prolapse of the uterus (rare).

follow is: *Consider all cervices suspect. Obtain cytologic studies on all patients who come for examination. Perform an excision biopsy on every bleeding cervical lesion.*

Assigning a *clinical stage* to each cervical cancer before starting active treatment is a helpful routine. Staging the disease dictates the treatment to be employed and indicates the course the cancer will take and the chances of survival. Statistical studies of the clinical stages allow clinics to compare the results of different modalities of treatment.

Carcinoma of the cervix like cancer elsewhere does not remain confined to the site of original growth but spreads by direct extension and through the lymphatics. Friedell and Parsons, utilizing giant histologic sections of the pelvic viscera, demonstrated the spread of cervical cancer into the paracervical and paravaginal tissues. They found a *halo of carcinoma in situ* around the invasive portions and down the vagina. Lymph node involvement was shown in a minority of patients by this method of study. However, in the specimens removed by radical hysterectomy with pelvic node excision, Brunschwig and Daniel encountered positive lymph node involvement in the following percentages: 13% in stage I, 30% in stage II, 46% in stage III, and 53% in stage IV.

The ureter is particularly vulnerable to cervical malignancy. About 65% of all patients show some degree of ureteral obstruction at autopsy. Almost one third of the deaths from cervical carcinoma are from uremia. Infection, peritonitis, pelvic cellulitis, and septicemia account for about 40% of the deaths. Distant metastases, although uncommon, may occur to any part of the body.

■ Symptoms

There are no early symptoms of cervical carcinoma. As a rule the cancer reaches a clinical stage II before producing signs. Bleeding or bloody discharge, often initiated by coitus or douching, is the first symptom; this means the growth has progressed to the point of ulceration. As the cancer grows, bleeding becomes almost constant until frank hemorrhage appears. Pain is encountered only in the late clinical stages when the carcinoma encroaches upon the sciatic plexus. Pain from carcinoma of the cervix should be looked upon as a symptom of approaching death.

■ Diagnosis

Although cytologic findings and clinical appearance may strongly suggest carcinoma of the cervix, *the diagnosis can only be made by the study of tissue taken from the lesion.* In the presence of what appears to be an obvious carcinoma, tissue may be easily secured using punch biopsy. If the pathologic diagnosis on tissue obtained by punch biopsy is anything but invasive cancer, a conization is required. The reason becomes apparent if it is recalled that in situ carcinoma, dysplasia, or chronic cervicitis is usually present at the periphery of an invasive lesion and that the punch may secure this tissue rather than the cancer. To supply the pathologist with sufficient material to assess the lesion and rule invasive cancer in or out, it is then mandatory to take a cone biopsy.

▪ Colposcopy

The colposcope is an instrument especially designed to study the cervix uteri. It provides a strong light and binocular magnification of ten to twenty times. A wide variety of additional information is obtained by studying all cervices in this manner. It is a great

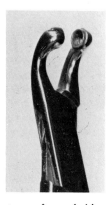

Fig. 43-6. One type of punch biopsy forceps that may provide adequate tissue to establish a diagnosis of invasive carcinoma of the cervix.

aid in localizing the best area to take a biopsy specimen in problem patients. As women successfully treated for cervical cancer advance in years, cytologic studies may reveal abnormalities which suggest the presence of carcinoma somewhere in the vagina, although gross inspection of the vault contributes little or no information. Areas of malignancy or advanced dysplasia are inconsistent in their reaction to iodine staining (Schiller positive). Further, epithelium beyond points of cellular unrest fail to take the stain in a predictable fashion. Richart found toluidine blue a reliable stain for delineating areas of exposed cervix in need of accurate tissue study. Colposcopic examination and toluidine blue stain provide a dependable means for clinical observation of both cervix and vagina.

Colposcopy in combination with exfoliative cytologic studies yields the highest return in screening for cervical cancer.

▪ Treatment

Carcinoma in situ. The need to treat noninvasive carcinoma is indicated by its acknowledged position in the genesis of invasive cervical cancer. The fact that it is generally found in young women raises issues that ordinarily need not be considered in older women with invasive cancer. Treatment is predicated on the recognized behavior of the lesion and is qualified by the patient's age, parity, and somewhat by her wishes.

Carcinoma in situ is in no sense a therapeutic emergency. Hard and fast rules for

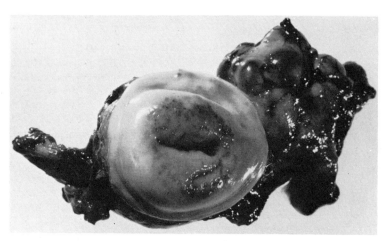

Fig. 43-7. Early carcinoma (invasive) of the posterior lip of the cervix. The shallow ulcer is easily seen. The anterior lip shows chronic cervicitis without atypical features.

intervention cannot be given, but careful, individualized consideration of every factor is required.

Disconcerting problems have a way of inserting themselves into the management of in situ cervical cancer. For example, the physician might well support the wishes of a childless woman under 35 years of age who desires more time to conceive, as well as those in the same age range who have one or two children but desire more. In so doing, the patient must be aware that invasive changes may take place momentarily and be cognizant of the risk involved.

Women assuming this risk must be carefully observed. Cytologic smears are necessary at least every 3 to 6 months. The well-trained cytologist with a few baseline smears may note cellular changes suggesting a shift toward invasive cancer. Alterations such as these call for repeat cone biopsy at once.

After a patient has her family or reaches 30 years of age, carcinoma in situ should be surgically removed. The preferable operation is vaginal or abdominal total hysterectomy, with the removal of about 3 cm. of vaginal cuff. Ovaries are not removed since there is no known relationship between squamous cell cancer and ovarian function.

Cervical carcinoma in situ complicating pregnancy presents intrinsically the same problem as in nonpregnant women. Almost all noninvasive lesions found during pregnancy have been diagnosed by conization tissue studies when indicated by abnormal smears. The patient in whom invasive cancer has been ruled out by conization is observed closely throughout her prenatal course. Repeat cytologic smears are taken every 2 months, and progressive cellular changes constitute an indication for a repeat conization.

Cervical dilatation in labor is a traumatic process and results in cervical injury. Delivery by elective cesarean section to prevent this trauma might seem reasonable if definitive treatment is to be delayed to permit a patient with carcinoma in situ to have more children. However, there is no information to suggest that vaginal delivery influences the course of carcinoma in situ of the cervix. Elective cesarean section and total hysterectomy as a combined procedure is recommended for those who desire no more children.

Follow-up care. Treatment does not end with surgical removal of a cervix harboring carcinoma in situ. Follow-up examination at regular 6-month intervals is an essential part of the therapeutic program. Neither the usual hysterectomy nor a more radical procedure is the complete answer to the treatment of carcinoma in situ. Operation does not protect against the development of carcinoma in the vaginal mucosa. Whether this occurs because noninvasive cancer in the cervix is part of an epithelial field of cellular unrest or because it is one lesion among multiple foci is not known. A woman treated for carcinoma in situ has a greater chance of developing cancer somewhere in her vagina or on her vulva than a patient who has never had a stage 0 cervical growth. These women must have regular cytologic examinations throughout the remainder of their lives.

Invasive carcinoma. Although invasive cervical carcinoma can be treated either by radiation therapy or by radical operation, the former is generally more applicable to the therapeutic problem. However, no other major pelvic lesion receives such offhand, inadequate therapy. Those responsible for treatment frequently put no requirements on therapy beyond the employment of roentgen rays and radium. As a result, random dosage, careless techniques, and inadequate machines in the hands of poorly trained therapeutic radiologists continue to be a major block to effective cancer therapy. Lest we appear unduly critical of the less-than-adequate therapeutic radiologist, we hasten to point out that many gynecologists and general surgeons compound the errors by their inadequate and poorly executed surgical attacks on cervical cancer. Since there are many centers with complete radiologic equipment and an expert staff, there is no reason why women with carcinoma of the cervix should not receive their benefits. It has been well established by comparative survival figures that a team approach to therapy in a treatment center has many advantages over treatment by a single individual. This is particularly true when that individual has only a casual acquaintance with cancer therapy.

A chronologic study and treatment program is initiated once a diagnosis of invasive cancer has been established. After the usual baseline studies the patient is examined by a team of gynecologists and therapeutic radiologists. General agreement is reached

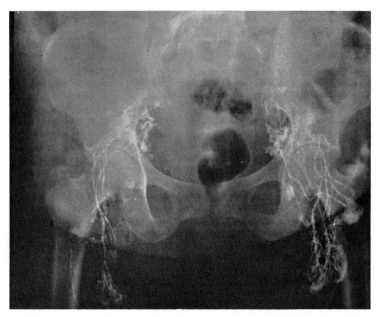

Fig. 43-8. Lymphoangiogram. Note irregular defects in the lymph nodes. The "moth-eaten" appearance suggests embolic carcinoma to the nodes.

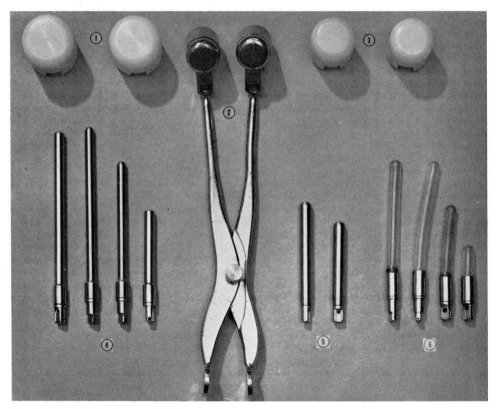

Fig. 43-9. Applicators used in intracavitary radium therapy. **1** and **3,** Large and medium sleeves to fit over **2,** the basic Fletcher applicator. **4** and **5,** Various-sized steel tandems. **6,** Plastic tandems.

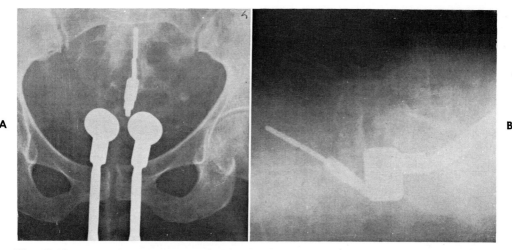

A   B

Fig. 43-10. Intracavitary radium tandem in the uterine canal and the Fletcher vaginal applicator with its two ovoids against the lateral fornices. **A,** Anteroposterior view. **B,** Lateral view.

Table 11. Radiation therapy for carcinoma of the cervix showing dosage limits for combining external radiation and intracavitary radium

Stage	Whole pelvis (rads)	Maximum hours	Milligram hours	Parametrial (rads)
1—less than 1 cm.		72, rest 2 weeks, 72	8,000 to 10,000	
1—greater than 1 cm.		72, rest 2 weeks, 72	8,000 to 10,000	3,000 to 3,500
IIA	2,000 to 3,500	48, rest 2 weeks, 72	8,000 to 9,000	1,000 to 1,500
IIB	3,500 to 4,000	48, rest 2 weeks, 48 to 72	4,500 to 6,500	500 to 1,000 on involved side
IIIA	4,000 to 5,000	48, rest 2 weeks, 24 to 48 or 72	4,000 to 6,500	1,000 to 1,500 on involved side
IIIB	5,000 to 6,000	72	3,000 to 4,000	

regarding the clinical stage of the lesion. The urinary tract is investigated by cystoscopy and pyelography not only to determine whether there is encroachment of the tumor on the bladder or ureters but to establish functional capacity as well. The bowel is evaluated by proctoscopic and sigmoidoscopic examinations. Lymphangiograms may be helpful in determining the extent of nodal involvement.

Radiotherapy, which usually includes both external and internal radiation therapy, is initiated after the evaluation studies. Early stage I (and early stage II in aged patients)

may be treated by radium alone. The radium is given in two applications 2 weeks apart for a total period of 3 to 6 days, using the Fletcher applicators in the so-called Manchester system. The number of milligrams varies from 50 to 80. It should be emphasized that the radium application is the major factor in the success of the treatment.

External radiation therapy is currently administered with supervoltage or telecobalt equipment, giving total pelvic radiation, radiation to the parametria, or a combination of these two, depending on the stage of disease. Ordinarily the external therapy treatments are given daily and last about 4 to 6 weeks. Radium insertions are suitably spaced in this period (Table 11).

Reactions, consisting mainly of diarrhea during the last half of the treatment, are few and easily controlled. Patients undergoing external radiation are customarily treated as outpatients. During this time the radiologist and gynecologist must examine each patient at weekly intervals, carefully noting response to therapy. Aside from clinical examinations, pertinent studies are to be carried out when indicated. Cytologic evaluation of the cervical smears is essential in cancer patients undergoing treatment and in the years subsequent to therapy. The physician is not indulging a scientific whim when he takes cytologic smears at each visit but is recording the cellular changes consistent with recovery and maintenance of good health.

Follow-up care. Women who have been radiated or operated upon for cervical cancer require medical observation for the remainder of their lives. The basic reasons for lifelong follow-up are (1) to study and record the tumor's response to treatment, and (2) to assist the patient in maintaining the best health possible by regular physical examinations and early treatment of other problems that may develop.

In the first 6 months after treatment a small percentage of women will give evidence that their tumor has not responded to therapy. Cytologic smears remain positive or at least suspicious, whereas rectal and vaginal examinations indicate tumor growth. Paracervical areas, uterosacral ligaments, and the base of the broad ligaments take on more of a ligneous feel. These facts will become apparent if the patient is studied every month by a gynecologic-radiologic team. Before the disease progresses beyond a treatable stage, radical operation (discussed later) must be offered the patient.

The majority of women treated for cervical cancer will, at the end of the first 6 months, show satisfactory response. Their cytologic smears will be normal and the cervix small, somewhat more mobile, and flush with the vaginal fornices. The supporting structures and paracervical and paravaginal areas will be smooth and more or less fibrotic. The time between follow-up appointments is then gradually lengthened, so that about 2 years from the completion of

treatment, examinations are on a semiannual basis. Although the initial response to therapy is satisfactory, the follow-up examiners must remain vigilant. Recurrence or regrowth may appear at any time.

The semiannual follow-up examination of a treated cancer patient should include an interval historic note and a reasonably complete physical examination. Taking a smear for cytologic evaluation is essential.

Five percent of women being followed after treatment for one malignant growth develop another primary cancer. It obviously follows that the entire body must not be forgotten in our zealous concern for the patient treated for cancer. I have observed the development of as many as five primary malignant lesions in a woman who first came under my care with a pelvic cancer.

Fortunately, every year more women are successfully treated for carcinoma of the cervix. As a consequence there is an increasing number of women in our follow-up clinics who have been observed over a longer period of time. A number of these, 10 to 15 years postradiation, develop worrisome cytologic changes, particularly in the upper vagina. These cellular alterations, unless due to a developing carcinoma in situ, are created by the atrophic effects of radiation admixed with secondary infection. In order to circumvent these troublesome features of treatment and age, the patient is advised to take conjugated estrogen (Premarin), 1.25 to 2.5 mg. daily, from the beginning of therapy.

Result of radiation therapy. There is a vast literature tabulating the results of therapy in carcinoma of the cervix. The most accurate figures are those dealing with absolute survival rate and without correction for those who die of conditions other than the cancer for which they were treated. Those living 5 years after treatment make up a valid survivor rate. A stage-by-stage comparison of those living 5 years after treatment gives the most reliable "cure rate."

Projected results that can be obtained are shown in Table 12. The enviable survival rates of patients treated by Fletcher and associates are directly attributable to detailed planning and administration of radiation. For the most part, results such as these are attainable in specially equipped centers.

Treatment by surgery. In about 1900

Wertheim in Vienna described his radical operation for the treatment of carcinoma of the cervix. It consisted of removing the uterus, upper vagina, adnexa, and glands. The operative mortality was between 20% and 25% with a fairly low "cure rate." Bonney in England did over 500 of these with a mortality of 15% and a "cure rate" of 28%. Following the results with radium and x-ray treatment, the radical operation was largely abandoned in the United States and Canada. On the continent of Europe, however, there are still many clinics that employ the old Wertheim technique, whereas others use a radical vaginal extirpation operation described by Schauta.

Since 1940 there has been a slight re-

surgence in the United States of the surgical treatment of carcinoma of the cervix. Meigs became dissastified with his results with radiation and revived the radical operation. Several clinics in this country have undertaken a reevaluation of this treatment on an experimental basis only. In 1951 Meigs reported 100 cases from his original experiment and was able to show a 78% 5-year salvage in stages I and II. Those with positive nodes, however, presented a 26% survival rate.

Brunschwig and Daniel have surgically treated a significant number of patients with cervical cancer. They prefer to remove a "cancerous organ together with adjacent lymph nodes rather than treat the cancer in situ." Table 13, showing their results and those reported by Fletcher and co-workers, compares radiation and surgery. These results, although from current sizable series, are difficult to compare. For example, Fletcher and co-workers considered adenocarcinoma and carcinoma of the cervical stump separately, whereas Brunschwig and Daniel included such patients in their series. Further, large endocervical carcinomas and stage IIB patients not responding to treatment were operated upon by Fletcher's group, but the number receiving this treatment is not given. Both series were to some extent selective.

All factors considered, radiation may be safely and effectively used in a greater number of women than radical surgery. Radical surgery has a definite place in the therapeutic program, however, even in clinics where optimum radiologic therapy prevails. There

Table 12. Survival rates for 2,200 radiotherapy patients with squamous cell carcinoma of the uterus*

5-year survival rate	
Stage	Percent
I	91.5
IIA	83.5
IIB	66.5
IIIA	45.0
IIIB	36.0
IV	14.0
Overall: 62.5	

*Adapted from Fletcher, G. H., and Rutledge, F. N.: Overall results in radiotherapy for carcinoma of the cervix, Clin. Obstet. Gynec. 10:958, 1967.

Table 13. Comparison of end results (5-year survivals) of patients treated by surgery and radiation for carcinoma of cervix

Stage	Surgery* (minimal selection)		Radiation† (minimal selection)	
	No. treated	Percent survival 5 years	No. treated	Percent survival 5 years
I	164	76.2		91.5
II	163	52.0		75.0
III	37	27.0		40.5
IV	40	15.0		14.0
All stages	409	55.0	2,220	62.5

*Based on data from Brunschwig, A., and Daniel, W. W.: The surgical treatment of cancer of the cervix, Amer. J. Obstet. Gynec. 82:60, 1961.
†Based on results from the M.D. Anderson Hospital and Tumor Institute in Houston, Texas.

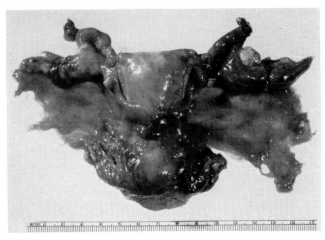

Fig. 43-11. Operative specimen of a radiation-resistant case of cervical carcinoma. Note the width and depth of dissection necessary to remove the parametrium and supporting structures.

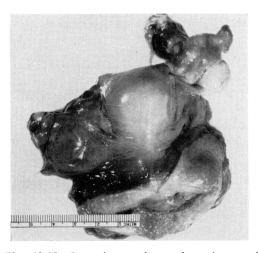

Fig. 43-12. Operative specimen of carcinoma of the cervix. Note the amount of vagina that must be removed.

will be a small number of patients in whom the lesion shows little response to radiation or in whom the tumor appears to have responded, but smears and/or biopsy remain positive. If the tumor does not respond satisfactorily, a surgical procedure should be performed. The type of operation must fit the particular lesion. If decisions are not too late in coming, many unresponsive patients may be successfully operated upon, using nothing more than a radical hysterectomy with complete removal of all supporting structures and pelvic lymph nodes. The fact that a full course of radiation has been ad-

ministered prior to surgery is no deterrent.

Just as there is supervoltage x-ray treatment, there is also super-radical surgery for the treatment of advanced cervical cancer. In such instances an exenteration procedure may be indicated. This consists in removing all the reproductive organs, the pelvic lymph nodes, the rectum, and the bladder. Circulation to the lower extremities and buttocks is maintained. A colostomy is, of course, necessary, and the ureters are placed either in the bowel, or a substitute bladder is made of bowel.

The exenteration operation carries a sizable primary surgical mortality and is obviously crippling. Under these circumstances the patient must be completely informed of her condition, the risk involved, her chances of survival, and the crippling effect. The final choice must be hers, not the surgeon's.

Complications. Problems incident to surgery for carcinoma in situ are no different from those encountered with hysterectomy for other disease. Operative and postoperative complications resulting from radical hysterectomy and lymph node dissection for invasive cervical cancer occur frequently and may be lethal as well as annoying. Hemorrhage, infection, and urinary fistula formation are the most common problems encountered.

Radiation therapy also is attended by complications. For the most part, these affect the skin, large and small bowel, urinary tract,

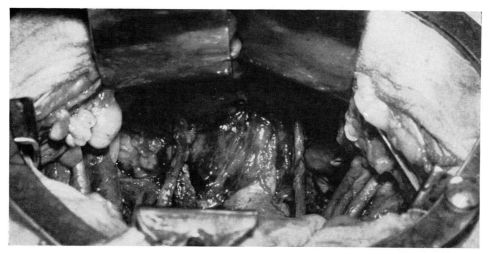

Fig. 43-13. The pelvis after a radical operation (Wertheim) for carcinoma of the cervix. Note the ureters and lateral blood vessels. The depth and width of dissection are easily seen.

and fistula formation. Complications, whether associated with surgery or radiation, occur least often when treatment is carried out in a well-equipped center, staffed by qualified, well-trained individuals.

■ Pregnancy complicating carcinoma of the cervix

The incidence of cervical carcinoma encountered during pregnancy is subject to wide variation, depending on the socioeconomic status of patients involved. The generally accepted incidence of 0.017% makes cervical cancer a rare complication of pregnancy. However, as a result of cytologically screening a large obstetric clinic population at Temple University Medical Center, *15.3% of the cervical carcinomas diagnosed during 1961* complicated pregnancy.

As previously stated, proved in situ carcinoma requires no definitive treatment during pregnancy. On the other hand, invasive cervical cancer must be treated following the principles previously outlined. With few exceptions the pregnancy is disregarded. Fetal death during radiation treatment, followed by spontaneous abortion or premature labor, is to be expected. An attempt to salvage the fetus by hysterotomy would be in order if the cervical cancer were diagnosed at or near 28 weeks' gestation. Radiation is started on the third postoperative day, following the plan of therapy most applicable to the stage of the disease.

■ Care of patients with advanced disease

The best that can be hoped for at present is a 63% 5-year salvage when considering all stages of cervical cancer. Obviously, in 37% of all carcinomas of the cervix treatment fails. As this disease advances throughout the pelvis, many nerve tracts are involved with maximal invasion of the sciatic plexus. Pain in the lower back, the sacroiliac region, and along the sciatic nerve distribution is to be anticipated. Sedation and opiates are best for these suffering women. There seems little sense to minimal use of these drugs. It is pointless to be concerned with drug addition at a time when these patients need sympathetic, kindly care and relief from pain.

■ Carcinoma of the cervix— a preventable disease

It is apparent that a great challenge is contained in the words, *invasive cancer of the cervix is preventable.* These are not idle words from the dream world of the theoretic gynecologist. They reflect a practical, workable idea that calls for cooperative patients interested in their own health and physicians who practice medicine as they were taught in medical school, using their normal skills and cytologic-screening techniques.

Long ago, Macfarlane and co-workers took the first long step in this direction by demonstrating the practical value of periodic examinations. If to that established basic point of good medical practice is added modern cytology and understanding of the genesis of invasive cervical carcinoma, the preventable factors are obvious. Areas of dysplasia would be generally destroyed before they progressed to anything more serious. At most, women on this program would not get beyond the carcinoma in situ stage before appropriate treatment was instituted.

References

Beecham, C. T., and Andros, G. J.: Cervical conization in pregnancy, Obstet. Gynec. 16:521, 1960.

Beecham, C. T., and Beiler, D.: Preferable treatment for cervical carcinoma, Postgrad. Med. 39:412, 1966.

Bonney, V.: Treatment of carcinoma of cervix by Wertheim's operation, Amer. J. Obstet. Gynec. 30:815, 1935.

Brunschwig, A., and Daniel, W. W.: The surgical treatment of cancer of the cervix, Amer. J. Obstet. Gynec. 82:60, 1961.

Butcher, H. R., Sugg, W. I., McAfee, C. A., and Bricker, E. M.: Ileal conduit method of ureteral urinary diversion, Ann. Surg. 156:682, 1962.

Fletcher, G. H., and Rutledge, F. N.: Over-all results in radiotherapy for carcinoma of the cervix, Clin. Obstet. Gynec. 10:958, 1967.

Friedell, G. H., and Parsons, L.: The spread of cancer of the uterine cervix as seen in giant histological section, Cancer 14:42, 1961.

Gray, L. A., Barnes, M. L., and Lee, J. J.: Carcinoma in situ and dysplasia of the cervix, Amer. J. Surg. 151:951, 1960.

Hinselmann, H., and Schmitt, A.: Colposcopy and colpophotography, Wuppertal, 1954, Girardel.

Jones, E. G., MacDonald, I., and Breslow, L.: A study of epidemiologic factors in carcinoma of the uterine cervix, Amer. J. Obstet. Gynec. 76:1, 1958.

Jones, H. W., Katayama, K. P., Stafl, A., and Davis, H. J.: Chromosomes of cervical atypia, carcinoma in situ and epidermoid carcinoma of the cervix, Obstet. Gynec. 30:790, 1967.

Macfarlane, C., Fetterman, F. C., and Sturgis, M. C.: Experiment on cancer control; preliminary report on periodic pelvic examinations of 1,000 well women, Amer. J. Obstet. Gynec. 39:983, 1940.

Marsh, M., and Fitzgerald, P. J.: Carcinoma in situ of the human uterine cervix in pregnancy, Cancer 9:1195, 1956.

McKay, D. G., Terjanian, B., Poschyachinda, D., Younge, P. A., and Hertig, A. T.: Clinical and pathologic significance of anaplasia of the cervix uteri, Obstet. Gynec. 13:2, 1959.

Meigs, J. V.: Wertheim operation for carcinoma of cervix, Amer. J. Obstet. Gynec. 49:542, 1945.

Niebergs, H. E., Stergus, I., Stephenson, E. M., and Harbin, B. L.: Mass screening of a total female population of a county for cervical carcinoma, J.A.M.A. 164:1546, 1957.

Papanicolaou, G. N., and Traut, N. F.: Diagnosis of uterine cancer by vaginal smears, New York, 1943, The Commonwealth Fund.

Peale, A. R.: Pathologic aspects of carcinoma in situ of the cervix, Obstet. Gynec. 13:657, 1959.

Pereyra, A. J.: The relationship of sexual activity to cervical cancer, Obstet. Gynec. 17:154, 1961.

Perez-Mesa, C., and Spjut, H. J.: Persistent postirradiation carcinoma of cervix uteri, Arch. Path. 75:462, 1963.

Richart, R. M.: A clinical staining test for the in vivo delineation of dysplasia and carcinoma in situ, Amer. J. Obstet. Gynec. 86:703, 1963.

Richart, R. M.: A radioautographic analysis of cellular proliferation in dysplasia and carcinoma in situ of the uterine cervix, Amer. J. Obstet. Gynec. 86:925, 1963.

Rubin, I. C.: The pathological diagnosis of incipient carcinoma of the uterus, Amer. J. Obstet. Dis. Wom. Child. 62:668, 1910.

Song, J., and Turner, J.: Lymphatic spread of carcinoma in situ of uterine cervix, Arch. Path. 75:1, 1963.

TeLinde, R. W.: Cancer-like lesions of the uterine cervix, J.A.M.A. 101:1211, 1933.

TeLinde, R. W., and Galvin, G.: The minimal histological changes in biopsies to justify a diagnosis of cervical cancer, Amer. J. Obstet. Gynec. 48:774, 1944.

Wallace, S., Jackson, L., Schaffer, B., Gould, J., Greening, R. R., Weiss, A., and Kramer, S.: Lymphangiograms; their diagnostic and therapeutic potential, Radiology 76:179, 1961.

Way, S., Hennigan, M., and Wright, V. C.: Some experiences with pre-invasive and micro-invasive carcinoma of the cervix, J. Obstet. Gynaec. Brit. Comm. 75:593, 1968.

Wilbanks, G. D., Richart, R. M., and Terner, J. Y.: DNA content of cervical epithelial neoplasia studied by two-wavelength Feulgen cytophotometry, Amer. J. Obstet. Gynec. 98:792, 1967.

Vaginitis and leukorrhea

Leukorrhea, a term applied to any non-bloody discharge from the vagina, may consist of physiologic secretions, or it may be produced in response to irritation or infection of the genital organs. A certain amount of vaginal discharge, made up of secretion of the cervical glands, endometrial debris, effusions from the vaginal mucosa, and exfoliated vaginal epithelium, is always present, but it is not obvious to most women. Normal secretions are nonirritating and usually are not profuse, although it is surprising how many women are completely unaware of the presence of a copious discharge.

The adult vagina is lined by stratified squamous epithelium, the activity, thickness, and glycogen content of which are controlled primarily by variations in the level of estrogenic hormone. The pH of the vaginal secretions in the adult is between 3.5 and 4.5, the acidity being produced by the conversion of cellular glycogen to lactic acid by Döderlein's

bacilli, which are normal vaginal inhabitants. Before the menarche and after the menopause, when estrogen production is low, the epithelium is inactive and only a few cell layers thick; the cells contain no glycogen, the Döderlein bacilli are absent, and the pH is between 6 and 7. The inactive unstimulated mucosa is especially susceptible to infection, whereas the estrogen-stimulated vagina during the years of menstruation is rarely invaded by pathogenic bacteria.

The volume of secretions in the normal vagina varies throughout the menstrual cycle. In the immediate postmenstrual phase, when the estrogen level is low, the mucosa is thin and relatively inactive and there is little secretion from the cervical glands. As estrogen production increases, the vaginal cells proliferate and exfoliate more rapidly and the cervical glands secrete more and more mucus. At ovulation, when estrogen production is maximum, cervical mucus is profuse and watery, and vaginal desquamation reaches a peak. Some women are aware of discharge only at this time. The secretions then diminish until just before the onset of menstruation.

Secretions of the genital organs are also influenced by psychic stimuli. Many women are aware of increased vaginal discharge during periods of emotional stress, and leukorrhea is a frequent complaint in women with pelvic congestion syndrome. The most powerful psychic stimulant to genital tract secretion is sexual excitement. Until recently vaginal lubrication before and during coitus was believed to come from an outpouring of secretions from cervical and Bartholin glands, but Masters observed the formation of a smooth, shiny, lubricating covering for the vagina during sexual stimulation that started as a transudation of droplets of fluid from the vaginal wall during the excitement phase and rapidly coalesced into a uniform coating.

Abnormal discharge is most often caused by infection of the vagina or the cervix, but it can be the result of chronic irritation, hyperemia, or endocrine disorders that are accompanied by excessive estrogen production.

■ Trichomoniasis

Vaginitis caused by *Trichomonas vaginalis* is a common cause of leukorrhea in adults, but it is seldom encountered during

	Newborn	Month-old child	Puberty	Sexually mature	Post-menopause
Estrogenic hormone	+	−	Appears	+	−
Epithelium ↓ ↓	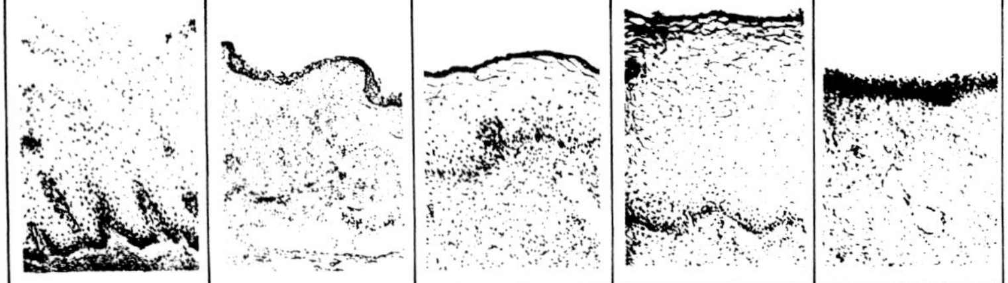				
Glycogen ↓	+	−	− to +	+	−
Acidity ↓	Acid pH 4-5	Alkaline pH 7	Alkaline ↓ acid	Acid pH 4-5	Neutral or alkaline pH 6-7
Flora ↓	Sterile Döderlein's bacilli (secretion abundant)	Sparse, coccal, and varied flora (secretion scant)	Sparse, coccal, ↓ rich bacillary	Döderlein's bacilli (secretion abundant)	Varied flora (secretion scant)

Fig. 44-1. Changes in the vagina and its flora and secretions at various ages. (From Davis, M. E., and Pearl, S. A.: Amer. J. Obstet. Gynec. **35**:77, 1938.)

the prepubertal period. It has been suggested that the symptoms attributed to trichomoniasis actually are caused by bacterial invaders rather than the parasite itself; however, a typical vaginitis can be produced by introducing pure cultures of the organisms into normal vaginas. The presence of trichomonads does not always indicate an active infection because they can sometimes be demonstrated in the vaginal secretions of women who have no symptoms.

The methods by which the infection is acquired are not obvious, but since trichomoniasis can be produced by introducing organisms into normal women, it must be assumed that it is in some degree contagious. Although it is possible that the infection can be acquired from contaminated toilet seats and towels, it seems much more likely that the organism is implanted in the vagina during sexual intercourse. Trichomonads have been found in the male urethra and prostate, and the highest incidence of positive cultures occurs in women who have had frequent exposure to numerous sexual partners. Buxton, Weinman, and Johnson could not culture the organism from any of 157 female college students. Positive cultures were ob-

tained in 6.9% of 575 women attending a private gynecologic clinic and in 15% of 715 inmates of a mental institution. Quite in contrast, cultures were positive in 70% of 221 inmates of a women's prison. These women undoubtedly had more sexual contacts than the average housewife.

Psychologic factors are important in certain instances, because persistent and severe symptoms are found in some patients in whom the degree of infestation is slight, and exacerbations of symptoms are often associated with difficulties of adjustment to life situations.

The primary complaint of most women with trichomoniasis is of moderate to profuse discharge, accompanied by intense itching and irritation of the vagina and vestibule. The intial symptoms often begin during or just after a menstrual period, and after the infection is established both the discomfort and the discharge usually increase during the premenstrual phase of each cycle.

The vestibule, vagina, and cervix are intensely inflamed, and punctate red "strawberry spots" can be seen scattered over the vaginal and cervical mucosa. The vagina contains a large amount of discharge that characteristically is thin, greenish yellow, and bubbly in appearance. The diagnosis is confirmed by identifying trichomonads in the secretion. A drop of pus is mixed with a small amount of warm saline solution in a test tube, and 2 or 3 drops of the suspension are placed on a clean glass slide and examined under the microscope at once without staining. Numerous motile trichomonads and pus cells can be seen. Culture is more accurate than the microscopic examination of vaginal secretions in confirming the diagnosis, but it is not readily available.

Treatment methods based upon attempts to eradicate the organisms by local treatment of the vagina are not always satisfactory. Cleansing douches, powders, suppositories, creams, and tablets have all been used, but recurrences or reinfections are common. The unpleasant symptoms of vaginitis can usually be controlled temporarily by almost any form of treatment, but permanent cures have not always been possible.

Metronidazole (Flagyl), a trichomonacidal drug that is effective when taken orally, will kill the organisms in both men and women. The trichomonads can be eradicated with more certainty if both partners are treated because the infection surely will recur unless foci in the male urethra and prostate are eliminated. The dosage schedule is 250 mg. three or four times daily for 10 days for the female and 250 mg. two or three times daily for 10 days for the male. The husband should wear a condom during intercourse until treatment is completed. In about 15% retreatment is necessary.

Transient relief from itching can be obtained with acid douches of vinegar (2 tablespoonfuls in 1 quart of warm water) once or twice daily. Other effective local agents are Floraquin (a diiodohydroxyquinoline), Tricofuron (a nitrofuran derivative), and silver picrate. Local treatment must usually be continued during menstruation because exacerbations usually occur at this time. Treatment must be continued for several months, even though the symptoms disappear and no organisms can be identified in the secretions. Patients should be advised to resume local therapy during each of the first three or four menstrual periods after daily treatment is stopped. The most important of the reasons for failure with these forms of treatment are that patients use the medi-

cations irregularly after the symptoms improve and that they are reinfected.

■ Candidiasis

Candidiasis, which is also called *moniliasis* or *yeast infection,* occurs most frequently during pregnancy and in women with diabetes mellitus. In recent years many women under treatment with antibiotic preparations have developed vaginitis from yeastlike organisms, even though they are not pregnant and do not have diabetes. Candidiasis also may develop in women using combined oral contraceptives. *Candida albicans* is responsible for almost all vaginitis of this type. Thrush in infants may be contracted during delivery if vaginal contents containing the organisms enter the mouth.

The typical symptoms, watery discharge accompanied by intense itching of the vagina and vulva, appear at any time during pregnancy. In many women the infection recurs with each pregnancy and may appear soon after the first period is missed. The external genitals usually are intensely inflamed and irritated, and the vagina is fiery red and contains a considerable amount of thin, watery discharge as well as a thick, white cheesy exudate that may be adherent to the vaginal walls.

The diagnosis is confirmed by culture or by demonstrating mycelia and spores in a dried smear of the secretion stained with Gram's stain. A simple and accurate culture method consists of the inoculation of a commercially prepared slant of Nickerson's medium with a specimen of discharge picked up on a dry sterile cotton applicator. The cap is replaced and the inoculated tube is kept at room temperature. If yeastlike organisms are present, they will appear as isolated brown or black colonies within 48 hours. Bacteria will not grow on Nickerson's medium.

Antibiotics that are effective against fungi have been developed. *Mycostatin vaginal tablets* (100,000 units of mystatin and 0.93 Gm. of lactose) or *Sporostacin (chlordantoin)* vaginal cream inserted into the vagina once or twice daily for 2 weeks will usually relieve the symptoms promptly. They often recur in pregnant women, and usually treatment must be continued until they deliver. Candidiasis associated with the use of oral contraceptives is treated the same way, but

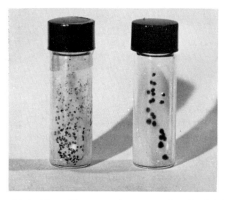

Fig. 44-2. Yeastlike organisms growing in Nickerson's medium.

in addition a change to another type of pill may be helpful. Occasionally the infection is so persistent that it is necessary to discontinue this form of contraception. Mycostatin may also be given orally to eradicate yeastlike organisms from the intestine.

Propionic or *ricinoleic acid jellies, 1% aqueous gentian solution* or *gentian violet cream,* and *povidone-iodine (Betadine) vaginal gel* and *douches* can also be used with good results.

■ Atrophic vaginitis

The pale, thin, smooth atrophic mucosa that lines the vagina in postmenopausal women is easily infected; even minor injuries may permit the entry of bacteria.

The patient usually complains of irritating vaginal discharge, pruritus, and often of swelling and pain. The vagina is red and inflamed and may be covered with "strawberry spots" similar to those observed with trichomoniasis. The discharge is purulent and often profuse; in some women it is blood tinged. *If the patient has a bloody discharge, cancer must be suspected even though the physician can see a vaginal source for the bleeding.* Even after the possibility of cancer has been eliminated by cytologic examination, curettage, and cervical biopsy, the physician should not diagnose atrophic vaginitis with certainty until he also has eliminated fungous infections and trichomoniasis as causes.

Estrogenic therapy will convert the atrophic mucosa to a thick, stratified squamous layer that is resistant to infection. Ordinarily no other medication is necessary.

Local treatment with stilbestrol suppositories, 0.5 mg. in the vagina nightly for 3 weeks, or stilbestrol tablets, 0.5 to 1 mg. orally daily for 3 weeks, will usually be effective. Other estrogenic preparations in comparable doses are equally satisfactory. In most patients the infection and the symptoms will recur if the medication is stopped after the initial period of treatment. There is no reason why estrogenic therapy cannot be continued indefinitely to prevent recurrent atrophy of the vagina and the accompanying infection. If atrophic vaginitis is not treated, the consequent adhesions and shrinkage of the vagina may prevent its use sexually.

■ Chemical and allergic vaginitis

The vaginal mucosa may become irritated, inflamed, and even secondarily infected in response to the introduction of certain chemicals such as gentian violet, potassium permanganate, and creosote solutions. Vaginitis for which there is no obvious cause may be an allergic reaction to locally applied or systemic medications. The symptoms, type of discharge, and the end result are all determined by the extent of the tissue injury. With mild irritation the symptoms clear rapidly and the tissues return to normal as soon as the irritant is removed. On the other hand, potassium permanganate or creosote can produce extensive local damage and even death. Chemical vaginitis should be suspected when the introduction of a substance into the vagina produces an irritating reaction that gradually subsides. Occasionally, for instance when a *Candida* infection is being treated with gentian violet, the discomfort increases rather than improves. The symptoms of the infection are so like those produced by the medication that the irritant effect of the latter may not be recognized for some time.

Treatment consists of recognizing the cause and discontinuing the use of the irritating preparation. Warm, plain water or saline solution douches may aid in relieving irritation. An antihistaminic preparation, either taken orally or applied locally as ointment, may be helpful if the reaction is primarily an allergic one.

■ Other causes of leukorrhea

Cervicitis, one of the most common causes of leukorrhea in adults, is discussed in Chapter 42. Among the less common causes are foreign bodies (tampons, pessaries, etc.), carcinoma of the cervix, endometrium, or tube, and certain rare infections of the genital organs.

References

Acter, R. L., Jones, C. P., and Carter, B.: Treatment of mycotic vaginitis with propionate vaginal jelly, Amer. J. Obstet. Gynec. **53:**241, 1947.

Buxton, C. L., Weinman, D., and Johnson, C.: Epidemiology of trichomonas vaginalis vaginitis, Obstet. Gynec. **12:**699, 1958.

Masters, W. H.: The sexual response cycle of the human vagina; vaginal lubrication, Ann. N. Y. Acad. Sci. **83:**301, 1959.

Trussel, R. E.: Trichomonas vaginalis and trichomoniasis, Springfield, Ill., 1947, Charles C Thomas, Publisher.

Wilson, D. G.: Vaginal candidiasis during pregnancy, Western J. Surg. **64:**180, 1956.

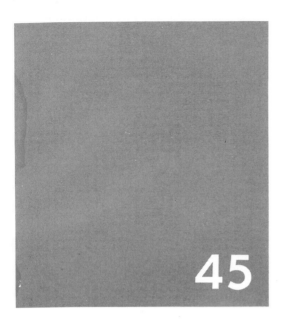

45

Diseases of the vulva

Allergy, dermatologic diseases, inflammatory conditions, and neoplasia give rise to vulvar disorders that extend from petty annoyances to those capable of destroying life.

■ Lesions of the vulvar glands

Bartholinitis. Infection of the vulvovaginal glands is a common entity. The duct of each gland opens on the inner aspect of the labium minus just in front of the hymen at 7 and 5 o'clock. The infection may be in the ducts and/or gland on one or both sides. Although a wide variety of pathogenic organisms have been isolated as etiologic agents, *Escherichia coli* and the gonococcus are common. Once infected, the gland becomes red, swollen, and acutely painful. Fluctuation soon follows, and if prompt drainage is not instituted, spontaneous rupture occurs. A broad-spectrum antibiotic is a helpful adjunct to treatment.

Chronic bartholinitis also occurs. The patient may have experienced one or more attacks of acute infection that subsided spontaneously or after drainage. Eventually the infection subsides and the only residual is a firm, possibly tender, enlargement of the gland. Occasionally, acute exacerbations occur at frequent intervals. The patient may be unaware of the presence of the enlarged gland except during acute attacks. Recurring acute infections are eliminated by keeping the gland open—marsupialization operation.

Bartholin cyst. This lesion is more properly called a Bartholin duct cyst because the latter structure, rather than the gland itself, is usually involved. The main duct, or one of its accessories, is occluded and gradually enlarges as the secretion, which cannot be discharged, accumulates. A cyst usually follows one or more attacks of infection, but some develop without previous disease.

Bartholin duct cysts vary in size and may reach a diameter of 6 or 7 cm. They often produce no symptoms unless they become infected, in which event an abscess develops. Asymptomatic cysts need no treatment, but those that are troublesome, either because of size or repeated infections, should be treated by marsupialization. Epithelium lining the cyst is sutured to the skin after the duct orifice has been incised. As a rule the artificial opening remains unobstructed, natural secretions are restored, and the cyst does not recur.

Solid tumors of Bartholin's gland. Carcinoma is uncommon but should be suspected whenever a firm, irregular mass is detected in the region of a Bartholin gland. These usually are adenocarcinomas, but squamous and transitional cell cancers also develop. Sarcoma, fibrosarcoma, and fibroadenoma occur occasionally. The preferable treatment for malignant lesions is radical excision. Recurrences are common.

Sebaceous cysts. Most body skin will develop sebaceous cysts, and the vulva is no exception. Occluded ducts permit the accumulation of sebaceous material, which may create an annoying enlargement or act as a nidus of recurrent infection; these are treated by excision.

Apocrine gland tumors—hidradenoma. Hidradenoma is a rare neoplasm of the vulva, occurring most often in white women and appearing as a raised, red, sessile mass about 3 to 4 cm. in diameter with an abrasion

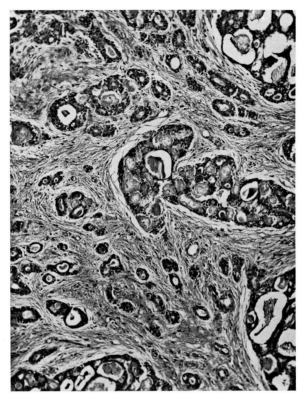

Fig. 45-1. Photomicrograph of an adenocarcinoma of Bartholin's gland. The pattern resembles multiple adenomas. (×142.)

on its summit. Wide local excision is usually adequate for this benign growth.

■ Skin changes

Pigmentation changes. Vulvar epithelial cells contain more melanin than do cells in other parts of the body. As a consequence the vulva darkens during pregnancy when production of melanocyte-stimulating hormone (MSH) is increased by the stimulus of the high concentration of estrogen.

Dermatitis. Dermatologic lesions that develop in skin of other parts of the body can also occur on the vulva. The most common of these are folliculitis, furunculosis, intertrigo, herpes, fungous infections, and seborrheic dermatitis. They are diagnosed and treated as they are when they occur elsewhere.

■ Vulvitis

Vulvovaginitis. A number of lesions affecting the vulva have one symptom in common: pruritus or vulvar itching. The most common

of these diseases is actually a vulvovaginitis caused by either or both of *Candida albicans* and *Trichomonas vaginalis*. The vulva appears swollen and red, and at times there may be superficial ulceration. Treatment is discussed in Chapter 44.

Allergic vulvitis. Pruritus unaccompanied by vaginal infection or vulvar skin changes suggests an allergy as the underlying cause. The reaction often represents a response to undergarments made of synthetic fibers or to the detergents used for washing them. Allergic vulvitis may also be caused by medications, either those applied locally or those administered systemically.

A spray or an ointment containing cortisone usually affords prompt relief, but it will be temporary unless the cause is eliminated. Women suspected of having allergic vulvitis should wear cotton panties, or preferably none at all, until a cause is found.

Diabetic vulvitis. Women with undetected diabetes complain of itching and burning long before there are demonstrable vulvar

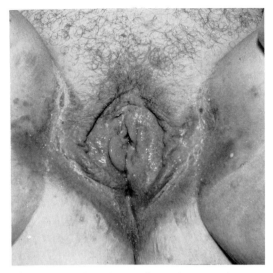

Fig. 45-2. Diabetic vulvitis with superimposed vaginal moniliasis.

skin changes. Vulvar skin, with the chronic assault of glycosuria and underlying metabolic disturbance, takes on a bluish red discoloration. The accompanying pruritus and excoriation (from scratching) that follow are understandable. Uncontrolled and untreated women, at or beyond menopause, usually have severe vulvar atrophy due to lack of estrogen in addition to their diabetes. Careful metabolic supervision with estrogen replacement improves this irksome problem.

Chronic vulvitis. Chronic vulvar infections occur at all ages but are particularly common in climacteric and postmenopausal women with atrophic tissues, and in women whose life situations create sexual frustrations, such as widows and divorcees.

The outstanding symptom is pruritus vulvae, which may be intractable. The itching is usually more troublesome at night after the patient has gone to bed than during the daytime when her thoughts are diverted from her genital organs. The vulva may appear normal, but more often it is inflamed and edematous. If the pruritus has been so intense that the patient scratches herself until she injures the skin, the vulva will be excoriated and secondarily infected.

Many cases of chronic vulvitis are secondary to long-standing *Trichomonas* or *Candida* vulvovaginitis, to cervicitis with profuse irritating discharge, or to atrophic vaginitis, but in others there is no obvious vaginitis or cervicitis. When the vagina and cervix are normal, the chronic condition may develop as a result of local infection from repeated fecal contamination, particularly if the tissues are atrophic, from secondarily infected allergic vulvitis, or from infection of excoriated areas in women with psychogenic pruritus.

Treatment consists of symptomatic control with cool starch sitz baths (4 handfuls of starch in about 4 inches of water in the tub), antibiotics, zinc oxide ointment, or cortisone preparations until the basic cause can be detected and eliminated. When this is possible, the symptoms can usually be relieved permanently. Those cases with a psychogenic background are more difficult to treat; in many instances local infection can be eliminated and the excoriated areas healed, but intractable itching persists. Some of these women will respond to superficial psychotherapeutic assistance from an understanding physician. Intractable psychogenic pruritus vulvae, however, usually indicates a serious psychsexual problem, which can best be managed by a psychiatrist.

Subcutaneous injection of local anesthetics or alcohol and various operative procedures have been recommended. These measures are seldom necessary for the patient whose chronic vulvitis has a pathogenic cause and are ineffective in those whose condition has a psychogenic origin.

■ Infections of the vulva

Tuberculosis. Tuberculous lesions of the vulva are caused by an abrasion having become infected through contact with a tuberculous discharge from the uterus or vagina, through genitourinary tuberculosis in the husband, or through contact with contaminated fingers or clothes, or it is transmitted by way of the blood or lymph.

Vulvar tuberculosis starts as a small nodule near the meatus, clitoris, or posterior commissure. The nodule breaks down into an ulcer with a hard margin, an irregular base, and an area of infiltration about it. The ulcer tends to become chronic, extending deeper and deeper until finally fistulas are formed. Rectovaginal, perineovaginal, vesicovaginal, and even peritoneal fistulas are thus created by this perforating ulcer. If tuberculous lesions are diagnosed on the vulva, the upper genital tract must be carefully investigated, since most tuberculous infections spread from above downward.

Treatment is highly effective and similar to that used in other forms of tuberculosis. The administration of cycloserine (Seromycin) 250 mg. twice daily, isoniazid 100 mg. three times daily, and sodium aminosalicylic acid 5 Gm. three times daily supplemented by pyridoxine 50 or 100 mg. daily is an effectual program. Should drug intolerance or resistance develop, the following can be substituted for any of the preceding agents: streptomycin 1 Gm. intramuscularly twice a week, kanamycin 1 Gm. intramuscularly twice a week, or ethionamide (Trecator) 250 mg. three times daily. Adverse drug reactions and possible toxic effects from these agents must be understood, and due precautions are in order (Chapter 40).

Chancroid. Chancroid is a genitoinfectious disease characterized clinically by necrotizing ulcerations at the site of inoculation. The genital lesions are frequently accompanied by an inflammatory swelling and suppuration of the regional lymph nodes. Chancroid is often referred to as *ulcus molle,* or *soft chancre,* and by the patient as soft sore. The infectious agent, *Haemophilus ducreyi,* is a fine, short, gram-negative bacillus with rounded ends.

The incubation period is thought to be 3 to 5 days. The mode of infection is predominantly venereal except for accidentally acquired chancroid on the fingers of doctors, nurses, and orderlies. Prostitutes are the main source of this infection, which occurs most often in the southeastern section of the United States, Morocco, Italy, and the Mediterranean area.

Chancroid begins as a vesicopustule, which quickly breaks down to an irregular, dirty ulcer. The ulcer is moist, with ragged, undermined edges and is covered by a gray exudate. Removal of the exudative covering causes slight bleeding. The ulcer is surrounded by a reddish halo. Pain and tenderness are quite severe. Autoinoculation allows for the rapid development of multiple lesions. The usual primary site of chancroid is anywhere on the external genitals, but the thigh and abdomen may become involved by autoinoculation.

Inguinal adenitis (bubo) appears about 2 weeks after the primary infection. These enlarged glands are often matted together to form a painful, acute inflammatory process.

Suppuration and spontaneous rupture may occur, and the ulcerated gland area looks much like the primary ulcer except that it is larger.

The diagnosis of chancroid is made by using Gram's stain on the exudate obtained from the edges of the ulcer. Although culture may yield much mixed infection, *Haemophilus ducreyi* is reportedly grown in a high percentage of cases.

Chancroid responds readily to oral oxytetracycline, 250 mg. four times daily supplemented by daily intramuscular injections of 250 mg. The length of treatment depends on the course of the disease but usually lasts no more than 6 days.

Granuloma inguinale. Granuloma inguinale is a granulomatous venereal disease, usually occupying the inguinal region. The disease is contagious, progressive, and autoinoculable, with a tendency toward chronicity. Deibert and Greenblatt regard granuloma inguinale as a precancerous process.

The incubation period is given as anywhere from 8 days to 12 weeks, indicating one of the areas of uncertainty surrounding this disease. Granuloma inguinale is found predominantly in blacks. The disease is indigenous to the United States.

The onset of granuloma inguinale is insidious; it appears without symptoms or constitutional upset. The first sign of the disease is a nodule, papule, or vesicle, which in turn becomes excoriated, leaving an ulcer with a red, granular base and a sharply defined margin. The primary lesions are painless and usually located on the vulva or in the vagina. If traumatized, the ulcer bleeds readily. The inguinal component of granuloma inguinale is secondary to the genital sore.

Granuloma inguinale spreads slowly by continuity and contiguity. As the lesion advances, the granulation tissue rolls over the bordering epithelial surface. Although spontaneous healing has been noted, the ulcerative process usually remains stationary for years.

Granuloma inguinale is diagnosed when Donovan bodies are demonstrated on spread or biopsy. Although treatment with Chloromycetin, streptomycin, and Aureomycin has been highly effective, oxytetracycline in a dosage of 1 Gm. daily for 6 days has been almost uniformly successful in eradicating the disease.

Lymphopathia venereum. Lymphopathia, another venereal disease, is uncommon in the North but endemic in southern states. This disease, caused by a filtrable virus, is characterized by a small initial lesion somewhere on the genitals. Regional lymphadenitis follows, and eventually rectal stricture and vulvar elephantiasis with or without ulceration may develop.

The primary lesion appears from 5 to 21 days after infective coitus. The inguinal adenitis follows quickly. The initial lesion is usually found on the posterior vaginal wall near the fourchet, although it can occur on the external genitals. It is a small erosion, a papule, or a herpetiform vesicle or ulcer. A lymphopathia venereum ulcer has clean-cut edges with a red, indurated zone surrounding it. The initial lesion is so painless that few patients are aware of the primary focus.

Hyperplasia and hypertrophy of the vulvar connective tissue, with local lymph stasis and dilatation of the lymph channels cause elephantoid growths and ulceration of the vulva and perianal region. Before antibiotic therapy, vaginal and/or rectal strictures with fistula formations were common. These complications in pregnancy were so formidable at times as to make cesarean section mandatory.

Lymphopathia venereum is diagnosed by the intradermal injection of 0.1 ml. of *Frei antigen*. An inflammatory nodule 5 to 6 mm. in diameter with a surrounding zone of erythema present at the end of 48 to 72 hours indicates a positive diagnosis.

Treatment for lymphopathia venereum is the same as that recommended for granuloma inguinale. Vulvectomy may be necessary for the chronic hypertrophic vulvar lesions.

■ Degenerative changes of the vulva

New understanding of vulvar dystrophy has revealed a distinct weakness in the time-honored diagnostic entities kraurosis vulvae and leukoplakia. Although the clinician has regarded these as separate entities, significant histologic differences cannot be discerned. Histologic variations are more a matter of degree of degeneration; coexistence of both in the same patient is usual. As a consequence the older terms have given way to *primary vulvar atrophy* and *lichen sclerosus et atrophicus* as interchangeable terms more suitable in describing microscopic variants.

Primary vulvar atrophy (kraurosis). Primary vulvar atrophy is limited to the skin surface of the vaginal vestibule and labia minora. Curiously enough the midline structures (perineum, urethral meatus, and clit-

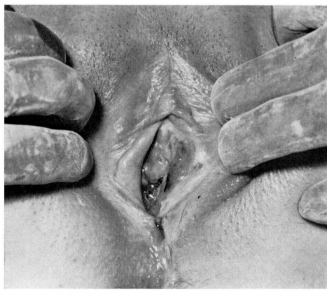

Fig. 45-3. Primary vulvar atrophy. Note extreme degree of atrophy with almost complete effacement of the labia minora and majora.

oris) are not usually involved in the process. Effacement of the labia minora with vulvo-vaginal stenosis results. Extreme changes cause whitening of the surface epithelium. Individual response to postmenopausal estrogen deficit seems to be the underlying cause of primary vulvar atrophy.

Severe pruritus and dyspareunia are the symptoms of consequence. The entire picture of vulvar senescence will improve with administration of oral conjugated estrogen (Premarin), 1.25 mg. daily. Topical corticosteroids such as Aristocort, betamethasone, or Decadron are important adjuncts affording prompt local relief.

Lichen sclerosus et atrophicus (leukoplakia). Since primary vulvar atrophy and lichen sclerosus et atrophicus are variants in epithelial response to degenerative change, they may coexist in the same patient as manifestations of the same condition. The appearance of the whitened vulvar skin surface in lichen sclerosus is hypertrophic rather than atrophic; microscopically, the epithelial and keratin layers are piled up and rete pegs are lengthened.

Although the exact etiology of lichen sclerosus et atrophicus is uncertain, it appears to be another change in the aging process. Alterations in metabolism that accompany estrogen deficiency are the likely cause.

Women with lichen sclerosus et atrophicus complain of itching, pain, and dyspareunia, but these are not always progressive. Periods occur when the condition seems to flare up and then subside into an asymptomatic state.

The greatest concern is over the association of lichen sclerosus and carcinoma. Gynecologic teaching in the past stressed the high incidence of malignant change; however, time has shown that there is a threat of cancer only in those areas demonstrating atypical basal activity. The likelihood of malignant change is no more than 10% over a period of 25 years.

Before any treatment of lichen sclerosus et atrophicus is undertaken, representative biopsies, particularly from fissured or ulcerated areas, should be taken. Collins, adapting Richart's toluidine blue study (on cervical dysplasia) to vulvar dystrophy, found a useful technique for determining the need of and selecting the site to biopsy. He found vulvar lesions stained with 1% toluidine blue and decolorized with 1% acetic acid retained blue stain in areas of inflammation or malignancy. The basis for a positive stain rests

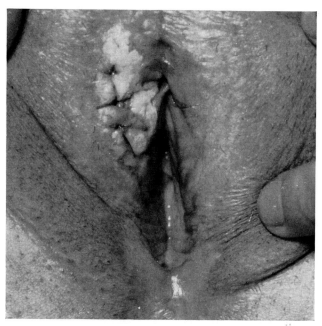

Fig. 45-4. Lichen sclerosus coexisting with primary vulvar atrophy. Early carcinoma was found in the center of the white area.

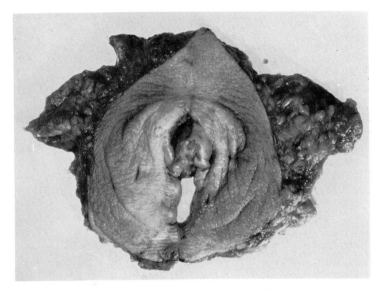

Fig. 45-5. Carcinoma of the vulva involving the clitoris.

with nucleated cells on an ulcerated surface absorbing the dye.

Treatment of vulvar dystrophies should include the elimination of all possible irritants, such as vaginal infections, glycosuria, local allergic factors, and menopausal epithelial atrophy. Corticosteroids and estrogen replacement are most helpful in relieving symptoms, even though they may not reverse the skin change.

Vulvectomy should be performed when the symptoms cannot be controlled by conservative therapy or when there is histologic evidence of dangerously overactive epithelium.

Follow-up examinations every 3 to 6 months are essential in all "white lesions" of the vulva.

■ Tumors

SOLID BENIGN TUMORS OF THE VULVA

Urethral caruncle. The most common solid benign tumor is the urethral caruncle. These small, red, single or multiple, polypoid growths are visible at the external urethral meatus. Caruncles are at times quite sensitive. Treatment is excision and electrocoagulation of the base.

Fibroma of the vulva. Fibromas of the vulva are relatively uncommon but are much the same as fibromas in other parts of the body. They are made up of edematous

fibrous tissue and a small amount of muscle. Sarcomatous degeneration can occur. The treatment is surgical excision.

Other types of rare tumors to be seen on the vulva are lipoma, hemangioma, lymphangioma, myxoma, neuroma, osteoma, chondroma, and myoblastoma.

Papillomas. True papilloma of the vulva is very rare. This is a slow-growing tumor occurring largely in middle-aged women. Microscopically, the growth is the same as papilloma seen elsewhere.

Condylomas. Condylomata acuminata are common vulvar lesions and are often mistakenly called venereal warts. They may follow venereal discharge or vaginal discharge of an irritating nature combined with uncleanliness. On the other hand, warts of the vulva occur in the most fastidious women in whom no discharge or other etiologic factors can be found. The treatment is always aimed at the underlying pathology, and if none is found or the warts persist, podophyllin ointment, 25%, or electrocoagulation will eliminate them rapidly.

CARCINOMA OF THE VULVA

Vulvar cancer makes up about 3.5% of all genital malignancy. Persons of all ages have been reported to have this carcinoma, but the average incidence is about 60 years of age.

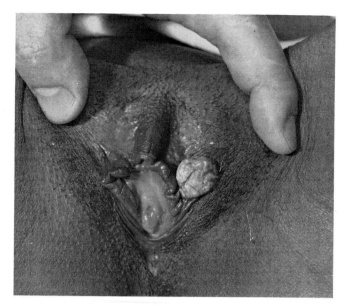

Fig. 45-6. Well-differentiated carcinoma of the vulva.

Cancer of the vulva is generally of the squamous cell type, although adenocarcinoma and melanocarcinoma have been reported. The growth may arise anywhere on the external genitals, including the vulvovaginal junction. Lichen sclerosus et atrophicus, papillomas, syphilis, and lymphogranuloma venereum are considered to be etiologic factors in some instances.

Pruritus is the most frequent early symptom of cancer of the vulva. The patient might be aware of a lump or small ulcer reasonably early in the disease or note a slight bloody discharge. These symptoms, coupled with the fact that every woman touches the vulva several times a day in cleaning herself, should lead to the early diagnosis of vulvar malignancy. Such is not the case. Women with vulvar cancer delay an average of 20 months after knowing that something is wrong before seeking medical attention. Indeed, studies of delay factors in pelvic cancer reveal the greatest patient delay in this accessible area.

The diagnosis is made by biopsy, and the treatment is radical surgical removal. Although many of the patients with carcinoma of the vulva are aged and many have serious medical complications, the necessary surgery is usually well tolerated. The operation consists of radically removing the entire vulvar area, from above the symphysis to the anus

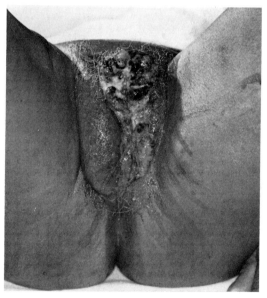

Fig. 45-7. Advanced carcinoma of the vulva, involving the entire vagina, urethra, and rectum. A total exenteration was necessary to remove the growth.

and laterally to the thighs. The superficial glands, fatty tissue, and deep gland-bearing areas of the inguinal, femoral, and retroperitoneal spaces are removed. Radiation of this carcinoma has little effect and ordinarily plays no part in the treatment.

References

Collins, C. G., Hansen, L. H., and Theriot, E.: A cinical stain for use in selecting biopsy sites in patients with vulvar disease, Obstet. Gynec. 28:158, 1966.

Creadick, R. N.: Severe chronic pruritus vulvae, J. Florida Med. Ass. 42:1007, 1956.

Deibert, A. V., and Greenblatt, R. B.: Malignancy and lymphogranuloma venereum, Amer. J. Syph., Gonor. Ven. Dis. 26:330, 1942.

Green, T. H., Ulfelder, H., and Meigs, J. V.: Epidermoid carcinoma of the vulva; an analysis of 238 cases, Amer. J. Obstet. Gynec. 75:834, 1958.

Greenblatt, R. B., Wammock, V. S., Dieust, R. B., and West, R. M.: Chloromycetin in the therapy of granuloma inguinale, Amer. J. Obstet. Gynec. 59:1129, 1950.

Hanson, S. M., and Beecham, C. T.: Myoblastoma of the vulva, Amer. J. Obstet. Gynec. 71:190, 1956.

Jacobson, P.: Vulvovaginal (Bartholin) cyst treatment by marsupialization, Western J. Surg. 58:704, 1950.

Janovski, N. A., and Ames, S.: Lichen sclerosus et atrophicus of the vulva, a poorly understood disease entity, Obstet. Gynec. 22:697, 1963.

Jeffcoate, T. N. A.: Chronic vulval dystrophies, Amer. J. Obstet. Gynec. 95:61, 1966.

Jeffcoate, T. N. A.: Dermatology of the vulva, J. Obstet. Gynaec. Brit. Comm. 69:888, 1962.

Novak, E., and Stevenson, R.: Sweat gland tumors of the vulva, Amer. J. Obstet. Gynec. 50:641, 1945.

Palmer, J. P., Sadugar, M. G., and Reinhard, M. C.: Carcinoma of the vulva, Surg. Gynec. Obstet. 88:435, 1949.

Symmonds, R. E., Pratt, J. H., and Dockerty, M. B.: Melanoma of the vulva, Obstet. Gynec. 15:543, 1960.

Taussig, F. J.: Cancer of the vulva, Amer. J. Obstet. Gynec. 40:764, 1940.

46

Benign uterine enlargement

The benign lesions that most often enlarge the uterus are multiple leiomyomas, symmetric hypertrophy of the muscular walls, and adenomyosis. Of these, leiomyomas are by far the most common.

■ Leiomyomas of the uterus

Benign uterine leiomyomas, also called myomas, fibromyomas, or more commonly fibroids, can be found in the uteri of at least one fifth of all women past 30 years of age. They appear at an earlier age and grow more luxuriantly in black than in white women, and although they are often encountered in nulliparas, many women with fibroids are highly fertile.

PATHOLOGY

The tumors develop from immature smooth-muscle cells of the uterine wall. The smallest ones are made up almost entirely of muscle, but strands of fibrous tissue appear between the bundles of unstriated muscle as the tumor enlarges. The fibrous tissue probably represents a degenerative change in the muscle itself rather than a primary proliferation of fibroblastic elements. In some tumors the fibrous tissue predominates. The muscle bundles develop in a whorl-like fashion, which is quite characteristic of the tumor. They have no true capsule, but the compressed uterine muscle surrounding each neoplasm forms a pseudocapsule.

The tumors may occur singly, but they more often are multiple. They vary in size from those that are only visible under the microscope to huge masses that almost fill the abdominal cavity. They may occupy any portion of the uterine wall, and when sectioned, they are firm and white in color, and the whorled, trabeculated muscular bundles are quite characteristic.

The tumor types are designated according to their position in the uterine wall. *Submucous* tumors lie beneath the endometrium and protrude into the uterine cavity. If there are many fibroids in this area or if they are large, the endometrial cavity may be tremendously enlarged and distorted. *Intramural* or *interstitial* tumors occupy the central portion of the uterine wall, whereas those of the *subserous* variety lie beneath the peritoneal covering and protrude into the abdominal cavity. If the tumors are predominantly intramural or subserous, they may grow to a remarkable size without altering the size and shape of the uterine cavity. *Cervical* fibroids develop from the musculature of the cervical portion of the uterus. Tumors that grow laterally between the leaves of the broad ligament are called *intraligamentous*.

The submucous, subserous, and cervical tumors can all become pedunculated, and occasionally a subserous growth loses its connection to the uterus completely and becomes a *wandering* or *parasitic* fibroid, deriving its blood supply from the omentum or some other extrapelvic source.

Degenerative changes. The blood supply that comes through the pseudocapsule from the vessels in the uterine wall often becomes inadequate as the tumor enlarges, and as a result degenerative changes are common. In *hyaline degeneration,* the type most often observed, the fibrous and muscle tissues are partially or completely replaced by hyaline tissue, which grossly is smooth, relatively soft, and lacks the usual whorl-like appear-

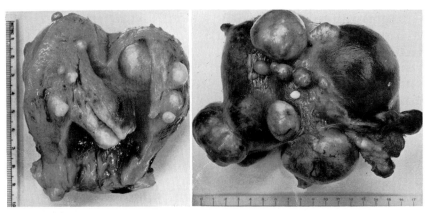

Fig. 46-1   Fig. 46-2

Fig. 46-1. Types of fibroid tumors. Large submucous tumor projects into the cavity of the opened uterus, and a smaller one can be seen near the left cornu. Several intramural tumors are also visible.

Fig. 46-2. Subserous fibroids of varying sizes on the surface of an unopened uterus that also contains large intramural tumors.

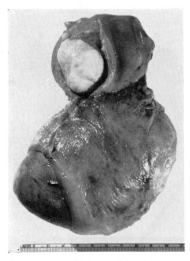

Fig. 46-3. Large cervical fibroid. The small opened uterus containing a white submucous tumor can be seen at the top of the specimen. The large mass is a cervical fibroid that can be seen protruding through the dilated external os at the left.

ance. Under the microscope the hyalinized areas are homogeneously pink stained and may be completely acellular. *Cystic degeneration* or *liquefaction* occurs when the hyaline material breaks down from a further reduction in blood supply. With *calcification* the tumor may be stonelike because of a deposition of calcium; these can often be detected by x-ray examination. *Fatty degeneration* is rare.

Necrosis of a tumor may occur if its blood supply is compromised. This is most often encountered when pedunculated tumors twist on their pedicles, completely occluding the vessels, but it may also happen in rapidly growing leiomyomas of other types. Necrotic tumors, particularly the submucous types, often become secondarily *infected*.

Red or *carneous degeneration* occurs during pregnancy and affects at least one half of all fibroids in gravid women. When sectioned, the tumor bulges out of its bed, and the characteristic dark red color produced by hemorrhage into the tissue is obvious.

Sarcomatous degeneration occurs in less than 0.5% of leiomyomas. The cut surface is pink and soft and has been compared to the appearance of raw pork. Later the tissue may become friable with ragged cavitation in the center.

ETIOLOGY

The etiology is unknown, but the growth of the tumor is in some way related to stimulation by the ovarian hormones. These neoplasms are rarely seen before the ovaries have functioned for several years, and growth usually ceases after the menopause. Some authorities believe that long-term estrogen therapy stimulates the growth of myomas, but this idea is not universally accepted. There seems to be little question, however, that some of the new and highly potent

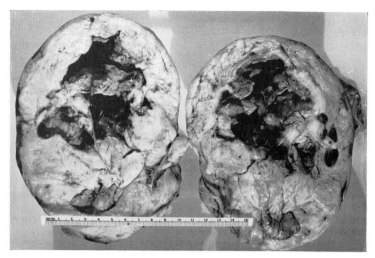

Fig. 46-4. Cystic degeneration in a large pedunculated fibroid.

progestogens do promote rapid enlargement of the tumors when they are administered for long periods of time and in large doses, as in the treatment of endometriosis. It seems likely that the muscle cells that are destined to become tumors have some special growth potential and are activated by steroid hormones.

SIGNS AND SYMPTOMS

The symptoms vary with the size and location of the tumors. Some huge growths cause no discomfort or disturbance of the menstrual pattern, whereas much smaller ones may produce severe pain or exsanguinating hemorrhage.

Bleeding. An alteration in menstrual bleeding is the most frequent single symptom produced by uterine fibroids. As the tumor grows, the duration and amount of bleeding gradually increase, whereas the interval between menses remains the same. Abnormal bleeding is almost always caused by submucous tumors that enlarge and distort the uterine cavity. Subserous tumors, even the largest ones, which do not alter the size and shape of the endometrial cavity, are ordinarily not accompanied by abnormal bleeding. The source of the bleeding is the endometrium, and the mechanism is the same as that which is responsible for menstruation in the normal uterus. The endometrial glands and stroma respond to the changes in ovarian hormone levels as do those in normal women, but the increased amount of blood lost is at least in part due to the increased endometrial

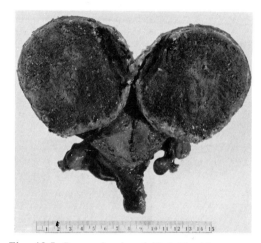

Fig. 46-5. Large, hard, calcified fibroid.

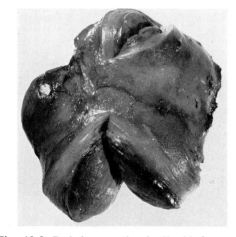

Fig. 46-6. Red degeneration in fibroids in a postpartum uterus. Note the dark color and how the cut surface of the tumor bulges out.

surface in the uterus containing a number of large submucous tumors.

Irregular bleeding may occur if submucous fibroids become infected or ulcerated, but *uncomplicated leiomyomas do not cause intermenstrual or postmenopausal bleeding.*

Pressure and pain. As the tumors grow, they may exert pressure on nearby organs and disturb their function. Frequency of urination and difficulty with bowel movements are common complaints in women with fibroids. Pain may indicate that the tumor itself is degenerated or infected or that it is pressing on another organ or on the pelvic nerve roots. Small tumors may cause more symptoms than large ones if they are located where they can exert pressure on sensitive areas.

Dysmenorrhea. Severe, cramping, labor-like pains may occur as the uterus attempts to expel a pedunculated submucous tumor. Dysmenorrhea, however, is not usually a characterstic symptom of fibroids.

Infertility. Many women with leiomyomas are infertile, but it is not always possible to relate the presence of the tumors to the failure to conceive because others with tumors of equal size or larger are normally fertile. Occasionally the growths distort the fallopian tubes or disturb their function, but more often the lumina are patent. Some women have experienced long periods of infertility before small fibroids can first be detected, making the presence of the tumors an unlikely etiologic factor. It is possible that the same basic disturbance that is responsible for the failure to become pregnant predisposes to the subsequent development of fibroids.

DIAGNOSIS

The diagnosis is made by abdominal and bimanual palpation of the tumors growing in the uterine wall. They are firm, smooth, and nontender unless degenerated or infected, and of varying size. The uterine mass may be fixed or freely movable, depending upon the size and location of the neoplasms.

Differential diagnosis. There are several pelvic lesions that are at least superficially similar to uterine fibroids.

Cancer. Endometrial and cervical carcinoma cause irregular intermenstrual bleeding and develop in fibroid uteri as often as in those that are normal. Benign uterine tumors do not predispose to the development of cancer. Necrotic, bleeding, pedunculated, submucous tumors protruding through a normal but dilated external os may appear much like cervical carcinoma. Malignancy should be excluded by cytologic examination, dilatation and curettage, and cervical biopsy in women with irregular or postmenopausal bleeding before they are treated for fibroids.

Pregnancy. Large, soft leiomyomas, particularly those growing on the fundus of the uterus, may simulate pregnancy, and women with uterine fibroids may conceive. Most errors in diagnosis are made because the history of amenorrhea and the softening of the cervix and the lower part of the uterus are ignored. If there is even a remote possibility of pregnancy, it should be eliminated by laboratory tests, fetal electrocardiography, and x-ray examination for evidence of a fetal skeleton before the patient is operated upon.

Ovarian neoplasms. These tumors usually are separate from the uterus, but it may be difficult to differentiate a pedunculated fibroid from a solid ovarian neoplasm. The symptoms produced by an ovarian neoplasm or a pedunculated leiomyoma twisting upon its pedicle are similar, and degenerated or cystic fibroids may simulate cystic ovarian tumors. Neoplasms of the ovary usually do not alter the menstrual cycle, whereas increased bleeding occurs frequently with uterine fibroids.

TREATMENT

There are several methods for treating women with uterine fibroids, and the one selected will be determined by the age, parity, and physical condition of the patient, the size of the tumors and the symptoms they produce. Cancer must always be suspected if the bleeding is irregular, intermenstrual, or postmenopausal and can be excluded by dilatation and curettage and cervical biopsy. Anemia can be corrected by iron therapy or if it is profound enough, by blood transfusion.

Observation. As a general rule, leiomyomas need not be treated unless they are producing symptoms because they do not predispose to malignancy, seldom undergo malignant degeneration, and do not interfere with the functions of other pelvic organs. Active treatment can be instituted at any time if symptoms develop or if the tumors begin to enlarge rapidly. Women with fibroids should be examined at least every 6 months; in the majority, active treatment never becomes necessary.

Observation is particularly indicated in women near the menopause because after ovarian function ceases the uterine mass will usually become smaller. Fibroid tumors in postmenopausal women rarely need to be removed unless they continue to grow or unless they are first discovered at this time. If a large tumor is found in a woman past the menopause, the physician, by physical examination alone, cannot always be sure it is a benign uterine fibroid rather than a sarcoma or an ovarian neoplasm.

Surgical removal. Large fibroids and those that produce symptoms should usually be removed. *Myomectomy* or the removal of individual tumors from the uterine wall should be considered for young women in whom it is desirable to maintain both menstruation and reproductive function. This operation is of particular value in the management of pedunculated subserous and submucous tumors. Myomectomy occasionally corrects infertility, but it should be reserved for those in whom all other possible factors have been eliminated. The removal of the tumors alone, except the pedunculated submucous variety in an otherwise normal uterus, may not alter excessive bleeding. If bleeding occurs irregularly and if curettage a few days prior to an anticipated period of bleeding is productive of proliferative endometrium or of benign hyperplastic endometrium (dysfunctional bleeding), hysterectomy usually is a preferable procedure because the bleeding is probably caused by an endocrine disorder rather than by the tumors. Small fibroids that are overlooked and left in place sometimes grow, making another operation necessary after several years. This seldom occurs and should not deter the physician from performing myomectomy in selected patients.

Hysterectomy, or removal of the uterus, is the operative procedure most often selected for the treatment of fibroid tumors. It is indicated for large and multiple tumors producing considerable distortion of the uterine cavity, for those that have grown rapidly, for those accompanied by profuse and irregular bleeding, and for those producing pressure symptoms. In young women one or both ovaries should be left in place if they appear normal.

Radiation castration. Radium or deep x-ray therapy terminates ovarian function and precipitates an artificial menopause, thereby inhibiting growth of the tumors. Although castration will control bleeding, it will not relieve symptoms produced by the size or position of the tumors. Its use, therefore, is restricted to women at or near the menopause with small tumors that produce no symptoms except bleeding. If the patient is a good surgical risk, operation is usually preferable to radiation.

SPECIAL PROBLEMS IN TREATMENT

Pedunculated submucous fibroids. Pedunculated submucous fibroids occasionally grow to a diameter of 10 to 12 cm., and they often undergo necrosis and become infected. The patient may experience severe, cramping, laborlike pains during the menses as the uterus attempts to expel the tumor. If the infected tumor protrudes through the cervix, it should usually be removed vaginally after preliminary treatment with an antibiotic preparation and, when necessary, blood transfusion. If there are no other fibroids in the uterus, further treatment may not be necessary, but if hysterectomy is required, it usually should not be performed until the residual uterine infection has been eliminated.

Degeneration and infection. Degenerative changes and subsequent infection usually develop because of interference with the blood supply to the tumor. If the blood flow is obstructed, antibiotic preparations cannot reach the tumor. Consequently removal is necessary before the surrounding intra-abdominal structures become involved in the inflammatory process.

Sarcomatous degeneration. Malignant degeneration in a fibroid tumor seldom occurs, but it should be suspected whenever a rapid increase in size is detected. Prompt removal of rapidly growing tumors is indicated.

■ Hypertrophy of the uterus

Another type of uterine enlargement is that termed *diffuse symmetric hypertrophy;* in it the uterus is smooth, heavy, enlarged, and frequently retrodisplaced. Menstruation is often excessive, and the patient may experience moderate to severe discomfort and

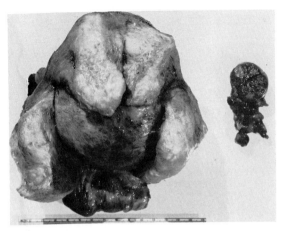

Fig. 46-7. Diffuse symmetric hypertrophy of the uterus. Note the thickness of the walls and the absence of fibroids. The uterus was removed because of persistent excessive bleeding.

pressure, particularly when the pelvic structures are congested before and during menses.

Because this syndrome is usually encountered in multiparous women, the uterine enlargement has been attributed to chronic subinvolution. That this is not always the case is indicated by the fact that the same change occasionally occurs in nulliparous women with chronic retrodisplacements. Taylor has termed this the congestion-fibrosis syndrome and believes that an emotional disturbance plays an important part in the genesis of the symptoms.

Dilatation and curettage usually is indicated to eliminate the possibility of carcinoma and small submucous fibroids, and the procedure may sometimes control the bleeding, at least temporarily. If the patient is given an opportunity to talk, she may bring up emotional factors such as sexual disturbances, fear of pregnancy, family problems, etc., which may contribute to her symptoms. Psychotherapy may improve the symptoms. If the bleeding and discomfort cannot be controlled by relatively simple means, hysterectomy may be warranted.

■ Adenomyosis

Adenomyosis uteri, which is discussed in Chapter 9, may also cause uterine enlargement and abnormal bleeding.

References

Curtis, A. H.: Hypertrophy of the uterus, Amer. J. Obstet. Gynec. **50:**748, 1945.
Faulkner, R. L.: Red degeneration of uterine myomas, Amer. J. Obstet. Gynec. **53:**474, 1947.
Hunter, W. C., Smith, L. L., and Reiner, W. C.: Uterine adenomyosis; incidence, symptoms, and pathology in 1,856 hysterectomies, Amer. J. Obstet. Gynec. **53:**663, 1947.
Kelly, H. A., and Cullen, T. S.: Myomata of the uterus, Philadelphia, 1909, W. B. Saunders Co.
Lewis, P. L., Lee, A. B. H., and Easler, R. E.: Myometrial hypertrophy, Amer. J. Obstet. Gynec. **84:**1032, 1962.
Taylor, H. C., Jr.: Vascular congestion and hyperemia; their effect on structure and function of the female reproductive system, Amer. J. Obstet. Gynec. **57:**2, 1949.

47

Malignant lesions of the corpus uteri

Corpus carcinoma is about one half as common as cervical malignancy. Randall, using data from the Department of Health of the State of New York, reports that there are 26.7 cervical, 14.6 corpus, and 11.3 ovarian malignancies per 100,000 women. He further revealed the death rates to be 14.3 in cervical, 7.4 in corpus, and 10.4 in ovarian malignancies per 100,000 female population.

Although carcinoma of the endometrium may occur at any age, it is most common near the menopause, the average age incidence being 55 years. Because this disease occurs in an older age group it often is complicated by degenerative conditions such as hypertensive cardiovascular disease, obesity, and diabetes. These medical complications along with a host of others add immeasurably to the problem of establishing an adequate treatment program.

■ Etiology

Many attempts have been made to implicate estrogenic hormones in the pathogenesis of carcinoma of the endometrium, but there is still a question as to their actual role. Hertig and Sommers observed changes, particularly *cortical stromal hyperplasia,* in the ovaries of many women with endometrial cancer. They postulated that estrogen, produced by the ovaries in response to abnormal pituitary stimulation, was responsible for the progressive endometrial changes leading to invasive cancer. Roddick and Greene doubt that such a relationship exists; their belief is supported by the fact that no correlation between carcinoma of the endometrium and amount of urinary estrogen can be established. It has been suggested that the incidence of endometrial cancer is higher in women with estrogen-producing ovarian tumors, but most investigators cannot confirm this. Furthermore, there has been no increase in the incidence of endometrial cancer despite the increasing use of estrogens as replacement therapy in climacteric and postmenopausal women.

Although a definite case cannot be made against estrogen as a cause for endometrial cancer, it seems likely that it develops in response to some dysfunction in endocrine metabolism. The lesion often develops in obese women with diabetes and hypertension, and many of these women also have had ovarian dysfunction, as demonstrated by infertility, abnormal bleeding often associated with anovulation, profuse and irregular climacteric bleeding, and late menopause. Peterson, studying 32 women under age 40 with carcinoma of the endometrium, found 8 with diabetes, 5 with hypertension, 26 who were overweight (20 weighing more than 200 pounds), 16 who had never been pregnant, and 26 with grossly irregular or anovulatory bleeding.

Dilman and co-workers have exhaustively surveyed gonadotropins, estrogens (classic and phenolic steroids), free fatty acid levels, and cholesterol levels in premenopausal and postmenopausal women with endometrial carcinoma. Their findings do not differ at all from other reports except for estrogen-like phenolic steroids. Here they found a substantial increase due primarily, they theorize, to hypothalamopituitary activity. Phenolic steroids are little understood and gen-

erally regarded as metabolic products of
classic estrogens—estradiol, estrone, and estriol. The consistency of evidence implicating
metabolism accumulates; the factors in this
complex metabolic process that will eventually prove out continue to be elusive.

■ Pathology

Cancer of the endometrium is like malignant lesions in other anatomic areas in that
it does not start as malignancy per se. Tissue
changes comparable to the shifting dysplasia
observed in basal cells preceding invasive

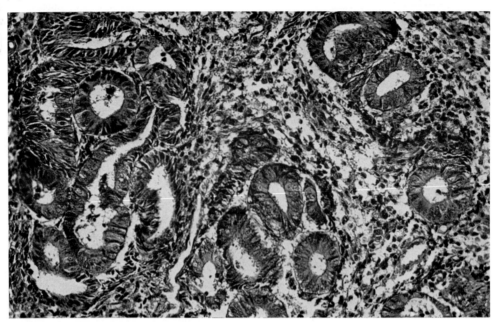

Fig. 47-1. Adenomatoid hyperplasia of the endometruim. Note dilated glands in their characteristic back-to-back position.

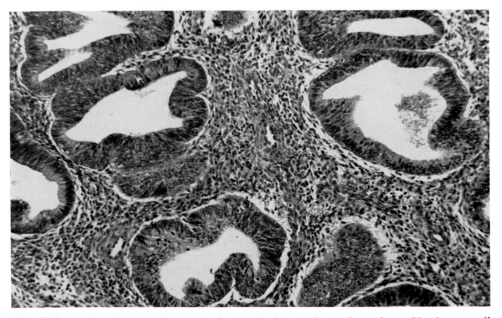

Fig. 47-2. Atypical hyperplasia or carcinoma in situ of the endometrium. Glands are well
formed and show no secretory activity. Glands have large cells, some cellular disorientation,
and disparity in size.

cervical cancer can usually be detected. The earliest change leading to carcinoma of the endometrium is called *adenomatoid hyperplasia*. The gland cells are overactive, and the glands, which lie back to back, may be dilated or irregularly shaped, with papillary projections into the lumina. The individual cells are fairly well oriented to each other, but the nuclei may be hyperchromatic, and mitoses may be present. As the process advances, more cellular evidences of malignancy can be detected. At the stage of *atypical hyperplasia* or *carcinoma in situ* the cells are larger and more disoriented and the nuclei often are eccentrically placed and irregular in size and in staining characteristics. There is no change in the stromal cells. It is not long after these abnormalities appear that the stage of invasive cancer is reached. Atypical hyperplastic endometrium and adenoacanthoma have been found by Katayama and Jones to have a diploid chromosomal count, whereas numerical and structural aberrations are noted in anaplastic carcinoma.

With few exceptions malignancy of the uterine body is an adenocarcinoma. As a rule these cancers do not develop and metastasize as rapidly as does cervical carcinoma. They metastasize by the lymphatics, and these fortunately are not abundant in the upper half of the uterus, but lymph vessels coursing under the tube in the mesosalpinx quite frequently carry the cancer to the ovary and the aortic nodes. Another area to which the tumor often metastasizes is the upper vagina; this likewise is by the lymphatics.

There are two types of invasive cancer, *circumscribed* and *diffuse*. In the more common circumscribed adenocarcinoma (Fig. 47-3) malignancy starts as a small local growth and invades the myometrium faster than it spreads along the endometrium. In diffuse adenocarcinoma of the corpus (Fig. 47-4) the growth starts as a superficial and almost uniform condition and may penetrate the myometrium slowly. It often is almost entirely removed by diagnostic curettage. This type of cancer will lead to an earlier enlargement of the uterine body than will the circumscribed neoplasm.

All degrees of anaplasia are seen in corpus carcinoma. In some there is a complete loss of glandular pattern, whereas in others the degree of malignancy may be so low as to make it difficult for the pathologist to determine whether he is dealing with atypical

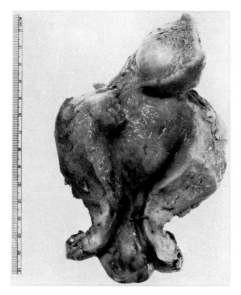

Fig. 47-3

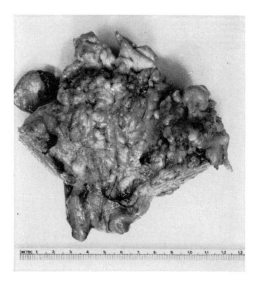

Fig. 47-4

Fig. 47-3. Circumscribed adenocarcinoma of the corpus; the superficial raised area 2.5 cm. in diameter is at the right cornu.

Fig. 47-4. Diffuse, far advanced carcinoma of the endometrium.

hyperplasia or a low-grade adenocarcinoma. All degrees of malignancy between these two extremes are seen.

An interesting type of adenocarcinoma is *adenoacanthoma*. Ewing used this term to designate squamous cell metaplasia occurring with glandular cancer. It is found in a very limited number of corpus carcinomas. We have seen metastases of the squamous cell elements with their curious keratin formation along with adenocarcinoma.

On rare occasions *secondary carcinoma* of the corpus uteri develops from metastases from carcinoma of the ovary, breast, or gastrointestinal tract. Women with carcinoma of the stomach may present no symptoms other than uterine bleeding from a metastatic lesion.

Sarcoma. Sarcoma of the uterus is rare and may arise either in fibroids or in otherwise normal muscle. About 0.5% of myomas are said to undergo this type of malignant change. Here are seen unripe or undifferentiated muscle cells. Novak and Anderson advise counting the mitoses in twenty high-power fields since this gives an important prognostic figure. They believe that over five mitotic figures indicates a very poor prognosis.

Carcinosarcoma is a rare and highly ma-

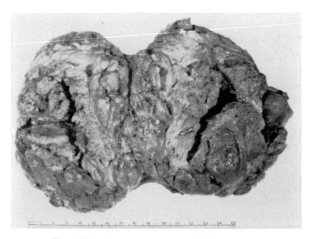

Fig. 47-5. Leiomyosarcoma of the uterus.

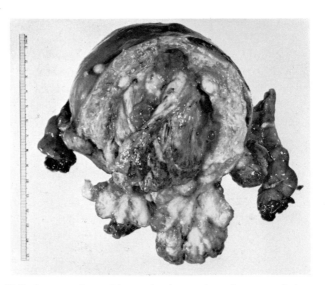

Fig. 47-6. Sarcoma botryoides—mixed mesodermal tumor of the uterus.

lignant uterine tumor. The histologic pattern of sarcoma and carcinoma growing side by side provokes frequent arguments among pathologists. No intermediate cells are found, and it seems clear that there is no transition of one cell type to the other. Two distinct cell types from a carcinosarcoma have been grown in tissue culture. Metastatic lesions may show either carcinoma or sarcoma rather than the mixed pattern of the primary tumor.

Müllerian stroma is capable of giving rise to a variety of highly malignant tumors whose histologic pattern runs a spectrum of mesodermal deviation. For this reason it is often suggested that all these growths be grouped together and referred to as *tumors of mixed mesodermal origin.* A highly malignant polypoid growth, *sarcoma botryoides,* is referred to by at least two other names (carcinosarcoma and mixed mesodermal tumor), depending on the pathologist making the diagnosis. On the other hand, cartilage must be found in these tumors before some pathologists will use the term *mixed mesodermal.*

Stromal endometriosis is a rare and strange malignant uterine growth that still provokes discussion. This unfortunate term has been used by some authors to designate a slow-growing tumor with a monotonous cellular pattern not unlike endometrial stroma. These growths are often multiple, tend to recur, and are lethal. Of undoubted mesodermal origin, they should be regarded as sarcomatous.

■ Clinical stages

Clinical stages are as useful in malignancy of the corpus as they are in cervical lesions. Unfortunately the clinical stage can only be determined after the patient has been operated upon and the tissue examined. It is therefore less helpful in planning initial treatment than is the clinical staging of cervical cancer.

Clinical stages of carcinoma of the corpus uteri, adopted by the International Federation of Gynaecology and Obstetrics (F.I.G.O.) in 1961, are as follows:

Stage 0. Histologic findings of malignancy but not proved.
Stage I. The carcinoma is confined to the corpus.

Stage II. The carcinoma has involved the corpus and the cervix.
Stage III. The carcinoma has extended outside the uterus but not outside the true pelvis.
Stage IV. The carcinoma has extended outside the true pelvis or has obviously involved the mucosa of the bladder or rectum.

Note: In rare cases it may be difficult to decide whether the cancer actually is a carcinoma of the endocervix or carcinoma of the corpus and endocervix. If a clear decision cannot be made at the fractional curettage, an adenocarcinoma should be considered as carcinoma of the corpus and an epidermal carcinoma as carcinoma of the cervix.

■ Symptoms

Endometrial cancer often produces early symptoms, the first of which usually is a serous, malodorous discharge. All too frequently it is not regarded seriously by the patient. It is not long before the watery leukorrhea is replaced by a bloody discharge, intermittent spotting of blood, or steady bleeding. If these symptoms are disregarded, the bleeding will ultimately become frank hemorrhage. All of these symptoms indicate progressive growth of the cancer and enlargement of its area of ulceration.

■ Differential diagnosis

The diagnosis of carcinoma of the corpus is immediately suggested when abnormal uterine bleeding occurs in any woman near the menopause or when it recurs in those who have already ceased menstruating. The average age at which corpus carcinoma is diagnosed is 55 years, but it is found frequently in premenopausal women. Peterson found 32 women under age 40 years, the youngest 17 years, in the group of women treated for endometrial carcinoma at the University of Michigan Hospital. Although only 20% of postmenopausal bleeding is due to pelvic carcinoma, a high index of suspicion must be maintained at all times or delays in diagnosis will result. It is unwise to assume that a cervical polyp, a fibroid, chronic cervicitis, or any other benign lesion is the cause of abnormal bleeding. The physician cannot make a definite diagnosis until he has examined the patient under anesthesia, performed a curettage, and made a biopsy of the cervix.

Since the diagnosis can only be made upon curettage, problems of differentiation have mainly to do with pathologic interpretation of the various hyperplasias. Exfoliative cytology and endometrial aspiration are of great help in screening for endometrial carcinoma, and the expert may even detect atypias by these methods, but the percentage of error is so high we must rely on actual curettage.

■ Treatment

It has been customary in most clinics to employ radiation in one form or another as a preliminary step to definitive surgery for endometrial carcinoma. Whether the uterus is radiated by multiple-radium sources from within the cavity or by external x-ray or telecobalt radiation makes little difference in survival figures. Gynecologists are agreed that surgery is essential for the cure, yet debates continue regarding the importance of preliminary radiation. So far, no one has published figures proving that preliminary radiation has advanced the cure rate over surgery alone. The issue cannot be resolved until a controlled, randomized series, using surgery on the one hand and radiation plus surgery on the other, is reported.

Surgery. The operation most often indicated in the treatment of endometrial carcinoma is hysterectomy and bilateral salpingo-oophorectomy. Most gynecologists advise a procedure in which the paracervical and broad ligament structures and the upper third of the vagina are all removed. Radical vaginal hysterectomy may be preferable to an abdominal operation in extremely obese women.

Corpus cancer often occurs in women with diabetes, hypertension, and cardiovascular disease. It is particularly important that each patient be completely evaluated preoperatively and that medical conditions be corrected or controlled before the operation is performed. With proper care the operative mortality should be no more than 0.5%.

Radiation. As previously stated, a variety of medical complications are encountered in women with endometrial carcinoma. Some of these women are in no condition for surgery, and their entire treatment must be by radiation. A preliminary course of telecobalt therapy followed by intrauterine radium applied in Heyman's capsules gives the best result. The uterus is tightly packed by the multiple-radium sources.

With extremely obese patients in whom it is impossible to perform anything but a standard hysterectomy, preliminary telecobalt, 5,000 rads, seems to improve the chances of a cure. The same may be said for women with high-grade, completely anaplastic adenocarcinoma. Cure rates are lowest in highly undifferentiated growths; consequently, what may be overtreatment is preferable—namely, external and internal radiation plus radical surgery.

Postoperative radiation. Far-advanced carcinoma of the endometrium may extend directly through the uterus at any point. Generally this occurs near the lower uterine segment and involves the parametrial and/or broad ligament areas. This kind of tumor spread may preclude the necessary wide dissection; in fact, the gynecologist may be forced to cut across the tumor at some point. Other patients with advanced carcinomas may be free of direct extension but have one or more positive lymph nodes. Preoperative radiation is preferable under these circumstances, but when it has not been given, the delivery of 4,000 to 5,000 r by means of telecobalt or high-voltage deep x-ray treatment uniformly throughout the pelvis may improve salvage.

Treatment of vaginal metastases. Vaginal metastases may follow an inadequate operation, but they often occur because the tumor already has extended beyond the uterus by the time the operation is performed. One of the major benefits of preoperative radiation appears to be that the incidence of postoperative vaginal metastases is less than that following a primary surgical procedure.

Metastases are best treated by radium in a mold; occasionally radium needles are preferable.

Treatment with progestogens. Kelly and Baker's report on the benefits of high dosages of progesterone in the treatment of metastatic endometrial carcinoma led to the employment of 17-alpha-hydroxyprogesterone (Delalutin) and medroxyprogesterone acetate (Provera). A well-controlled study in which these agents are used before and after operation has not been reported. The effect of progesterone in producing remission is most pronounced on pulmonary metastases, but control of local pelvic recurrence has also been observed. Progesterone therapy must be considered as palliative rather than curative.

■ Results of treatment

The 5-year salvage for endometrial carcinoma depends on the stage of the disease when treatment was instituted and on the adequacy of surgery. Stage I growths yield the greatest salvage, reported to be as high as 95%, although 85% is nearer the usually attained rate. The *overall salvage* in most clinics averages about 55%. This does not necessarily indicate an inadequate treatment program but may reflect the quality of patient material. Many women with endometrial cancer are poor risks for any form of treatment, and others have disease that is too extensive to eradicate.

References

Anderson, D. G.: Management of advanced endometrial adenocarcinoma with medroxyprogesterone acetate, Amer. J. Obstet. Gynec. 92:87, 1965.

Anderson, D. G.: Progestins in the treatment of endometrial carcinoma, Surg. Forum 16:398, 1965.

Beecham, C. T., Messick, R. R., and Wiley, J. H.: Primary surgical therapy for adenocarcinoma of the endometrium. In Lewis, G. C., et al.: New concepts in gynecological oncology, Philadelphia, 1966, F. A. Davis Co.

Boss, J. H., Scully, R. E., Wegner, K. H., and Cohen, R. B.: Structural variations in the adult ovary; clinical significance, Obstet. Gynec. 25:747, 1965.

Carter, E. R., and McDonald, J. R.: Uterine mesodermal mixed tumors, Amer. J. Obstet. Gynec. 80:368, 1960.

Charles, D., Bell, E. T., Loraine, J. A., and Harkness, R. A.: Endometrial carcinoma—endocrinological and clinical studies, Amer. J. Obstet. Gynec. 91:1050, 1965.

Dilman, V. M., Berstein, L. M., Bobrov, Y. F., Bohman, Y. V., Kovleva, I. G., and Krylova, N. V.: Hypothalamopituitary hyperactivity and endometrial carcinoma, Amer. J. Obstet. Gynec. 102:880, 1968.

Hertig, A. T., and Sommers, S. C.: Genesis of endometrial carcinoma, Cancer 2:946, 1949.

Hunter, W. C., and Mohlgren, J. E.: Stromal endometriosis or endometrial sarcoma, Amer. J. Obstet. Gynec. 72:1072, 1956.

Katayama, K. P., and Jones, H. W.: Chromosomes of atypical (adenomatous) hyperplasia and carcinoma of the endometrium, Amer. J. Obstet. Gynec. 97:978, 1967.

Kelley, R. M., and Baker, W. H.: Progestational agents in the treatment of carcinoma of the endometrium, New Eng. J. Med. 264:216, 1961.

Kistner, R. W.: Histological effects of progestins on hyperplasia and carcinoma in situ of the endometrium, Cancer 12:1106, 1959.

McLennan, C. E.: Treatment, Amer. J. Obstet. Gynec. 81:1104, 1961.

Novak, E., and Anderson, D. F.: Sarcoma of the uterus, Amer. J. Obstet. Gynec. 34:740, 1937.

Novak, E. R., and Nalley, W. B.: Uterine adenocanthoma, Obstet. Gynec. 9:396, 1957.

Peterson, E. P.: Endometrial carcinoma in young women, Obstet. Gynec. 31:702, 1968.

Randall, C. L.: Results of treatment of ovarian carcinoma, Trans. Amer. Ass. Obstet. Gynec. Abdom. Surg. 62:206, 1951.

Roddick, J. W., Jr., and Greene, R. R., Jr.: Relation of ovarian hyperplasia to endometrial carcinoma, Amer. J. Obstet. Gynec. 73:843, 1957.

Rubin, A.: The histogenesis of carcinosarcoma (mixed mesodermal tumor) of the uterus as revealed by tissue culture studies, Amer. J. Obstet. Gynec. 77:269, 1959.

Tammes, A. R.: Carcinosarcoma of the uterus, Arch. Path. 70:343, 1960.

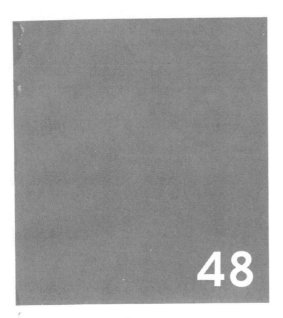

48

Ovarian neoplasms

According to Ricci, the earliest work devoted entirely to ovarian cysts was Justus Theodorus Schorkopff's doctor's thesis at the University of Basel in 1685. He seems to have been the first to differentiate between follicles and simple or retention cysts. Schorkopff also wrote of ovarian abscesses. From that time on writings increased, and large, single volumes devoted entirely to the ovary have been written. Extirpation of normal ovaries was first reported by Percival Pott in 1756. This famous London surgeon removed the gonads found in hernial sacs.

It remained for an American physician, Ephraim McDowell of Danville, Kentucky, to remove the first ovarian tumor in 1809. McDowell's operation ranks high among the monumental accomplishments of the medical profession. Certainly he opened the way for all modern surgery in the abdominal cavity by proving that an operation was not necessarily fatal. This great event cannot be passed without paying tribute to the patient also. Mrs. Jane Todd Crawford was thought to be pregnant by two physicians who, in turn, called Ephraim McDowell in consultation. He had this to say, "Upon examination, per vaginam, I found nothing in the uterus; which induced the conclusion that it must be an enlarged ovarium. Having never seen so large a substance extracted, nor heard of an attempt or success attending any operation, such as this required, I gave to the unhappy woman information of her dangerous situation. She appeared willing to undergo an experiment, which I promised to perform if she would come to Danville (the town where I live), a distance of sixty miles from her place of residence . . . she performed the journey in a few days on horseback."* Mrs. Crawford made an uneventful recovery. McDowell successfully removed two other large ovarian tumors before publishing his results.

Huge ovarian neoplasms of the type encountered by McDowell are no longer common, but patients with benign and malignant ovarian tumors make up about 2% to 3% of the admissions to a busy gynecologic service.

■ Classification

A wide variety of benign and malignant tumors develop in the ovary, and because our knowledge of embryology is still imperfect it is difficult to construct a precise classification. Two logical classifications are those based upon Novak's grouping of the lesions and that proposed by Abell.

CLASSIFICATION AFTER NOVAK

Benign ovarian tumors
  I. Cystic
    A. Nonneoplastic
      1. Follicle cysts
      2. Lutein cysts
      3. Germinal inclusion cysts
      4. Endometrial cysts
    B. Neoplastic

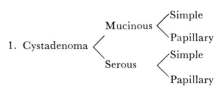

      2. Cystic teratoma

---

*From McDowell, Ephraim: Three cases of extirpation of diseased ovaria, The Eclectic Repertory and Analytical Review, vol. 7, Philadelphia, 1817, Medical and Philosophical Publishing Co.

Benign ovarian tumors—cont'd

II. Solid
    A. Fibroma, osteoma, chondroma, and many other rare forms
    B. Brenner tumors
    C. Adrenal tumors (masculinovoblastoma)

Malignant ovarian tumors

I. Primary cystic tumors
    A. Mucinous cystadenocarcinoma
    B. Serous cystadenocarcinoma

II. Primary solid tumors
    A. Adrenocarcinoma
    B. Fibrosarcoma, carcinosarcoma
    C. Gonadal stroma tumors
        1. Granulosa-theca cell
        2. Arrhenoblastoma
        3. Gynandroblastoma
    D. Germ cell tumors
        1. Choriocarcinoma
        2. Dysgerminoma
        3. Malignant teratoma
    E. Congenital rest tumors
        1. Adrenal cortical carcinoma
        2. Mesonephromas

III. Metastatic tumors

ABELL CLASSIFICATION

I. Neoplasms of germ cell origin
    A. Germinoma
    B. Embryonal teratoma (embryonal carcinoma)
    C. Partially differentiated teratoma (malignant teratoma, solid teratoma)
    D. Mature teratoma (benign cystic teratoma)
    E. Mixed germ cell neoplasms (teratocarcinoma)
    F. Carcinoma or sarcoma arising in a mature teratoma

II. Neoplasms of coelomic (germinal) epithelium and its derivatives
    A. Serous (tubal cell) type
        1. Benign
            a. Cystadenoma
            b. Papilloma
            c. Cystadenofibroma
            d. Adenofibroma
        2. Malignant
            a. Papillary cystadenocarcinoma
    B. Mucinous (cervical cell) type
        1. Benign
            a. Cystadenoma
            b. Cystadenofibroma
            c. Adenofibroma
        2. Malignant
            a. Cystadenocarcinoma
    C. Endometrioid (endometrial cell) type
        1. Benign
            a. Cystadenoma
        2. Malignant
            a. Cystadenocarcinoma
            b. Acanthoadenocarcinoma
    D. Brenner tumors
    E. Mixed and unclassified cell types

III. Neoplasms of specialized gonadal stroma (sex cords and mesenchymal)
    A. Granulosa-theca cell group

        1. Granulosa cell tumor
        2. Theca cell tumor
        3. Granulosa-theca cell tumor
    B. Sertoli-Leydig cell group
        1. Sertoli cell tumor
        2. Leydig cell tumor (hilus cell)
        3. Arrhenoblastoma
    C. Luteomas
    D. Gynandroblastoma

IV. Neoplasms of nonspecialized stroma and heterotopic elements
    A. Fibroma–fibrosarcoma
    B. Leiomyoma–leiomyosarcoma
    C. Angioma–angiosarcoma
    D. Adrenal cortical adenoma–adrenal cortical
    E. Mesonephric cystadenoma–mesonephric
    F. Lymphoblastoma

■ Benign ovarian tumors
NONNEOPLASTIC CYSTS OF THE OVARY

Follicle cysts. Follicle cysts are normal components of the ovary and are formed by the graafian follicle failing to rupture under the ebb and flow of pituitary stimulation. Since as a rule only one follicle matures during each menstrual cycle, the vast majority die somewhere in their developmental stage and remain for a while as a small cystic collection. The average normal ovary contains many of these cystic structures without ova. It is rare for these follicle collections to exceed 5 cm. in diameter. The cavity may be lined by either granulosa cells or theca interna or by both of these. On rare occasions when the cyst is large and the capsule stretched, only thin theca cells mixed with fibrous connective tissue can be seen. Large single-follicle cysts usually have no hormonal activity. Abnormal numbers of follicle cysts are associated with an endocrine imbalance, often leading to hyperestrinism and menometrorrhagia. However, amenorrhea, sterility, and virilism often occur with polycystic ovaries of the Stein-Leventhal type.

Lutein cysts. Luteinization may occur in either granulosa or theca cells. The usual corpus luteum develops from the granulosa layer, whereas in pregnancy the theca cells also are luteinized. Because of excessive amounts of chorionic gonadotropin associated with hydatidiform mole and choriocarcinoma, increased luteinization causes large cystic ovaries. These are referred to as theca-lutein cysts.

At rare intervals the corpus luteum may fail to involute because of some minor hormonal imbalance. This delays the onset of

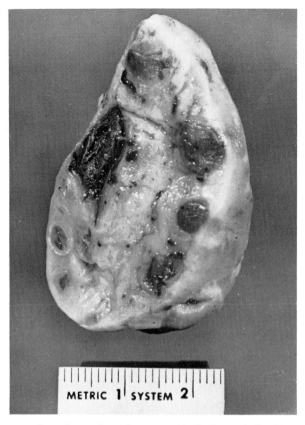

Fig. 48-1. Wedge resection of a polycystic ovary (Stein-Leventhal). Note the thick capsule, edema throughout, and multiple follicle cysts.

the period or produces incomplete amenorrhea. The history and the palpable small mass (the persistent corpus luteum) suggests the diagnosis of an ectopic pregnancy. Some physicians believe that this is not a valid diagnosis but that the persistent corpus is in fact the result of pregnancy which fails to continue.

Germinal inclusion cysts. From middle life on, small microcysts, caused by infoldings of the germinal layer, are likely to form on the surface of the ovary. It is a pathologist's diagnosis and of no importance clinically.

Endometrial cysts. The frequency with which endometriosis is encountered has led many investigators to consider it as a likely background for the development of ovarian tumors. Few will dispute the assumption that ovarian serosa may retain its embryologic potential from coelomic epithelium, making possible differentiation into various

tissues. Since benign and malignant derivatives may arise in all tissues, it is not reasonable to exclude endometriosis.

NEOPLASTIC CYSTS OF THE OVARY

Mucinous cystadenoma. The mucinous cystadenoma is more common than the serous variety. Its behavior is unpredictable and its size may reach spectacular proportions. Cysts of this type weighing over 300 pounds have been reported. It is quite probable that the tumor Ephraim McDowell removed from Jane Crawford was mucinous.

The outward appearance of the mucinous and serous cystadenomas are so much alike that Pfannenstiel suggested the names to convey some idea of their contents, hoping to aid in differentiation. On the external surface will be seen convolutions and indentations indicating the multiple locules that lie within. The surface coloring is a pearly gray, which may take on a darker

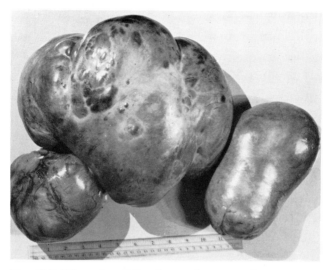

Fig. 48-2. Bilateral, multilocular mucinous cystadenoma.

hue if bleeding occurs inside the cyst. If the cyst is papillary, such proliferative features may be seen on the surface. Free peritoneal fluid often accompanies the papillary variety of mucinous cystadenoma.

A histologic picture of tall, columnar cells with basal nuclei and light cytoplasm, swollen by secreted mucin, characterizes the mucinous cystadenoma. There is a pronounced activity to nonspecific esterases and 5-nucleotidase; alkaline phosphatase activity, on the other hand, is lacking in mucinous cystadenomas. Although the resemblance to intestinal epithelium has been noted, a number of histogenetic possibilities have been offered. It seems likely that the tumor arises from coelomic epithelium, but it may develop from teratomas.

The behavior of the mucinous cyst is on rare occasions quite different from that of other benign cysts. Numerous examples have been reported of the metastasis of benign mucinous cysts to distant organs, sometimes many years after the removal of the primary growth. Rarely one of these cysts may rupture, and the adhesive, gluelike contents can be seen clinging to intestines, peritoneum, and other organs. In a short time free fluid will form, and large plaques of growing mucinous material are to be found within the peritoneal cavity. This condition is called *pseudomyxoma peritonei* and from a histologic standpoint is benign, yet the peritoneal implants grow and the patients die in ca-

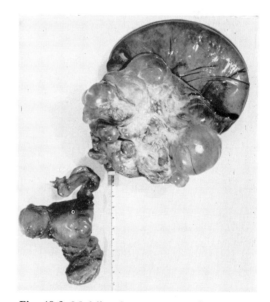

Fig. 48-3. Multilocular serous cystadenoma.

chexia as with advanced cancer. About 2% of mucinous cystadenomas are said to become malignant.

Serous cystadenoma. The serous cystadenoma, slightly less common than the mucinous variety, has a far higher incidence of malignant change. It is generally a pearly gray multilocular tumor mass, with brown or bloody coloring only when there is hemorrhage into the cyst. There may be papillary excrescences in some of these tumors, and the resemblance to cancer is striking. These

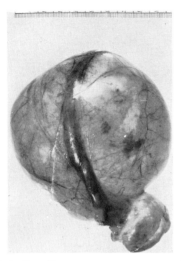

Fig. 48-4. Interligamentous serous cystadenoma. Note the tube stretched out over the tumor.

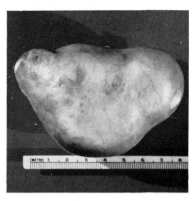

Fig. 48-5. Benign cystic teratoma with a corpus luteum cyst on the left.

cysts may be either unilateral or bilateral, small or large; they are confined within the folds of the broad ligament or swing freely on a long pedicle.

Histologic features are usually quite different from those of the mucinous cyst. The serous cystadenoma is lined by a cuboidal epithelium. When the papillary form exists, the cellular arrangement in a characteristic treelike pattern can be seen. Enzymatic histochemical reactions show most serous cystomas to have alkaline phosphatase activity, 5-nucleotidase rarely, and nonspecific esterases uncommonly. The specialized covering epithelium of the ovary, peritoneal in origin and similar to müllerian duct epithelium, is the source of serous cystadenomas.

Benign cystic teratoma. Collectively the benign cystic tumors of epithelial origin (mucinous and serous) have a higher incidence than the benign cystic teratoma (dermoid). About 15% of all neoplastic ovarian growths are the benign cystic teratoma type. Derivations of ectodermal elements predominate in the histologic picture, although well-differentiated mesodermal and endodermal constituents are found. The suggestion made by Hertig and Gore that the tumor derives from primordial germ cells in the line of their migration is reasonable. Their theory is supported by chromosomal studies showing benign cystic teratomas to have a female karyotype—obviously from an endogenous cell line.

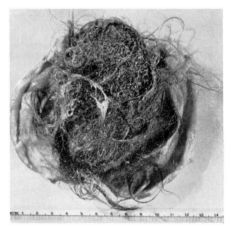

Fig. 48-6. An opened benign cystic teratoma, the contents of which are mainly hair and sebaceous material.

Benign cystic teratoma may be found at any age but is more commonly discovered in young women. It is not at all unusual for the tumor to be diagnosed at the first prenatal examination of a young primigravida.

The cyst generally assumes a slightly lumpy, round shape, rarely more than 10 cm. in diameter. The structure is usually unilocular and possesses a somewhat oily sheen, and yellowish areas of keratin may be visible through the cyst wall. Dermoids contain an oily, flaky sebaceous fluid, generally with a mass of matted hair. Teeth, cartilage, bones, or other evidences of disarranged

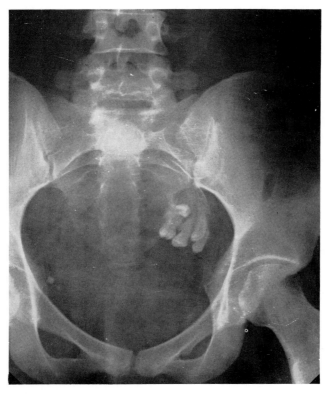

Fig. 48-7. Well-developed teeth within a benign cystic teratoma demonstrated by x-ray examination.

gonad development may complete this odd display. Enzymatic patterns follow those of normal homologous body structures. A troublesome and frequently serious chemical peritonitis results from rupture of a benign cystic teratoma. Malignancy is exceptionally rare in these cysts. If it occurs, a squamous cell carcinoma results.

Struma ovarii is an uncommon teratoid aberration in which thyroid tissue dominates the tumor. It is generally a smooth, dark red to yellowish brown, essentially solid tumor. Thyrotoxicosis has been reported to be caused by this tumor.

SOLID BENIGN TUMORS

Solid benign ovarian tumors are rather uncommon; many are pathologic curiosities.

Fibroma. The fibroma is the most frequently encountered solid benign tumor. As the name suggests, it is a dense tumor, predominantly solid but occasionally containing areas of cystic degeneration in the center, much like uterine fibroids. Meigs has pointed out an interesting association of ascites and hydrothorax with ovarian fibroma. The term *Meigs' syndrome* has been given to this association of ovarian fibroma and hydrothorax, although it is known that fluid can collect in both the peritoneal and pleural cavities when other types of ovarian tumors are present. There is as yet no clear explanation for the development of pleural effusions.

Brenner tumors. Until recently, Brenner tumors were diagnosed as fibromas of the ovary and considered quite rare. Though uncommon, they are no longer pathologic curiosities. According to Greene they probably have several different modes of origin; some develop from surface epithelium of the ovary, others from rete ovarii or ovarian stroma. These neoplasms are slow growing and show little inclination to undergo malignant degeneration. Generally they are removed after the menopause because of their late discovery. Histologically one sees nests of epithelial cells surrounded by fibromatous connective tissue.

Other solid benign tumors. The group of solid benign ovarian tumors has many

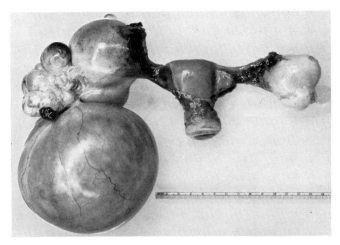

Fig. 48-8. Bilateral fibroadenoma of the ovary. Areas of cystic degeneration are visible.

other rare and interesting growths, such as angioma, chondroma, fibroadenoma, lymphangioma, and papilloma.

SYMPTOMS OF BENIGN TUMORS

Ovarian tumors as a rule produce few symptoms. The nonneoplastic ovarian cysts have often been held responsible for lower abdominal discomfort, which is really from intestinal spasm or some other emotional problem. Undoubtedly in some extreme cases the overabundance of follicle cysts stretching the germinal epithelium to a great degree might produce pain in hypersensitive women.

On rare occasions, if ovulation opens an ovarian blood vessel, there may be *considerable intraperitoneal bleeding*. As might be expected, the pain then is quite severe and unremitting, and in an occasional patient the blood loss may be enough to produce shock. This condition can be confused with ectopic pregnancy. Laparotomy may be necessary to control bleeding.

The true tumors of the ovary are likewise associated with minimal symptoms, the most common being *abdominal enlargement* and a *sense of pelvic pressure*. It is by no means rare for a woman to come to the doctor perplexed because she is menstruating normally and regularly, yet her abdomen is enlarging and she thinks herself pregnant. Pressure symptoms are dependent upon the size of the tumor, its location, and adherence. Fixed or incarcerated ovarian neoplasms may produce *painful micturition, rectal tenesmus, and/or painful defecation. Menstrual dis-*

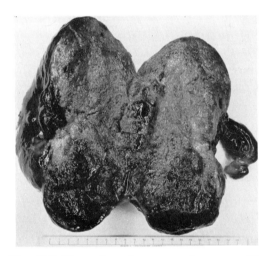

Fig. 48-9. Hemorrhage into an ovarian tumor. The tumor has been opened. The long pedicle on the right was completely occluded by a 360-degree twist.

turbances are not very common, occurring in about 10% to 15% of patients.

Accidental *twisting of the pedicle* carrying the blood supply to an ovarian cyst is not an uncommon occurrence. Moderate-sized tumors (8 to 12 cm.) are most likely to incur this fate. When the accident occurs, the patient experiences a sudden sharp pain that will subside when the twist is reversed. The attacks generally are recurrent and transitory, although at times a complete twist may remain, compromising the blood supply of the tumor, thereby causing necrosis and hemorrhage. These patients present signs of peritoneal irritation in addition to the tender cystic structure, and if allowed to go untreated, a widespread peritonitis results.

The diagnosis of ovarian neoplasms is made by complete abdominal and pelvic examination of all patients who have any abdominal complaints, no matter how trivial, and by periodic examination of presumably well women.

TREATMENT OF BENIGN TUMORS

Since a true ovarian neoplasm will continue to grow and may ultimately undergo malignant degeneration, the treatment is surgical removal. Operations for ovarian neoplasms should constitute no more than 6% of all pelvic surgical procedures. A careful selection of patients is necessary. In almost every instance if the ovary exceeds 5 cm. in diameter, the enlargement is the result of a true neoplasm and the removal is indicated. Although all ovarian neoplasms are at some time smaller than 5 cm. in diameter, they are rarely discovered at this stage because of the total lack of symptoms. If the physician has been examining a patient every 6 months, there is one finding of significance to aid in early diagnosis, that is, an ovary which was always freely moveable on previous examinations has become slightly enlarged and adherent to the cul-de-sac or posterior leaf of the broad ligament. This is cause for alarm and continued close scrutiny.

Since about 97% of ovarian enlargements under 5 cm. are nonneoplastic, immediate removal of slightly enlarged ovaries is contraindicated. Such an enlargement is usually temporary due to a normal follicle or corpus luteum, and at reexamination in 1 or 2 weeks it will have disappeared. Observation of these small cysts at 3 to 6 months is the only treatment required. Should they increase in size, a true neoplasm is to be suspected, and removal may then be considered. The low incidence of malignancy in these small tumors makes the risk from observation negligible.

Unilateral cystectomy or cystoophorectomy is the treatment of choice for young women with single benign lesions, but in each instance the opposite ovary must be carefully inspected, bisected, and a *biopsy* made in an effort to detect a small neoplasm that may grow later. Benign cystic teratomas are easily resectable, and much normal ovarian tissue

can be preserved. The high incidence of bilaterality and almost total lack of malignant change make conservative surgery a highly desirable practice for benign cystic teratomas in young women.

Benign serous cystadenomas are likely to occur bilaterally, hence bilateral cystoophorectomy frequently is necessary. In young women with a unilateral serous cystadenoma the normal ovary and the uterus can be left in place if bisection of the normal-appearing ovary reveals no tumor. If the excised tumor proves to be malignant, hysterectomy and removal of the other ovary should be considered.

Mucinous cystadenomas are usually unilateral, and the incidence of malignancy is far less than with the serous variety. It is usually possible, therefore, to remove the involved ovary and leave the normal-appearing one if it looks normal when bisected.

In women over 40 years of age with unilateral neoplasms, particularly serous cystadenomas, bilateral salpingo-oophorectomy and hysterectomy usually are indicated because of the increased possibility of malignancy.

Ovarian tumors diagnosed after the menopause are often malignant, and complete hysterectomy and bilateral removal of the adnexa are indicated. Ovarian neoplasms with torsion of the pedicle must be considered an acute surgical emergency, and immediate operative removal is indicated.

Oophorectomy for reasons other than neoplasms. Ever since Ephraim McDowell demonstrated that an ovarian tumor could be safely removed, the ovary has received enthusiastic surgical attack for reasons that are not altogether valid. It has been a common practice for a long time to remove the ovaries at the time of hysterectomy as prophylaxis against cancer. Some of the leaders in gynecologic teaching have gone so far as to say that a woman does not need her ovaries after 35 years of age.

Randall has brought reality in statistical form to this aspect of prophylactic surgery. He has this to say about the risk of ovarian cancer:

It seems practical to keep in mind the relative risk of ovarian cancer and carcinoma of the breast in the age groups most frequently considered. Between the ages of 20 and 25 years, for instance, we should expect to find an average of 1 case of cancer of the breast and 1 of cancer of the ovary per 100,000 women per year. Between the ages of 25 and 29 we should expect to find 5 malignancies of the breast and 2 carcinomas of the ovary per 100,000 women per year. The risk of malignancy in the breast increases rapidly as women grow older. It is 5 times more likely than ovarian malignancies in the thirties, and 6 times as frequent in the forties. In the fifties, when carcinoma of the ovary is most frequent, the ratio is again 4 carcinomas of the breast per 1 carcinoma of the ovary. After 60 the relatively greater frequency of malignancy in the breast continues, whereas the risk of ovarian malignancy decreases noticeably as women grow older.*

As a general rule the ovaries can be removed at the time of hysterectomy in women who are approaching the menopause and certainly in those whose periods have ceased.

■ Malignant ovarian tumors

About 15% of all ovarian tumors are malignant and frequently bilateral. At Geisinger Medical Center, Danville, Pa., patients with primary ovarian malignancy constitute 10.5% of all female patients with pelvic cancer. New York State statistics (1966) indicate an overall incidence of 11.6 ovarian cancers per 100,000 women.

Although the average age incidence is

*From Randall, C. L.: Ovarian function and women after the menopause, Amer. J. Obstet. Gynec. **73:**1001, 1957.

50 years, these malignant tumors are found in older and younger persons alike. Insidious and asymptomatic growth results too often in a disseminated malignancy at the time of the first physical examination. In these situations a commonplace story is often related by the patient—an awareness for months of a lower abdominal mass, which suddenly enlarges and causes abdominal pain. The patient's decision to seek consultation is made when she experiences pain, and this is often too late for effective therapy. Other women with ovarian cancer may attribute their abdominal enlargement to pregnancy, and as a consequence see no urgency in the matter.

As a rule, except for hormonopoietic tumors, ovarian malignancies continue asymptomatic until normal intestinal function is interrupted by tumor growth. Intermittent cramps, constipation, and distention follow. About 10% of the patients exhibit uterine bleeding.

PRIMARY CYSTIC TUMORS

Cystadenocarcinoma. The largest group of ovarian malignant tumors are the cystadenocarcinomas. When their capsule is intact, they lack distinguishing features. The more common *serous* variety may be of any size, gray, and contain a thick, turbid, mucoid fluid. The interior of the malignant cystic

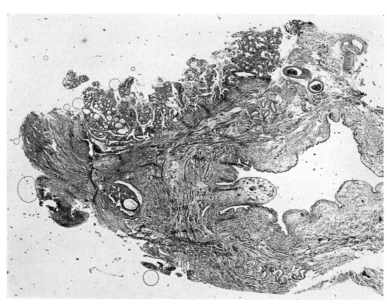

Fig. 48-10. Photomicrograph demonstrating *direct extension* of cancer to the tube wall from a cystadenocarcinoma with an intact, smooth capsule. Note incidental endometriosis and hydrosalpinx. (×17.3.)

tumor is rough and granular with papillary projections infiltrating the wall. Papillary foci of tumor cells metastasize to parietal peritoneum and omentum, although any abdominal or pelvic area may become involved. Metastases to the corpus uteri are common.

A discouraging feature of cystadenocarcinomas and all other ovarian cancer is the finding of malignant cells in peritoneal washings in spite of an intact, nonadherent capsule. Further, the surface of surrounding pelvic and abdominal structures as well as parietal peritoneum may show microscopic tumor involvement, although the malignancy has no obvious surface growth or adhesions (Fig. 48-10). Also, these ovarian cancer cells often make their way to the cervix, where they may be identified by cytologic examinations.

Several investigators in this field consider endometriosis a source of some cystadenocarcinomas. Unquestionably many of these neoplasms resemble adenocarcinoma of the uterus. On this basis it has been suggested that *endometrioid tumors* be added to present-day classifications.

In an attempt to add clarity to this concept, Long and Taylor studied the clinical behavior of malignant ovarian tumors in relation to nucleoli size. RNA-identified nucleoli were subjected to micromeasurements and found to be smaller in what is considered endometrioid carcinoma. These tumors have a higher survival rate with an obvious lower capacity for rapid growth and metastasis.

Explanation lies in RNA and its related enzyme systems—a major factor in protein synthesis and cellular growth. Anaplastic ovarian carcinomas show an intense alkaline phosphatase activity. Thus, according to Long and Taylor, smaller nucleoli have lower RNA activity and less extensive disease. Consistent with this work, Toews and co-workers have found well-differentiated ovarian carcinomas to demonstrate a diploid mode, whereas undifferentiated ovarian carcinomas are triploid.

PRIMARY SOLID TUMORS

There are different types of primary solid carcinoma of the ovary, but adenocarcinoma is by far the most common. Fibrosarcoma, the malignant aberration of the fibroma, and carcinosarcoma are rare entities. These tumors all tend to be irregularly round with smooth surfaces that are rather hard upon cutting. Depending on the amount of fibrous tissue or blood present, the tumors will be varying shades of gray to reddish. It is conceded that nearly all ovarian carcinomas come to surgery late because implants on the surrounding pelvic viscera and peritoneum are usually found. Local peritoneal metastases are common, and the omentum becomes involved quite early. Lymph nodes seem to be a relatively late area for spread.

Gonadal stromal tumors. The *granulosa-theca cell tumor* is the most common growth arising from cortical ovarian stroma. Typically it occurs at or beyond the menopause,

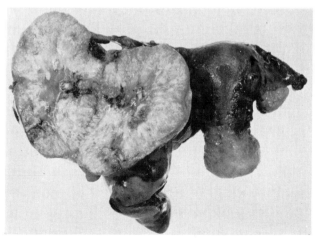

Fig. 48-11. Solid adenocarcinoma of the ovary. The malignancy is shown divided. The opposite ovary is normal.

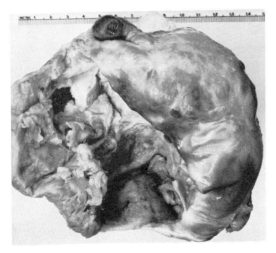

Fig. 48-12. Huge granulosa-theca cell tumor of the ovary.

although it is sometimes found in very young girls. Large quantities of estrogen produced by this hormonopoietic neoplasm have a feminizing effect. Infants and young girls experience premature sex development and uterine bleeding. The excessive amounts of estrogen produce hypertrophy of the uterus and hyperplasia of the endometrium. As a rule, in older women the hyperplasia may take on some atypical features and prove worrisome to the pathologist. An association between feminizing tumors and endometrial carcinoma was suggested in early reports; however, support for this tenuous relationship has not been forthcoming.

Only about 20% or 30% of granulosa cell tumors are malignant; consequently they should usually be treated as benign lesions.

The counterpart of the feminizing tumor is the masculinizing ovarian neoplasm *arrhenoblastoma*. The arrhenoblastoma grows slowly and possesses a low degree of undifferentiation. The developing masculinizing growth produces increasing amounts of male sex hormone, which in turn cause a progressive defeminization of the patient. With the development of amenorrhea, the voice takes on a huskier quality, breasts atrophy, facial and body hirsutism appears, and the clitoris usually enlarges. These secondary sex changes will usually reverse themselves after the tumor is removed.

A rare and strange tumor with mixed tissues resembling both arrhenoblastoma and granulosa-theca cell tumors is called a *gynan-*

droblastoma. The histologic picture is bizarre and the clinical behavior equally odd. Hormone levels are at times normal yet may vary to a point of virilism. Women with these tumors have borne children. The gynandroblastoma is considered malignant.

Germ cell tumors. Presumably, germ cell tumors come from primordial germ cells before they differentiate. *Primary choriocarcinoma,* an exceedingly rare ovarian neoplasm, may be within a teratoma or alone as a primary growth. It is rapidly fatal. These usually do not respond to Methotrexate as do trophoblastic tumors with an identical histologic appearance.

Germinoma, an ovarian malignancy arising in the primordial germ cell, is most commonly found in young girls during the early reproductive years. The solid, grayish red features are hardly distinctive; however, the individual dysgerminoma cell is large and polygonal with nuclear DNA content about twice that found in lymphocytes, according to Asadourian and Taylor. They have recorded a 10-year survival rate of 88.6% in cases of unilateral involvement. This alone justifies conservative surgical therapy when preservation of ovarian function is desirable. Recurrent tumor responds favorably to high-voltage radiation.

Teratoma differs from the dermoid in that it is solid in contrast to a cystic growth, and it is highly malignant. All three primitive layers may be seen in a heterogeneous mass with areas of cystic degeneration and broken capsule (Fig. 48-13).

Congenital rest tumors. *Adrenal rest tumors* may be benign or malignant. A variety of names (adrenocorticoid, luteoma, etc.) have been applied to these little-understood neoplasms. As would be expected, symptoms are those of virilization. Improvement follows oophorectomy.

Another rare and highly malignant growth is the *mesonephroma,* sometimes called clear-cell carcinoma. As the name implies, this tumor arises from mesonephric rests.

METASTATIC CARCINOMA

Secondary carcinoma of the ovary is fairly common. The primary carcinomas are generally in the gastrointestinal tract, although instances of breast carcinoma metastasizing to the ovary are to be found. About 5% of the early carcinomas of the corpus uteri will

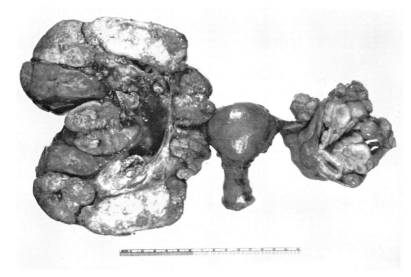

Fig. 48-13. Malignant teratoma.

be found to have secondarily involved the ovary. A classic example of ovarian involvement is the Krukenberg tumor, secondary to gastrointestinal malignancy. The histology of this metastatic lesion is characteristic, with the formation of the "signet ring cells," which are the mucus-producing cells, their nuclei pressed against the cell wall forming a crescent. Other types of cancer metastasizing to the ovary will produce cells similar to those of the primary cancer. Removal of massive metastatic lesions in the ovary adds materially to the comfort of the patient and is recommended as a palliative measure.

■ Stage grouping on primary carcinoma of the ovary*

The staging should take into consideration the findings at clinical examination and surgical exploration.

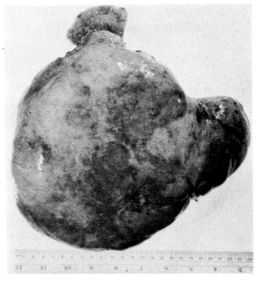

Fig. 48-14. Krukenberg tumor, metastatic from the stomach.

Stage   I.   Growth limited to the ovaries.
        Ia. Growth limited to one ovary.
        Ib. Growth limited to both ovaries.
        Ic. Growth limited to one or both ovaries with ascites showing malignant cells.

Stage   II. Growth involving one or both ovaries with pelvic extension.
        IIa. Extension and/or metastases to the uterus and/or tubes.
        IIb. Extension to other pelvic tissues.

Stage III. Growth involving one or both ovaries with wide-spread intraperitoneal metastasis to upper half of abdomen (the omentum, the small intestine, and its mesentery).

Stage IV. Growth involving one or both ovaries with distant metastasis outside the peritoneal cavity.

Note: The presence of ascites will not influence the staging for stages II, III, and IV.

*From the Cancer Committee of the International Federation of Gynecology and Obstetrics.

TREATMENT OF MALIGNANT OVARIAN NEOPLASMS

It is virtually an accident to discover an ovarian carcinoma early. This being the case, a warranted pessimism surrounds the treatment. Initial therapy should consist of removing the uterus, both tubes and ovaries, the omentum, and other involved areas if they are easily resectable. At times the cancer may be so extensive that the entire abdominal and pelvic cavity seem to be involved. To do more than take a biopsy and close the abdomen would be futile. Supervoltage radiation is called for in such instances. Regression sometimes follows radiation, making surgical removal of the bulk of the tumor possible at a second laparotomy.

Except in stage Ia, all patients operated upon for ovarian malignancy should receive external radiation even though the capsule was intact and there was no spill during operation. Survival figures clearly reveal the benefits to be gained by adequate surgery followed by total abdominal radiation. Depending on residual disease, 4,000 to 5,000 rads of tumor dose by telecobalt should be delivered to the total pelvis. The upper abdomen should receive, with kidney shielding, 2,000 to 3,000 rads of tissue dose.

Several chemotherapeutic agents have been used in the treatment of ovarian cancer. Cytoxan, nitrogen mustard, L-phenylalanine mustard, triethylenethiophosphoramide (Thio-TEPA), and radioactive colloidal gold have shown cytotoxic effects but little in the way of specific action. Objective response has been observed using all of these agents. Thio-TEPA seems to have a slight advantage over the others. It may be used in doses of 0.8 mg./kg. of body weight, but particular attention must be paid to the possibility of bone marrow depression. Oral, intravenous, or intraperitoneal routes of administration are applicable for Thio-TEPA. It appears to help reduce ascitic fluid in patients with far-advanced ovarian cancer.

PROGNOSIS FOR MALIGNANT OVARIAN NEOPLASMS

Ovarian carcinoma no longer merits the gloomy picture that prevailed for so many years. Munnell's absolute cure rate of 70% where complete removal was possible and 61% in those conservatively managed compares favorably with overall results obtained in other pelvic malignant lesions. These figures are significantly supported by Villa-Santa and Bloedorn's 60.6% survival rate.

References

Abell, M. R.: The nature and classifications of ovarian neoplasms, Canad. Med. Ass. J. **94:** 1102, 1966.

Asadourian, L. A., and Taylor, H. B.: Dysgerminoma, an analysis of 105 cases, Obstet. Gynec. **33:**370, 1969.

Beecham, C. T.: The behavior of pseudomucinous cystadenoma, Amer. J. Obstet. Gynec. **61:**755, 1951.

Brenner, F.: Das Oophoroma Folliculare, Frankfurt. Z. Path. **1:**150, 1907.

Emge, L. A.: Functional and growth characteristics of struma ovarii, Amer. J. Obstet. Gynec. **40:**738, 1940.

Emig, O. R., Hertig, A. T., and Rowe, F. J.: Gynandroblastoma of the ovary, Obstet. Gynec. **1:**135, 1959.

Erdmann, J. F., and Spaulding, H. V.: Papillary cystadenoma of ovary, Surg. Gynec. Obstet. **33:**362, 1921.

Greene, R. R.: The diverse origins of Brenner tumors, Amer. J. Obstet. Gynec. **64:**878, 1952.

Herrera, J. R.: Carcinoma of the uterine cervix, endometrium and ovary, Chicago, 1962, Year Book Medical Publishers, Inc.

Hertig, A. T., and Gore, H.: Tumors of the female sex organs. III. Tumors of the ovary and fallopian tube, Section IX, Fasc. 33, Washington, D. C., 1961, Armed Forces Institute of Pathology.

Hundley, J. M., Jr.: Krukenberg tumors of the ovary and other secondary ovarian carcinomas, Southern Med. J. **24:**579, 1931.

King, J. E.: Pseudomyxoma peritonaei, Amer. J. Obstet. **80:**426, 1919.

Long, M. E., and Taylor, H. C., Jr.: Endometroid carcinoma of the ovary, Amer. J. Obstet. Gynec. **80:**936, 1965.

McDowell, E.: Three cases of extirpation of diseased ovaria, The Eclectic Repertory and Analytical Review, vol. 7, Philadelphia, 1817, Medical and Philosophical Publishing Co.

Morris, J. M., and Scully, R. E.: Endocrine pathology of the ovary, St. Louis, 1958, The C. V. Mosby Co.

Morris, J. M.: The syndrome of testicular feminization in male pseudohermaphrodites, Amer. J. Obstet. Gynec. **65:**1192, 1953.

Munnell, E. W.: Is conservative therapy ever justified in Stage I (IA) cancer of the ovary? Amer. J. Obstet. Gynec. **103:**641, 1969.

Novak, E.: Granulosa-cell ovarian tumors as cause of precocious puberty, witht report of 3 cases, Amer. J. Obstet. Gynec. **26:**505, 1933.

Peterson, W. F.: Malignant degeneration of benign cystic teratomas of the ovary, Obstet. Gynec. Surv. **12:**793, 1957.

Pfannenstiel, H. J.: Die Erkrankungen des Eierstockes und Nebeneirstockes. In Veit's Handbuch der Gynäkologie, Wiesbaden, 1908, J. F. Bergmann.

Randall, C. L.: Ovarian function and women after the menopause, Amer. J. Obstet. Gynec. **73:** 1000, 1957.

Reagan, J. W.: Histopathology of ovarian pseudomucinous cystadenoma, Amer. J. Path. **25:**689, 1949.

Ricci, J. V.: The genealogy of gynaecology, New York, 1943, Blakiston Division, McGraw-Hill Book Co.

Schreier, P. C., and Alexander, A. M.: Conservative surgery for large ovarian cysts, Southern Med. J. **54:**948, 1961.

Serr, D. M., Padeh, B., Mashiach, S., and Shaki, R.: Chromosomal studies in tumors of embryonic origin, Obstet. Gynec. **33:**324, 1969.

Toews, H. A., Katayama, K. P., and Jones, H. W., Jr.: Chromosomes of normal and neoplastic ovarian tissue, Obstet. Gynec. **32:**465, 1968.

VillaSanta, U., and Bloedorn, F. G.: Operation, external irradiation, adioactive isotopes, and chemotherapy in treatment of metastatic ovarian malignancies, Amer. J. Obstet. Gynec. **102:**531, 1968.

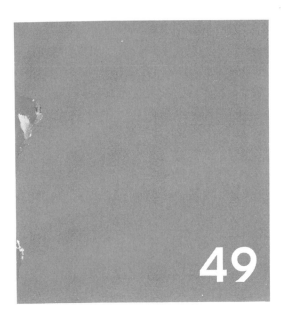

49

The climacteric and the menopause

The reproductive phase of life fades out with a gradual decline in ovarian function. This transitional period between the childbearing phase and the phase of senescence is spoken of as the *climacteric,* or "change of life"; it is an epoch analogous in many respects to adolescence. Just as menarche (onset of menstruation) is the outstanding event of adolescence, *menopause* (cessation of menstruation) is the most important manifestation of the climateric. In other words, *menopause is to the climacteric what menarche is to adolescence.*

■ Menopause

The cessation of menstruation usually occurs between the ages of 47 and 50 years. Some women may stop menstruating at 35 years of age and others may continue to 55 years of age, but both of these age limits are most unusual. Many factors have been held responsible for either an abnormally early or late menopause, including climate,

race, childbearing, general health, and heredity. Of these, the last is probably the most significant. It has been stated that the earlier the menarche, the later the menopause. The validity of this dictum is open to considerable question.

MECHANISM OF THE MENOPAUSE

Changes in body structure and function that commence with the climacteric and continue for the remaining years follow a decrease in ovarian function resulting from normal gonadal aging. The ovary gradually loses its ability to make graaffian follicles and corpora lutea. It decreases in size, first becoming wrinkled, then smooth with no evidence of macroscopic cysts. Microscopic examination gives proof of considerable cortical thinning and a relative thickening of the medulla from increased fibrous connective tissue. Early in the climacteric, primordial follicles and small cystic follicles may be noted; as the aging process continues, these disappear, with only occasional atretic follicles or corpora albicantia to be seen. The blood vessels of the hilum and medulla become progressively sclerotic. These structural changes in the ovary lead to anovulation, cessation of progesterone production, and great reduction in estrogen.

The decline in ovarian function is accompanied by several endocrine changes, particularly those related to trophic hormones produced by the pituitary gland. Most prominent is the overproduction of gonadotropins. Postmenopausal women excrete 90 to 100 I.U. of follicle-stimulating hormone (FSH) in 24 hours, whereas women in the third decade of life excrete 5 to 30 I.U. In addition, luteinizing hormone (LH) averages 95 I.U. in the postmenopausal years as against 6 to 10 I.U. in the third decade of life. Hormone assays have shown this overproduction of FSH and LH to extend over several years.

The duration of major steroid synthesis (estrogen, progesterone, and androgen) has not been clearly established for the postmenopausal period. Although continued gonadotropin secretion results in minimal estrogen production, a capacity for testosterone creation by ovarian stroma has been demonstrated by Mattingly and Huang. Their "low yield of estrone and estradiol from Δ^4-androstenedione suggests ovarian stroma has a limited capacity to aromatize androgen precursors to estrogen." That the menopausal ovary may have an important role in steroid precursors is a further suggestion. Mechanisms involved between the adrenal and the ovarian stroma remain to be established.

■ Climacteric
PELVIC CHANGES

With the gradual withdrawal of the tissue-stimulating effect of the estrogenic hormone, significant regressive changes occur in the genital system, particularly in the vagina

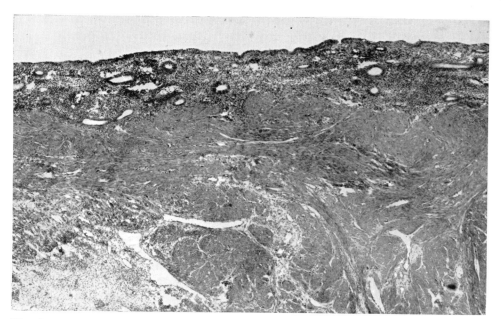

Fig. 49-1. Atrophic endometrium. The endometrium is thin, the stroma is compact, and the glands are few in number, narrow, and straight. (×60.)

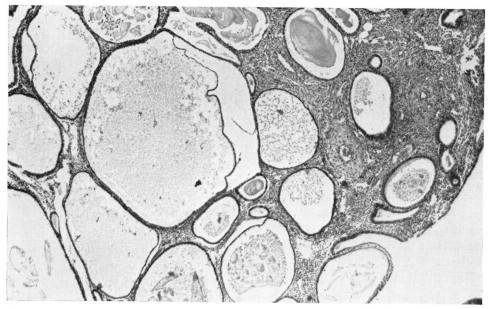

Fig. 49-2. Retrograde hyperplasia. Senile cystic endometrium. Note the resemblance to Swiss cheese hyperplasia. Stroma in this condition is more fibrous, and the lining cells of the glands are low cuboidal or flattened. (×60.)

and uterus. The vagina gradually becomes smaller, the fornices become shallower, and the mucosa becomes progressively thinner. The vaginal smear reflects this change by the absence of cornified cells and, eventually, by the appearance of basal layer cells typical of the "estrogen-deficiency smear."

The supporting structures of the uterus, bladder, and rectum lose much of their tone and premenopausal strength. These changes accompanying atrophy of the vaginal wall contribute to the development of cystocele, rectocele, and uterine prolapse. The cervix gradually decreases in size, but this may not be evident for some years; however, there is a great diminution in the secretory activity of the cervical glands very early in the climacteric. The mucus becomes scant and viscid, and the arborization phenomenon is either absent or greatly reduced.

As a result of thinning of the myometrium, the uterus gradually becomes smaller in size and eventually becomes extremely tiny, resembling the uterus of the prepubertal girl. The endometrium as a rule becomes thin and atrophic, but various forms of retrogressive hyperplasia may be found in response to extragonadal estrogen stimulation.

GENERAL BODY CHANGES

Biochemical and physiologic research, particularly in nutrition, continues to uncover new basic facts concerning estrogen and other steroids. One of the most important postmenopausal changes is the rapidity with which *atherosclerosis* develops after castration or complete ovarian failure. This point is further developed in considering age levels at which women and men develop coronary occlusion. Premenopausal women have a negligible amount of coronary disease, whereas in the late postmenopausal period the incidence in men and women is essentially the same.

Starting with the menopause, there is a steady decline in body bone mass. This has been referred to as *osteoporosis,* but there is a growing tendency to employ a new term, *osteopenia*. A number of theories have been offered as to basic etiology; none entirely explains the events. In simplest terms there is a decline in osteoblastic activity corresponding with the fall in estrogen level. These bone changes are permanent; although

their progress is stopped by estrogens, the process cannot be reversed.

Estrogen, by activating two carbohydrate enzymes, hexokinase and glucokinase, aids in the mobilization and distribution of glucose reserves. In this manner carbohydrate metabolism is affected by the climacteric; indeed, estrogen deprivation may be a factor in the production of diabetes.

SYMPTOMS

It is often assumed that inasmuch as spontaneous cessation of ovarian function is a physiologic process, it is unattended by symptoms of consequence. In a few women this might be true, but usually the great hormone imbalance coupled with regressive changes creates a number of symptoms.

Vasomotor (hot flush). The most common subjective symptom is the *hot flush,* described as a sensation of heat over the body, especially over the face and neck, accompanied by reddening of the skin of these areas. This is often followed by profuse perspiration and chilliness. These vasomotor disturbances may occur only once or twice a day or as often as every half hour. They are most distressing when they recur during the night and interfere with the patient's rest. The frequency and severity of vasomotor symptoms are subject to wide variations. They are mild to moderate in most women and severe in only a few.

The cause of the hot flush has been the subject of much speculation and debate. Since the menopause is primarily due to lack of ovarian function, this would seem to be the logical explanation for the symptom. There are, however, several objections to this theory. Prepubertal girls, who have no circulating estrogen, do not suffer from flushes, nor do women with estrogen deficiency secondary to pituitary hypofunction. The more reasonable explanation is that the vasomotor disturbance is related to high levels of gonadotropic hormone. Several investigators have demonstrated a definite relationship between the titer of FSH in the blood and urine and the severity of the hot flushes. This is true not only in climacteric women but also in patients of reproductive age who develop ovarian failure as a result of surgery or radiation. There are, however, several objections to this theory as well:

1. An increase in gonadotropins has been

observed in menopausal women who have not complained of flushes.

2. The administration of large doses of gonadotropic hormone preparations does not produce vasomotor symptoms.

3. The hot flushes may be favorably influenced by doses of estrogen too small to inhibit the anterior pituitary gland. Hot flushes are rarely seen in the male climacteric. It would appear, therefore, that there may be other unknown factors operating to produce the vasomotor symptoms. One of these might be the hyperactivity of other glands involved in the endocrine upheaval of the climacteric, notably the thyroid and the adrenal glands. Also, one cannot entirely overlook the emotional factor as at least an accessory in the production of vasomotor symptoms. It is a common observation that flushes are usually more severe in the anxious, neurotic woman and invariably intensified in the average woman when she is subjected to unusual stress.

Nervous and psychic symptoms. During the climacteric a woman frequently suffers from headache, dizziness, and insomnia. These symptoms, as well as variable degrees of depression, with feelings of hopelessness, worthlessness, and self-condemnation are most often seen in women who have tended to be psychoneurotic in their premenopausal years. There are, however, instances of mild to severe emotional disturbances in women who previously had been considered to be quite stable. There is little doubt that the endocrine upheaval of the climacteric may be responsible for a measure of psychic disturbance. This is certainly the case in many adolescents. But we believe that the degree of psychic involvement at the climacteric is predetermined largely by the patient's personality. The specter of advancing years and impending old age is dramatically and suddenly revealed to every woman at this period of her life. Whether she reacts with relative equanimity and calm or with anxiety and depression depends on many factors, not the least of which is her own estimate of herself as a person. Her life situation and important environmental factors, however, do play a definite role. A most somber mental outlook is often conditioned by the general misinformation obtained from well-meaning friends and relatives regarding the dire consequences of the menopause.

Loss of libido is a common complaint during the climacteric and becomes more of a problem with advancing years. On the other hand, some women, once the menopause has been well established and the fear of pregnancy has been removed, tend to become more interested in sex. The relative increase in androgenic activity, occasionally present in menopausal women, may also be a factor in increased libido.

Genital symptoms. The loss of ovarian function results in the gradual atrophy of the genital organs. This is especially evident in the vagina. The mucosa shrinks and thins greatly; the vaginal secretion becomes scant and less acid. These changes render the vaginal tissues more susceptible to trauma, inflammation, and infection. Atrophic vaginitis, pruritus vulvae, and dyspareunia develop with increasing frequency as the postmenopausal phase progresses.

Muscle strength, both voluntary and involuntary, is affected by estrogen loss. In some women cystocele, rectocele, and even uterine prolapse first occur after the menopause. This may happen even in virginal women. In others whose tissues already are relaxed, symptoms first appear after the periods cease. Frequency, urgency, and stress urinary incontinence may appear or become much worse after the menopause. This undoubtedly is a result of muscle changes in the tissues surrounding the vesicle neck.

Skeletal symptoms. Pain and stiffness in the joints is a common complaint in climacteric women and is referred to as *menopausal arthralgia*. Physical and x-ray examinations do not disclose any arthritic changes. Discomfort is caused by some type of obscure change in the soft tissue surrounding joints. It is often confused with true arthritis.

Osteoporosis involves most of the bone mass. It is particularly noticeable in the spine, with the formation of "dowager's hump" (dorsal kyphosis). Pain occurs only with fractures that ultimately result.

DIFFERENTIAL DIAGNOSIS

The amenorrhea of the early climacteric period frequently arouses the suspicion of pregnancy. A pelvic examination and a demonstration of arborization of cervical mucus will ordinarily rule out this possibility. In doubtful cases a test for pregnancy may be necessary.

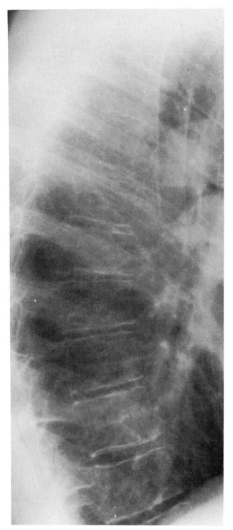

Fig. 49-3. Osteoporosis with resultant dorsal kyphosis in a 28-year-old woman who had been castrated (bilateral oophorectomy) at 20 years of age. She had not received estrogen replacement.

Not infrequently the physician sees women in their forties who are still menstruating regularly but who complain of headache, dizziness, insomnia, fatigue, and some degree of mental depression. The temptation to blame these symptoms on the menopause is very strong, and unfortunately too many physicians succumb to it. Most often the patient is suffering from a psychoneurosis or perhaps an organic disease that is totally unrelated to estrogen deprivation. The physician should hesitate to make a diagnosis of "menopausal syndrome" in patients who are still menstruating regularly,

especially if vasomotor phenomena are not prominent features of the illness.

TREATMENT OF THE CLIMACTERIC PATIENT

All women should be under the care of a physician at this critical period. The patient should be encouraged to see her doctor at least once a year. The periodic checkup should include a careful physical examination, with palpation of the breasts, inspection of the cervix, and a smear for cytologic examination. It also should provide an opportunity for the physician to allay the patient's fears and anxieties regarding the supposed dire consequences of the "change of life" and to counteract the baneful influence of well-intentioned but often misinformed lay advisers.

Psychotherapy. A careful examination and an unhurried discussion of the meaning and manifestation of the menopause is the first and perhaps most important step in the psychotherapy of the climacteric patient. This provides authoritative guidance as well as reassurrance to the middle-aged woman who at this time finds herself in need of both. No woman can blithely disregard the change in her appearance, loss of attractiveness, and prospect of progressive aging. A well-adjusted, emotionally secure woman can be encouraged to draw psychic strength from her past successes in home building and child rearing. Relieved of these responsibilities, she may turn her energies and resources to endeavors outside the home and thus maintain her feeling of usefulness and productivity.

Careful periodic reexamination, reeducation, reassurance, and mild manipulation of the patient's environment constitute the methods of superficial psychotherapy that are available to all interested physicians. Such measures plus estrogen replacement therapy will be sufficient for the vast majority of climacteric women. The patient who presents profound changes in personality or who becomes extremely depressed should be referred to a psychiatrist for more specialized treatment.

Hormone therapy. Although there remain a few physicians who oppose treatment for the climacteric women, their number decreases steadily. Most endocrinologists and gynecologists agree that estrogen replacement therapy is beneficial.

Estrogens. The most convenient and least

expensive method of employing estrogens is by the oral route. A bewildering number of effective preparations are available. These differ in their derivation, potency, duration of action, and cost. The physician should regulate the dosage by the degree to which hot flushes are relieved, insomnia corrected, and a feeling of well-being produced. In addition, the vaginal mucosa should be maintained in a healthy premenopausal state.

The preparations most often used are sodium estrone sulfate (Premarin) in daily dosages of 0.625 to 1.25 mg., ethinyl estradiol 0.05 to 0.2 mg., or diethylstilbestrol 0.5 to 1 mg. Many physicians suggest using estrogens in a cyclic manner: 3 weeks on the hormone followed by 1 week of rest in order to prevent constant tissue stimulation. Vasomotor symptoms are likely to recur during the rest period, as is withdrawal bleeding. We know of no reason why estrogen cannot be administered continuously after a dosage level adequate to prevent symptoms has been established.

UTERINE BLEEDING. Postmenopausal women being treated with estrogens occasionally develop uterine bleeding. When this happens, the estrogen is best withheld for 1 month. Bleeding should subside promptly, but in the event it continues more than 7 days, curettage is indicated. Although the bleeding is usually caused by estrogenic stimulation, a thorough search for pelvic neoplasia should be made.

ESTROGENS AFTER TREATMENT FOR CANCER. Estrogen replacement has been withheld from women who have been treated for endometrial breast or ovarian cancer on the supposition that the hormone would stimulate the growth of residual or disseminated cancer cells. Since the adrenal continues to secrete estrogen, even after oophorectomy, and since the survival rates for these tumors are improving, it does not seem likely that estrogen influences their growth significantly. It may therefore be prescribed for those women who need it.

Androgens. Whenever repeated episodes of uterine bleeding follow the administration of estrogen, the physician might employ an androgen-estrogen combination. Premarin is available with either 5 or 10 mg. of testosterone added. Estrogen-androgen combinations have been found particularly effective in the management of postmenopausal osteoporosis.

Drug therapy. In patients with many functional complaints associated with but not caused by ovarian senescence, Milprem (meprobamate, 200 to 400 mg., in combination with conjugated estrogens, 0.4 mg.) is particularly helpful. In selected cases small doses of phenobarbital (15 to 30 mg.) may be found of more help to the patient than steroids and/or tranquilizers.

References

Albright, F.: Studies on ovarian dysfunction; menopause, Endocrinology 20:24, 1936.

Fluhmann, C. F.: The management of menstrual disorders, Philadelphia, 1956, W. B. Saunders Co.

Fluhmann, C. F., and Murphy, K.: Estrogenic and gonadotropic hormones in the blood of climacteric women and castrates, Amer. J. Obstet. Gynec. 38:778, 1939.

Glass, S. J., and Shapiro, M. R.: Androgen-estrogen therapy in menopause, GP 3:39, 1951.

Greenblatt, R. B.: Estrogen therapy for postmenopausal females, New Eng. J. Med. 272:305, 1965.

Greenblatt, R. B., Mahesh, V. B., Rigas, L. C., and Shapiro, S. T.: Physiologic and clinical aspects of ovarian hormones, Arch. Derm. 89: 846, 1964.

Griffith, C. G.: Oophorectomy and cardiovascular tissues, Obstet. Gynec. 7:479, 1956.

Hamblen, E.: The use of estrogen in obstetrics and gynecology, Clin. Obstet. Gynec. 3:1021, 1960.

Kirkpatrick, H. F. W., and Robertson, J. D.: Biochemistry and physiology of nutrition, vol. II, New York, 1953, Academic Press, Inc.

Masters, W. H.: Sex steroid influence on the aging process, Amer. J. Obstet. Gynec. 74:733, 1957.

Mattingly, R. F., and Huang, W. Y.: Steroidogenesis of the menopausal and postmenopausal ovary, Amer. J. Obstet. Gynec. 103:679, 1969.

Stoddard, F. J.: The postmenopause, Obstet. Gynec. Surv. 10:801, 1955.

Wuest, J. H., Dry, T. J., and Edwards, J. E.: The degree of coronary atherosclerosis in bilaterally oophorectomized women, Circulation 7:801, 1953.

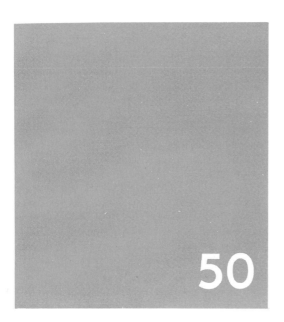

50

Clinical uses of sex hormones and related substances in gynecology

The medical treatment of reproductive tract disorders has undergone revolutionary changes in the 1960's. This has occurred because of the development and application of a large number of synthetic analogs of the sex hormones and several antagonists. It can be estimated that in 1969 well over 8 million women in the United States were utilizing one variety or another of "the pill" as ovulation inhibitors for contraceptive purposes alone, and in 1970 the trend toward even more widespread use is clearly evident. At the opposite pole, development of antagonists such as antiestrogenic substances of remarkable efficacy in inducing ovulation in the human has ushered in a new era in the treatment of certain previously hopeless types of infertility in the female. The physiologic action of the sex hormones and their clinical application have been discussed in the chapters on normal menstruation, menstrual disturbances, and infertility. The material in this chapter is intended to serve as a brief summary of practical hormone therapy in gynecologic conditions.

Most of these hormones have a similar cyclic nucleus designated as the cyclopentanoperhydrophenanthrene nucleus (Fig. 50-1). Estradiol-17β is the major estrogenic hormone in the ovary. Estrone is the principal circulating form, and estriol is the major estrogen produced by the fetoplacental unit and excreted in the urine largely in the conjugated form.

■ Gonadal steroid hormones

The gonadal steroids, estrogen, progesterone, and androgen, are available in pure crystalline form and may be produced synthetically or may be extracted from biologic sources. They are stable and contain no foreign protein that might act as an allergen when ingested or injected.

ESTROGENS

The follicular hormones are C-18 steroids, which differ in structure from androgens in that the C-19 position is lacking (Fig. 50-2).

On the basis of the physiologic action of the estrogens they may be employed clinically not only in conditions in which there is a definite deficiency of the hormone but as effective agents to depress function of the anterior lobe of the pituitary gland. Estrogen therapy has proved to be of value in the following clinical conditions:

1. To relieve menopausal symptoms
2. To treat atrophic vaginitis and vulvovaginal atrophy
3. To treat postmenopausal osteoporosis (with calcium and occasionally androgen)
4. To control hemorrhage in dysfunctional uterine bleeding
5. To inhibit ovulation in dysmenorrhea
6. To produce pseudopregnancy in the treatment of endometriosis (with or without progestins)
7. To suppress lactation
8. To correct sexual infantilism or "hypopubescence" with amenorrhea
9. To reverse functional amenorrhea (with progesterone)

10. To stimulate increased secretion of cervical mucus

11. To inhibit excessive growth in female adolescents

Some patients experience untoward side effects such as *nausea* during estrogen therapy, especially when stilbestrol is employed, *uterine bleeding* during prolonged treatment or upon withdrawal of the hormone, *swelling* and *tenderness of the breasts,* and sodium retention with *edema.*

As a rule estrogens should not be prescribed for women who have had cancer of the breast or uterus or for those who give a strong family history of these lesions because of the occasional association of long-term uninterrupted estrogen therapy with the development of cancer. There is no firm proof

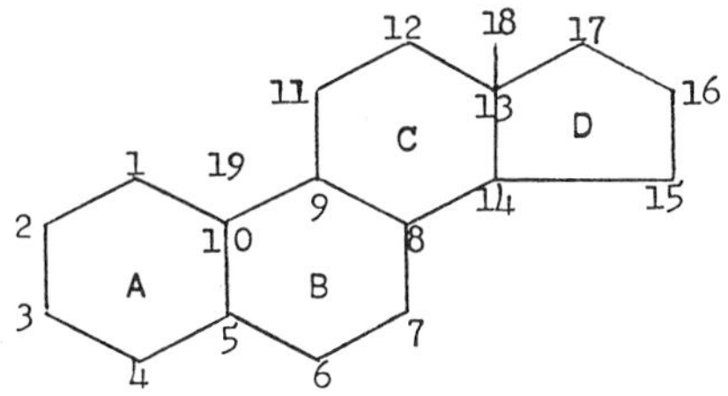

Fig. 50-1. Cyclopentanoperhydrophenanthrene nucleus.

that this occurrence represents a cause-and-effect relationship in humans. It is our opinion that most symptomatic postmenopausal or castrate women should not be denied the relief afforded by appropriate use of estrogens. Periodic examinations, including breasts, pelvis, and vaginal cytology, are indicated in these as in all postmenopausal women.

Route of administration. Estrogen preparations may be administered orally, parenterally, or topically. Oral preparations are quite effective, and there is usually little indication for parenteral therapy. Topical applications in the form of vaginal creams and suppositories are useful in the treatment of local conditions in the vagina.

Commonly employed estrogens. There are numerous commercial preparations of estrogens on the market, and to enumerate them all would only be confusing. Those most often employed by us will be discussed.

Conjugated estrogen. The oral preparation of conjugated estrogen (estrone sulfate) is effective in the management of climacteric symptoms and is marketed in dosages of 0.63, 1.25, and 2.5 mg. as Premarin, Amnestrogen, and Konogen. This material is also available for intravenous use. Premarin in 20 mg. ampules for intravenous injection may be

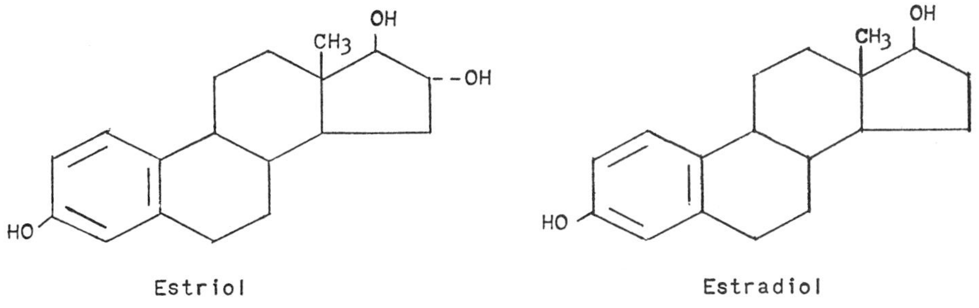

Estriol

Estradiol

Fig. 50-2. Follicular hormones.

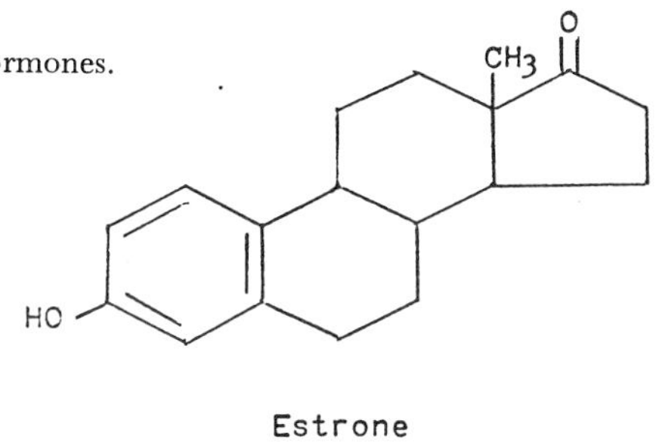

Estrone

used for temporary control of severe dysfunctional bleeding, but withdrawal bleeding must be anticipated.

Ethinyl estradiol. Ethinyl estradiol is one of the most potent estrogens available for oral administration. It is most effective in the treatment of menopausal symptoms in dosages varying from 0.02 to 0.05 mg. This preparation is on the market as Estinyl, Eticylol, and Lynoral.

Estradiol benzoate. Estradiol benzoate is a potent estrogenic substance available for intramuscular injection. If administered in dosages of 5 to 10 mg. 2 to 3 days before an expected ovulation, it may serve to increase secretion of cervical mucus and thus increase sperm receptivity.

Estradiol valerate. Estradiol valerate (Delestrogen) is a long-acting preparation for intramuscular use. Its action is prompt, and estrogenic effects are sustained for 3 weeks after a single injection of 10 to 20 mg. The solution contains 10 mg./ml. and is available in 1 and 5 ml. vials.

Diethylstilbestrol. Diethylstilbestrol (stilbestrol) is a nonsteroid stilbene compound that has marked estrogenic properties. It is widely used because it is relatively inexpensive and is therefore applicable in conditions in which high dosages of hormone are indicated as, for example, in the treatment of endometriosis. Stilbestrol is marketed in many dosages; tablets containing as little as 0.1 mg. and as much as 25 mg. are commercially available. Vaginal suppositories containing 0.5 mg. of the drug are often used in the management of atrophic vaginitis.

Dienestrol. Dienestrol is another synthetic nonsteroid estrogen that is quite potent and relatively free from adverse side effects. We have used it mainly as an intravaginal cream in the treatment of atrophic vaginitis.

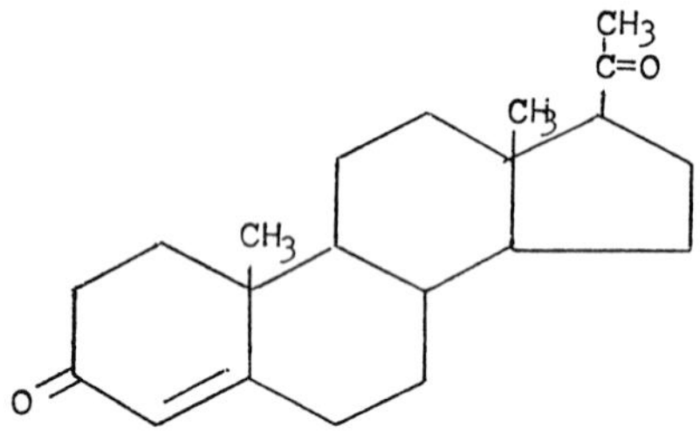

PROGESTERONE

Progesterone $(C_{21}H_{30}O_2)$ is a tetracyclic diketone produced by the corpus luteum, by the placenta, and by the adrenal cortex as a precursor of C-19 and C-21 corticosteroids (Fig. 50-3). This hormone is clinically useful in the treatment of (1) amenorrhea, (2) dysfunctional uterine bleeding, and (3) habitual abortion due to inadequate progesterone production.

In the treatment of secondary amenorrhea, progesterone is effective through its stimulating effect on both the estrogen-primed endometrium and the gonadotropic function of the pituitary gland. The withdrawal bleeding that follows a few days after the administration of progesterone has been called "medical curettage" and is applicable in the treatment of dysfunctional uterine bleeding as well as in the treatment of amenorrhea since it results in a complete shedding of the endometrium.

The administration of progesterone produces no adverse effects, and in contradistinction to estrogen there are no particular contraindications to its use.

Synthetic progestins. Several potent synthetic progestational agents are currently available. The long-acting progestational compound Delalutin is a synthetic esterified derivative of progesterone, effective only by

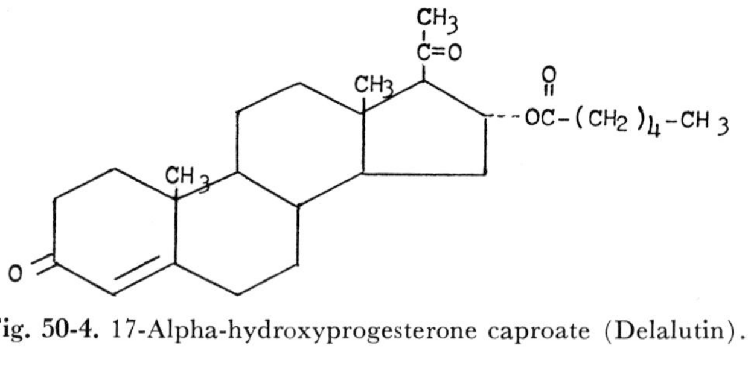

Fig. 50-3. Progesterone.

Fig. 50-4. 17-Alpha-hydroxyprogesterone caproate (Delalutin).

the parenteral route. It has very little, if any, androgenic effect. The metabolic pathway for this material is not clear since administration does not increase pregnanediol excretion. Each milliliter of this preparation contains 125 mg. of 17-alpha-hydroxyprogesterone caproate, and a single injection of 125 to 500 mg. is quite feasible. Local skin reactions occasionally occur with large doses. Since the effect of this material is sustained for 12 to 16 days, it becomes a most convenient method in the therapy of progesterone deficiency disorders of pregnancy. It should be emphasized that the efficacy of progesterone or any of its analogs in the treatment of threatened abortion is equivocal. In selected cases supplemental progesterone may be needed in order to provide a more favorable uterine environment for implantation and early growth and development of the embryo. In some cases myometrial activity from inadequate progesterone effect may be offset by timely administration of the hormone. Unfortunately, if the threatened abortion is not caused by progesterone deficiency, addition of this material substantially increases the chance of retention of the fetus as a missed abortion.

Oral synthetic progestins. Phenomenal numbers of orally active progestins have been produced in recent years. Applezweig reported 253 compounds derived from eight basic chemical structures. Only a small percentage of these are fully approved for clinical use. In the United States the most widely employed are as listed in Table 14.

Medroxyprogesterone acetate. Of the oral preparations in current use medroxyprogesterone acetate (Provera) is the most purely progesterone-like in action. Provera lacks estrogen activity, and none is added. It is an effective agent in testing endogenous estrogen production in patients with amenorrhea. When used for a long period of time, for example in the treatment of endometriosis, breakthrough bleeding frequently occurs at some point in the course of therapy unless small amounts of estrogen are added. If estrogen is not administered, Provera induces atrophic changes demonstrable in the vaginal smear after several months of uninterrupted use. The drug has no apparent androgenic activity and does not appear to inhibit either pituitary or adrenal hormone production. Tablets containing 2, 5, and 10 mg. are available. Parenteral Provera, 50 mg. (1 ml.), is equal in potency to 250 mg. of Delalutin, and

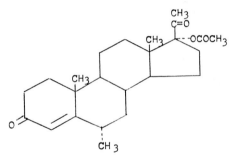

Fig. 50-5. Medroxyprogesterone acetate (Provera), in which no estrogen is added.

Table 14. Composition of synthetic progestational agents

	Acetoxy-progestins	
Trade name	*Progestin*	*Estrogen*
Delalutin	12 hydroxyprogesterone caproate	None
Provera	Medroxyprogesterone acetate 10 mg.	None
Provest	Medroxyprogesterone acetate 10 mg.	Ethinyl estradiol 0.05 mg.
Protex	Medroxyprogesterone acetate 5 mg.	Ethinyl estradiol 0.05 mg.
	19-Norprogestins	
Enovid	Norethynodrel 10, 5, and 2.5 mg.	Mestranol 0.15, 0.075, and 0.1 mg., respectively
Norlutin	Norethindrone 10 mg.	
Norlestrin	Norethindrone acetate 2.5 mg.	Ethinyl estradiol 0.05 mg.
Ortho-Novum	Norethindrone 10 and 2 mg.	Mestranol 0.1 mg.
Norinyl	Norethindrone 10 and 2 mg.	Mestranol 0.1 mg.
Lyndiol Gestanin	Allylestranol 5 mg.	Mestranol 0.15 mg.

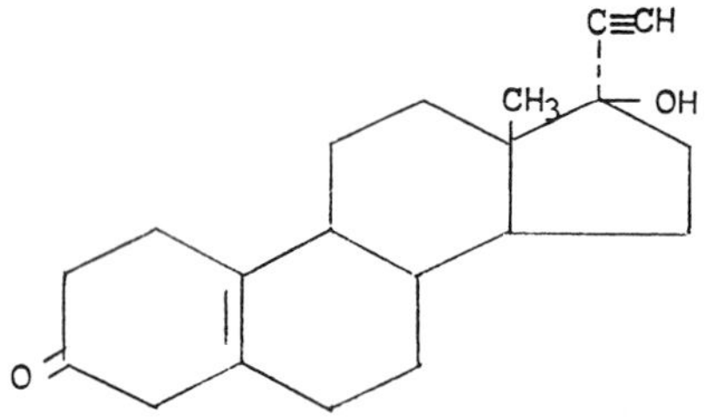

Fig. 50-6. Norethynodrel, Enovid (estrogen added) —0.15 mg. of ethinyl estradiol 3-methyl ether to 9.85 mg. of norethynodrel.

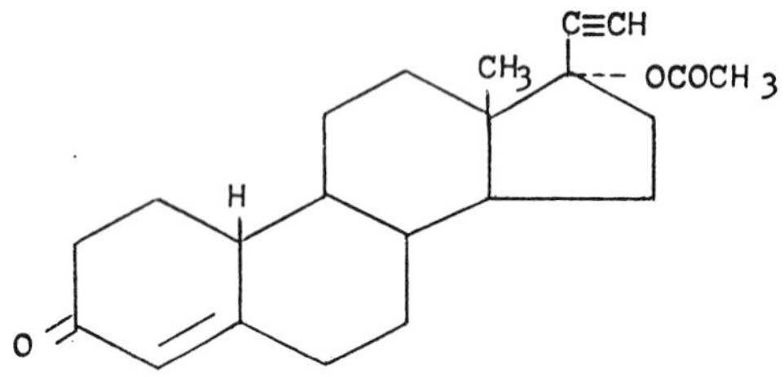

Fig. 50-7. Norethindrone acetate, Norlutate (estrogen added)—0.05 mg. of ethinyl estradiol to 4.95 mg. of norethindrone acetate.

its duration of action is approximately twice that of Delalutin.

Norethynodrel. Norethynodrel (Enovid) contains about 5% inherent estrogen activity as well as 0.15 mg. of ethinyl estradiol 3-methyl ether, which is added to 9.85 mg. of norethynodrel in preparing each 10 mg. tablet. It has little or no androgenic potency but produces slight pituitary gonadotropin inhibition, possibly because of its estrogen content. Side effects of nausea and occasionally acne may be noted.

Norethindrone acetate. Norethindrone acetate (Norlestrin) is a true 19-nortestosterone. It has a slight inherent estrogen activity, which is increased slightly by the addition of 0.05 mg. of ethinyl acetate to 4.95 mg. of norethindrone acetate per 5 mg. tablet. The progestational action is similar to that of Enovid. Norlestrin has increased inhibitory effect on pituitary activity and increased androgen activity.

The orally active progestins are of indisputable value in the treatment of *dysfunctional uterine bleeding,* especially when it is associated with endometrial hyperplasia and excessive flow so commonly seen in the premenopausal years. In the treatment of *endo-*metriosis, the pseudopregnancy induced by the oral progestins has almost replaced medical treatment with either estrogens or androgens.

Control of conception. The remarkable efficacy of oral progestins in control of conception has not been equalled by any other method. When used consistently from the fifth to the twenty-fifth day of the cycle, these agents appear to be 100% effective. Preparations containing 2 mg. of the progestogen and small amounts of estrogen are just as effective as larger dosages. The mechanism of action has been a matter of heated debate. Suppression of ovulation occurs in most but not in all instances; in approximately 3% to 5% of women, ovulation does occur. The critical action in inhibition of ovulation is an interference with synthesis or release of pituitary gonadotropins, luteinizing hormone (LH) being particularly affected. Changes in the cervical mucus and in the endometrium appear to be contributory in their efficacy.

Endometrial carcinoma. Progestins are used as adjuvant therapy in the treatment of endometrial carcinoma and in the management of recurrent or metastatic adenocarcinoma of the endometrium. The rationale is based on the ability of these drugs to inhibit pituitary activity and to induce endometrial glandular atrophy. Subjective relief is often striking, and although objective improvement is inconstant, therapeutic trial is worthwhile. Long-acting preparations, Depo-Provera or Delalutin described earlier, when administered in large doses for about 14 weeks per course, give objective improvement in about 30% of cases and subjective improvement in about 70%. All cases that show favorable response appear to do so by the end of the third month of treatment.

ANDROGENS

The tendency to induce masculinizing changes seriously limits the use of androgen therapy in the female. Virilizing signs include increased oiliness of the skin, acne and facial hirsutism, deepening of the voice, and enlargement of the clitoris. Androgens exhibit moderate inhibiting effect upon the production of pituitary gonadotropins. For this reason and in order to modify the action of estrogen on the endometrium and breasts, androgen therapy has been used in a wide

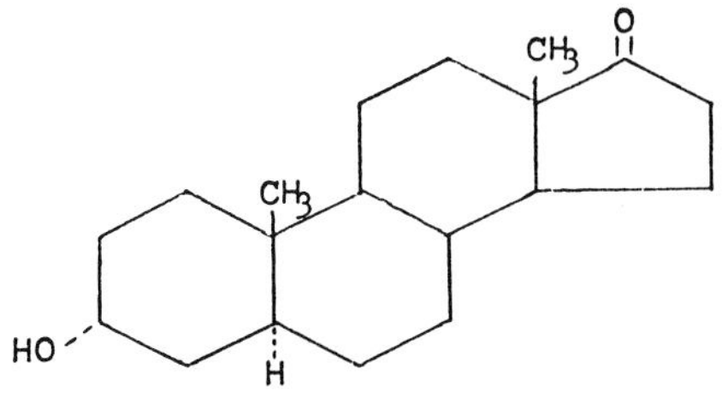

Androsterone

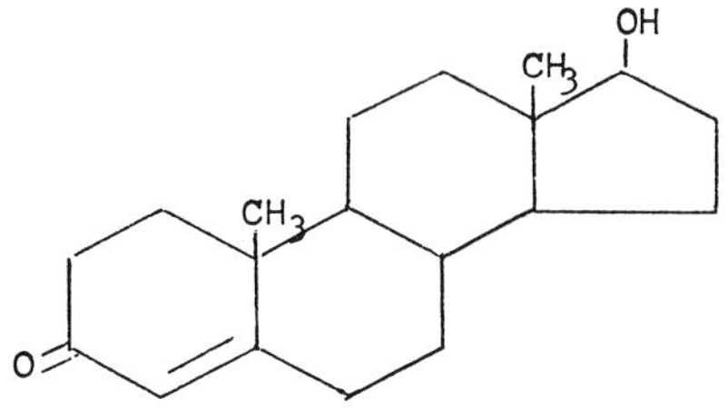

Testosterone

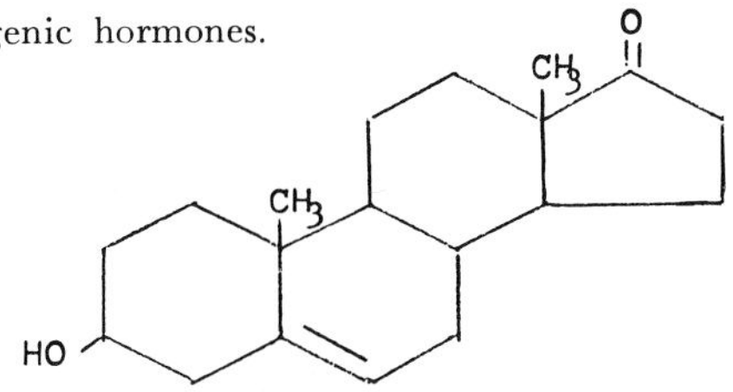

Fig. 50-8. Androgenic hormones.

Dehydroepiandrosterone

variety of menstrual disorders, particularly dysfunctional uterine bleeding and endometriosis. More effective orally active progestins have fortunately replaced androgens in the treatment of these disorders.

Androgens do, however, have a very important place in the therapy of breast cancer with bone metastasis. Testosterone propionate, 250 to 300 mg. per week is the usual dose. There is evidence that metastasis is delayed and discomfort is less on this regimen, although the virilizing symptoms appear when such large amounts must be given. Dromostanolone propionate (Drolban), an analog of testosterone, appears to induce fewer undesirable hormonal effects. The drug is administered in 100 mg. doses intramuscularly two to three times a week. Androgens may be administered orally as tablets of methyltestosterone, 10 or 25 mg. daily, but the oral administration appears to give less satisfactory results.

COMBINED ESTROGEN-ANDROGEN THERAPY

Combined steroid therapy was devised in an attempt to reduce the undesirable side effects of the two hormones by the administration of smaller dosages of each. The combination of these two hormones is available for oral and parenteral administration in a variety of dosage levels. The oral tablets usually contain methyltestosterone 5 to 10 mg., and estradiol 1 mg., or ethinyl estradiol 0.02 to 0.04 mg., whereas the parenteral preparations contain estradiol benzoate 1 mg. and testosterone propionate 20 mg. These drugs are particularly useful in the treatment of senile osteoporosis.

■ Gonadotropic hormones

The discovery of the gonadotropic hormones and the demonstration of their ability to stimulate follicular growth, ovulation, and corpus luteum formation in laboratory animals aroused the expectation that these substances would prove to be effective tools in the treatment of menstrual disturbances and infertility, but the results obtained with currently available commercial preparations such as equine gonadotropin have been disappointing. This material can stimulate follicular growth in the human ovary, but the addition of chorionic gonadotropin does not result in ovulation. Furthermore, equine gonadotropin is a complex protein and may cause serious allergic reactions in sensitized persons. However, human gonadotropic extracts currently under investigation show great promise.

Human pituitary gonadotropic extracts

have been prepared from autopsy material and studied chemically by Gemzell in Sweden. The quantity available is extremely small, but the successes reported by Gemzell and by Buxton and Herrmann in the United States are exceptional. Extracts of *postmenopausal urine* (*Pergonal*) prepared in Italy have also been successful and are more readily available. The human pituitary gonadotropin or the follicle-stimulating hormone (FSH) extracted from postmenopausal urine is given first. When it is estimated that sufficient follicular maturation is obtained, ovulation is induced with human chorionic gonadotropin (HCG).

Clomiphene. Clomiphene citrate (MRL-41) is an analog of the synthetic estrogen chlorotrianisene (Tace). It has an extremely potent ovarian stimulatory action and has been used mainly for this purpose in the treatment of infertility, primary and secondary amenorrhea, and dysfunctional uterine bleeding. Wall and his group showed that atypical endometria may revert to normal during treatment with clomiphene.

The mechanisms of action of the two drugs are not completely understood, but it is recognized that there are differences and that responses can be predicted on the basis of the patient's hormonal status. Neither is effective in patients with consistently high gonadotropic secretion suggestive of total ovarian failure. Clomiphene in particular is effective only in patients showing positive estrogenic activity as noted in anovulatory menstrual cycles, whereas Pergonal followed by HCG therapy is effective in some cases of secondary amenorrhea associated with relatively low estrogenic activity and moderately elevated pituitary gonadotropins.

Side reactions with the new gonadotropic substances and with clomiphene are important. All of them cause overstimulation with enlargement of the ovary and multiple ovulation. Because the cysts enlarge so rapidly these patients must be examined frequently during treatment. Ovarian enlargements persist for 3 to 13 weeks after the drug is discontinued, but all regress and operation is indicated only for rupture or torsion.

■ Adrenal hormones

Cortisone is the only specifically effective adrenal hormone used in the treatment of gynecologic disorders. This hormone has ini-

tiated ovulatory cycles in women with amenorrhea due to congenital adrenal hyperplasia. In this condition the excessive secretion of adrenal estrogen-androgen suppresses the production of pituitary gonadotropins, which results in ovarian failure. Cortisone, by depressing ACTH, decreases the stimulus to the adrenals, thus reducing adrenal androgen-estrogen production. The lowering of the level of these steroids permits resumption of anterior pituitary gonadotropic function and consequent normalization of ovarian activity. Cortisone may also be effectively employed in the differential diagnosis between adrenal hyperplasia and adrenal tumor. The excretion of 17-ketosteroids is elevated in both conditions. It is greatly reduced in adrenal hyperplasia by the administration of cortisone but is unaffected if an adrenal tumor is present.

Cortisol, prednisone, and other of the cortisone preparations have been used to reduce pelvic fibrosis associated with radiation therapy for pelvic cancer, pelvic inflammatory disease with scarring and occlusion of the fallopian tubes, and to hasten the preparation of the patient for correction of urinary or rectal fistula. Except for their effects on fistulas, the results have not been outstanding and scarcely warrant the use of these drugs. Hydrocortisone in topical form of 1% to 2.5% ointment or lotion is useful in treatment of pruritus vulvae and ani.

Since oral or parenteral cortisone can produce adrenal atrophy, it is important to question patients about previously taken medications before operation or delivery and to provide replacement if these drugs have been taken for any protracted period of time within the preceding 3 months.

■ Thyroid therapy

Menstrual disturbances and infertility may be the earliest manifestations of either mild hypothyroidism or the hypometabolic syndrome (hypometabolism). When there is clinical or laboratory evidence of such dysfunction, the administration of a potent thyroid preparation is an effective therapeutic tool. Our choice of thyroid preparation has been thyroid extract (Proloid) in dosages of 65 to 130 mg. (1 to 2 grains). The maintenance dose is an amount slightly less than that which produces untoward symptoms and should be continued for several months.

A crystalline thyroid compound (triiodo-thyronine) is available under the trade names Cytomel and Trionine. This preparation has the advantage of rapid therapeutic effect and quick dissipation of action upon withdrawal. It is particularly efficacious in cases of hypometabolism where there is faulty utilization of thyroid hormone by the individual tissue cells because of the inability of the tissue enzymes to deiodinate thyroxine to triiodothyronine. The drug may be administered in dosages of 25 to 100 μg daily. Fifty micrograms is equal to approximately 60 to 100 mg. of desiccated thyroid.

References

Applezweig, N.: Steroid drugs, New York, 1962, McGraw-Hill Book Co.

Bishop, P. M. F.: Hormones and cancer, Clin. Obstet. Gynec. 3:1109, 1960.

Buxton, C. L., and Herrmann, W.: Induction of ovulation in the human with human gonadotropins, Yale J. Biol. Med. 33:145, 1960.

Claesson, L., Högberg, B., Rosenberg, T., and Westman, A.: Crystalline human chorionic gonadotropin and its biological action, Acta Endocr. 1:1, 1948.

Dorfman, R. I.: Steroid hormones in gynecology; a review, Obstet. Gynec. Surv. 18:65, 1963.

Federal Drug Administration report on Enovid: Ad hoc advisory committee for the evaluation of a possible etiologic relation with thromboembolic conditions, J.A.M.A. 185:776, 1963.

Fishman, J., Bredlow, H. L., and Gallagher, T. F.: Oxidative metabolism of estradiol, J. Biol. Chem. 235:3104, 1960.

Garcia, C. R., Pincus, G., and Rock, J.: Effects of three 19-nor steroids on human ovulation and menstruation, Amer. J. Obstet. Gynec. 75: 82, 1958.

Gemzell, C. A.: Induction of ovulation with human pituitary gonadotropins, Fertil. Steril. 13:153, 1962.

Gold, J. J., Borushek, S., Smith, L., and Scommegna, A.: Synthetic progestins; a review, Int. J. Fertil. 10:99, 1965.

Goldzieher, J. W.: Dobule-blind trial of a progestin in habitual abortion, J.A.M.A. 188:651, 1964.

Johannisson, E., Tillinger, K. G., and Diczfalusy, E.: Effect of oral contraceptives on the ovarian reaction to human gonadotropins in amenorrheic women, Fertil. Steril. 16:292, 1965.

Kennedy, B. J.: A progestogen for treatment of advanced endometrial cancer, J.A.M.A. 184: 758, 1963.

Kistner, R. W.: The use of progestational agents in obstetrics and gynecology, Clin. Obstet. Gynec. 3:1047, 1960.

Leach, R. B., and Margulis, R. R.: Inhibition of adrenocortical responsiveness during progestin therapy, Amer. J. Obstet. Gynec. 92:762, 1965.

Pildes, R. B.: Induction of ovulation with clomiphene, Amer. J. Obstet. Gynec. 91:466, 1965.

Reerink, E. H., Scholer, H. F. L., Westerhof, P., Wuerido, A., Kassenaar, A. A. H., Diczfalusy, E., and Tillinger, K. C.: A new class of hormonally active steroid, Nature 186:168, 1960.

Roy, S., Greenblatt, R. B., Mahesh, V. B., and Jungck, E. C.: Clomiphene citrate; further observations on its use in induction of ovulation in the human and its mode of action, Fertil. Steril. 14:575, 1963.

Rudel, H. W., Martinez-Manautou, J., and Maqueo-Topete, M.: The role of progestogens in the hormonal control of fertility, Fertil. Steril. 16:158, 1965.

Ryan, G. M., Jr., Craig, J., and Reid, D. E.: Histology of the uterus and ovaries after long-term cyclic norethynodrel therapy, Amer. J. Obstet. Gynec. 90:715, 1964.

Southam, A. L., and Turksoy, R. N.: Induction of ovulation with clomiphene citrate, Bull. Sloane Hosp. Wom. 10:240, 1964.

Steiner, G. J., Kistner, R. W., and Craig, J. M.: Histologic effects of progestins on hyperplasia and carcinoma in situ of the endometrium, Metabolism 14:356, 1965.

Tyler, E. T.: Current status of oral contraception, J.A.M.A. 187:562, 1964.

Wall, J. A., Franklin, R. R., Kaufman, R. H., and Kaplan, A. L.: The effects of clomiphene citrate on the endometrium, Amer. J. Obstet. Gynec. 93:842, 1965.

Wallach, S., and Henneman, P.: Prolonged estrogen therapy in postmenopausal women, J.A.M.A. 171:1637, 1959.

Whedon, G. D.: Effects of high calcium intakes on bones, blood and soft tissues; relationship of calcium intake to balance in osteoporosis, Fed. Proc. 18:1112, 1959.

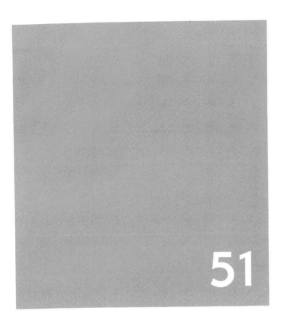

51

Preoperative evaluation and preparation; postoperative care; gynecologic operations

The best surgical results are obtained when a qualified surgeon operates upon and directs the postoperative care of a patient who has been prepared both physically and emotionally for the operation. Although there may be other physicians involved in the many aspects of preoperative and postoperative care, it is the surgeon's responsibility to see that such care is optimal.

■ Preoperative preparation

A surgical procedure should not be scheduled until adequate preliminary study and preparation have been carried out. A complete physical examination is so much a part of good medical practice that it seems redundant to mention it, yet this is too often carried out in such an offhand or incomplete manner as to constitute a real danger to the

patient. All abnormal findings that could possibly have an adverse effect on the patient during her surgical venture should be adequately studied. Full appreciation of the cardiac status is essential in older patients. A complete blood count, urinalysis, and a serologic test for syphilis constitute the bare minimum in preoperative laboratory studies.

It is best to avoid cathartics before surgery, and in general a cleansing enema the night before or the morning of operation is adequate unless gastrointestinal involvement is anticipated, in which case more detailed preparation is necessary. All food and liquids by mouth should be withheld from midnight on, regardless of the type of anesthesia to be used. A good night's sleep before surgery is desirable and should be ensured by the use of suitable hypnotic or analgesic drugs or both.

The evening before surgery is an excellent time for the anesthetist to become acquainted with his patient for the following day. This procedure not only allows the patient to discuss anesthesia with the individual who is to administer it, but also the answering of questions and a minimum of "small talk" pays large dividends in patient relaxation. The anesthetist also gains much in this meeting because he may wish to check certain physical findings as well as acquaint himself with the studies as noted on the chart.

Metabolism and nutrition. Women with diabetes require special consideration before surgery. Even though a diabetic patient is under full control at the time of admission, daily blood sugar determinations for a minimum of 2 days before operation are desirable, except in emergencies. Caloric requirements in the form of intravenous sugar with covering insulin should be given on the day of surgery and each day thereafter until oral feedings are tolerated. Obviously daily blood sugar determinations are essential postoperatively.

Many women come to an operation with tissues in poor condition because of a lifetime of poor dietary habits. Zealous as we may be in our attempts to correct malnutrition, it cannot possibly be done in a few days of preoperative care. High concentrations of vitamins, minerals, and proteins administered parenterally, however, are of considerable aid to wound healing. One of the most essential components is a high *ascorbic acid level*. With the cutting or injury of any tissue, there is an immediate mobilization of ascorbic acid to the point of injury. Maintaining high levels of this water-soluble vitamin requires steady high dosage, particularly in the malnourished person.

Blood transfusions. It is not wise to perform elective operations on women with a hemoglobin of less than 11 grams. Patients with anemia caused by chronic blood loss from the genital tract or from a nutritional cause are best prepared for surgery by daily transfusions of 500 ml. of blood; with repeated heavy losses of blood, 1,000 ml. a day may be necessary. Aside from the correction of anemia, blood will facilitate wound healing and help prevent wound infection.

There should be 1,000 ml. of compatible blood on hand for all patients scheduled for major gynecologic procedures. For those having radical surgery there must be 3,000 ml. of blood immediately available.

Urinary tract. A urinalysis should be performed before any operation; at times more complete diagnostic urologic studies are indicated. When operating for massive fixed lesions of all types, or with radical surgery for malignant disease, it is wise to be aware of the position of the ureters or of ureteral obstruction or narrowing beforehand. The surgeon may find it useful to have upper urinary tract catheters in place at the time of surgery to act as guides in selected patients. An indwelling catheter in the bladder to keep it empty during gynecologic laparotomy will facilitate the operation and reduce bladder injuries.

Fluid and electrolyte balance. In the average elective surgical patient there is no need for electrolyte studies unless there is a suggestion of derangement. Patients scheduled for radical procedures, however, should have complete base-line studies of their electrolytes as well as of the protein fractions. Preoperative blood volume studies are essential in these patients also.

Special colon preparation. When the surgeon is operating for carcinoma either of the uterus or ovary, particularly when a radical procedure is planned, it is necessary to have a fully prepared bowel, even though no bowel surgery is anticipated. Resections, ureteral transplants, or simple repairs may then be accomplished with greater use and safety. The following regimen is currently in use and seems satisfactory:

1. Castor oil, 60 ml., in the afternoon of the day before operation
2. Neomycin, 0.5 Gm., every 4 hours for 6 doses, the day before surgery
3. Colonic irrigations until clear the evening before operation
4. Low-residue diet liquids only at the evening meal just before operation
5. A soapsuds enema at 6 A.M. the day of operation

Preoperative medication. For sedation and to lessen bronchial secretions, morphine, 8 to 10 mg., and atropine or scopolamine, 0.4 mg., are administered subcutaneously about 45 minutes before anesthesia. For the occasional patient who is sensitive to morphine, Dilaudid, 1 to 3 mg., may be substituted.

■ Care during surgery

The surgeon is responsible for the welfare of the patient at all times during the operation, even though the anesthetist carries out his all-important duties. Selection of the operative procedure and the facility with which it is performed, the administration of the proper amounts of fluids and blood, and careful attention to the details of anesthesia all contribute to the end result.

■ Postoperative care

Fluids and electrolytes. A 5% glucose solution is generally given intravenously during an operation and allowed to continue when the procedure is completed. Intravenous therapy can be discontinued when the patient is able to take fluid by mouth without discomfort. The average patient does not require intravenous replacement after the second day following a major gynecologic procedure.

There is a tendency for water and sodium to be retained after any operation, and for this reason saline solutions should not be administered during the procedure or during the first 24 hours thereafter unless a special need exists. During the second postoperative day, if the full amount of fluid required (2 to 3 L.) must be given intravenously, 500 to 1,000 ml. of 0.85% saline in 5% glucose solution may be given if the patient has been vomiting or has perspired profusely. Patients who are losing fluid and electrolytes, for instance, those on gastrointestinal suction, need more than glucose. The basic needs can be maintained by replacing the drainage, volume for volume, with 0.85% saline or Ringer's solution.

Because of water retention on the day of operation and the first postoperative day, the urinary output often is not above 750 ml., but the physician should be concerned if the volume falls below 500 ml. On the second postoperative day and thereafter the urinary output should be at least 1,000 ml. a day.

Potassium replacement is essential in patients with diarrhea, intestinal fistula, constant intestinal suction, or ureteral transplants into the bowel. The daily requirement for potassium is met by adding 2.2 Gm. (30 mEq.) of potassium chloride to 1,000 ml. of 5% glucose solution. Administration time should be at least 1 hour. When serum potassium falls to 3 mEq. or lower, 10 Gm. of potassium chloride may be given over a 12-hour period. When the cellular potassium level is low, the patient complains of weakness and extreme lassitude, whereas the electrocardiogram often shows flat T waves that may even be inverted. Prolonged potassium deficiency leads to circulatory failure and myocardial necrosis. Paralytic ileus can be induced by the resultant decrease in tone of both skeletal and smooth muscle. An electrocardiographic study should be run in any postoperative patient demonstrating these symptoms even though the serum potassium level is normal because tissue potassium can be reduced while the serum level is maintained.

Blood and plasma. Essential as electrolyte balance is known to be, blood and plasma requirements also demand close observation. Blood volume measurements would indicate accurately the need for replacement, but since such determinations are not always possible or practical, we depend on measurements of blood loss, postoperative blood pressure, and the general condition of the patient. A simple way of estimating blood loss during the operation is to weigh sponges, the increased weight in grams being roughly the volume of blood in milliliters absorbed by the sponge, and add this to the amount in the suction bottle. The total is then increased by one third to account for the amount in the packs, drapes, and towels, etc., which cannot be weighed. It is important to calcu-

late blood loss in this manner because it is not possible to estimate it accurately, and in most instances the estimated blood loss is far less than the actual amount. Every patient who is operated upon does not need to be transfused, but excessive blood loss should be replaced, starting during the operation and continuing until the loss has been met. In patients for whom no replacement has been deemed necessary, a fall in blood pressure, signs of shock, or maintained hypotension suggests the need for blood.

Sedation. Pain-relieving drugs can be given safely if the dosage for each patient is individualized and if each patient is seen often enough during the postoperative period to observe the drug effect. Morphine in doses of 8 to 15 mg. (depending on the age and patient weight) and meperidine (Demerol), 50 to 100 mg., are the drugs of choice for pain relief. The use of various tranquilizing preparations in the postoperative period greatly lessens the need for sedative and analgesic drugs. Anxiety and fear are often reduced, if not abolished, by Librium, Compazine, or similar drugs. The soothing effects of these drugs are helpful when women have radium applicators in place and are required to lie essentially in one position for several days or in women with a vesicovaginal fistula repair, who in some instances must lie on their abdomen for about 10 days.

Activity and ambulation. The patient should be kept flat until she has reacted fully from the anesthetic. Constant observation (preferably in a recovery room) for vomiting, stabilization of blood pressure, and other vital signs is essential. When fully reacted, the patient must be encouraged to move in bed at least every hour. Elderly women may dangle their feet over the side of the bed 4 hours after surgery if they have reacted from the anesthetic and should be out of bed for short intervals starting 8 hours postoperatively. The average woman may be out of bed the first postoperative day and take some steps by the second day. The advantages of early ambulation are numerous; increase in diaphragmatic excursion, the prevention of venous stasis, and improved peristalsis leave no doubt as to the benefits from early movement. The older the patient is the earlier ambulation is desired.

Bladder care. Bed rest coupled with a pelvic operation frequently causes urinary retention. To forestall this complication a catheter is generally left in place until the end of the first postoperative day after hysterectomy. This not only allows for accurate measurement of output but does away with the discomfort of urinary bladder retention. As a rule the patient will void without difficulty when the catheter is withdrawn. With vaginal plastic operations the problem is generally more difficult since many patients are operated upon for stress incontinence as well as for other types of relaxations. There is little uniformity among gynecologists as to how long a retention catheter should be left in place after repair work or even whether one should be used. It seems to us that 5 days is about as soon as our patients will void well after a vaginal plastic operation, and for this reason we leave the catheter in place until then. The patient is checked for residual urine twice after she voids, and if she retains more than 100 ml. of urine, the catheter may be replaced for another 24 hours, or the residual may be checked three times during the next 24 hours, which will serve to empty the bladder completely and aid in its function. If she cannot void at all or passes only small amounts of urine, the catheter must be replaced. Gantrisin, 3 to 4 Gm. daily, is prescribed while the catheter is in place.

Complete anuria may be noted shortly after any gynecologic operation. This may result either from pathologic causes such as shock, lower nephron nephrosis or a cortical necrosis, or from mechanical blockage of the urinary tract, particularly the ureters. An exact diagnosis should be made within 12 to 18 hours; consequently cystoscopy and attempts to pass ureteral catheters are advisable. If the ureters are blocked, it generally means they are either ligated or cut and ligated; this must be corrected promptly. If the patient is in very poor condition and cannot stand another abdominal operation, bilateral nephrostomies can be done. This procedure is rarely necessary if the diagnosis is made early. In almost every patient with surgical ureteral obstruction the cut ends can be anastomosed or the severed ureter can be implanted into the bladder. The corrective procedures that may be carried out are detailed by Beecham.

Anuria from lower nephron nephrosis is treated in exactly the same manner after a surgical procedure as in any other patient.

Gastrointestinal tract. Peristalsis is usually heard on the second postoperative day, and if so it is safe to allow fluids by mouth. In case of doubt, fluid should be withheld until there is either auscultatory evidence of peristalsis or direct evidence of free passage of gas from the anus. A saline or mild soapsuds enema may be given on the third or fourth postoperative day. If given on the second day, the patient often has trouble expelling the fluid. Soft and solid foods may be added to the patient's diet as tolerated.

Adynamic ileus follows any type of abdominal surgery; the degree to which it becomes a problem depends on the amount of operative trauma, the amount of time tissues were exposed, the amount of handling and packing around the intestines, and the emotional balance of the patient. After the first postoperative day, adynamic ileus may be treated by the insertion of a rectal tube and the administration of an enema. If these are ineffectual, Prostigmin (1:2,000), 1 ml. every 3 hours for 3 doses, may be tried. Meperidine, 50 mg., and chlorpromazine (Thorazine), 25 mg., may be administered subcutaneously for pain relief. If the distention is still present, continuous gastric and intestinal drainage should be instituted with either a Levin or a Miller-Abbott tube. Intestinal obstruction is an unusual postoperative complication after pelvic operations, but the characteristic clinical and x-ray signs will usually be obvious.

Postoperative infection and wound dehiscence. Wound infection may follow any operation, even though meticulous technique is used. Infections mean that pathogenic organisms have been introduced into the wound during the procedure. When a wound infection does occur, the operating team, the nursing staff, and the technique should be studied in an attempt to determine the reason. Wound dehiscence may occur because the wound in a chronically malnourished, iron-deficient person cannot heal properly, but occasionally this complication is encountered in presumably normal women. Careful closure of the incision will keep dehiscence at a minimum.

Venous thrombosis and embolic phenomena remain an ever-present threat to the well-being of the postoperative gynecologic patient. Although the incidence of thrombophlebitis has been sharply reduced in recent years, it must be constantly searched for on daily rounds if we are to diagnose and treat embolization before a fatality occurs. Thrombophlebitis is treated as in other patients.

■ Gynecologic operations

No attempt will be made to describe the many operative procedures the gynecologist is prepared to execute. Excellent illustrations and descriptive text are provided in the works of TeLinde and Parsons and Ulfelder. We urge those interested in the various techniques to study these completed works.

MINOR OPERATIONS

Dilatation and curettage (D and C). Dilatation and curettage is the most common operative procedure employed in gynecology. The cervical canal is dilated to allow a curet to be passed into the uterus. The endometrial cavity is scraped, and the tissue obtained is sent to the pathologist for microscopic study.

Biopsy and conization of the cervix. When a dilatation and curettage is being performed, it is wise to take a biopsy of the cervix. This additional step does not complicate the procedure and may provide important information on unsuspected cellular dysplasia. If there is evident chronic cervicitis or if a more extensive study of the tissue is desired, the entire lesion on the portio, the squamocolumnar junction, and a portion of the lower cervical canal can be obtained by removing a cone-shaped portion of tissue with a knife. With this "cold conization" the tissue is not coagulated as it is during electrothermic conization. This type of biopsy is curative as well as diagnostic because the abnormal tissue is removed. Troublesome bleeding is best controlled by suture.

Dilatation and evacuation (D and E). Dilatation and evacuation is, as the name implies, an operation to empty the uterus of its contents. It often becomes necessary when treating incomplete or inevitable abortions. Since incomplete abortions make up the vast majority of these cases and dilatation of the cervix has already taken place, the procedure is actually one of evacuation. In addition to the evacuation, rewarding information often comes from taking quadrant cervical biopsies at the same time.

Cauterization of the cervix. Cauterizing a cervix is generally considered an office procedure for proved chronic cervicitis. It is reserved largely for young women with negative cytologic smears.

Trachelorrhaphy. Cervical plastic operations of many different types are referred to as trachelorrhaphies. These operations have been largely replaced by more understanding use of cautery or conization techniques. *Cervical amputation* is generally reserved for use with the Manchester-Fothergill vaginal plastic operation.

Bartholin gland marsupialization. A cyst in the vulvovaginal gland usually follows acute infection. It is best treated by marsupialization when it is quiescent.

Simple vulvectomy. When the entire epithelial surface of the vulva is removed, we speak of the operation as a simple vulvectomy; the labia majora, minora, and clitoris are usually also removed. The line of excision ends at the vulvovaginal junction or just within the canal. It is not necessary to remove much subcutaneous fat.

ABDOMINAL OPERATIONS

Hysterectomy. When both the corpus and the cervix of the uterus are removed, the operation is termed *complete* or *total hysterectomy*. In this operation the body of the uterus and the cervix are separated from their attachments to the ovarian ligaments, round ligaments, fallopian tubes, anterior and posterior leaves of the broad ligaments, bladder, and cardinal ligaments and are then removed by a circular incision around the superior vaginal fornices.

Supracervical, supravaginal, subtotal, or incomplete hysterectomy. Supracervical, supravaginal, subtotal, or incomplete hysterectomy are the terms used to designate an operation in which only the body of the uterus is removed, the cervix being left in place. This was the usual procedure until about 1945, when complete hysterectomy began to replace it. The change was brought about by a seemingly high incidence of carcinoma of the cervical stump and the annoyance of discharge and pain from chronically infected cervices left behind.

Vaginal hysterectomy. The uterus can be removed vaginally as part of the operative treatment of prolapse or when hysterectomy is indicated, even though the structure is well supported. Both the cervix and the corpus are excised. Although vaginal hysterectomy is easiest when the uterus is normal in size or only slightly enlarged, it can be performed when the organ is greatly distorted by myomas.

Fundectomy. With fundectomy, also called *defundation,* only the fundal portion of the uterus is removed. If enough endometrium is left, the patient may continue to menstruate scantily but regularly. This procedure is rarely used today.

Myomectomy. Myomectomy is the operative removal of fibromyomas from the uterine wall. Single tumors may be removed, or multiple myomectomy may be performed. If the defects are carefully closed, they heal well, and if all the fibroids can be excised, recurrences are rare. It is one of the most satisfying gynecologic operations and should be considered for young women with symptom-producing tumors, particularly those who have had no children.

Uterine suspension. Uterine suspension is mentioned only for completeness since it is rarely done today. There was a time when the uterus was suspended for a variety of reasons, none of which has stood the test of time. Today the operation is employed almost exclusively as part of the conservative surgical treatment of pelvic inflammatory disease or endometriosis when the uterus is bound down in the cul-de-sac.

Operations on the adnexa. *Oophorectomy* means the removal of an ovary, whereas *ovarian cystectomy* denotes the removal of an ovarian cyst. *Salpingectomy* refers to the operative excision of a fallopian tube, and *salpingo-oophorectomy* means the removal of one tube and ovary. Women often understand the term *complete hysterectomy* to mean the removal of the uterus, both tubes, and the ovaries, not knowing that the word hysterectomy refers to the uterus only. An operation in which the uterus and adnexa are removed is referred to as a total hysterectomy and bilateral salpingo-oophorectomy.

Ovarian resection is the procedure whereby a benign tumor such as a dermoid is dissected out of the ovary, leaving normal ovarian tissue. *Ovarian bisection* is a division of the ovary through its long axis, cutting toward the hilus. The ovary is thus opened much like an oyster, allowing close inspection of the stroma and the taking of biopsies.

Tubal ligation is a technique for permanent prevention of conception. *Tubal plastic* procedures are performed in an attempt to correct mechanical blockage of the tubes.

VAGINAL OPERATIONS

Colpotomy. Colpotomy is the operative procedure to open the posterior cul-de-sac from the vagina by making a transverse incision through the vagina and peritoneum behind the cervix at the superior point of the posterior fornix. This opening into the pelvic cavity permits the gynecologist to examine and even remove the tubes and ovaries. It is contraindicated in endometriosis and with old inflammatory disease because of the cul-de-sac adhesions. The operation is most useful for the diagnosis of tubal pregnancy and drainage of pelvic abscesses.

Vaginal plastic procedures. Cystocele, cystourethrocele, rectocele, and enterocele, prolapse of the uterus, or any combination of these defects are the main reasons for the correction of vaginal relaxation. The indications for the various procedures are discussed in Chapter 39.

RADICAL OPERATIONS FOR MALIGNANCY

Radical hysterectomy. Radical hysterectomy is frequently referred to as the Wertheim operation and includes the removal of the entire uterus, the upper 3 to 4 cm. of the vagina, the parametrium, the broad ligaments, and the uterosacral ligaments. If a complete lymph node dissection of the pelvis is carried out with the hysterectomy, it should be so stated, for it is not implied by the term *radical hysterectomy.*

Radical vulvectomy. Removing the vulvar area from about 4 cm. above the symphysis to the anal sphincter and laterally to the thigh, deep to the periosteum of the pubis and ischiorectal fossa, is referred to as a radical vulvectomy. When the glands of the inguinal area and the femoral triangle are included, it is further qualified by stating that a bilateral inguinal and femoral node dissection has been carried out.

Exenteration. Cancer of the uterus, vagina, or vulva involving the bladder, rectum, and/or pubis cannot be successfully treated with radiation. For these advanced cases, faced with certain death, we offer exenteration.

Briefly the operation consists in removing all pelvic viscera. Blood supply to the legs and gluteal area is carefully maintained, and the obturator nerve and sciatic plexus must not be damaged. Urinary diversion is ordinarily accomplished by constructing an ileal conduit with a stoma on the opposite side of the colostomy opening.

Under optimum conditions the operation carries about a 10% mortality, and there is no assurance of a cure. The 5-year salvage is in the neighborhood of 25%. These facts should be given the patient and her family so that she can decide whether or not she wishes the operation done. As a rule, most women, after the gynecologic surgeon answers her questions and has a full discussion of the relevant facts, choose the operation.

References

Beecham, C. T., editor: Complications of gynecologic surgery; clinical obstetrics and gynecology, vol. 5, no. 2, New York, 1962, Paul B. Hoeber, Inc., Medical Book Department, Harper & Row, Publishers.

Conger, K., Beecham, C. T., and Horrax, T.: Ureteral injury in pelvic surgery, Obstet. Gynec. 3:343, 1954.

Parsons, L., and Ulfelder, H.: An atlas of pelvic operations, ed. 2, Philadelphia, 1968, W. B. Saunders Co.

Taylor, G. W., and Nathanson, I. T.: Lymph node metastases, New York, 1942, Oxford University Press, Inc.

TeLinde, R. W.: Operative gynecology, ed. 3, Philadelphia, 1962, J. B. Lippincott Co.

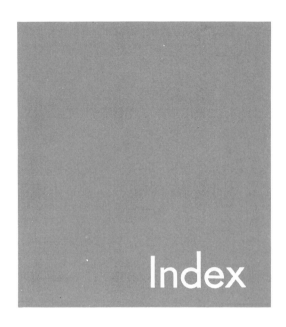

Index